History of the
Medical Society
of the
District of Columbia,
1817-1909

Also from Westphalia Press

westphaliapress.org

History of the
Medical Society
of the
District of Columbia,
1817-1909

by The Medical Society of
the District of Columbia

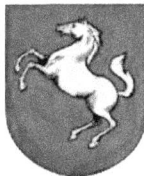

WESTPHALIA PRESS
An imprint of Policy Studies Organization

History of the Medical Society of the District of Columbia, 1817-1909
All Rights Reserved © 2016 by Policy Studies Organization

Westphalia Press
An imprint of Policy Studies Organization
1527 New Hampshire Ave., NW
Washington, D.C. 20036
info@ipsonet.org

ISBN-13: 978-1-63391-393-6
ISBN-10: 1-63391-393-7

Cover design by Taillefer Long at Illuminated Stories:
www.illuminatedstories.com

Daniel Gutierrez-Sandoval, Executive Director
PSO and Westphalia Press

Updated material and comments on this edition
can be found at the Westphalia Press website:
www.westphaliapress.org

HISTORY

OF THE

MEDICAL SOCIETY

OF THE

DISTRICT OF COLUMBIA

1817–1909

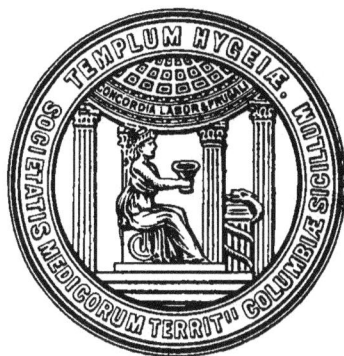

WASHINGTON, D. C.
PUBLISHED BY THE SOCIETY
1909

PREFACE.

On the 26th of September, 1866, Dr. J. M. Toner made an address before the Medical Society of the District of Columbia, the occasion being the forty-ninth anniversary of its formation, or more correctly, of the first meeting preliminary to its formation. The address was largely a history of the Society, and was the outcome of much laborious research. It is due to Dr. Toner to state that except for some fragments of history by a few other persons his is the only account of the first half century of the Society's existence. The address was published in 1869,* and was largely the basis of the addresses of Drs. Busey and W. W. Johnston at the seventy-fifth anniversary, February 16, 1894.†

Dr. Busey, in a note‡ to his address, says: "I take great pleasure in making the statement that I am indebted to Dr. J. M. Toner, a distinguished member of this Society, for many of the historical data cited in this address." And Dr. Johnston§ says: "The history and origin and early progress of the organization was told with a fullness and detail which will make the address of Dr. J. M. Toner a valued record for all time to come. I wish that he were

---

*Anniversary oration delivered before the Medical Society of the District of Columbia, September 26, 1866, by J. M. Toner, M. D.; Washington, 1869.

†Transactions and Proceedings of the Seventy-Fifth Anniversary of the Medical Society of the District of Columbia, celebrated February 16, 1894.

‡Transactions, etc., page 19.

§ *Ibid*, page 26.

standing in my place tonight and that you were again listening to the story of the olden time, which he has made so full of freshness and of life."

Dr. Busey, in his address at the announcement of Dr. Toner's death, October 21, 1896, stated that (See Busey's Souvenir, p. 370) "This Society will hold his memory in honored remembrance as the faithful historian who through years of painstaking and laborious investigation collated the early history of the profession in this District from municipal and national records, newspaper publications, family reminiscences, legend and tradition. He verified and arranged the data with such accuracy and completeness in an address delivered September 26, 1866, that it is now and always will be accepted as the standard history of the medical profession of this District prior to 1866.   .   .   . He was eminent and conspicuous as a patient, industrious and honest student.   .   .   .   He was eminently and acutely truthful."

The Presidential address of Dr. D. S. Lamb, December 18, 1901,* dealt mainly with the history of the Society, which, as he said "had been written more especially by Dr. J. M. Toner." Dr. Lamb, in his address† recommended that a committee be appointed to consider the question of publishing a full history of the Society, and report at its convenience. The recommendation was adopted by the Society, and a committee consisting of Drs. W. W. Johnston, A. F. A. King and E. L. Morgan was appointed. Dr.

---

* Transactions of the Medical Society of the District of Columbia, from January, 1901, to December, 1901 ; Washington, 1902, page 333.

† *Ibid*, page 357.

Johnston died March 21, 1902, and, April 16th, Dr. C. H. A. Kleinschmidt was appointed, Dr. King becoming chairman. It is known that Dr. Kleinschmidt made extensive researches, but the material that he collected is not at hand.

January 10, 1906, on request of the President of the Society, Dr. J. D. Morgan, he was given authority to enlarge the committee to five, and, January 17th, he appointed the following: Dr. A. F. A. King, Chairman, and Drs. D. S. Lamb, C. W. Franzoni, G. Wythe Cook and R. T. Holden. Dr. King resigned April 3, 1907, Dr. Lamb becoming chairman, and in August, 1908, Dr. L. Eliot was added to the committee.

As soon as appointed in 1906, the committee went to work, and, February 7th, made a report to the Society, outlining a plan of work and was given authority to issue a circular embodying the same. The Society also authorized the committee to prepare and publish the History and draw on the Treasurer for funds to defray the necessary expenses.

From time to time the subject was brought to the attention of the Society at its meetings and in the successive issues of the "Washington Medical Annals." The members were requested to furnish their personal sketches and photographs to the committee. A card catalogue of the entire membership was made in duplicate, and the personal sketches and photographs were gradually collected. At first it was thought to arrange the photographs in albums, but later it was decided to reproduce them as halftones in the book. November 28, 1906, the committee was authorized to print one thousand copies. October 7, 1908, it reported that the manuscript was nearly ready for the printer, and October 21st, the Society assessed each member $3.00 to meet the cost of publication. The printing began in January, 1909.

The sources from which information has been obtained in preparing the History are as follows:

1. The manuscript and typewritten records of the Society, including the volumes of transactions. The first volume of transactions of the Society, comprising the period from its beginning to January 1, 1838, has long been missing. At one time it was thought to be in the possession of the family of the late Dr. Thomas Sewall, but inquiry failed to discover it; it was then concluded to have been destroyed in the fire that burned the Washington Infirmary in 1861.

The second volume included the period from January 1, 1838, to October 31, 1866, and was fully indexed by the Recording Secretary, Dr. A. F. A. King. The third volume included the time from November 7, 1866, to November 3, 1869, and was indexed by the Secretary, Dr. Wm. Lee. The fourth from November 10, 1869, to December 18, 1872, was not indexed. The fifth from January 6, 1873, to July 21, 1874; sixth, from September 9, 1874, to May 17, 1876; seventh, from May 24, 1876, to December 20, 1878; eighth, from January 6, 1879, to September 21, 1881; all were indexed. The ninth was from September 28, 1881, to February 27, 1884; tenth, from March 5, 1884, to December 22, 1886; neither was indexed. The succeeding volumes were each for one year and were indexed, and many were typewritten.

There are also a few books in manuscript, such as were kept by the Corresponding Secretary, including copies of his correspondence.

2. The *printed* records of the Society, which include the occasional publication of the charter, constitution and by-laws and list of members under one cover. Such publications were made in 1820, following the first charter; in 1839, following the second charter; in 1854, 1861, 1867, 1870, 1882, 1894, 1897 and 1904. Several of these were necessitated by the numerous changes that had been made in the constitution and by-laws. To these must be added the catalogue published in 1885.

Some portion of the Society's transactions appeared in Volume II, of the "National Medical Journal," Washington. This journal was published, Vol. I, 1870-1, edited by Dr. C. C. Cox; Vol. II, 1871-2, edited by Drs. Busey and Lee. That portion of the Transactions from November 18, 1868, to December, 1870, appeared in the second volume.

"Transactions of the Society," published quarterly by the Society, from April, 1874, to December 20, 1878, inclusive; five volumes. This publication covered much of the work of the Society from 1865 to February, 1878.

The "National Medical Review," published in Washington by Walter Scott Wells; six numbers were published; December to May, 1878-9. A number of contributions to the Society were published in this journal.

"Walsh's Retrospect of American Medicine and Surgery," published in Washington; Volumes I to III, 1880 to 1882. Ralph Walsh and T. E. McArdle edited the first and Walsh the other volumes. Only a very few contributions to the Society appeared in this journal.

The "Maryland Medical Journal," Vols. IX to XIII, 1882-3 to 1885, contained much of the Society work from January 17, 1883, to June 17, 1885.

"Journal of the American Medical Association," 1882 to 1909.

"National Medical Review," Washington, D. C., 1892 to its suspension in 1901.

"Washington Medical Annals," the official publication of the Society's work, 1901 to 1909.

3. Besides the above mentioned publications the following have also been consulted:

Toner's Anniversary Oration, 1866. Dr. Toner compiled a list of members and officers (*ibid,* p. 19) from 1818 to 1838, from the "National Intelligencer" and other sources, chiefly made up, as he says, from publications authorized from time to time by the Society. He believed the list was correct.

"Toner's Medical Register of the District of Columbia," 1867.

Busey's four volumes, "Personal Reminiscences," &c., Washington, 1895; "A Souvenir," &c., Washington, 1896; "Pictures of the City of Washington," &c., 1898; "Annual Addresses," Washington, 1899.

"Index Catalogue of the Library of the Surgeon General's Office," two series.

"Transactions of the American Medical Association," 33 Vols.

"Congressional Globe" and "Congressional Record."

L. Eliot—"Historical Roster of the Medical Association, D. C., 1899."

The halftones were made by the Joyce Engraving Co. of Washington, and are arranged in the order of accession to membership in the Society. Some photographs received were not distinct enough to make good halftones. Two portraits were duplicated, appearing in both the Honorary and Active list—Drs. Antisell and Bedford Brown. Two others were duplicated through inadvertence—Drs. Ball and Hoover. Another, Dr. Garnett, was duplicated because the first photograph received was not as desirable as the second. In three cases there is misspelling in the names; Byrnes should be Byrns; Isadore (Bermann) should be Isidor; Phoebe (Norris) should be Phebe.

The thanks of the Society as well as the committee are due to the following persons for assistance in the work: To Dr. J. D. Morgan, and Miss Cordelia Jackson of Georgetown, for their general interest in the work and especially in obtaining personal sketches and photographs. To Drs. E. L. Morgan, H. A. Robbins and J. H. Yarnall, for similar aid. To Dr. Isabel H. Lamb, for comparing all the copy with the proof; and to Miss Alice Haslup, of Washington, for making photographs of places of meeting without any charge.

D. S. LAMB,

C. W. FRANZONI,

G. WYTHE COOK,

R. T. HOLDEN,

LLEWELLIN ELIOT,

September 1, 1909.   Committee on History.

TABLE OF CONTENTS.

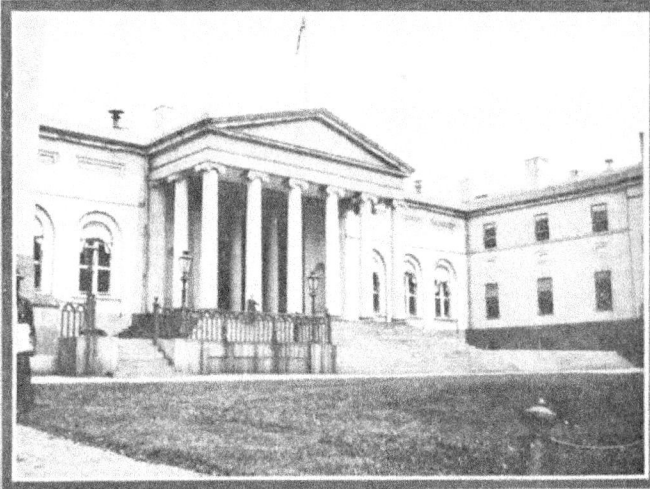

CITY HALL

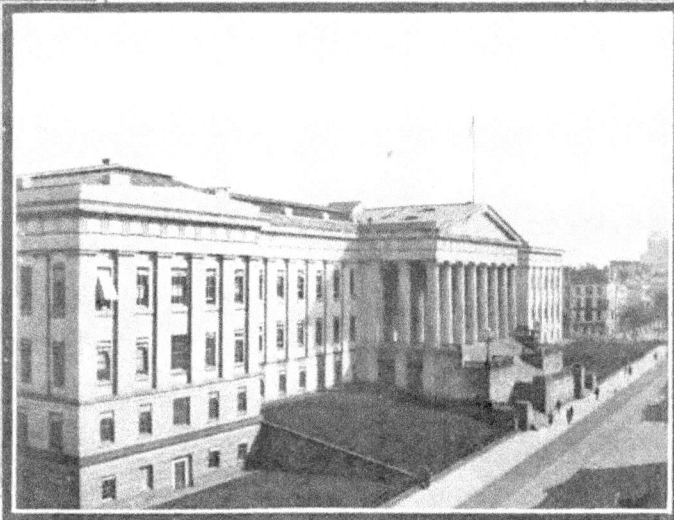

U. S. PATENT OFFICE

1

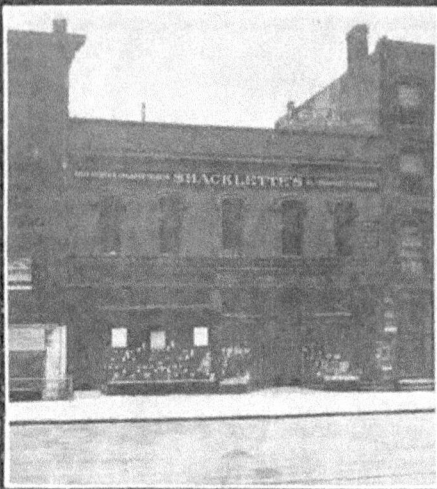

MEDICAL HALL
1002-4 F ST. N.W.

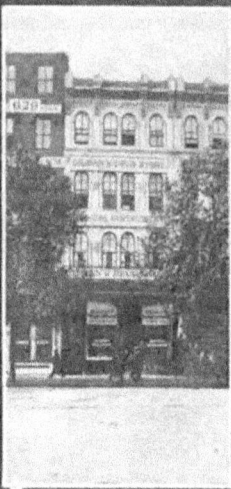

GILMAN'S
627 PENNA. AVE. N.W.

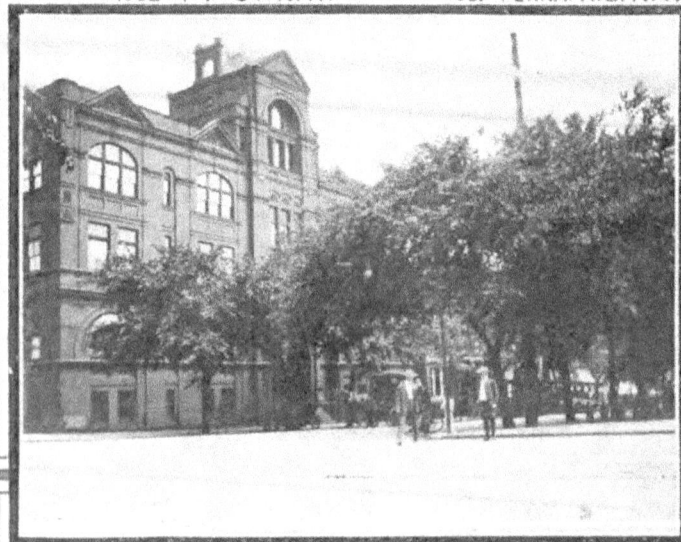

ASSEMBLY BUILDING
COLUMBIAN COLLEGE
15TH & H STS. N.W.

HISTORY.

On the 9th of July, 1790, the Congress of the United States passed a law establishing the seat of the National Government on the banks of the Potomac River. On the 16th of the same month the law was approved by President George Washington. September 19, 1793, President Washington laid the corner stone of the United States Capitol, and on the third Monday in November, 1800, Congress began its first session in the "City of Washington."

The new city was then but sparsely inhabited and there were few physicians. According to Dr. J. M. Toner* there were only nine physicians and two apothecaries in 1815. Today (1909) there are registered at the Health Office of the District of Columbia 1,581 physicians, 648 dentists and 597 pharmacists.

We are further told by Dr. Toner that the first assembling of physicians that took place in Washington was in 1813, and was called to take action on the death of Dr. Benjamin Rush, one of the signers of the Declaration of Independence, and known also as the "Founder of American Medicine."

According to Dr. S. C. Busey, the Medical Society of the District of Columbia was number twelve in the list of Medical Societies in the United States which in 1894 had reached the age of seventy-five years, and was probably the first scientific society chartered by Act of Congress. Ten of

*Oration, 1869, p. 37.

the founders of the Society were natives of Maryland, four were Virginians, two were from Massachusetts, three were born in the District of Columbia, and of two the nativities are unknown. The Society is a natural and direct heir of the Medical and Chirurgical Faculty of Maryland, and three founders of the Faculty became afterwards incorporators of the Medical Society of the District of Columbia. It may be added that of the twenty-one original incorporators of the Society, six were surgeons in the U. S. Army, two in the U. S. Navy, and one served in both—nearly one half the entire number of incorporators.

The eleven other societies referred to were as follows: New Jersey Medical Society, organized in 1766; Massachusetts Medical Society, in 1781; College of Physicians, Philadelphia, 1787; New Hampshire Medical Society 1791; Connecticut Medical Society, 1792; Medical and Chirurgical Faculty of Maryland, 1799; New York Medical Society, 1806; Albany (N. Y.,) Medical Society, 1806; New York County Medical Society, 1807; Rhode Island Medical Society, 1811; and Vermont Medical Society, 1814. *

It should be remembered that from 1790 until 1846 the city of Alexandria, Va., was included in the District of Columbia.

In the early days of the District there were many medical charlatans, who not only imposed on the citizens but worked a hardship, as such pretenders always do, to the regularly qualified physicians. This condition of things was largely the reason for the formation of the Medical Society. By a canvass of the regular physicians it was ascertained that there was a unanimous sentiment in favor of founding such a society. An advertisement was accordingly inserted in the principal Washington newspaper, the " National Intel-

*Trans. 75th Anniv. Med. Soc. D. C., p. 17.

ligencer," September 24, 1817, that "The physicians of Washington and Georgetown are requested to meet at Tennison's Hotel on Friday, the 26th instant, at 11 o'clock, for the purpose of taking into consideration the organization of a Medical Society."*

The meeting was held as advertised; sixteen physicians, including nearly all those practicing in Washington and Georgetown, attended. They were Drs. B. S. Bohrer, J. H. Blake, George Clark, Robert French, John Harrison, Thomas Henderson, Samuel Horsley, Henry Huntt, James T. Johnson, William Jones, J. P. C. McMahon, Alex. McWilliams, Thomas Sim, Peregrine Warfield and Charles and Nicholas Worthington. Dr. Charles Worthington was made chairman and Dr. Huntt, secretary. The object of the meeting was explained and the following resolution was unanimously adopted : "*Resolved*, that the physicians attending this meeting deem it important and expedient to organize at once a society in the District for the promotion of medical science."

Dr. W. W. Johnston describes this meeting as follows :

"In a small hotel or tavern, called Tennison's, situated on Pennsylvania Avenue near Fourteenth Street, on the morning of September 26, 1817, at 11 o'clock, there were gathered sixteen men. * * *

"They form an interesting group as they sit there. They were the descendants of that better class of settlers who came to America, some in the spirit of adventure (the Old World being too narrow for their ambition), some for conscience sake, seeking a new home from political or religious disaffection, but bringing with them the tastes, the courtesies and much of the wealth of the old European life. The ancestor of Dr. Thomas Sewall, who settled in Washington in 1820, crossed the ocean to America in 1814, plentifully provided with money and English servants, neat

---

* Toner. Oration. p. 8 *et seq.*

cattle and provisions, and with other things suitable for the
commencement of a plantation. Many were the heirs of
large estates, and inherited the gallant bearing and good
looks of their ancestry. Their names, too, tell us of what
stock they came—Worthington, Warfield, Henderson,
Blake, McWilliams, McMahon, are the same race which
has always been found equal to every emergency in Europe
or America.

"There was youth as well as hearty manhood in this
gathering: Worthington was 57; Blake, 50; Huntt, 35;
Bohrer, 29; William Jones, 28; and Weightman, 24*—
matured wisdom and judgment united to youthful fire,
qualities needed in a new enterprize like this. We can see
them there in Tennison's Tavern, as fine a looking body of
hale, handsome men as could be seen anywhere, with
strong faces, indicating the set purpose and the firm decision to do all that was possible for the advancement of their
profession in this, the new Capital of the Country."†

A committee of seven was selected to draft a constitution and by-laws for the government of the Society, which
was to be called the "Medical Society of the District of
Columbia." The committee consisted of Drs. Blake, Thos.
Sim, Henderson, Clark, Charles Worthington, Warfield and
Huntt. The committee reported November 3d; some
amendments were offered and some portions of the proposed
constitution and by-laws were adopted; the remainder were
adopted November 10th. The constitution and by-laws
were ordered to be copied in a book and signed by the
members. As this work required time, it was ordered that
the next meeting should be held January 5, 1818, and that
all physicians of the District should be invited to attend
and take part in adopting the constitution and by-laws as
a whole and in the election of officers.

At the meeting January 5th Charles Worthington was

---

*Weightman's name is not in the list of sixteen as given by Dr. Toner.
†75th Anniv. Trans. of Soc., 1894, p. 28.

elected President; Arnold Elzey and J. H. Blake, Vice Presidents; Henry Huntt, Corresponding Secretary; Thos. Henderson, Recording Secretary; Richard Weightman, Librarian; and Wm. Jones, Treasurer. "Thus," says Dr. Toner, "was launched on the waters of time a new craft that was destined to affect materially the social, intellectual, moral and sanitary character of the District. Meetings were held quarterly, at which papers were read and discussed, and sometimes adjourned meetings were also held. Some of the papers read were published."* Dr. Toner also states that as far as professional improvement was concerned the expectations of the members were more than realized, but that the expected relief from charlatans did not come. The members of the Society finally came to the conclusion that in order to obtain this relief it would be necessary to secure the enactment of some law that would prevent any but competent physicians from beginning the practice of medicine in the District of Columbia. Accordingly twenty-one members of the Society applied to Congress in 1818 for a charter or act of incorporation as a Medical Society. The charter was granted, approved by President Monroe, February 16, 1819. It was almost an exact copy of that of the Medical and Chirurgical Faculty of Maryland.

AN ACT TO INCORPORATE THE MEDICAL SOCIETY OF THE DISTRICT OF COLUMBIA.

Be it enacted by the Senate and House of Representatives of the United States of America, in Congress assembled, That Charles Worthington, James H. Blake, John T. Shaaff, Thomas Sim, Frederick May, Joel T. Gustine, Elisha Harrison, Peregrine Warfield, Alexander McWilliams, George Clark, Henry Huntt, Thomas Henderson, John Harrison, Benjamin S. Bohrer, Samuel Horseley, Nicholas W. Worthington, William Jones, James T. Johnson, Richard Weightman, George May, Robert French, and such persons as they may from time to time elect, and their successors, are hereby declared to be a community, corporation, and body politic, forever, by and under the name and title of the Medical Society of the District of Columbia; and by and under the same name and title

---

* Toner's Oration, p. 10.

they shall be able and capable in law to purchase, take, have and enjoy, to them and their successors, in fee or for lease, estate or estates, any land, tenements, rents, annuities, chattels, bank stock, registered debts, or other public securities within the District, by the gift, bargain, sale, demise, or of any person or persons, bodies politic or corporate, capable to make the same, and the same, at their pleasure, to alien, sell, transfer or lease and apply to such purposes as they may adjudge most conducive to the promoting and disseminating medical and surgical knowledge, and for no other purpose whatever : *Provided nevertheless*, That the said society, or body politic, shall not, at any one time, hold or possess property, real personal or mixt, exceeding in total value the sum of six thousand dollars per annum.

SEC. 2. *And be it further enacted*, That the members of the said society, above designated, shall hold, in the City of Washington, four stated meetings in every year, viz : on the first Mondays in January, April, July and October ; the officers of the society to consist of a President, two Vice-Presidents, one Corresponding Secretary, one Recording Secretary, one Treasurer and one Librarian, who shall be appointed on the second Monday in March, one thousand eight hundred and nineteen, and on the annual meeting in January forever thereafter, (not less than seven members being present at such meeting), and the society may make a common seal, and may elect into their body such medical and chirurgical practitioners, within the District of Columbia, as they may deem qualified to become members of the society ; it being understood that the officers of the society now elected are to remain in office until the next election after the passage of this act.

SEC. 3. *And be it further enacted*, That it shall and may be lawful for the said Medical Society, or any number of them attending, (not less than seven), to elect by ballot five persons, residents of the District, who shall be stiled the Medical Board of Examiners of the District of Columbia, whose duty it shall be to grant licenses to such medical and chirurgical gentlemen as they may, upon a full examination, judge adequate to commence the practice of the medical and chirurgical arts, or as may produce diplomas from some respectable college or society ; each person so obtaining a certificate to pay a sum not exceeding ten dollars, to be fixed on or ascertained by the society.

SEC. 4. *And be it further enacted*, That any three of the examiners shall constitute a board for examining such candidates as may apply, and shall subscribe their names to each certificate by them granted, which certificate shall also be countersigned by the President of the society, and have the seal of the society affixed thereto by the Secretary, upon paying into the hands of the Treasurer the sum of money to be ascertained, as above, by the society ; and any one of the said examiners may grant a license to practice, until a board, in conformity to this act, can be held ; *Provided*, That nothing herein contained shall authorize the said corporation in any wise to regulate the price of medical or chirurgical attendance, on such persons as may need those services.

SEC. 5. *And be it further enacted*, That after the appointment of the aforesaid medical board, no person, not heretofore a practitioner of medicine or surgery within the District of Columbia, shall be allowed to practice within the said District, in either of said branches, and receive payment for his services, without first having obtained a license, testified as by this law directed, or without the production of a diploma, under the penalty of fifty dollars for each offence, to be recovered in the county court where he may reside, by bill of presentment and indictment; one half for the use of the society, and the other for that of the informer.

SEC. 6. *And be it further enacted*, That every person who, upon application, shall be elected a member of the Medical Society, shall pay a sum not exceeding ten dollars, to be ascertained by the society.

SEC. 7. *And be it further enacted*, That the Medical Society be, and they are hereby empowered, from time to time, to make such by-laws, rules and regulations, as they may find requisite, to break or alter their common seal, to fix the times and places for the meetings of the board of examiners, filling up vacancies in the medical board, and to do and perform such other things as may be requisite for carrying this act into execution, and which may not be repugnant to the constitution and laws of the United States; *Provided*, That nothing herein contained shall extend to prohibit any person during his actual residence in any of the United States, and who, by the laws of the state wherein he doth or may reside, is not prohibited from practising in either of the above branches, from practising in this District; *Provided always*, That it shall and may be lawful for any person, resident as aforesaid, and not prohibited as aforesaid, when specially sent for, to come into any part of this District, and administer or prescribe medicine, or perform any operation for the relief of such to whose assistance he may be sent for.

SEC. 8. *And be it further enacted*, That Congress may, at any time, alter, amend, or annul this act of incorporation of said society at pleasure.

H. CLAY,
Speaker of the House of Representatives.
DANIEL D. TOMPKINS,
Vice President of the United States and President of the Senate.
JAMES MONROE.

Approved February 16, 1819.

A curious lapse in language occurred in the charter of the Medical Society. That of the Maryland Faculty, in enumerating the ways in which that Faculty might acquire property, stated that they might be by gift, bargain, sale, *devise* of any person or persons; but the charter of the Medical Society of this District uses the words " gift, bargain, sale, *demise*, or of any person or persons." The same lapse reappeared in the second charter, that of 1838.

On the 3d of the following March a notice appeared in the " National Intelligencer" that:

" By an act of Congress the Medical Society of the District of Columbia has been incorporated, and by a provision of the act the term of service of the officers expires on the 8th of March. A meeting of the Society is called on Monday next (March 8th) at 11 o'clock, at Strother's Hotel, where much business of great importance to the Society will be laid before the members, who are notified to attend precisely at the hour appointed.

"The Library Committee are requested to meet at the same place on the same day, at 10 o'clock, and prepare to make a report. (Signed) Thomas Henderson, Recording Secretary."

The meeting was held and officers were elected for the year. In addition to those provided for by the charter, three Censors were elected. The constitution and by-laws made no mention of any such officers, and it is not clear what were their duties. (See Board of Censors.)

Dr. Toner states that the members attended the four meetings of the year with much punctuality and showed great interest in the success of the Society.

"The papers read before it were well prepared and the discussions which followed were able and practical. A hall was rented in 1819 for the use of the Society and a library collected by donation and purchase. It seems, however, that the novelty of the meetings gradually wore away with the younger members, and some of the older ones became infirm and ceased to attend, or died. The interest in the proceedings and discussions gradually abated, and in a few years barely a quorum could be got together." He adds that "there was an absence of fraternal feeling among the younger members and the strangers who came to the city to practice; and that the opening of the Medical Department of Columbian College in 1821 added to the indifference, because it was a 'new source of professional entertainment.' "*

Still another adverse condition presented itself, namely, a dispute as to the need of a licensing body, since a diploma from a medical college was all that was required or contemplated by the provision of the charter.

-----
* Toner's Oration, p. 14 *et seq.*

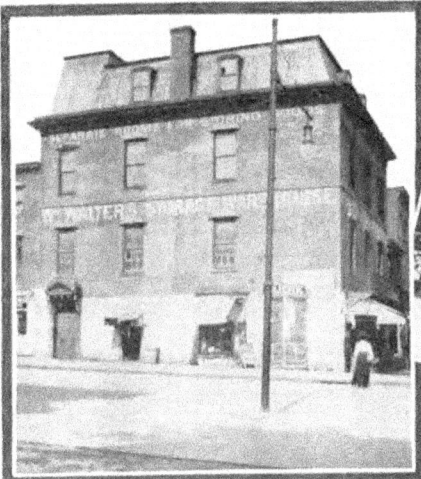

OLD MEDICAL SCHOOL
10TH & E STS N.W.

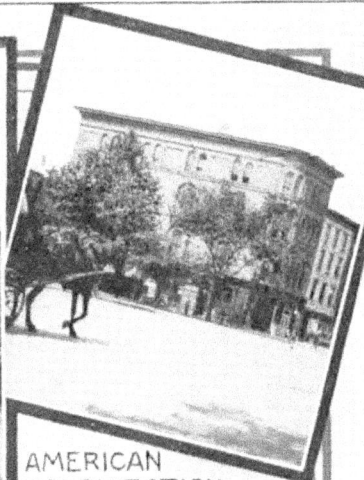

AMERICAN
COLONIZATION
SOCIETY BUILDING
4½ & PENNA. AVE.

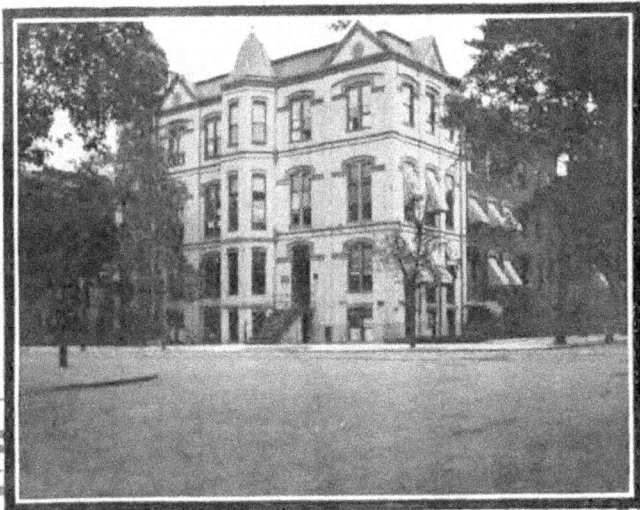

OLD LAW SCHOOL BUILDING
GEORGETOWN UNIVERSITY
6TH & F STS N.W.

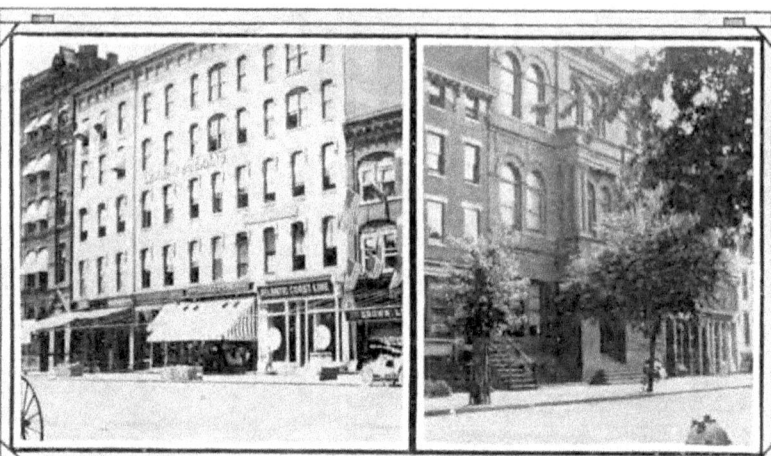

LENMAN BUILDING

GEORGETOWN LAW SCHOOL

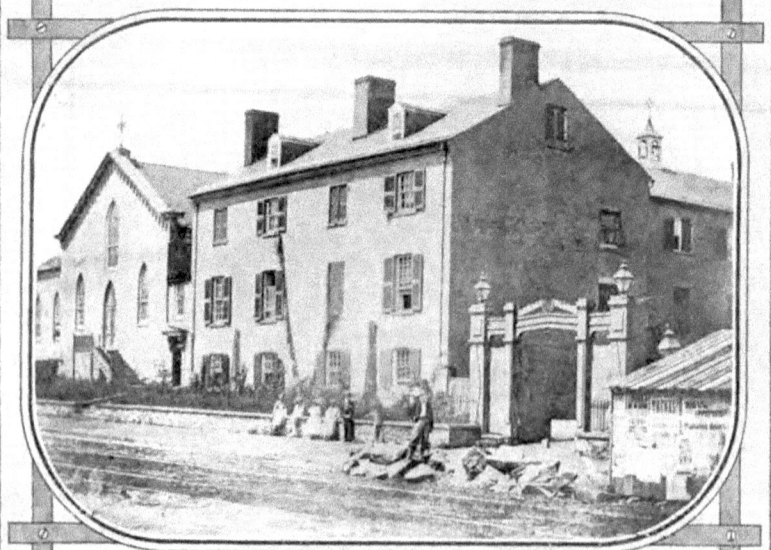

GONZAGA COLLEGE
F ST, BET. 9TH & 10TH
NORTH SIDE

4

"In 1825 and 1826, during a period of the most active discontent among the members,* a very determined effort was made by a few physicians of Washington and Georgetown to form a new medical society which should supersede the chartered organization. The profession was thoroughly canvassed and several meetings were held in the interest of the movement, which at first promised to be successful."

A notice appeared in the "National Intelligencer" April 5, 1826, as follows: "Notice.—A meeting of the physicians of Washington and Georgetown who have agreed to form a medical association is requested at the City Hall on Tuesday, the 6th, at 12 o'clock."

The meeting was held and, what seems strange to us, Dr. Frederick May was elected Chairman and Dr. Thomas Henderson, Secretary. Meetings were also held on the 10th and 11th of April. There was much diversity of opinion, and nothing was accomplished.

Again, in 1828, the following notice appeared in the "National Intelligencer" of January 23d :†

"Medical Society.—A meeting of the Medical Society of the District of Columbia will be held on Wednesday, the 23d instant, at the City Hall, the object of the meeting being to decide whether the Society shall in future hold its meetings."

The attempt to destroy the Society was not, however, sufficiently supported.

"The discordant views previously alluded to, with personal jealousies that unfortunately sprung up in the Society, prevailed to such an extent in 1831–3, that for want of a quorum at the annual meetings, the Society, it is believed, failed to elect officers; at least no record of elections can be found."‡

---

* Toner's Oration, p. 22.   †Toner Oration, p. 18.   ‡Toner Oration, p. 23.

A better feeling, however, began to manifest itself among the members in 1834–6, during which years meetings were held, officers elected, and the diseases incident to the territory and the best modes of treatment were discussed without the least suspicion that the charter had been forfeited. This disagreeable fact was not discovered by the Society until a case involving the powers and privileges of the Society was taken into court, when it was shown that the charter had been forfeited by neglect of duty, and therefore no penalty could be incurred for violation of its provisions.

In Cranch's *Reports* Vol. V, pp. 62 to 71, is the report of the trial of John Williams for practicing medicine in the District of Columbia without a license from the Medical Board of Examiners of the District. He professed to be an oculist, and practiced and received payment therefor. In the indictment, the specific date of violation of the law was December 15, 1836. The defence set up the contention that the Society had gone out of existence because for some years before 1834 it had failed to hold annual meetings as required by the charter, and therein had failed to elect the Medical Board as it should have done; that, therefore, the Board had been acting without any legal authority, and indeed had never since the charter was given, in 1819, been properly elected. The defence further claimed that some members had given out that they were no longer members, and it was also stated that it had been agreed that the property and effects of the Society were to be divided among the individual members. The minutes of the Board had been lost. The court consisted of Chief Justice Wm. Cranch, with Associate Justices Buckner Thruston and James Sewall Morsell. Francis Scott Key, the author of "The Star Spangled Banner," was United States Attorney and prosecuting officer. It is interesting to note that Justice Thruston gave it as his opinion that the Society had had authority only to license students and those about to begin practice, and not those already in practice. The jury was out two days and a night, and then rendered a verdict of acquittal.

At that time all but seven of the original incorporators were dead or had removed from the city; these seven, Drs. Frederick May, Alex. McWilliams, Henry Huntt, Wm. Jones, G. W. May, Peregrine Warfield and N. W. Worthington, with fourteen others who had joined the Society, petitioned Congress, on its assembling in 1837, for a revival of the charter with amendments.*

The new charter, or act of reincorporation, was approved by President Van Buren July 7, 1838. In the main it is the same as the first charter; there were some emendations.

ACT OF INCORPORATION.

AN ACT TO REVIVE, WITH AMENDMENTS, AN ACT TO INCORPORATE THE MEDICAL SOCIETY OF THE DISTRICT OF COLUMBIA.

Be it enacted by the Senate and House of Representatives of the United States of America in Congress assembled, That Frederick May, M. D., Alexander McWilliams, M. D., Henry Huntt, M. D., N. P. Causin, M. D., W. Jones, M. D., Richmond Johnson, M. D., Thomas Sewall, M. D., George W. May, M. D., Nicholas W. Worthington, M. D., Joshua Reily, M. D., James S. Gunnell, M. D., Harvey Lindsly, M. D., James C. Hall, M. D., Thomas Miller, M. D., Joseph Borrows, M. D., Alexander McD. Davis, M. D., Benjamin King, M. D., Noble Young, M. D., H. F. Condict, M. D., W. B. Magruder, M. D., Peregrine Warfield, M. D., J. B. Blake, M. D., and such other persons as they may from time to time elect, and their successors, are hereby declared to be a community, corporation, and body politic, forever, or until Congress shall by law direct this charter to cease and determine, by and under the name and title of the Medical Society of the District of Columbia; and by and under the same name and title they shall be able and capable in law to purchase, take, have and enjoy, to them and their successors, in fee or for lease, estate or estates, any land, tenements, rents, annuities, chattels, bank stock, registered debts, or other public securities within the District, by the gift, bargain, sale, demise, or of any person or persons, bodies politic or corporate, capable to make the same, and the same, at their pleasure, to alien, sell, transfer, or lease and apply, to such purposes as they may adjudge most conducive to the promoting and disseminating medical and

*Toner Oration, p. 18.

surgical knowledge, and for no other purpose whatever: *Provided, nevertheless,* That the said Society or body politic shall not, at any one time, hold or possess property, real, personal, or mixed, exceeding in total value the sum of six thousand dollars per annum.

SEC. 2. *And be it further enacted,* That the members of the said Society above designated shall hold, in the City of Washington, two stated meetings in every year, viz: on the first Monday in January and July; the officers of the Society to consist of a President, two Vice Presidents, one Corresponding Secretary, one Recording Secretary, one Treasurer and one Librarian, who shall be appointed on the first Monday in July, one thousand eight hundred and thirty-eight, and on the annual meeting in January forever thereafter, and who shall hold their offices for one year, and until others are chosen in their stead (not less than seven members being present at such meeting); and the Society may make a common seal, and may elect into their body such medical and chirurgical practitioners, within the District of Columbia, as they may deem qualified to become members of the Society, it being understood that the officers of the Society now elected are to remain in office until the next election after the passage of this act.

SEC. 3. *And be it further enacted,* That it shall and may be lawful for the said Medical Society, or any number of them attending, (not less than seven), to elect by ballot five persons, residents of the District of Columbia, whose duty it shall be to grant licenses to such medical and chirurgical gentlemen as they may, upon a full examination, judge qualified to practice the medical and chirurgical arts, or as may produce a diploma from some respectable medical college or society, each person so obtaining a certificate to pay a sum, not exceeding ten dollars, to be fixed on or ascertained by the Society.

SEC. 4. *And be it further enacted,* That any three of the examiners shall constitute a board for examining such candidates as may apply, and shall subscribe their names to each certificate by them granted, which certificate shall also be countersigned by the President of the Society, and have the seal of the Society affixed thereto by the Secretary, upon paying into the hands of the Treasurer the sum of money to be ascertained as above by the Society; and any one of the said examiners may grant a license to practice until a board in conformity to this act can be held: *Provided,* That nothing herein contained shall authorize the said corporation in anywise to regulate the practice of medical or chirurgical attendance on such persons as may need those services, nor to establish or fix a tariff of charges or fees for medical attendance or advice, or to interfere in any way with charges or fees for medical attendance or advice.

SEC. 5. *And be it further enacted,* That after the appointment of the aforesaid medical board no person, not heretofore a practitioner of medicine or surgery within the District of Columbia shall be allowed to practice within the said District, in either of said branches, without first having obtained a license, testified as by this law directed, or the production of a diploma from a respectable medical college or a board of examiners established by law: *Provided,* That the professors in such college, or the examiners in such board, be men regularly instructed in medicine and surgery, and the collateral branches of medical education, anatomy, chemistry, under the penalty of fifty dollars for each offense, to be recovered in the county court where he may reside, by bill of presentment and indictment, one-half for the use of the Society, and the other for that of the informer.

SEC. 6. *And be it further enacted*, That every person who upon application shall be elected a member of the Medical Society, shall pay a sum not exceeding ten dollars, to be ascertained by the Society.

SEC. 7. *And be it further enacted*, That the Medical Society be, and they are hereby, empowered, from time to time, to make such by-laws, rules, and regulations as they may find requisite; which by-laws, rules, and regulations shall, in their application and operation, be exclusively confined to said Society, as a Society, or body corporate, and not to its members individually, when not acting in a corporate character ; to break or alter their common seal ; to fix the times and places for the meetings of the boards of examiners ; filling up vacancies in the medical board ; and to do and perform such other things as may be requisite for carrying this act into execution, and which may not be repugnant to the Constitution and laws of the United States : *Provided always*, That it shall and may be lawful for any person, resident as aforesaid, and not prohibited as aforesaid, when specially sent for, to come into any part of this District and administer or prescribe medicine, or perform any operation for the relief of such to whose assistance he may be sent for : *And provided also*, That nothing in this act contained shall be so construed as to prevent any person, living within or without said District, from administering medicine, or performing any surgical operation, with the consent of the person or the attendants of the person to whom such medicine is administered, or upon whom such surgical operation is performed, without fee or reward ; nor to prevent the giving advice or assistance in any way to the sick or afflicted, upon charity and kindness ; nor to prevent the receipt of reward for the same, if voluntarily tendered or made ; nor to extend to midwifery by females ; and any person so administering medicine or performing any surgical operation, not authorized to practice physic and surgery agreeably to the provisions of this act, shall be prohibited from collecting any fee or reward for the same by any process of law : *And be it further provided*, That no person shall be admitted to an examination until he shall produce satisfactory evidence that he has studied physic and surgery three years, including one full course of medical lectures, as usually taught at medical schools, or four years without such a course of lectures.

SEC. 8. *And be it further enacted*, That Congress may at any time alter, amend, or annul this act of incorporation of said Society at pleasure.

JAMES K. POLK,
Speaker of the House of Representatives.
RD. M. JOHNSON,
Vice President of the United States and President of the Senate.
M. VAN BUREN.

Approved July 7, 1838.

Since that time the Society has not failed to meet to elect officers except possibly in the years 1862 and 1863, during the civil war. The Treasurer made no report from January 7, 1861, until January 4, 1864.

Dr. Toner states that in 1826 a " Washington Medical Society" was formed by the professors and students of the

Medical Department of Columbian College and met at the
College.   Eventually the Society admitted other physicians.
It seems to have ceased to exist in 1832.*

The present MEDICAL ASSOCIATION OF THE DISTRICT
OF COLUMBIA was formed in January, 1833.   Its object
was to provide a code of ethics and fee bill, both of
which were denied to the Medical Society by its charter,
sections I and IV.   It has been held by some members
of the Society that by its charter it is prevented from disciplining its members for any offence committed outside of
its actual meetings.   As an example it may be mentioned
that a charge of bribery in which there was a public scandal was brought against a member of the Society in 1868.
The Society ordered an investigation which was duly made.
The investigating committee made a report recommending
that the offending member be reprimanded by the President
of the Society.   The Society approved the recommendation
and the reprimand was duly administered.   But Dr. S. C.
Busey strenuously objected to any action being taken in
the case, claiming that the charter forbade it.   His efforts
and those of a few others, however, failed to prevent the reprimand.

After the second charter had been approved, the Society
held a meeting, July 30, 1838, and the following resolution
was adopted:

" *Resolved* that, whereas the Act of Congress entitled An Act to revive with amendments an Act to incorporate the Medical Society of the District of Columbia,
passed 7 July, 1838, did not finally pass both branches of
Congress and receive the approval of the President until
five days after the first Monday in July, 1838, the day designated in the charter for the first meeting of the Society;
therefore this day has been assumed for the first meeting,

* Toner's Oration. p. 23.

it being the earliest period after the passage and approval of the Act at which the members of the Society could be notified and assembled. This course has been adopted from the necessity of the case, and as in accordance with the design of the charter."

The next meeting was held August 8th, and eight members attended. A committee was appointed to revise the constitution, by-laws and rules; it consisted of Drs. Thos. Sewall, J. C. Hall, H. Lindsly, N. Worthington and O. Fairfax (of Alexandria). Monday, January 8, 1839, the annual meeting was held at the City Hall, at which there was just a quorum. Officers were elected for the year. The Committee on Revision of the Constitution made report which was adopted. The Society ordered that the report should be printed and a copy of the revised document sent to each member. From this time for many years the minutes show little more than that the Society met, that there were so many members present at the meeting, and that officers were elected; occasionally some other statement is inserted; as, for instance, that there was " no quorum." July 3, 1843, a letter from Dr. J. B. S. Jackson, of Harvard Medical School, was read, giving an account of the results of the autopsy made on Hon. Hugh S. Legare, late Secretary of State.

" The first breeze which ruffled the calmness of the Society's existence is noted in the records as occurring at the meeting of January 13, 1849. Dr. J. C. Hall, the president, suggested the propriety of taking some action in regard to the appointment of delegates to the American Medical Association, whereupon Dr. Lindsly offered a resolution authorizing the president to appoint five members as delegates. Dr. Young offered an amendment instructing the president to make his selection from the profession at large, as distinguished from the professors of colleges, on which amendment there were two ayes, four noes, three members not voting. A reconsideration of the amendment was moved, this was laid on the table and the original motion was carried without amendment. This incident illustrates a phase of feeling which has all but passed away. The rivalry between the colleges is a generous one, without any feeling or jealousy, and the profession at large so outnumbers the professors in colleges that they need never fear being controlled by them. The Society may be said to have passed through its "storms and stress" period and to have reached the open sea of generous feeling, broad aims and united purpose."*

From 1838 to 1864 the Society met at the time of the regular semi-annual meetings, and occasional special meetings, mostly memorial meetings to deceased members, were also held. With 1864, however, a new régime came in, and during that year fifteen meetings were held. The difference is shown by the minutes. The first volume of the Transactions of the Society under the second charter is a manuscript volume of 330 pages with an excellent index, made up by Dr. A. F. A. King. The volume covers the period from January, 1838, to October 31, 1866—both dates inclusive—over twenty-eight years. The first 169 pages carry the record to May 30, 1865, twenty-seven years, leaving the remaining 161 pages for the remaining seventeen months. This striking difference in space indicates the difference in the activity of the Society in its scientific work. The 161 pages constitute the record made during the Secretaryship of Dr. King.

PLACES OF MEETING OF THE MEDICAL SOCIETY.

During the ninety-one years of its existence the Society has met at many different places. As already stated, the first meeting, preliminary to the formation of the Society, was held in Tennison's Hotel, on Pennsylvania Avenue,

*Johnston, in Trans. 75th Anniv., p. 44.

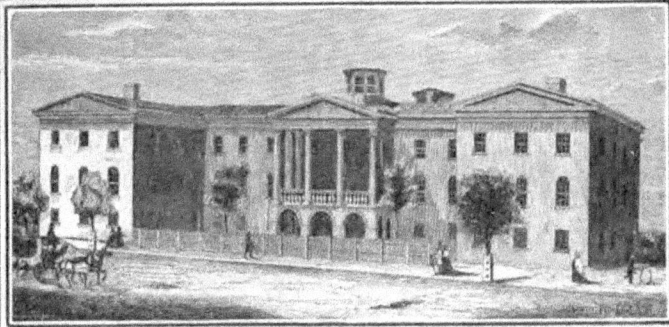

WASHINGTON INFIRMARY

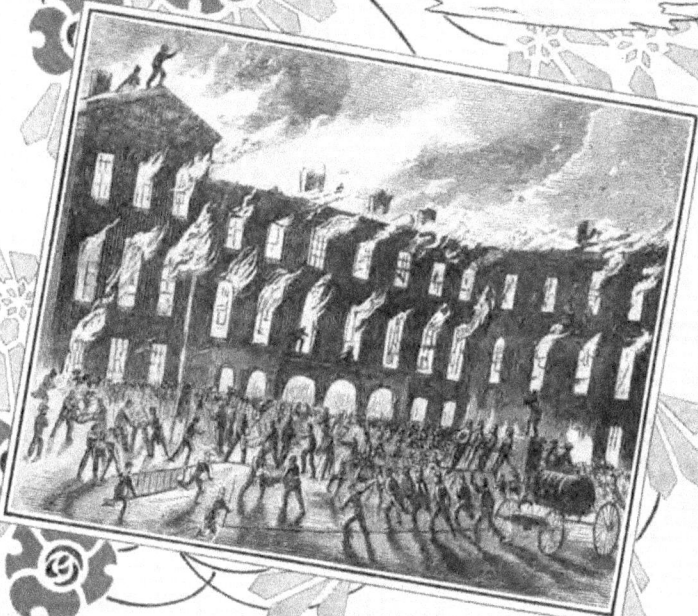

Praeses et Quaesitores Societatis Medicorum

IN TERRITORIO COLUMBIANO

Omnibus et singulis has literas visuris

SALUTEM

NOTUM SIT. John E. Walsh

*Medicinae et Chirurgiae doctum peritumque ejus scientiae examine rite habito, nos comprobavi*mus

Itaque auctoritate nobis societatis decreto collata *eidem* John E. Walsh *jus potestatemque artes medendi et Chirurgicae exercendi damus et exedimus*

Cujus rei testimonio sigillum Societatis commune huic monimento afferimus et et nomina nostra sunt subscripta.

(*Datum*) Washington Oct 7. Anno Domini Millesimo Octingentesimo nonagesimo *Reipublicae fundatae Centesimo decimo quarto Itaque salus SOCIETATIS instituta Ano et quinquagesimo*

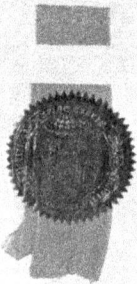

Fred W. Purcell M.D. (*Praeses*)

E.M. Clements Smith M.D.
Thomas F. Adams M.D.
J. ___ Simmons M.D.
Llewellyn Eliot M.D.
S.R. Acker M.D.

6

near Fourteenth Street, N. W. The next place mentioned was where the meeting was held March 8, 1819, after the incorporation, namely at Strother's Hotel, corner of Fourteenth Street and Pennsylvania Avenue, N. W., where Willard's Hotel is now. October 1st a room was rented for meetings, known as McPhail's, afterward's as Haskell's schoolroom, on Sixteenth Street, between H and I Streets, N. W., just north of St. John's Episcopal Church. It was called the "Medical Hall," and was rented for one year. The Society afterwards "went wandering about, and met wherever it could find accommodations." Sometimes it met at Strother's, sometimes at Tennison's, sometimes at the office of Dr. Huntt or Dr. Causin; occasionally at the rooms of the City Councils in the building on Eleventh Street, between C and Pennsylvania Avenue, N. W., owned and occupied by the Washington Library Company. Later on, when the City Councils occupied the rooms of General Richard Weightman, on Sixth Street, N. W., afterwards a part of the National Hotel, the Society met there. The advertisements also show that it met in the room over the United States Engine House, E Street, between Seventh and Eighth, N. W., on the grounds afterwards occupied by the General Post Office. Sometimes it met in a room in the U. S. Patent Office.

After 1827 it occasionally met at the Columbian Medical College, northeast corner Tenth and E Streets, N. W. After the completion of the City Hall the meetings were generally held there; the Society met there January 8, 1839, after the second incorporation. January 6, 1840, it met again at the Medical College, Tenth and E Streets, and continued to meet there till January 6, 1845, when it held its first meeting at the City Hospital in Judiciary Square, afterwards known as the Washington Infirmary, and to which the College had moved. July 6, 1846, is the first

2

date on which the Infirmary is mentioned in the minutes of the Society, which continued to meet there until October 1, 1861. The Infirmary was destroyed by fire (November 4, 1861), and it is believed that some of the Society's minutes and other records were then consumed.

January 6, 1862, the Society met at the rooms of the Medical Department, Georgetown College, which was then on F Street east of Twelfth, south side. It continued to meet there until March 8, 1865, when it held its first meeting in the building 627 Pennsylvania Avenue, N. W., the first floor of which was and still is occupied by Gilman's drug store.

March 20, 1867, the Society returned to the rooms of the Medical Department of Georgetown College (removed to Tenth and E Streets, N. W., in 1867), and continued to meet there until the Medical Hall at 1002-4 F Street, N. W., was ready for occupancy. The first meeting at this hall was held January 29, 1869. The Society remained there nearly two years; then, January 2, 1871, it met for the first time at the American Colonization Society Building, Southwest corner Pennsylvania Avenue and Four-and-a-half Street, N. W. October 2, 1872, it met for the first time at Gonzaga College, on F Street, N. W., between Ninth and Tenth, east of the old St. Patrick's Church.

October 12, 1881, the Society met for the first time in the Lenman Building, 1425 New York Avenue, N. W. In the early part of 1884 it removed to the old Georgetown University Law Building, southeast corner Sixth and F Streets, N. W., and about November 25, 1891, to the new Georgetown University Law Building, 506-8 E Street, N. W. February 7, 1906, it removed to the assembly room of the Columbian University, southeast corner Fifteenth and

H Streets, N. W., and has continued to meet there till the present date.*

THE MEDICAL BOARD OF EXAMINERS OF THE DISTRICT OF COLUMBIA.

The above was the title prescribed by the first charter of the Society, but in the second charter the Board was designated simply as the " examiners" and " Medical Board." The constitution and by-laws under the first charter made no mention of the Board ; under the second charter it is called "The Board of Examiners," and a section of the by-laws prescribed its duties. The Board ceased to exist in 1896 by operation of the Medical Practice Act passed by the Congress of the United States.

As will be seen by consulting the first charter, sections 3 to 5, the Board consisted of five members, residents of the District of Columbia, who were to be elected by ballot by the Medical Society ; the dates of election were not fixed by the charter, which, however, required that a quorum should be present at the meeting at which the members were elected.

The duty of the Board as prescribed by both charters was to examine and license those gentlemen† who desired to practice medicine in the District of Columbia. A candidate who could show a diploma from some respectable college or society was not required to be examined, but if he was unable to show such diploma, the Board was required to give him a "full examination" to determine if he was

*Of the places of meeting above named those buildings that are still standing are represented pictorially in this history ; and also Gonzaga College, that was torn down and replaced by stores, and the Washington Infirmary, that was burned. Efforts were made to secure pictures of other buildings that have disappeared, but without success. The Committee on History is indebted to Father Himmel, the President of Gonzaga College, for the photograph of the old college building, and to Dr. A. F. A. King for the photograph of the Washington Infirmary.

†As the word "gentlemen" was literally construed by the Board, it excluded women from its provisions.

"adequate (in the second charter 'qualified') to commence the practice of medicine and chirurgical arts." If a satisfactory diploma was shown or a satisfactory examination passed, the Board gave a license or certificate. The charters provided that any three examiners should constitute the Board, and until the Board could be assembled to act upon applications, any examiner could temporarily grant a license.

The charter of 1838 provided that no one should be admitted to the examination unless he could present satisfactory evidence that he had studied physic and surgery three years, including one full course of medical lectures as usually taught at medical schools, or four years without such a course of lectures. The charter also provided that the professors in the college granting the diploma, or the examiners in any Board granting a diploma (a Board established by law), should be men regularly instructed in medicine and surgery and the collateral branches of medical education, anatomy and chemistry.

The charters required that the license certificate should be signed by at least three examiners, be countersigned by the President of the Society, and have the Society seal affixed by the Secretary of the Society. As there were both a Corresponding and a Recording Secretary, there arose a question as to which should affix the seal; the dispute was finally settled by making the Corresponding Secretary the custodian of the Seal.

Previous to the seal being affixed, the candidate was required to pay to the Treasurer of the Society a fee not to exceed ten dollars, the amount to be determined by the Society.

The penalty for practicing without a license was fifty dollars for each offense, one-half to the Society, the other half to the informer. The fine was to be recovered by bill of presentment and indictment in the court.

The charter authorized the Society to fix the times and places of the meetings of the Board and fill vacancies therein.

After the reincorporation in 1838 the Society adopted a by-law concerning the Board of Examiners. Curiously, the charter did not require the members of the Board to be members of the Society, simply that they should be residents of the District; but the Society itself saw to it that only its own members should be on the Board. The fee was at first fixed at five dollars. The senior practitioner on the Board was the chairman. The Board was required to keep a record of its proceedings and make a report at the annual meeting of the Society. The fee was increased to ten dollars in 1867. In 1871 the Board was authorized to elect its own chairman, the granting of temporary licenses was discontinued, and the Board was required to meet on the first Wednesday of each month at such hour and place as it might determine.

Of course, one of the most important acts of the Society when it met March 8, 1819, was to elect a " Board." Drs. J. T. Shaaff, Charles Worthington, Thos. Sim, Frederick May and Thomas Semmes were the first Board. It devised a form of license or certificate, engraved on parchment. The engraved plate was 13 by 15 inches. The text was in Latin and read as follows:

Praeses et Quaesitores Societatis Medicorum in Columbiae Territorio omnibus et singulis has literas lecturis salutem:

Notum sit, examinatione habita ———— ———— virum doctumque Medicinae et chirurgiae satis peritum nos comprobare.

Itaque auctoritate nobis collata ex Societatis decreto,

eidem ———— ———— jusque potestatem artemque salutarem et Chirurgiam exercendi damus et concedimus.

Cujus sigillum communi huic membranae affixum
nominaque nostra subscripta testimonio sint.

Datum ————, Anno Domini Millesimo Octingentesimo
et Republicae Septuagesimo ———— et hujusce Societatis
institutae ————.

(Signed by) Praeses (and) Quaesitores.

The translation is: "The President and Examiners of
the Medical Society of the District of Columbia to all and
singular who may read these presents, greeting: Be it
known that upon examination held, we approve ————
———— as a man sufficiently skilled in medicine and surgery. Therefore by the authority conferred on us by the
decree of the Society, we grant and confirm to the said
———— ———— the right and authority of practicing therapeutics and Surgery. In witness whereof the seal of the
Society is affixed to this parchment and our names subscribed. Given at ————, Anno Domini 18—, and of the
Republic the ————, and of the establishment of the
Society the ————. Signed by the President of the Society and the members of the Board.

The Board went promptly to work, as appears from a
notice in the "National Intelligencer," March 17, 1819:

"The Medical Board of Examiners elected under the law
of Congress incorporating the Medical Society of the District of Columbia, will hold their first stated meeting in the
City of Washington on the first Monday in April. Applicants for licenses to practice medicine or surgery in the
District of Columbia will then attend, and in the meantime
may obtain a special license from any member of the Board.'
Signed by the five members of the Board.

November 3, 1875, Drs. A. F. A. King, T. M. Healey and
C. H. A. Kleinschmidt were appointed a committee to consider the wording of the license, which was said to be incorrect. February 9, 1876, the committee reported, recom-

mending that a new plate with the necessary corrections be made. The committee was instructed to ascertain the cost of the plate. December 13th the Society ordered the new plate. The corrected form was as follows:

Praeses et Quaesitores Societatis Medicorum in Territorio Columbiano.
Omnibus et singulis has literas visuris salutem. Notum sit ——— ——— Virum Medicinae et Chirurgiae doctum peritumque, ejus scientiae examinae rite habito, nos comprobare.
Itaque, auctoritate nobis, societatis decreto collata, eidem ——— ——— jus potestatemque artis medendi et chirurgiae exercendae damus et concedimus.
Cujus rei testimonios sigillum societatis commune huic membranae affixum est et nomina nostra sunt subscripta.
Datum Washington Anno Domini Millesimo octingentesimo, ——— Republicae fundatae ———, hujusce autem societatis institutae ———.
(Signed) ——— ——— Praeses.
——— ——— Quaesitores.

September 24, 1879, Dr. D. W. Prentiss moved to print the licenses in English; this was opposed by Drs. King, J. W. H. Lovejoy and J. T. Sothoron, and October 1 the subject was referred to the Board of Examiners. The question came up again January 14, 1880. Drs. Prentiss, E. M. Schaeffer and W. H. Triplett favored the English, Drs. Toner, R. Reyburn, Lovejoy, J. Ford Thompson and Kleinschmidt the Latin, and so the motion failed.

As stated above, the Board expired by law June 3, 1896. Its records prior to 1869 cannot be found.

THE SEAL OF THE SOCIETY.

A seal*, provided for in the charter, was adopted by the Society presumably at its first meeting or soon afterward. It was engraved on a circular die, $2\frac{1}{2}$ inches in diameter.

---

* See title page.

In the center is a figure of the goddess Hygeia on an elevated altar in her temple ; she holds in her hand a cup extended toward a serpent, the emblem of wisdom, which is
twined around a pillar and has its head raised as if to place
medicine in the cup. Over the altar are the words "Con-
cordia, labor, frugali" (concord, labor and frugality), and
around the margin the words "Templum hygeiae," and
"Societatis medicorum territ Columbiae sigillum" (Seal
of the Medical Society of the District of Columbia).

The first seal disappeared in some way not stated, and
the Recording Secretary was directed, January 4, 1847, to
have a new one made; it cost $22.00. Again, May 23,
1883, the old seal being much worn, the Society directed
that a new one be procured, which was done.

From time to time the question arose as to who should
have charge of the seal, and was not settled till March 31,
1869, when an amendment to the by-laws was adopted,
giving the custody to the Corresponding Secretary.

NATIONAL AND INTERNATIONAL SOCIETIES.

The relations of the Medical Society to National and
International Societies have been many and important.
One reason for this is the fact that Washington is so frequently selected as the place of meeting of these societies.
As early as April, 1819, soon after its first incorporation, a
delegation from the Society was elected to a "Convention
of the Middle States" that met in Philadelphia, June 1 of
that year, to frame and publish an "American Pharmacopoeia." Drs. Shaaff, Sim and Huntt were the delegates.

Delegates were also sent to the "National Convention of
Physicians" that met in the Capitol at Washington, January 1, 1820, at which the "United States Pharmacopoeia"
was adopted and a committee appointed to attend to its

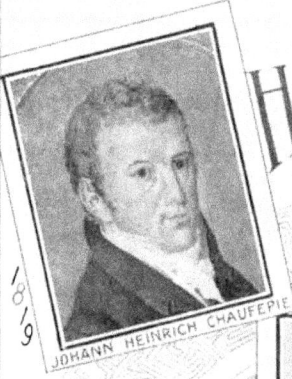

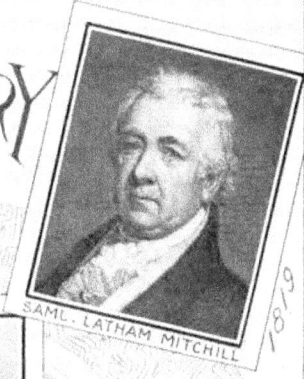

HONORARY

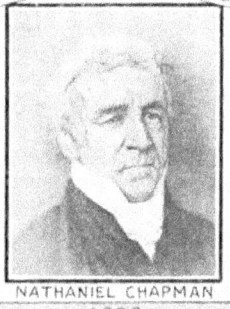

1819 JOHANN HEINRICH CHAUFEPIE

SAML. LATHAM MITCHILL 1819

NATHANIEL CHAPMAN
1820

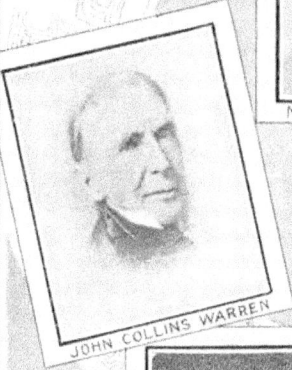

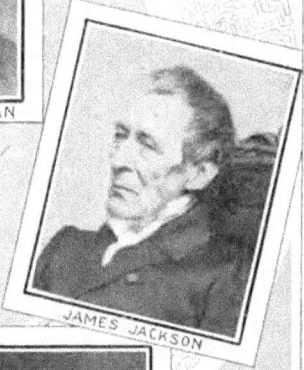

JOHN COLLINS WARREN

JAMES JACKSON

18

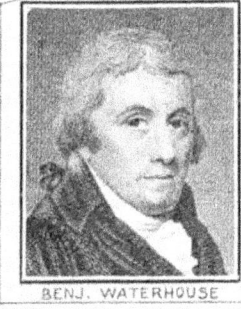

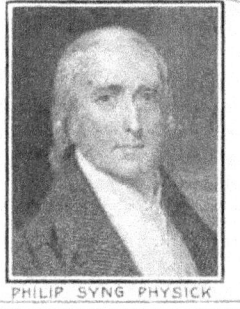

21

BENJ. WATERHOUSE

PHILIP SYNG PHYSICK

7

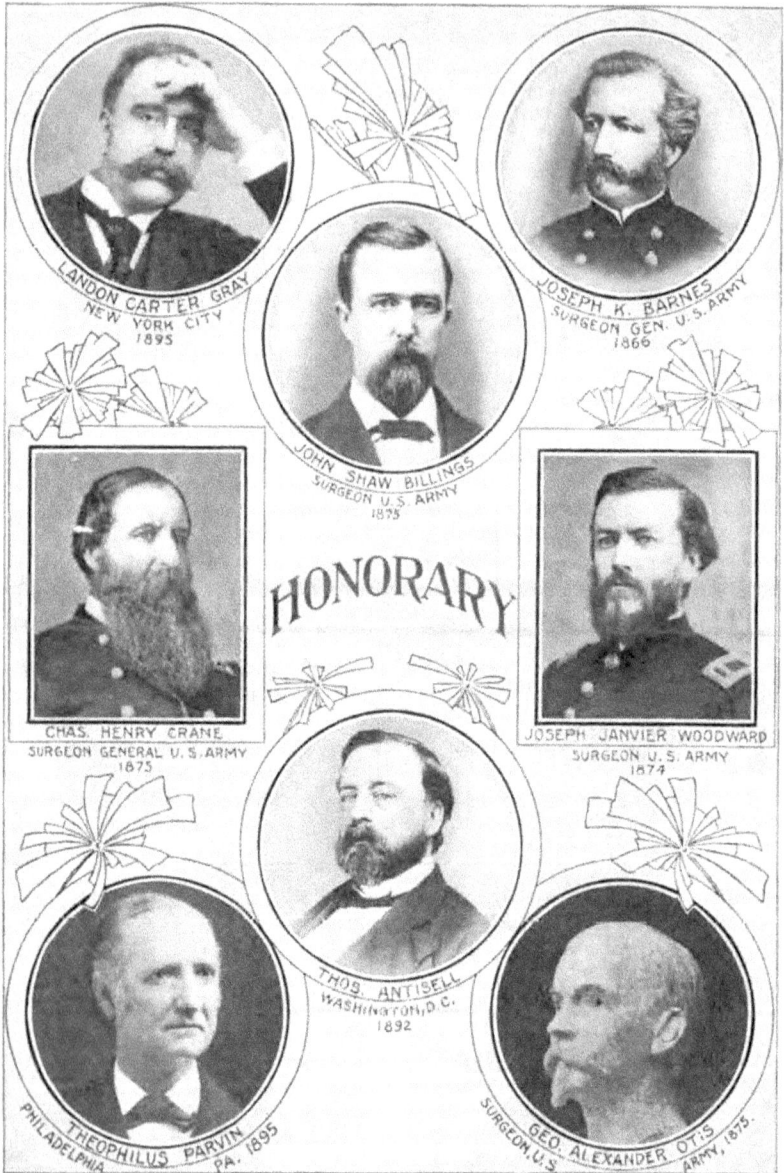

LANDON CARTER GRAY
NEW YORK CITY
1895

JOSEPH K. BARNES
SURGEON GEN. U.S. ARMY
1866

JOHN SHAW BILLINGS
SURGEON U.S. ARMY
1875

HONORARY

CHAS. HENRY CRANE
SURGEON GENERAL U.S. ARMY
1875

JOSEPH JANVIER WOODWARD
SURGEON U.S. ARMY
1874

THOS. ANTISELL
WASHINGTON, D.C.
1892

THEOPHILUS PARVIN
PHILADELPHIA, PA. 1895

GEO. ALEXANDER OTIS
SURGEON U.S. ARMY, 1875

8

publication. This meeting was the first of the decennial meetings for revising the pharmacopoeia.

The Medical Society was deeply interested in the formation of the American Medical Association. January 4, 1847, three delegates were elected to the first meeting of that body, H. Lindsly, F. Howard and J. Borrows; Dr. Borrows did not attend. The meeting was held in Philadelphia May 5th of that year, under the name of the "National Medical Convention." It should be stated that a preliminary meeting had been held in New York City May 5, 1846. The organization was completed at Philadelphia and the name changed to "American Medical Association." Under the new name the first meeting was held in Baltimore May 2, 1848, where the Medical Society of this District was represented by Drs. Noble Young, T. B. J. Frye, J. M. Thomas and F. Howard. Dr. J. C. Hall was elected, but did not attend.

The election of delegates to the American Medical Association was generally attended with some evidence of partisanship and personal feeling. Sometimes the Society elected them, at other times it appointed a committee to select them. Sometimes the President (1853 and 1854) was authorized to appoint delegates, and he was usually authorized to fill vacancies. Apparently some advantage must have been taken of election as delegates to acquire a little notoriety, for, January 7, 1856, the Society ordered that the names of delegates should not be published in the local newspapers.

Each year the number of delegates increased with the increase in membership of the Society, so that in time the number became quite large. January 5, 1852, an effort was made to have the Society pay the traveling expenses of its delegates, but the effort failed and apparently was never afterward renewed. The American Medical Association met in Washington May 4, 1858, at which time Dr. Harvey Lindsly, of Washington, was elected President for the session of 1859.

April 19, 1865, the Society ordered that, in view of the political and social condition in Washington at that time, its delegates to the American Medical Association should not invite that body to meet in Washington. June 5, 1867, however, a committee of arrangements was appointed to attend to the meeting which was to be held in 1868 in Washington.

The committee consisted of Drs. Grafton Tyler, Chairman; Harvey Lindsly, W. P. Johnston, F. Howard, L. Mackall, Wm. Marbury, J. M. Toner and T. F. Maury, with Dr. J. W. H. Lovejoy as Secretary.

At the suggestion of Dr. Toner, April 7, 1869, the Society offered to house and care for the proposed library of the American Medical Association. Dr. Toner succeeded in securing a room in the Smithsonian Institution. Dr. Robt. Reyburn was then the Librarian, succeeded in 1871 by Dr. F. A. Ashford, in 1873 by Dr. Wm. Lee, and in 1883 by Dr. C. H. A. Kleinschmidt. The library was eventually removed to Chicago.

It may be mentioned here that among the earlier officers of the Association, besides Dr. Harvey Lindsly, who was President in 1859, Dr. Grafton Tyler was a Vice President in 1856, Dr. W. P. Johnston in 1866 and Dr. Noble Young in 1869; Dr. J. M. Toner was President in 1874; Dr. S. C. Busey a Vice President in 1877. In 1859, when the Association met in Washington, Dr. A. J. Semmes was Secretary; Dr. Lovejoy was Assistant Secretary in 1868 at the meeting in Washington, and in 1870, at the next meeting in Washington, Dr. Wm. Lee was Assistant Secretary. Dr. A. Y. P. Garnett was President in 1888. This District and this Society have been, therefore, well represented in the higher offices of the Association. Several members have been chairmen of sections, while others have been selected to deliver special addresses.

November 12, 1890, Dr. H. L. E. Johnson offered the following resolution :

" The Medical Society of the District of Columbia, having learned that the Trustees of the American Medical Association have under consideration a plan for the permanent publication of the Journal, *Resolved*, That in the opinion of this Society the Capital of our common country affords the only proper place for the publication of the Journal of an association representing every State in the Union, and that we respectfully urge the Trustees to guarantee equality of influence in the Journal management by its publication in this neutral territory, where every State medical association in affiliation shall have equal consideration.

" *Be it further resolved*, That in case the Trustees shall adopt this view we agree in all proper and honorable means to further the interests of the Journal. The Society desires further to inform the Trustees that there is now no medical journal published in the Capital, and that in its opinion the financial prosperity of the Journal, instead of being jeopardized by the change of place of publication, would be materially advanced."

After discussion the motion was lost by a vote of twelve to thirteen.

SMALLPOX AND VACCINATION.

Dr. Toner states that in 1828 the Society held extra meetings and discussed measures to arrest the spread of smallpox.

January 19, 1846, a meeting was held to take measures to allay the excitement caused by the prevalence of smallpox in the District. A committee consisting of Drs. Thos. Miller, J. C. Hall and W. P. Johnston was appointed to consider the matter and make report. A resolution was also adopted to coöperate with the Board of Health in its effort to suppress the disease.

March 14, 1864, Dr. D. R. Hagner read a paper on vaccination, which was referred to a committee, which reported April 5th, and the paper was ordered to be printed in pamphlet form.

May 22, 1865, Dr. Toner read a paper on smallpox. The Society adopted resolutions stating that its views were in accord with those of the Committee of the American Medical Association on the value and necessity of universal vaccination ; some measures should be inaugurated by the city authorities by which every person within the limits of the city should be vaccinated and kept protected by revaccination, and that a committee should be appointed in conjunction with the Auxiliary Committee of the American Medical Association to represent to the Mayor and other corporate authorities of Washington and Georgetown the advantages of early and universal vaccination and occasional revaccination.

November 25, 1868, a committee was appointed, consisting of Drs. J. Eliot, W. P. Johnston and F. A. Ashford, to consider the best means of introducing into use pure vaccine virus and preserving it for the use of members of the Society. Drs. Garnett and Busey were added to the committee January 20, 1869.

"The committee reported February 10, recommending the establishment of a Vaccine Institute, under the sole control of the Society, to be managed by a Board of three members of the Society to be elected annually. This Board should examine or inspect all vaccine virus presented to or bought by the Institute, before disposing of it to those entitled to it. One member of the Board should be the curator, having charge of all the virus in the Institute and dispensing it or disposing of it under the supervision of the Board.

The curator should act as secretary of the Board, and keep a record of its proceedings. The virus should be distributed gratuitously to the members of the Society ; a charge of $2.00 should be made to non-members ; the money to go to the treasurer of the Society and to be used to buy virus when needed and pay the current expenses of the Institute. The members of the Society, at the Wednesday meetings, should deposit the virus in their possession with the presiding officer who should deliver it to the Board. The curator should adopt the most improved methods of preservation. In order that a constant and fresh supply of the virus might be maintained, the members of the Society should vaccinate all infants delivered by them, within forty days after birth."

It does not appear that the Institute ever materialized.

October 23, 1872, the Society discussed the question of the accuracy of the report of the Board of Health in regard to the actual number of cases of smallpox in the District.

February 21, 1877, Dr. Garnett stated that a case which he had diagnosed as syphilis had been sent to the smallpox hospital by the Board of Health. He asked that a committee be appointed to examine into the matter. Drs. Garnett, G. L. Magruder and F. A. Ashford were appointed. March 14 the committee reported that the case was one of syphilis; that the physician in charge of the smallpox hospital had so pronounced it; but the patient had been admitted during this physician's absence from the hospital.

October 31, 1894, a committee was appointed to investigate a recent introduction and dissemination of smallpox in the city, and the committee was instructed to impress upon the community the importance of vaccination as a prophylactic. Drs. S. S. Adams, W. W. Johnston, Kleinschmidt, G. Wythe Cook and J. D. Morgan were the committee. It does not appear that the committee reported to the Society.

MEDICAL ETHICS.

Elsewhere it is stated that the Medical Association of the District of Columbia was formed to provide a fee bill and code of ethics, because both were denied to the Society by its charter, which says, section 4, " Provided that nothing herein contained shall authorize the said corporation in any wise to regulate the price of medical or chirurgical attendance." The charter of 1838 adds these words " nor to establish or fix a tariff of charges or fees for medical attendance or advice, or to interfere in any way with charges or fees for medical attendance or advice."

Both charters, in section 1, state the object of the Society to be " the promoting and disseminating medical and surgical knowledge," and add the words " and for no other purpose whatever." The charter of 1838 goes further ; section 7, after empowering the Society to make such by-laws, rules and regulations as it may find requisite, limits this power by the words " which by-laws, rules and regulations shall in their application and operation be exclusively confined to said Society as a society or body corporate, and not to its members individually when not acting in a corporate character." As previously stated, it has been held by some members that these clauses forbid the Society disciplining a member for any offense committed outside the actual meetings of the Society, and mention was made of a case occurring in 1868, in which a member was charged with bribery, that caused a public scandal (see page 14).

On several other occasions the Society has taken action in regard to statements made by members outside the meetings, where the purpose or effect of the statements was to injure the Society. But no extreme measures have ever been taken—nothing beyond a vote of censure. In one case this vote was followed by the resignations of the members ;

in another, the moral effect of the Society investigation was sufficient, and no further action was taken.

It was necessary, however, at the very beginning that there should be some ethical understanding among the members, and in the first publication made by the Society, in 1820, in connection with the charter, constitution, by-laws and rules, we find the following:

"*Rules and regulations for the purpose of establishing etiquette and professional intercourse among the members of the Medical Society of the District of Columbia:*

"Any member of the Medical Society of the District of Columbia who may violate any of the following rules and regulations, and upon conviction thereof before the said Society, shall, for the first offense, be fined a sum not exceeding twenty dollars; for the second offense he shall be *expelled*, and his expulsion shall be published in one or more newspapers in this District; and no member of said Society shall consult with, or voluntarily meet in a professional way, or aid, or abet, any practitioner of medicine who may have suffered the penalty of expulsion.

"ARTICLE I. If a physician be called to any member of a *family* in the absence of the family physician, on the arrival of the latter the patient shall be resigned by the former.

"ARTICLE II. When a physician engaged to attend a case of midwifery is absent and a second delivers the woman, the latter shall receive the fee and relinquish the patient to the first on his arrival. If the first arrive while the second is present, and before the woman is delivered, the second shall retire and resign the patient to the first.

"ARTICLE III. No physician shall directly or indirectly interfere in the practice of a brother physician or surgeon; or give opinion in any manner concerning a case knowing him to be in attendance, unless it be during his absence and in cases of emergency.

"ARTICLE IV. In consultation it shall be the duty of the consulting physician to enter the sick room and investigate the case in *company* with the attending physician, and shall leave the room immediately after having obtained such information as may be required to decide on the case. All directions agreed upon shall be left to the charge of the attending physician. No statements or discussions of the case shall take place in the *presence of the patient or his friends*, and no opinions at variance with the plan agreed upon shall ever be promulgated. Punctuality shall always be observed in the visits, and no visits shall be made by the *consulting physician*, but in concert or by mutual consent, except in cases of emergency when the attending physician cannot be readily procured.

"ARTICLE V. No member of the Society shall publicly advertise for sale any medicine the composition of which he keeps a secret; or shall offer, either publicly or through his friends, to cure diseases by any such secret medicine, or otherwise.

"ARTICLE VI. No member of this Society shall either *casually* or *formally* prescribe for or visit *professionally* any case *gratuitously* when the circumstances of the patient will justify a charge, except in cases of practicing physicians, or their families, and regular ministers of the Gospel of every denomination.

"ARTICLE VII. No member of this Society shall make any previous contract with any person or family for a definite sum as a remuneration for his annual attendance on said person or family."

There is no actual evidence existing, only the probability, that these ethical rules were made by the Society itself, and whether the Society deliberately violated the provision of its charter may never be known. Of course, when the Medical Association of the District of Columbia was formed, in 1833, its members adopted a code of ethics by which they were to be governed, and that of the Society was no longer needed.

April 6, 1887, Dr. Busey moved to refer certain charges which had been made by one member against another to the Standing Committee of the Medical Association, and

HONORARY

1895

WM OSLER.
BALTIMORE MD.

GEO. MILLER STERNBERG
SURG. GEN.
U.S.A.

JAMES RUFUS TRYON
SURG. GEN.
U.S. NAVY

WALTER WYMAN
SUPERVISING
SURG. GEN.
U.S.M.H.S.

FREDERICK CHEEVER SHATTUCK
BOSTON MASS.

THOMAS ALMOND ASHBY
BALTIMORE MD.

MOSES WADLEIGH RUSSELL
CONCORD N.H.

BEDFORD BROWN
ALEXANDRIA VA.

9

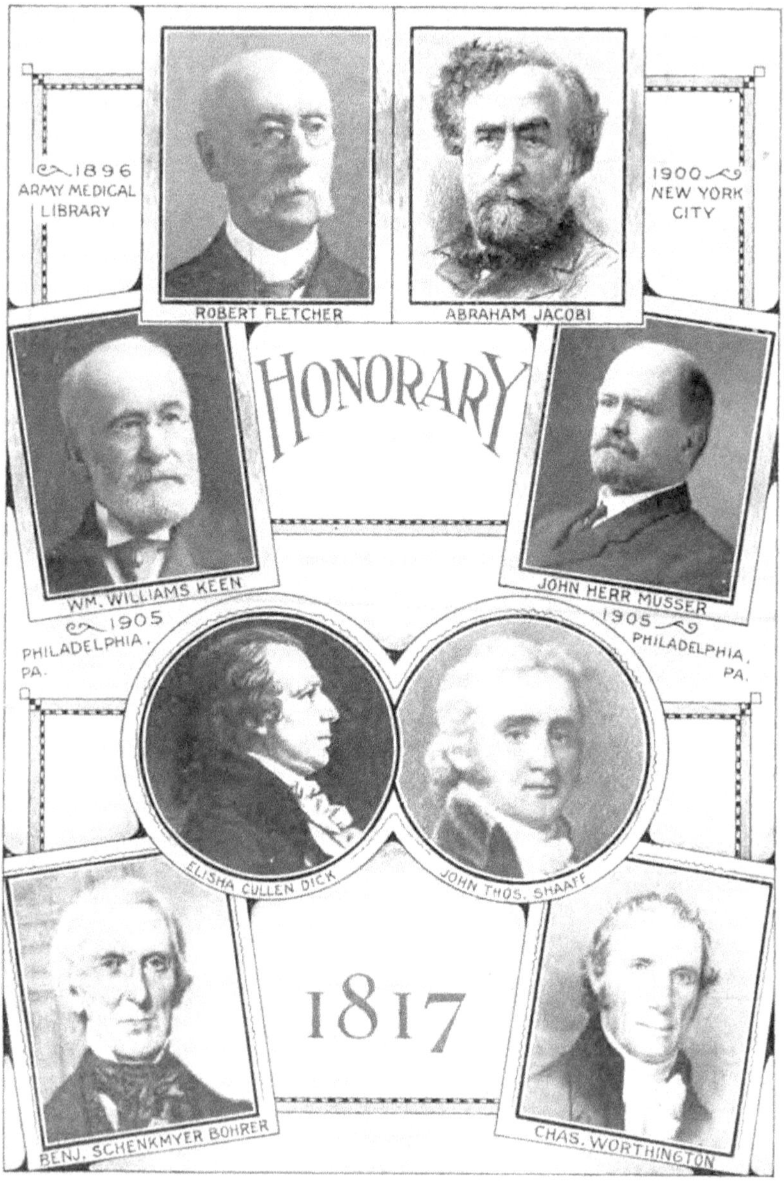
1896
ARMY MEDICAL LIBRARY
ROBERT FLETCHER
ABRAHAM JACOBI
1900
NEW YORK CITY
HONORARY
WM. WILLIAMS KEEN
1905
PHILADELPHIA, PA.
JOHN HERR MUSSER
1905
PHILADELPHIA, PA.
ELISHA CULLEN DICK
JOHN THOS. SHAAFF
1817
BENJ. SCHENKMYER BOHRER
CHAS. WORTHINGTON

stated that the Board of Censors had decided that the charges were outside its jurisdiction. The charges were so referred.

October 5, 1892, the attention of the Society was called to the fact that a member had written to a Congressional committee a letter which reflected upon the Society. The matter was referred to the Board of Censors, and the Board reported, November 23d, that the said member had stated that he had been in error in what he had written and would so inform the Congressional committee. The report was accepted, and no further action was taken.

THE HOSPITALS AND DISPENSARIES OF THE DISTRICT OF COLUMBIA.

The first public hospital in the District of Columbia was that connected with the poor house, situated then in the square between Sixth and Seventh and M and N Streets, N. W., and called the Washington Infirmary. About 1846 the Washington Asylum, on Nineteenth Street southeast, near the Anacostia river, was completed and the poor house and hospital inmates removed thereto.

During the cholera epidemic in 1832 temporary hospitals were established. After the epidemic ceased the Board of Health petitioned Congress from year to year to establish a public hospital. The Medical Society became interested, and January 11, 1841, appointed a committee consisting of Drs. Thos. Sewall, Alex. McWilliams, Thos. Miller, Wm. Jones and Harvey Lindsly to petition Congress for a national hospital. August 29, 1842, Congress passed a law giving authority for the old jail in Judiciary Square to be altered and fitted up as an insane asylum and hospital for sick, disabled, infirm seamen, soldiers or others; but in 1844 Congress decided that the site and building were unsuitable for such purpose. "At this juncture the Medi-

3

cal Faculty of Columbian College applied to Congress for the use of the building for an infirmary and for other purposes." The other purposes were "medical instruction and scientific purposes." The application met with favor, and Congress passed a law, June 15, 1844, to that effect, but required a bond from the incorporators for the return of the property in good condition when demanded. This institution was also called the *Washington Infirmary*. In 1853, by an appropriation from Congress, the building was much enlarged. At the outbreak of the civil war in 1861 the U. S. Government took possession of the building for military hospital purposes; November 3d of that year it was entirely destroyed by fire. (See Toner's Oration.)

In 1852 Congress made an appropriation for an *insane asylum*. The location proposed encountered some objections, and the Society held a special meeting November 19th of that year, at which a committee was appointed "to take into consideration the policy of interference in regard to the location of the lunatic asylum and the appointment of the physician thereof." The committee consisted of Drs. Fred. May, H. Lindsly, J. Borrows, F. Howard and A. Y. P. Garnett. November 20 the committee asked to be, and was, excused from the further consideration of the subject by the Society. A resolution was then offered by Dr. J. C. Hall,

"that the Medical Society of the District of Columbia, actuated solely by motives of humanity and a desire that the liberal appropriation made by Congress for the erection and support of an insane asylum be employed in a manner most conducive to the wellbeing of the unfortunate objects of its bounty, respectfully suggests to the President of the United States that a committee of resident physicians of this city, appointed by this Society, be permitted to confer with him in relation to the healthiness and suitableness of a proposed site for the said asylum."

This resolution was laid on the table, and so the matter ended. The asylum was located, as is well known, on a hill south of the Eastern Branch. Dr. Charles H. Nichols was appointed its Superintendent, and, about July 7, 1856, was elected a member of the Society.

In consequence of the U. S. Government taking possession of the Washington Infirmary in 1861, the necessity of a public hospital led to the establishment of *Providence Hospital* the same year, and mainly through the efforts of Dr. Toner. It was opened in June, 1861.

The *Columbia Hospital for Women and Lying-in Asylum* was established in 1866, mainly through the efforts of Dr. J. Harry Thompson, who was for ten years the surgeon in charge ; it was situated at the northwest corner of Massachusetts Avenue and Fourteenth Street, N. W., in the building that was occupied during the civil war as the Desmarres and afterwards the Ricord General (Military) Hospitals.

The Society was represented more or less on the staff of each of the hospitals in the District and naturally was interested in the work done in them. October 23, 1867, the Society directed that a request be made of the officers in charge of the hospitals and asylums in the District to make quarterly reports to the Society, and March 10, 1869, the Committee on Essays was instructed to request such reports either quarterly or annually. The minutes show that some reports were received and discussed.

January 20, 1869, a committee was appointed to consider the feasibility of establishing a Dispensary under the auspices of the Society itself. The committee reported February 10th, recommending that a dispensary be established at the new Medical Hall with branches elsewhere as might be thought desirable. It was proposed that the Dispensary should secure to the sick poor competent medical ser-

vice and medicine gratuitously. It should be under a
" Board of Control and Consultation," composed of seven
members of the Society, to be appointed annually. This
Board should make the necessary rules and regulations for
the government of the Dispensary, provide ways and means
for its management, and disburse the funds. There should
be three departments—medical, surgical and diseases of
women and children. There should be a superintendent
and two or more assistants for each department, to be
appointed from members of the Society, by the Board of
Control. There were other details in regard to service,
consultations, apothecaries, &c. The report was referred
back to the committee February 24th for further consideration, was never discussed by the Society, and, May 12th,
the committee was discharged and no further action taken.

Although this project failed to materialize, as indeed
might have been expected, the discussion of the subject
was not without results. Some members of the Society
went to work, more especially Drs. G. L. Magruder and H.
H. Barker, and started the *Central Dispensary*, which was
opened May 1, 1871, in the Medical College building,
Tenth and E Streets, N. W. About 1880, mainly through
the efforts of Dr. Barker, an emergency department was attached to the Dispensary, so that the title became *The Central Dispensary and Emergency Hospital.* The hospital
had then been moved to a building on Tenth Street, between D and E, N. W.

In May, 1874, Drs. L. W. Ritchie and C. H. A. Kleinschmidt of the Society, who lived in Georgetown, started
a hospital there and called it the *General Hospital of the
District of Columbia.* For want, however, of sufficient support it was compelled, two years afterwards, to close its
doors.

Through the efforts mainly of Dr. F. A. Ashford of the Society, *Garfield Memorial Hospital* was founded. Dr. Busey in his "Reminiscences," p. 221 *et seq.*, gives a full account of the movement that finally ended in the opening of the hospital in 1882. Many of the medical profession of the District supported the movement, and the Medical Society, May 10, 1882, passed the following resolutions commending it :

" *Whereas* the medical profession of this District have long felt the need of a general hospital, and, in a very largely attended meeting before the late civil war, had, with great unanimity, formed a project for the establishment of such a hospital, the movements for which were unfortunately interrupted and rendered abortive by that unhappy event; and *Whereas* the necessities for such an institution are unquestionable and have, since that time, not diminished, but increased more than sevenfold ; therefore

" *Resolved*, That this Society has learned with great pleasure that certain patriotic and benevolent ladies and gentlemen are now earnestly coöperating in the endeavor to procure the establishment of a general hospital to be known as the Garfield Memorial Hospital.

" *Resolved*, That no more appropriate method of honoring the memory of our late brutally murdered President can be conceived of than the erection of such a monument ; an ever active institution for the relief of humanity, suffering in so many various forms ; a source for the acquirement and development of knowledge in those branches of scientific study most nearly directed to the immediate relief of many ; and an everlasting and inexhaustible well-spring of charity and benevolence which in the minds of all men of right feeling must be esteemed far above the tablets of brass or mere monuments of bronze or marble.

" *Resolved*, That this Society desires to assure all concerned that the proposed measure meets with its entire approbation, to express the extreme interest which is felt in the success of so good a benevolence, and to offer its cordial coöperation in efforts to obtain so desirable an object."

Contagious Diseases Hospital.—January 18, 1893, the Society appointed a committee, consisting of Drs. W. W. Johnston, J. H. Bryan and S. S. Adams, to confer with the Conference Committee of Congress and urge the passage of the bill appropriating money to establish a hospital for contagious diseases in the District of Columbia. May 17th a letter was received from the Board of Directors of the proposed Contagious Diseases Hospital, signed by Mr. Archibald Hopkins, asking advice and assistance in connection with the project of putting up buildings for the isolation and treatment of contagious diseases. The Society appointed a committee—Drs. W. W. Johnston, J. Ford Thompson, J. W. H. Lovejoy, E. A. Balloch and B. G. Pool—to consider the matter and report. The committee reported May 24th, recommending that such hospital should not be located within the city limits nor in any thickly settled portion of the suburbs; should have ample grounds around it; in fact, should be preferably in the country, away from dwelling houses, but still accessible; in such case there would be little or no fear of dissemination of disease. The committee recommended a location near the Eastern Branch; the only objection seemed to be the prevalence there of malaria. The report was much discussed and opposed, but finally adopted. The hospital, however, has never been built.* One result however of this movement was the erection of buildings at Garfield Hospital for contagious diseases patients, through the efforts of the Daisy Chain Guild, and at Providence Hospital a contagious ward was opened.

February 19, 1902, Dr. W. W. Johnston, as Chairman of the Executive Committee of the Society, read letters in regard to a recent communication of the Board of Charities

*See " Nat. Med. Rev.," 1892-3, I, p. 22; and Busey's " Souvenir," p. 291 *et seq.*

concerning a proposed *municipal* hospital.* The Society authorized the Committee to send the letters to the District Commissioners.

The municipal hospital has so far materialized that a site was bought on Varnum Street, between Seventh and Fourteenth, N. W., and an appropriation was made by Congress to erect a building for tuberculous patients. With regard to this hospital the Society, January 10, 1906, formally approved the efforts of the committees of Congress on the District of Columbia. June 26, 1908, the *Tuberculosis Hospital* was formally opened. Dr. G. M. Kober was mainly instrumental in establishing the hospital.

The Freedmen's Hospital and other civil hospitals in the city, the Children's Hospital, the Episcopal Eye and Ear Hospital, the Georgetown University Hospital, the Columbian University Hospital, the Woman's Dispensary at Four-and-a-half Street and Maryland Avenue, S. W., Woman's Clinic at 1237 T Street, N. W., and others, although they were all founded by members of the Medical Society and Medical Association of the District, the Society as a body took no action therein. The *Freedmen's Hospital* was an outgrowth of the medical side of the Freedmen's Bureau. The *Children's Hospital* was an outcome of the Department of Diseases of Children at the Columbia Hospital for Women ; was inaugurated in 1870 by Drs. Busey, F. A. Ashford, W. B. Drinkard and W. W. Johnston, after a conference with the lady managers of the Washington City Orphan Asylum followed by a public meeting of citizens. The *Episcopal Eye, Ear and Throat Hospital* was founded mainly through the efforts of Dr. E. O. Belt. The University hospitals were established, of course, through the activity of the medical faculties thereof. The *Woman's Dispensary* was founded by Drs. Annie Rice and

*See the Minutes of the Society, p. 689, and WASHINGTON MED. ANNALS, 1902, I, p. 147.

Jeannette Sumner; the *Woman's Clinic* by Drs. Ida J.
Heiberger, D. S. Lamb and others; the *Lutheran Eye, Ear
and Throat Infirmary* mainly by Dr. W. K. Butler; *Sibley
Hospital* mainly by a gift from Wm. Sibley, of Washington, as a memorial to his deceased wife; the *Eastern Dispensary and Casualty Hospital* by Drs. J. F. Hartigan,
J. T. Winter, G. B. Harrison, L. Tyler, L. Eliot and others;
the *Washington Hospital for Foundlings* by the will of
Joshua Pierce, in 1869, although the buildings were not
completed and opened until 1887; Mr. and Mrs. Wm.
Stickney and Dr. Z. T. Sowers were most active in the
matter. The *Washington Home for Incurables* was founded
in 1889 by Mrs. H. F. Everett, Mrs. E. S. Bell and Mr.
E. F. Riggs; it admits cases of cancer, and cares for both
adults and children.

The *Homeopathic Hospital* was founded by physicians
and laymen of that method of medical practice. There is
also a hospital for officers and soldiers of the U. S. Army,
on the old arsenal grounds at the foot of Four-and-a-half
Street, S. W., and an army dispensary at 1720 H Street,
N. W.; two naval hospitals, the old one at Ninth Street
and Pennsylvania Avenue, S. E., the new one on the old
Observatory Hill, Twenty-third and E, N. W. With none
of these, however, has the Society anything directly to do.

THE LIBRARY OF THE SOCIETY.

As we might suppose, the idea of a Medical Library early
occurred to the members of the Society. Indeed, the first
charter provided for a Librarian as one of the officers, and
at the meeting of organization, January 5, 1818, Dr. Richard
Weightman was elected Librarian. The notice of the
meeting of March 8, 1819, included a request that the Committee on Library should meet at the same time. What

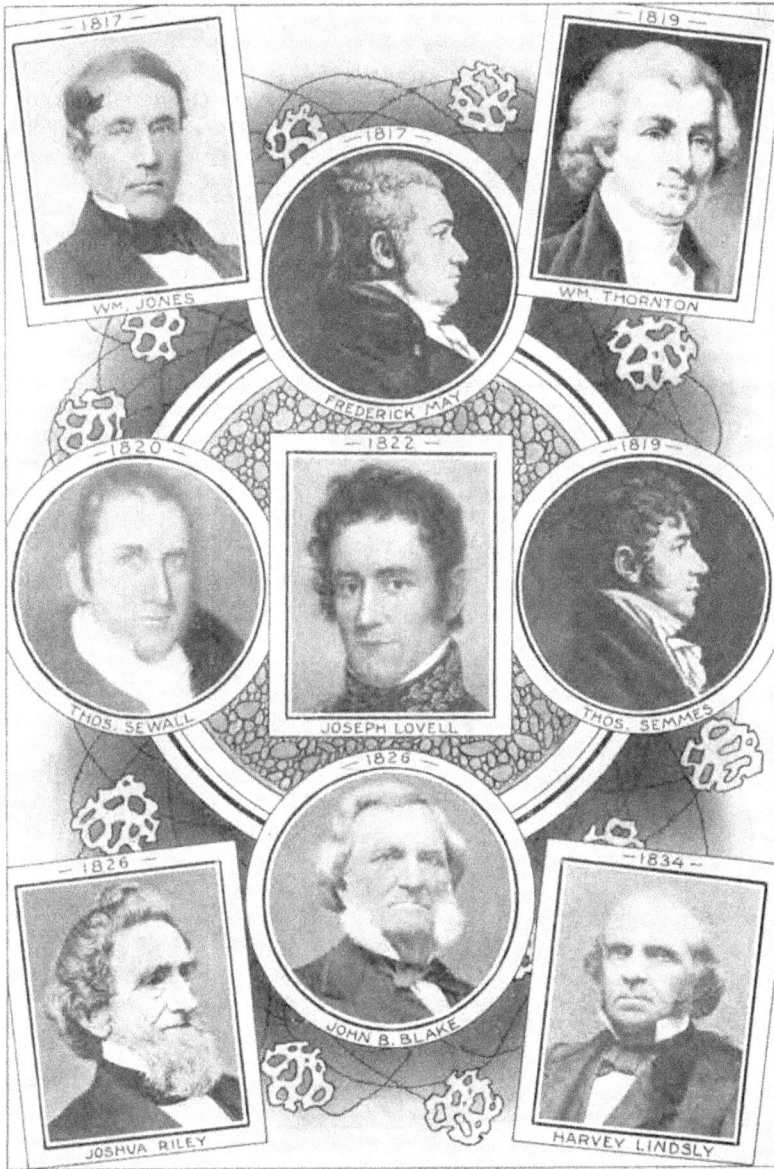

— 1817 — WM. JONES

— 1817 — FREDERICK MAY

— 1819 — WM. THORNTON

— 1820 — THOS. SEWALL

— 1822 — JOSEPH LOVELL

— 1819 — THOS. SEMMES

— 1826 — JOSHUA RILEY

— 1826 — JOHN B. BLAKE

— 1834 — HARVEY LINDSLY

11

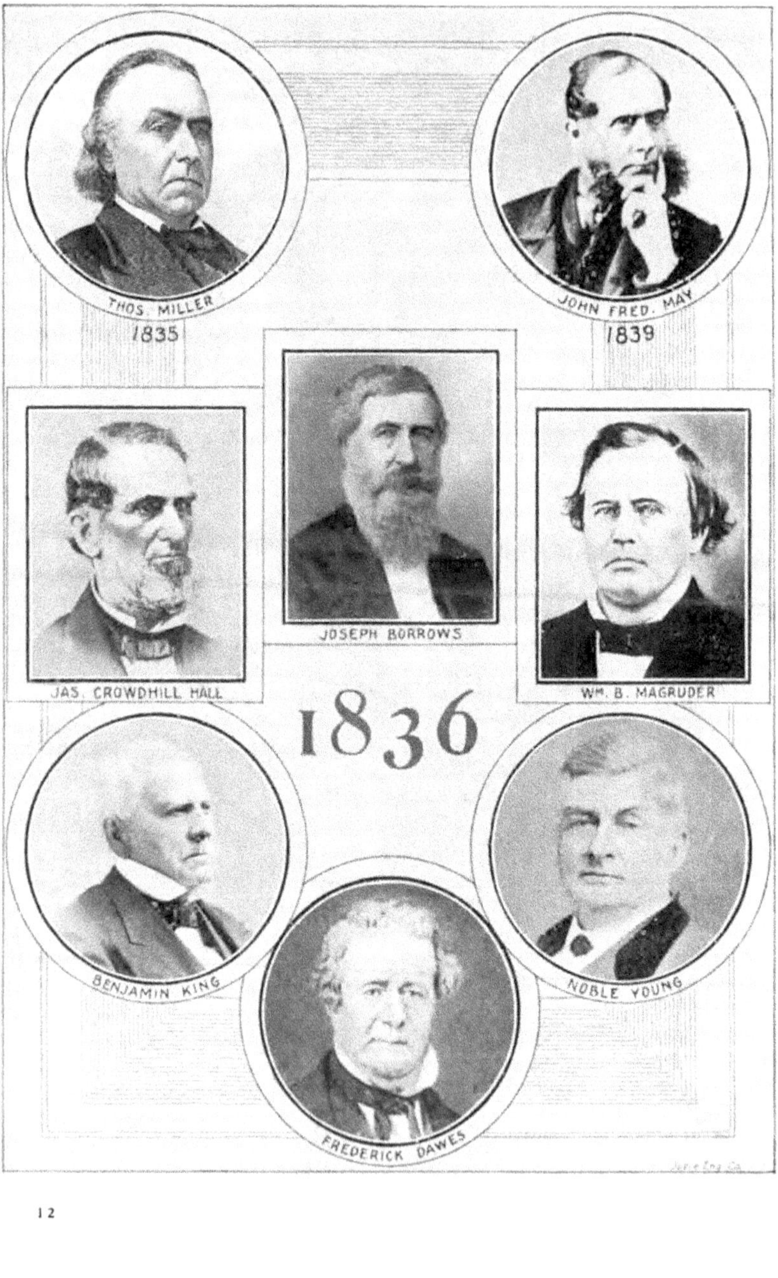

THOS. MILLER
1835

JOHN FRED. MAY
1839

JAS. CROWDHILL HALL

JOSEPH BORROWS

WM. B. MAGRUDER

1836

BENJAMIN KING

FREDERICK DAWES

NOBLE YOUNG

were the duties of this Library Committee does not appear. At the meeting just mentioned, Dr. N. W. Worthington was elected Librarian.

The duty of the Librarian (see section 6, by-laws) was to take charge of and preserve for the use of the Society all the Society property except the moneys; to keep a list of the donors; and report to the Society when desired to do so. The duties today are the same as they were over ninety years ago.

Dr. Toner states that a library was collected by donation and purchase, a portion of the yearly dues being set aside for that purpose, but when he made his anniversary address, September 26, 1866, there was only one book left, namely, Quincey's Lexicon, which had been presented to the Society July 1, 1818, by Dr. Thomas Henderson. It is easy to understand that as the Society had no permanent home, but moved about, the Library, especially, suffered in the moving.

July 1, 1844, it was ordered that the Librarian should subscribe for standard medical works and periodicals to the amount of ten dollars and that the necessary shelving should be put up. January 3, 1848, the subscription was discontinued. The next mention of the Library was January 10, 1861, when Dr. Lovejoy presented a copy of Copeland's Dictionary of Practical Medicine "as a nucleus for the formation of a medical library;" at the same time Dr. Harvey Lindsly presented "Rayer on Diseases of the Skin." These gifts aroused the Society to request the members to contribute books and pamphlets. February 21st following, Dr. Lovejoy gave three more books, and at the same meeting the Society ordered that the official papers should be preserved by the Librarian. March 21st, a bookcase and shelving were ordered ; and it was also ordered that the pamphlets so far received should be bound. May 16th, Dr.

Thomas Miller presented a hundred pamphlets and a book. September 12th, Dr. Thos. Antisell gave four books. October 3d, the Society ordered a subscription to the New Sydenham publications.

By January 9, 1867, Dr. Toner, the retiring Librarian, was able to report 152 books and pamphlets in the Library.

March 10, 1869, a Committee on Library was appointed, consisting of Drs. W. P. Johnston, J. M. Toner, T. Antisell, L. Mackall and W. B. Drinkard. What the committee did does not appear. Another committee was appointed November 9, 1870, Drs. Mackall, C. H. Liebermann and Wm. Marbury, to confer with a committee of the "Journal Club" * * * [this club was formed in 1869 and was a part of the Society in that its members were required to be members of the Society] with the view of establishing a reading room and library. The committee reported November 16th, recommending that a room be rented and furnished for the meetings of the Society and the care of the journals of the club. December 29th, rooms were obtained at the American Colonization Building, and January 11, 1871, it was ordered that shelving should be put up in the Library room and the use of the room be granted to the Journal Club.

There was no special mention of the Library again until September 28, 1881, when Dr. T. C. Smith moved that the Library, which consisted "only of old books which nobody ever consulted," be sold at auction. As this motion was not seconded he moved next to turn the books over to the Library of the Surgeon General's Office. This motion also failed to receive a second, and there the matter dropped for a time.

March 21, 1883, because the Society thought it was paying too much for the rooms it was occupying, it considered the question of giving up the library room and removing the library; but where to move it does not appear.

In his Presidential address December 18, 1901, Dr. D. S. Lamb recommended that the library be disposed of, and the Society ordered that a committee, consisting of the President, Recording Secretary and Librarian arrange to carry out the recommendation.

January 22, 1902, the committee reported that a portion of the library had been donated to the Surgeon General's Library and the remainder would be given to the Carnegie Public Library of Washington. April 2d the Librarian was instructed to report to the Society the titles of books and any other effects remaining after these donations.

Later on the Librarian, Dr. E. L. Morgan, made a report in which he recommended that, if possible, a room be secured at the Carnegie Library, in which the books given by the Society might be arranged and the room used as a reading room for the members of the Society. To carry out this suggestion a committee, consisting of Drs. D. S. Lamb, E. L. Morgan and F. P. Morgan, the Recording Secretary, was appointed March 18, 1903. Thus far the committee has not succeeded in making the desired arrangement.

April 22, 1903, the Librarian was instructed to retain in the Library one copy of each publication of the Society.

OBITUARIES.

Sometimes, more especially in the case of a member who had taken a prominent part in the work of the Society, an entire meeting was given, and oftentimes a special meeting was called, for the adoption of appropriate resolutions in regard to the deceased. In the case of less well-known members usually a part of a regular meeting was devoted to this purpose, and this custom has prevailed in later years.

For many years it was the custom not only to pass resolutions, but for the members to attend the funeral in a body; of course, this was much more readily done when the number of members was small, deaths were few and every one knew every one else. It was the custom, also, to wear a badge of mourning on the left arm for thirty days, but this has long since ceased. The Society also usually appointed several members to take charge of the funeral arrangements; this has also long since ceased. But these customs were in vogue as late as 1876.

So far as this history is concerned, where a memorial meeting was held or resolutions passed, a note of the fact has been made in the biographical sketch of the member, so that it is unnecessary to give any list of obituary notices. It will be interesting, however, to state that the first recorded notice of the kind was April 1, 1845, for Dr. Thomas Sewall; the next was January 25, 1847, for Dr. Frederick May; the third, July 31, 1849, for Dr. N. W. Worthington; the fourth, April 1, 1850, for Dr. Alexander McWilliams. Other members had died, but so far as the record shows no notice was taken of the death. In a few cases notice was taken of the death of a celebrated physician not resident in the District of Columbia; as, July 4, 1853, when a meeting was held in honor of Dr. Nathaniel Chapman, of Philadelphia, and May 3, 1865, in honor of Dr. Valentine Mott, of New York City.

November 1, 1876, Dr. Busey called attention to the irregularities of attendance of members of the Society at funerals of deceased members and thought that there should be some definite rules to guide such attendance. No action, however, was taken.

May 30, 1877, the Society took action on the death of Dr. Henry Powers Ritter, of Norfolk, Va., who at one time practiced medicine in Washington, although he never joined the Medical Society or Association. While visiting the city he died, May 29, 1877. May 15, 1878, the Society also took action on the death of Professor Joseph Henry, Secretary of the Smithsonian Institution, who, although not a physician nor a member of the Society, had shown many courtesies to the Society.

September 21, 1881, the Society adopted the following resolution on the death of PRESIDENT GARFIELD :

"*Resolved*, That in view of the great calamity which has befallen the country in the untimely taking off of our Chief Magistrate, and partaking as we do as citizens and patriots of the sorrow and grief which pervade every part of our land, this Society do now adjourn and this resolution be entered upon the journal."

April 11, 1883, the Society took action on the death of Surgeon General Joseph K. Barnes, U. S. A., and October 11th, of the same year, on the death of his successor, Surgeon General Charles H. Crane, U. S. A. Both of these were honorary members. November 21st, of the same year, action was taken on the death of Dr. J. Marion Sims; this was published in *Gaillard's Medical Journal*, for February, 1884, and republished as a pamphlet.

March 13, 1886, the Society took action on the death of Dr. Alexander Y. P. Garnett, Jr. Dr. Garnett had applied for membership, July 6, 1885, but his name was not reported on at the time of election, October 7th. He died March 12th, 1886, and was never, therefore, a member, although supposed to be by many of the Society.

January 31, 1895, the Society took action on the death of Dr. Alfred L. Loomis, of New York City.

October 2, 1901, the Society passed the following resolution :

"The Medical Society of the District of Columbia, desiring to manifest its appreciation of WILLIAM McKINLEY, late President of the United States, directs the Recording Secretary to place upon a memorial page this tribute of respect to the memory of a faithful public servant, worthy citizen, loyal and brave soldier, unselfish and pure statesman, efficient President and upright, honorable, Christian man, whose exemplary and consistent devotion to duty in every position which he was called upon to fill endeared him to his fellow citizens throughout the entire land. His virtues are worthy of emulation, his memory worth cherishing."

December 31, 1902, the Society held a memorial meeting in honor of Dr. Walter Reed, Surgeon, U. S. Army, and a member by invitation, who had achieved fame as the discoverer of the "carrier" of the yellow-fever germ, and had also, as Curator of the Army Medical Museum, shown many courtesies to the Society.*

On the death of Dr. A. B. Richardson, Superintendent of the Government Hospital for the Insane, D. C., the Society adopted appropriate resolutions, November 4, 1903.† And February 24, 1904, on the death of Dr. E. A. de Schweinitz, of the Department of Agriculture.‡ Drs. Richardson and de Schweinitz were also members by invitation.

October 15, 1907, action was taken on the death of Dr. James Carroll, Major and Surgeon, U. S. A., and Curator of the Army Medical Museum. He was one of the members of the U. S. A. Yellow Fever Commission, and a member of the Society by invitation.

CORONERS' INQUESTS.

July 7, 1856, a committee, consisting of Drs. Noble Young, A. J. Semmes and Grafton Tyler, was appointed to confer with the proper authorities concerning coroners' inquests. January 5, 1857, the committee reported progress and was continued. There is no further record in regard to the matter.

QUACKERY IN THE DISTRICT OF COLUMBIA.

The prevalence of quackery in this District lay at the foundation of the original formation of the Society. Dr. Toner speaks of " The frequent injury and injustice which had been perpetrated upon citizens of the District by charlatans and pretended doctors." The Society undertook to inform the public as to who were qualified to practice the healing art and were worthy of the confidence of the public. "It found, however, that it could do its work more successfully by incorporating and going to Congress for authority ; and, accordingly, the charter was applied for and granted."

May 9, 1860, the Society held a meeting to consider the case of a man named J. E. E. Ealin, calling himself a doctor, and claiming to be a celebrated aurist ; the same man had practiced in Nashville, Tenn., as a " corn doctor." Drs. Fred. May, H. P. Howard and J. Borrows were appointed a committee to consult with the District Attorney, with a view to take such action as would be legal and desirable.

September 15, 1880, the Corresponding Secretary was directed to communicate with the editor of the *Philadelphia Press* and obtain the names of those persons in the District of Columbia who held bogus diplomas, so that they might be exposed. September 28th the Secretary reported the names of several persons.

May 21, 1884, the Board of Examiners was requested to take measures to rid the community of traveling quacks. The Board reported May 28th that this was not a part of its duties. The Society then appointed a committee, Drs.

Reyburn, Lovejoy, Kleinschmidt, Franzoni and W. H. Taylor, to attend to the matter. This committee reported July 7th, stating that as a preliminary step it had taken legal advice as to the authority of the Medical Society over the practice of medicine in the District. The District Attorney, after careful attention to the matter, had stated his opinion that the charter of the Society was still in force and there would be no difficulty in enforcing the penalties provided for therein against all persons practicing medicine in the District without a diploma. But the penalty could not be inflicted if the person had a diploma from a regular medical college. The proper method of procedure would be to summon the offending party before the police court, and thence to the grand jury, for a bill of indictment. The District Attorney would aid, in every possible way, to secure conviction.

The chairman of the committee corresponded with the Secretary of the Homeopathic Medical Society of the District, who stated that that Society had not and would not license any irregular practitioner. The committee recommended that a circular letter should be prepared by the proper officers of the Medical Society and be sent to all the irregular practitioners of the District, requiring them to state by what authority they were practicing in the District, and calling their attention to the law.

In the discussion of the report Dr. Lovejoy stated that he did not agree with the District Attorney that the possession of a diploma was sufficient; but that, under the law, the individual should present said diploma to the Board of Examiners.

The report was accepted, and the Corresponding Secretary was directed to prepare and send out the circular letter indicated, and to report results to a committee appointed to receive them.

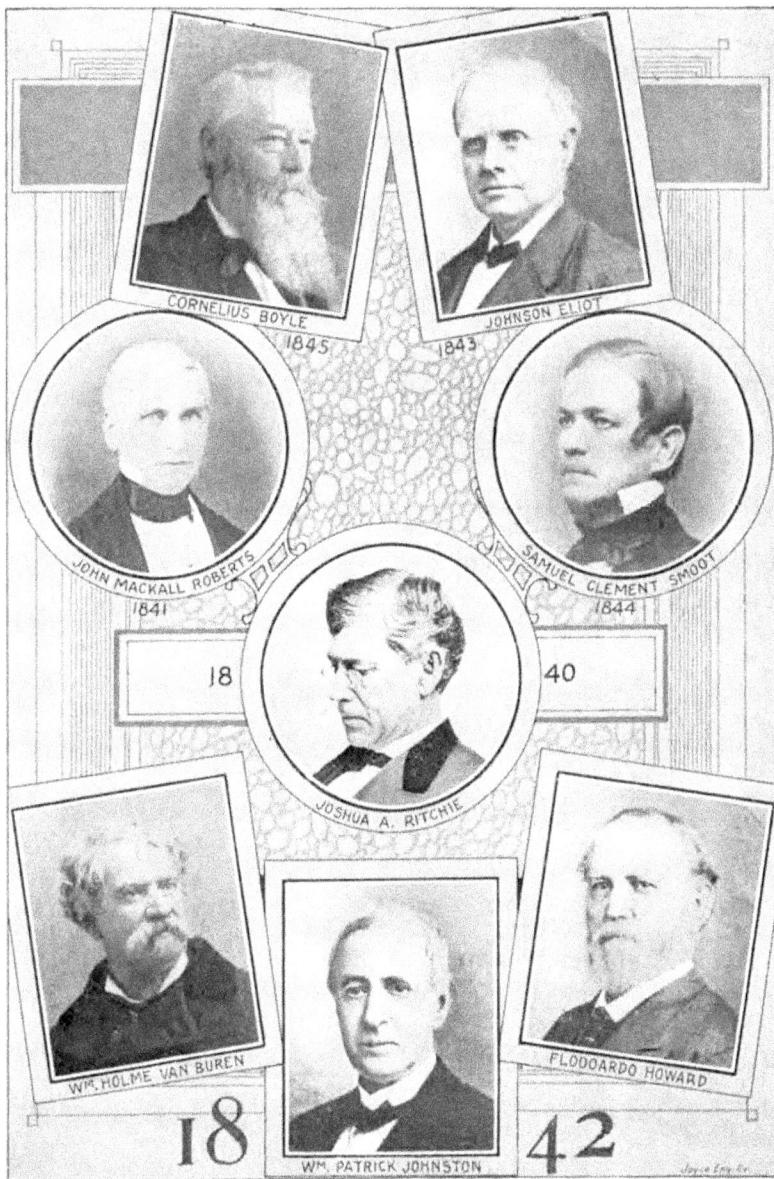

CORNELIUS BOYLE
1845

JOHNSON ELIOT
1843

JOHN MACKALL ROBERTS
1841

SAMUEL CLEMENT SMOOT
1844

18   40

JOSHUA A. RITCHIE

WM. HOLME VAN BUREN

WM. PATRICK JOHNSTON

FLODOARDO HOWARD

18   42

13

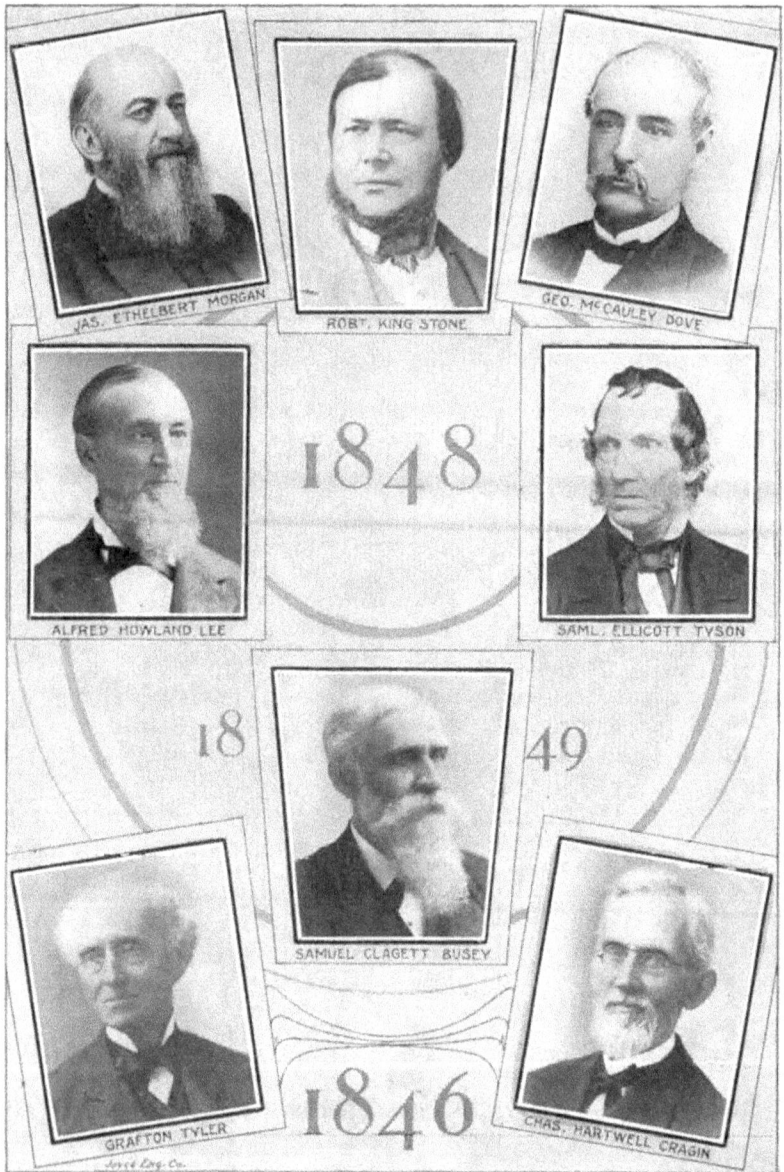

JAS. ETHELBERT MORGAN   ROBT. KING STONE   GEO. McCAULEY DOVE

ALFRED HOWLAND LEE   1848   SAML. ELLICOTT TYSON

18   SAMUEL CLAGETT BUSEY   49

GRAFTON TYLER   1846   CHAS. HARTWELL CRAGIN

14

This committee consisted of Drs. D. C. Patterson, H. D. Fry, J. Taber Johnson, T. E. McArdle and Kleinschmidt. September 17th, the Corresponding Secretary reported that he had done as directed; and his report was given to the appropriate committee, with instructions to confer with the Health Officer in regard to the registration of physicians.

The committee reported, October 15th, that as the result of the letter of the Corresponding Secretary quite a number of persons had applied to the Board of Examiners, and one person had been licensed. The District Attorney, however, had expressed grave doubts as to the validity of the law or his ability to collect fines under it, but said that if any one would make up a case he would prosecute it. With a prosecuting officer in doubt as to the soundness of his case, and in a community always ready to raise the cry of persecution, it was a question if the chances of success would be equal to the danger of failure. Some of those receiving the circular of the Corresponding Secretary claimed the right to practice under the regulations of the Health Office. The committee believed this claim to be without foundation, and while the Health Officer deemed it his duty to allow any one to register who showed his diploma from some college or a certificate of membership in a respectable medical society, he did not regard that act as conferring any legal right whatever to practice medicine. He was asked if he could not so far change his order in regard to registration as to require every one proposing to register to first obtain a license from the Board of Examiners. This he declined to do, taking the ground that he had no authority under the law to require this as a preliminary to registration. The committee was inclined to think that most, if not all, respectable physicians in the District were willing and anxious, when they came to understand the law, to take out this license, and that they would do so in due time. But if they declined to do so after a proper time, it would be the duty of the members of the Society to refuse to consult with them. It was believed that this would be much more effective than a resort to legal pro-

4

ceedings. After a careful review of the whole subject and after consultation with the Board of Examiners, the committee was of the opinion that the Board would be obliged under existing laws to license all who made application, if they furnished a diploma from a respectable medical college or passed a satisfactory examination. This would give many disreputable persons the very standing in the community which above everything else they most desired, namely, a recognition by the Medical Society of the District, and they would no doubt immediately advertise as licentiates of the Medical Society. In view of all the circumstances of the case, the uncertainty as to the results of legal proceedings, the danger to the Society in case of failure, and last, but not least, the obloquy which would justly attach to the Society should the Board of Examiners be forced to license every charlatan who might be fortunate enough to hold a diploma from some respectable medical college, the committee respectfully recommended that the further consideration of the matter should be indefinitely postponed.

The report was accepted and committee discharged, but a motion to concur in the report was laid on the table.

February 28, 1894, the Society adopted the following resolution :

WHEREAS, The *Washington Post*, of this city, enters a large number of our homes and is read by a large number of our sons and daughters; and whereas, we have no desire to deprive our families of the benefits arising from the perusal of this newspaper ; and whereas, this paper has, in our opinion, some most objectionable advertisements, such as the following : "one male in every five is afflicted with varicocele ; they are the great impediment to marriage ; I am the only physician on earth that can cure a varicocele without operation or pain ;" the above advertisement being in bold type and occupying a whole column, thus rendering it very conspicuous. Also the advertisements of " sexual impotency," "seminal losses," "the curing of syphilis in from 30 to 90 days," " pennyroyal pills," " results of self-abuse in youth," "nocturnal emissions," "sexual exhaustion," and many other objectionable announcements of like character. And whereas, we believe these statements to be false ; calling attention to subjects which should not occupy the minds of the young ; suggesting to them the impure, rather than the pure ; and thus both directly and indirectly tending to promote crime, disease and licentiousness ; therefore

"*Resolved:* That a committee of three be appointed by the Chair to report to this Society what action, if any, should be taken in the matter."

Drs. C. H. Stowell, T. E. McArdle and P. S. Roy were appointed the committee ; it reported March 14th as follows:

" WHEREAS, It is the duty of the medical profession to protect the community from all things which menace health ; and whereas, the public press contains many advertisements which advise people to purchase nostrums and consult charlatans ; and whereas, many of these advertisements are both indecent and immoral, tending to excite curiosity in the young and calling attention to those subjects which by common consent are deemed productive of disease, vice and crime, and whereby many individuals are thereby led to think themselves suffering from some serious disease so enticingly, but incorrectly, described by said charlatans : and whereas, a bill has been introduced in the House of Representatives, known as Bill No. 4732, a copy of which is here appended, the purpose of which is to correct these existing evils, to wit :

"*Be it enacted by the Senate and House of Representatives of the United States of America in Congress assembled:* That Section 3893 of the Revised Statutes of the United States be, and the same is hereby, amended so as to read as follows :

"SEC. 3893. Every obscene, lewd, filthy, indecent or lascivious book, pamphlet, picture, paper, letter, writing, print, or other publication of an indecent or filthy character, or devoted to the publication or principally made up of criminal news, police reports, or accounts of criminal deeds, or pictures or stories of immoral deeds, lust, or crime, and every article or thing designed or intended for the prevention of conception or procuring of abortion, and every article or thing intended or adapted for any indecent or immoral use, and every written or printed card, letter, circular, book, pamphlet, advertisement, or notice of any kind, giving information directly or indirectly, where, or how, or of whom, or by what means any of the hereinbefore mentioned matters, articles, or things may be obtained or made, or advertisement contained in any newspaper, pamphlet, or circular giving information where or by whom abortions may be performed, or where pills, medicines, nostrums, or advice for the prevention of conception or for abortion may be obtained, or advertisements of medicines, drugs, nostrums or apparatus for the cure of private or venereal diseases, whether sealed as first-class matter or not, are hereby declared to be non-mailable matter, and shall not be conveyed in the mails nor delivered from any post-office nor by any letter carrier; and any person who shall knowingly deposit or cause to be deposited for mailing or delivery, anything declared by this section to be nonmailable matter, and any person who shall knowingly take the same, or cause the same to be taken from the mails for the purpose of circulating or disposing of or aiding in the circulation or disposition of the same shall, for each and every offence be fined upon conviction thereof not more than five thousand dollars or imprisoned at hard labor not more than five years, or both, at the discretion of the court; and all offences committed under the section of which this is amendatory, prior to the approval of this act, may be prosecuted and punished under the same in the same manner and with the same effect as if this act had not been passed; and the Postmaster General shall have full authority to declare what matter is nonmailable under this act so far as the transportation in the mails is concerned: *Provided,* That nothing in this act shall authorize any person to open any letter or sealed matter of the first class not addressed to himself; *And provided further,* That upon the continued mailing of newspapers or periodicals containing advertisements or other articles or items forbidden by this act to be transmitted in the mails, the Postmaster General is hereby authorized to declare said publication, including future issues thereof, nonmailable.

" Therefore, your committee recommends the passage of the following resolution ; *Resolved*, that the Medical Society of the District of Columbia, in behalf of the health and morality of this community, gives its hearty support and unqualified approval to the House bill No. 4732, and that we hereby urge upon Congress the passage of the same."

The report was adopted and a copy ordered to be sent to the House Committee on Post Offices.

April 18, 1894, the Society appointed a committee, consisting of Drs. T. E. McArdle, S. O. Richey, J. H. McCormick, G. Wythe Cook and W. C. Woodward, to consider what steps should be taken to suppress quackery in the District. To this committee was referred the section of the Pharmacy Act in regard to illegal dispensing of medicines. It does not appear that the committee made any report.

THE SCIENTIFIC WORK OF THE SOCIETY ; THE ESSAYS READ ; THE PATHOLOGICAL SPECIMEMS AND PATIENTS PRESENTED ; AND THE DISCUSSIONS THEREON.

There would be no advantage in listing the many essays that have been read before the Society. Their name is legion and their scope is the whole domain of medicine and surgery, and the collateral sciences. Very many have been published and thus made accessible to the profession at large. They may be said to have had the average value of Medical Society papers; some, perhaps many, showed originality and observation.

Dr. Toner * * * (Anniv. Oration, page 68) gives a list of papers contributed by members to medical journals in the early history of the Society ; the following three, at least, were read before the Society : " On ovarian disease and abdominal steatomata ;" read by Dr. Thomas Hender-son, July, 1818. By Dr. Henderson also, " Report on the diseases of Georgetown ; report for 1820 and 1821 ;" read in 1821. By Dr. N. P. Causin, " An essay on autumnal bilious epidemic of the United States ;" read in April, 1823.

The minutes of the Society up to 1838 were either lost or destroyed by fire. For many years after 1838 the titles of papers read before the Society did not appear in the minutes; indeed, were we to judge by the scanty minutes themselves the scientific side of the Society would seem to have been almost entirely neglected. The first record of any essay read is of one by Dr. D. R. Hagner, March 14, 1864, on " Vaccination ;" it was referred to a committee and was ordered printed ; there is no record of its having been discussed. The next record is July 4, 1864, when Dr. Charles Allen read a paper, expressing the desire that special meetings should be held to promote a more friendly relation between the members and to consider and promote subjects connected with medicine. August 8th, Dr. John-son Eliot was appointed to ask Dr. Harvey Lindsly to read a paper on Asiatic cholera. August 22d, the time appointed, Dr. Lindsly failed to appear, and Dr. Eliot himself read the paper; and it is stated that there was considerable discussion. The same evening Dr. J. E. Morgan was ap-pointed to read a paper on diphtheria, with Dr. F. Howard as alternate ; September 5th, Dr. Morgan being absent, Dr. Howard opened a discussion on this subject. September 19th, Dr. N. S. Lincoln read a paper on typhoid fever, which was discussed, and the discussion continued over the next meeting. October 25th, Dr. Wm. Marbury read one on placenta praevia. November 15th, Dr. J. Ford Thompson read one on syphilis. November 28th, Dr. Eliot read one on the bromides in epilepsy ; and Dr. L. Mackall, on the use of permanganate of potassium in diphtheria. The use of digitalis and sulphuric ether in delirium tremens was also discussed. December 12th, epilepsy was discussed. Thus ended the essays for 1864.

The good example of 1864 was imitated in 1865, and a few of the papers read may be mentioned. May 3d, Dr. R. K. Stone read an account of the death of President Lincoln and the results of the autopsy. May 30th, Dr. A. F. A. King read a paper on menstruation, which he claimed to be a disease. October 4th, Dr. L. Mackall, Jr., read a paper which had been published by his father, Dr. Louis Mackall, in 1862, on the philosophy of muscular action. This paper was much criticised, and Dr. Mackall replied to the criticism January 31, 1866. December 20, 1865, Dr. Toner read a paper on the history of the medical profession in this District. He lamented that up to that time no full record of the Society's transactions had been made, and no history of the various epidemics that had prevailed. He wanted a medical library and museum and also a permanent home for the Society. This address was presumably the basis of his oration September 26, 1866.

In 1866 a Committee on Evening Arrangements was appointed, whose duty it was to propose subjects for discussion. From this time an increase of interest in the scientific work of the Society was noted.

In the early part of 1883 the Society ordered that postal cards should be sent to members, giving information of papers to be read. Dr. J. T. Howard says that in 1863 and 1864 notices of the meetings were mailed by the President [Dr. Borrows] himself to the members, over his signature, and on a card two by three inches, duly stamped. Dr. Howard maintains that President Borrows was the founder of the postal-card system in this city. October 31st, the Society again ordered that cards should be sent to

members, announcing the titles of papers to be read and
names of authors.   January 7, 1884, the Society adopted
an amendment to Art. III of the by-laws, that the Corresponding Secretary should notify members, by mail, of the
meetings and the titles of papers and the authors' names.

January 29, 1890, the Committee on Essays recommended that the President of the Society be authorized
and requested to appoint essayists whose duty it should be
to read papers before the Society on the first Wednesday
in each month; also to appoint an alternate, to supply a
paper when an essayist was unable to do so.   The committee also recommended that during the month of
December of each year the President should deliver an
address, the date to be left to his convenience.   February
5th, the recommendations were adopted.   At the meeting
October 7th, the President appointed the essayists for the
remainder of the year 1891 and the first session of 1892;
July 4, 1892, for 1892–3; July 3, 1893, for 1893–4; December 5, 1894, for 1894–5; July 1, 1895, for 1895–6;
October 28, 1896, for the year 1897; and since then the
essayists for the ensuing year have been announced, either
at the December meeting, when the President delivered
his annual address, or at the first meeting in the following
January.   According to By-law I, the appointment should
be made at the "commencement of the year."

January 16, 1895, the Society ordered that discussion
on a paper should be closed on the evening that the paper
was read, unless carried over by a two-thirds vote; also
that the regular essayist of the evening should read his
paper immediately after the presentation of pathological
specimens.   February 6th, the Society created the office of
Assistant Recording Secretary, his duty to make a stenographic report of all medical discussions and, after consultation with the members concerned therein, make the

BENJ. FANEUIL CRAIG

JOHN CAMPBELL RILEY

1853

WM. JAS. C. DuHAMEL

WM. GRAY PALMER

18   50

HEZEKIAH MAGRUDER

ALEX. Y. P. GARNETT
1851

SAML. A. H. McKIM
1854

18   52

MARTIN VAN BUREN BOGAN

Joyce Eng. Co.

15

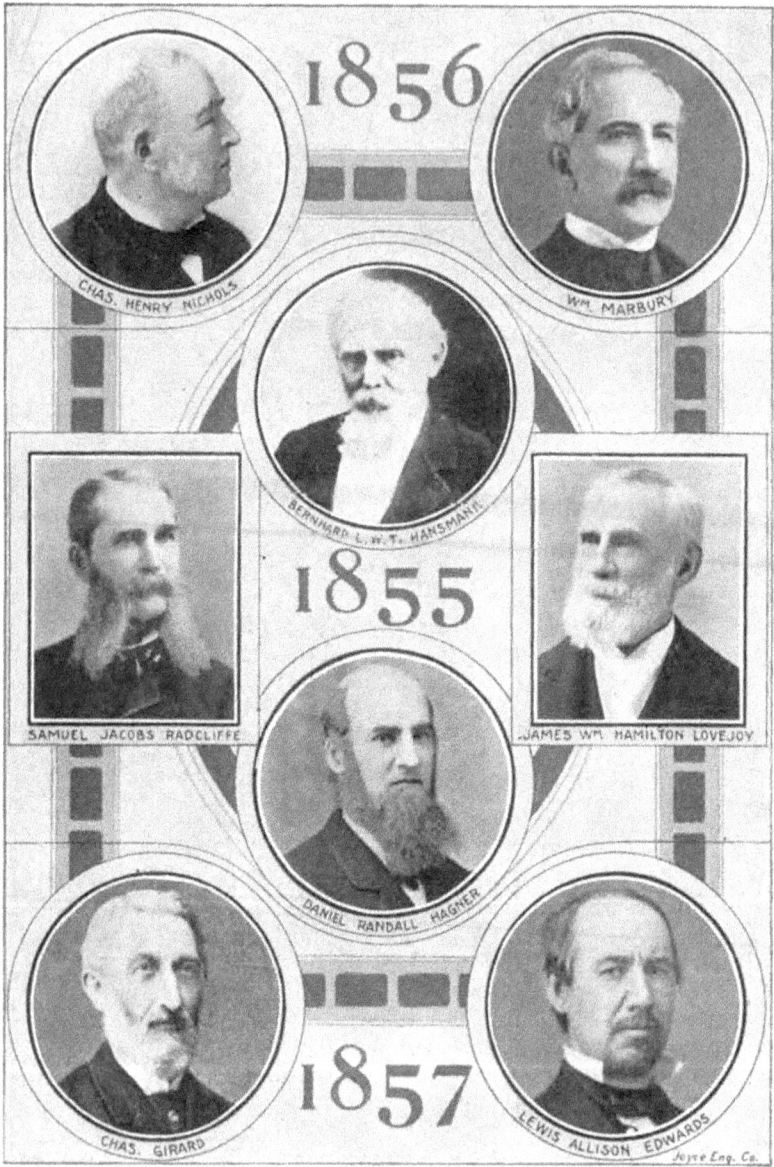

1856

CHAS. HENRY NICHOLS

WM. MARBURY

BERNHARD L. W. T. HANSMANN

1855

SAMUEL JACOBS RADCLIFFE

JAMES WM. HAMILTON LOVEJOY

DANIEL RANDALL HAGNER

1857

CHAS. GIRARD

LEWIS ALLISON EDWARDS

Joyce Eng. Co.

necessary corrections in the report; these to be verified by a committee, consisting of the President, Recording Secretary and Assistant Secretary, and when any alteration had been made not accepted by said committee, the fact should be reported to the Society at the meeting next succeeding that at which the discussion took place, for final vote by the Society. The office of Assistant Secretary lapsed February 2, 1898, and with it the above provision.

The record of many cases of disease and injury reported to the Society fails to show whether or not the pathological specimens were also presented; probably in most of these cases they were not. The first case reported was one by Dr. Antisell, July 19, 1865, a fracture of the skull, with abscess of brain. The second recorded case was August 30th, the same year, by Dr. S. A. H. McKim; laceration of the liver by shot wound. September 30th, Dr. J. Ford Thompson reported two cases of fracture of the skull. December 20th, Dr. G. Tyler reported a case of malformation in a stillborn infant. December 27th, Dr. Thomas Miller reported another malformation.

It is not worth while to continue this list. Suffice it to say that from this time it became quite common to report such cases.

Presentation of pathological specimens.—The first recorded instance of the presentation of a pathological specimen was April 19, 1865, when Dr. D. R. Hagner showed a specimen of ossification (?) of the mitral valve. The second instance was July 19th; Dr. Antisell showed a specimen and reported the case of perforation of the vermiform appendix. The third instance was August 30th, when Dr. Johnson Eliot showed a bone to illustrate how the cranium is made secure after trephining. March 7, 1866, Dr. S. S. Bond showed a specimen of great distension of the colon in a man reputed to be 105 years old. March 21st, Dr. J.

Ford Thompson showed a specimen of thickened and contracted bladder.   After this time specimens were shown
with comparative frequency, so much so, that the Society
ordered the purchase of an anatomical tray.   May 16th, Dr.
J. Harry Thompson showed a hypertrophied heart weighing 28 ounces, and cirrhosis of the liver and kidneys, the
kidneys weighing, respectively, 13 and 14 ounces; from a
case of death from Bright's disease in a man who weighed
500 pounds and had eight inches of fat over his abdomen.
October 17th, Dr. J. H. Thompson showed an ovarian
tumor.

It would be of no advantage to continue the record.
Such specimens have been frequently shown and discussed;
but it was not until January 12, 1870, that any provision
for them was made in the order of business; their presentation was then indicated after "Miscellaneous business."
Curiously enough, there have been members who looked
with scant favor on this part of the evening program, but
to the majority, probably, the specimens have proved interesting and instructive.

March 26, 1873, the Society ordered the purchase of
another tray, or waiter; December 8, 1875, a washstand
with basin and pitcher; November 30, 1887, plates and
towels were ordered; and December 7th, Dr. C. E. Hagner
presented the Society with a dissecting case.   March 5,
1902, the Society ordered that one Wednesday in each
month should be devoted exclusively to pathological specimens, but this rule soon passed into "innocuous desuetude."

The presentation of the patients themselves.—The first
recorded presentation of the patient himself to the consideration of the Society was May 14, 1856, when the
famous Alexis St. Martin, of gastric fistula fame, was
examined and discussed.   A special meeting was called for

the purpose. In spite, however, of the extraordinary character of the case, the meeting was but poorly attended.

The next record of the patient himself being presented was February 5, 1859. This case was less famous, but was equally unusual; it was that of Dr. Groux, who had a congenital fissure of the sternum; the action of the heart, aorta and lungs was demonstrated. A special meeting was called for the purpose.

The third record is on August 30, 1865, when Dr. C. M. Ford showed a patient with fracture of the skull.

So far as the record shows, ten years more now elapsed before another patient was presented.

The reading of papers or exhibition of specimens by others than active members of the Society.—The first recorded instance of this was May 9, 1866, when Drs. C. A. Lee, of New York, and L. M. Linton, of St. Louis, discussed the subject of Asiatic cholera and Dr. Marsden's quarantine system. The same month, May 30th, Dr. N. W. Hubbard, of Ohio, showed a patent hernia truss of his own invention. Next came Dr. J. J. Woodward, U. S. A., January 21, 1874; Dr. John S. Billings, U. S. A., February 28, 1877; Dr. Paul F. Mundè, of New York City, April 26, 1882; Capt. T. W. Simonds, U. S. A., April 21, 1886; Dr. I. W. Blackburn, Pathologist to the Government Hospital for the Insane, November 3d; Dr. W. W. Godding, Superintendent of the same hospital, and who afterwards became a member of the Society, December 1st; Dr. E. O. Shakspeare, of Philadelphia, who had just returned from an investigation of cholera abroad, March 16, 1887; and Dr. M. G. Ellzey, May 4th.

May 11, 1887, Dr. T. C. Smith, as Corresponding Secretary, asked to be instructed as to how far he might go on his own responsibility in inviting gentlemen not members or licentiates of the Society to address the Society on some live topic. He had been asked to invite a gentleman to do so, but in talking the matter over with a member Dr. Smith found that there was some opposition to this person, and he wanted to know if he should extend any invitation without first consulting the Society. The discussion showed that the consensus of opinion was that the Corresponding Secretary might extend invitations on his own responsibility, but it would be expected that he would exercise discretion. No formal action, however, was taken.

November 23d, Dr. Blackburn again addressed the Society, and May 3, 1888, Dr. William A. Hammond, retired Surgeon General, U. S. A.

January 30, 1889, Dr. Smith again raised the question of non-members reading essays before the Society. He wanted to know whether the Committee on Essays was authorized to secure papers from prominent medical men visiting the city, and, to settle the question, moved that the committee be instructed to secure papers from said persons. The matter was postponed until February 13th, when the Essay Committee was instructed to secure papers from medical gentlemen, eminent in the profession, from a distance, who might be visiting the city, but the committee should not extend invitations under other circumstances.

Dr. J. B. Mattison, of Brooklyn, N. Y., addressed the Society, January 21, 1891 ; Dr. George B. Penrose, resident physician at Barnes Hospital, D. C., March 2, 1892; Dr. L. Emmett Holt, of New York City, March 30th ; and Dr. Elmer Lee, of Chicago, December 7th; Dr. Herman Canfield, of Bristol, R. I., May 24, 1893 ; Dr. J. J. Kinyoun, of the Marine Hospital Service, March 7, 1894; Dr. John S. Billings, U. S. A., October 24th ; Dr. Joseph Price, of Philadelphia, November 28th; Dr. Kinyoun again, January 9, 1895 ; Dr. Wm. P. Mason, of Troy, N. Y., January 30th ; Dr. W. J. McGee, of the Bureau of American Ethnology, Washington, February 6th. On this date the Society ordered that men eminent in medicine, not members of the Society and not exceeding four in number, might be invited annually to address the Society.

March 6, 1895, Surgeon General George M. Sternberg, U. S. A., addressed the Society; March 27th, Dr. C. W. Stiles, of the Department of Agriculture; April 10th, Dr. Andrew H. Smith, of New York City; May 1st, Dr. Wm. Osler; May 15th, Dr. Bedford Brown, of Alexandria, Va.; May 29th, Dr. Walter Reed, Surgeon, U. S. Army, and Curator of the Army Medical Museum; November 27th, Dr. Abraham Jacobi, of New York City.

May 6, 1896, Dr. C. H. Alden, Assist. Surg. Gen., U. S. A.; May 13th, Dr. V. A. Moore, of the Department of Agriculture; November 25th, Dr. C. F. Dawson, of the same Department.

February 24, 1897, General Sternberg again; March 17th, Dr. D. L. Huntington, Assist. Surg. General, U. S. A., and in charge of the Army Medical Museum and Library; March 24th, Dr. Walter Wyman, Supervising Surgeon General, Marine Hospital Service.

January 19, 1898, Dr. Stiles again; February 2d, Dr. E. A. de Schweinitz, of the Department of Agriculture; April 20th, Dr. E. M. Gallaudet, President of the Deaf Mute College, D. C.; April 27th, Dr. Robert Fletcher, of the Army Medical Library; October 5th, Mrs. Armstrong Hopkins, of India.

February 22, 1899, Dr. E. L. Munson, U. S. A.; April 12th, Dr. G. T. Vaughan, U. S. Marine Hospital Service; April 26th, Drs. L. A. LaGarde, W. C. Borden and E. L. Munson, U. S. A.; May 17th, Dr. Harvey Wiley, of the Department of Agriculture; October 11th, Mr. G. E. Gordon, of the Walker-Gordon Laboratory, Washington;

October 25th, Dr. Borden again ; November 1st, Dr. La-Garde again.

January 10, 1900, Dr. Jacobi again; January 17th, Dr. W. O. Atwater, of Wesleyan College, New Haven, Conn., Dr. Charles Smart, Asst. Surg. Gen., U. S. A., and Mr. C. F. Langworthy; April 11th, Dr. E. B. Behrend, of Washington; October 3d, Dr. Borden again ; October 17th, Dr. Stiles again ; November 14th, Dr. LaGarde again.

May 8, 1901, Mr. L. H. Warner, of New York City ; May 29th, Dr. Walter Reed again ; November 6th, Dr. Stiles again.

February 26, 1902, Dr. V. P. Gibney, of New York City ; March 26th, Dr. Robert Fletcher again ; April 30th, Dr. Jacobi again ; October 1st, Dr. Borden again ; December 4th, Dr. Adolf Lorenz, of Vienna, Austria.

March 11, 1903, Dr. E. L. Keyes, Jr., of New York City ; March 16th, Dr. W. C. Gorgas, Asst. Surg. Gen., U. S. A. ; April 22d, Dr. Wiley again ; April 29th, Dr. de Schweinitz again and Dr. D. V. Salmon, of the Department of Agriculture ; May 15th, Dr. J. B. Murphy, of Chicago.

March 16, 1904, Dr. W. W. Keen, of Philadelphia ; March 23d, Dr. Keyes again ; October 26th, Dr. Sternberg again ; November 9th, Dr. J. H. Musser, of Philadelphia, and Dr. E. B. Dench, of New York City.

January 11, 1905, Dr. James J. Walsh, of New York City; April 20th, Dr. W. F. Grenfell, of the Labrador Coast; October 11th, Dr. Blackburn again; November 29th, Dr. A. Hrdlicka, of the U. S. National Museum.

January 24, 1906, Dr. Vaughan again; January 31st, Drs. Blackburn and Stiles again ; February 21st, Mr. Charles Truax, of Chicago; March 14th, Dr. Robert Abbe, of New York City ; October 12th, Dr. A. E. Wright, of London, England.

January 23, 1907, Dr. E. M. Santee and Messrs. K. F.

Kellerman, T. D. Beckwith and G. M. Whitaker, Dept. Agriculture, and Dr. Turner, Health Dept., D. C.; February 13th, Dr. Theodor Schott, of Bad Nauheim, Germany; February 27th, Dr. J. C. Wise, U. S. Navy; March 27th, Dr. B. K. Ashford, U. S. A., and Dr. C. W. Stiles again; April 10th, Dr. Blackburn again; April 17th, Dr. W. S. Halsted, of Johns Hopkins; May 29th, Dr. Wm. A. White, Supt. Government Hospital for the Insane, D. C.; November 6th, Dr. Hrdlicka again.

February 19, 1908, Major Spencer Cosby, U. S. A.; Mr. F. F. Longley; Drs. M. J. Rosenau, L. L. Lumsden and Mr. J. H. Kastle, Marine Hospital Service; and Drs. Harvey Wiley, B. M. Bolton and Mr. C. B. Lane, U. S. Dept. Agriculture; March 18th, Dr. J. M. T. Finney, Baltimore, Md.; April 8th, Dr. T. A. Williams; April 29th, Dr. J. C. DaCosta, Philadelphia, Pa.; November 4th, Dr. R. A. Hamilton of Washington; December 2d, Dr. Williams again.

January 13, 1909, Dr. Geo. Ben Johnston, Richmond, Va.; February 17th, Dr. T. M. Rotch, Boston, Mass.; March 10th, Dr. L. L. Flick, of Philadelphia, and General Sternberg; March 24th, Dr. Wm. P. Spratling, Baltimore, Md.; and March 31st, Dr. White again.

In 1905, several members were appointed to read reviews on important subjects, and annually since then, the President has announced a list of "Reviewers" for the year. There is no record of any action having been taken by the Society; the custom, however, appears to be established.

THE SOCIETY AND THE DISTRICT OF COLUMBIA GENERALLY.

At a very early period in its history the Society showed an interest in public matters—disease, sanitation, etc., as affecting the District of Columbia. Whenever the occasion has required, the Society has met its opportunity and generally succeeded in making itself felt in the community.

Dr. Toner, in his oration, 1866, said that—

" The benefits of the Medical Society of the District of Columbia to this community have never been fully appreciated by them, and perhaps not to the full extent it deserves by the members themselves.   *   *   *   It is a mistake to suppose that the benefits of a medical association are limited, or chiefly important, to its members. The skill and proficiency of the medical profession is but a legacy held in trust for the use and benefit of the community. The interest of the public and the profession in this respect is almost identical. Each is benefited, but the public most, by whatever measure advances and disseminates a knowledge of the healing art and the prevention of disease.   *   *   *   But there are other duties of a more public nature, which belong to the profession in its associate rather than in its individual capacity. With special reference to these this Society was originally constituted."

February 1, 1864, in view of the prevalence of smallpox, the Society appointed a committee, consisting of one member from each ward of Washington and two from Georgetown, to consider the sanitary condition of the District. Dr. T. Antisell was made chairman ; the other members were Drs. W. G. H. Newman, F. Howard, Wm. Marbury, J. Eliot, G. W. McCoy, J. M. Roberts and J. E. Morgan. March 7th, the committee reported; the report was adopted and ordered printed. The printed report covered ten pages, besides twelve pages of appendices. It related mainly to precautions against smallpox, but also considered insanitary matters generally, and especially recommended a skeleton of a constitution and duties of a Board of Health.

Three committees were appointed to carry out the recommendations : Drs. Liebermann and W. P. Johnston to

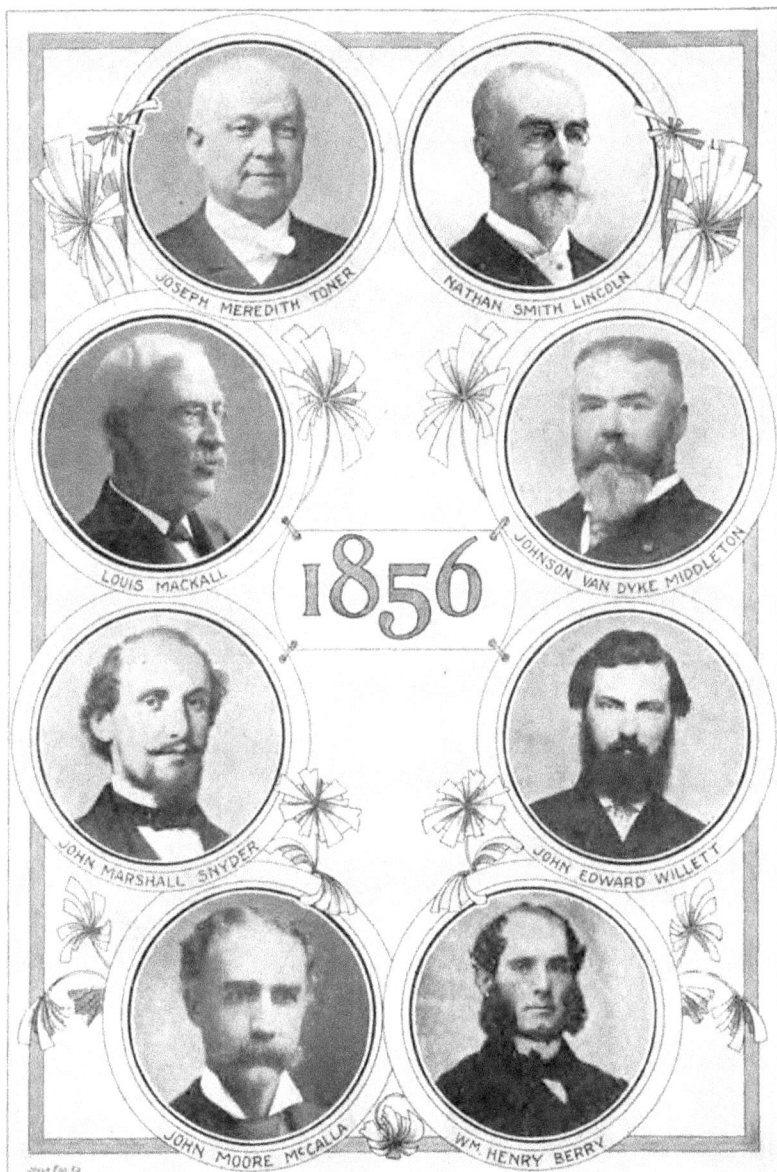

JOSEPH MEREDITH TONER

NATHAN SMITH LINCOLN

LOUIS MACKALL

1856

JOHNSON VAN DYKE MIDDLETON

JOHN MARSHALL SNYDER

JOHN EDWARD WILLETT

JOHN MOORE McCALLA

WM. HENRY BERRY

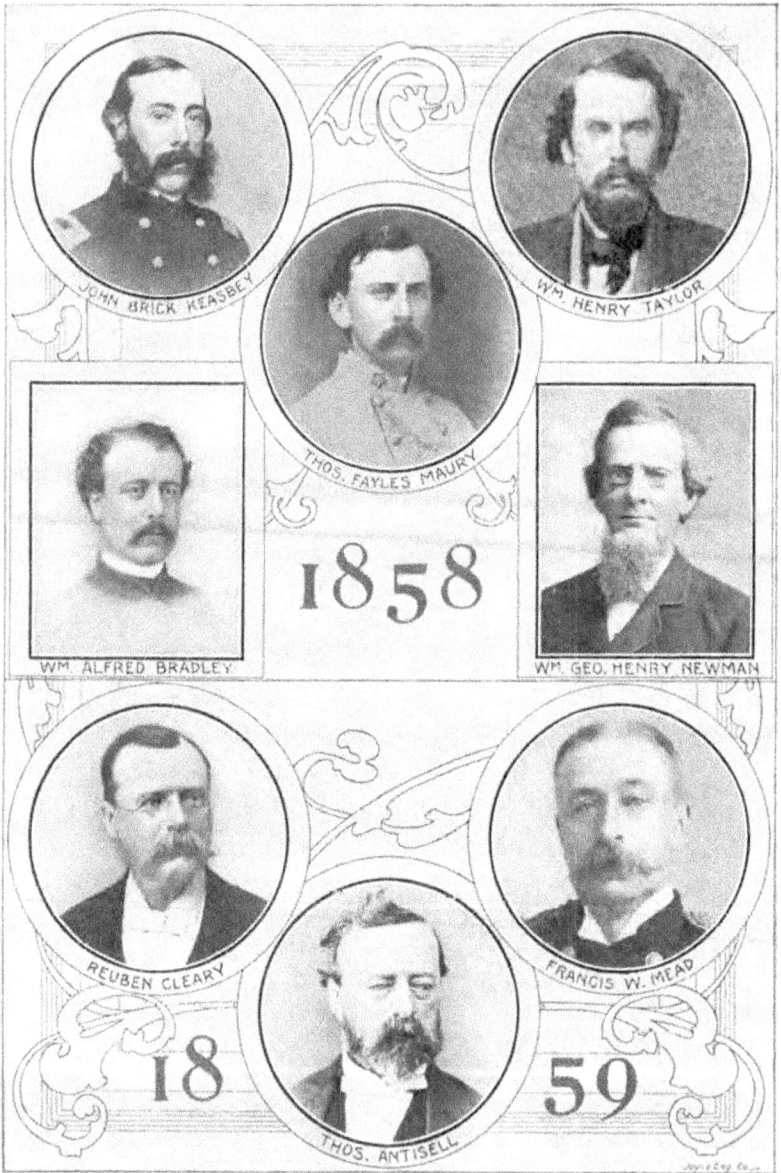

JOHN BRICK KEASBEY

WM. HENRY TAYLOR

THOS. FAYLES MAURY

WM. ALFRED BRADLEY

1858

WM. GEO. HENRY NEWMAN

REUBEN CLEARY

FRANCIS W. MEAD

18

THOS. ANTISELL

59

18

see the Secretary of War; Drs. Wm. Jones, F. B. Culver and Marbury to see members of Congress; and Drs. Morgan, J. Borrows and Howard to see the municipal authorities. January 9, 1865, Dr. Antisell made a report, which was accepted, and the committee was instructed to submit the matter to Congress. January 23d, Dr. Antisell reported that a bill had been introduced into Congress and referred to a committee.

March 28, 1866, Dr. J. Phillips read a paper on the sanitary condition of Washington, in which he recommended surface drainage, removal of garbage, daily sweeping of streets and removal of sweepings; also rigid ordinances regarding .privies, preventing the waste from running hydrants, and filling the canal; and the appointing of proper medical inspectors and attendants to the poor.

April 7, 1897, the Society ordered that a memorial be prepared and sent to the U. S. Senate favoring a bill (House bill 9142) that had passed the House at a previous session, regulating the disposal of animal excreta [see Senate Documents, 1897, No. 14].

Further information in regard to certain subjects of sanitation will be found under the respective headings in this publication. Those interested are also referred to the address of Dr. Busey before the Washington Academy of Sciences, December 14, 1898, published in his volume of addresses, pages 135 to 173, with four plates; also in the *Trans. Med. Soc.* for 1898, pages 182, 198; and in *National Med. Review*, 1898–9, VIII, pages 502 to 518.

January 31, 1866, a committee, Drs. Howard, Morgan and Borrows, was appointed to inquire into the expediency of organizing a society in the District for the relief of widows and orphans of medical men. The committee made no report, and the subject was never again brought before the Society.

5

ASIATIC CHOLERA.

The subject of cholera has been discussed by the Society a number of times. Washington had a serious visitation of the disease in 1832, but what the Society did as a society, in that epidemic, does not appear.

The approach of the epidemic of 1865–6 induced Dr. Toner, November 22, 1865, to offer the following, which was adopted :

"WHEREAS, the threatened approach of cholera from Europe, and its probable appearance among us at no very remote time, is likely to disturb and injuriously excite the public mind and be aggravated by members of the profession inconsiderately giving publicity to their opinions through the newspapers of the city; to prevent this evil and to give dignity and efficiency to the skill and efforts of the profession, *Therefore, be it resolved*, That the Society disapprove of any newspaper publications or notices whatever upon the subject of cholera, by any of its members, not previously authorized by this body ; and that a committee upon epidemics be appointed, to consist of the President of this Society, one member from each ward and one from Georgetown, to take into consideration the subject of epidemics and their probable influence upon the community, and report to this body at their earliest convenience."

It does not appear that the committee made any report.

November 29, 1865, Drs. Toner and Thos. Miller were appointed a committee to ascertain from Prof. Henry, of the Smithsonian Institution, whether the Society might be permitted to hold a monthly meeting at the Smithsonian, and see there and examine the new books on medicine and the collateral sciences. The reply was favorable, and December 6th a resolution was adopted to have an informal scientific reunion of the members at the Smithsonian on the first Monday evening of each month.

THE PUBLICATION OF THE TRANSACTIONS
OF THE SOCIETY.

Many papers read before the Society were published in the ephemeral medical literature of the early part of the last century. The question of publication by the Society itself was early discussed, but naturally and promptly opposed on the ground of expense, and as long as the Society was comparatively small in number of members the objection was serious. Later, when the membership had much increased, the force of the objection was much diminished.

As early as December 20, 1865, Dr. Toner, in an address before the Society on the history of the medical profession and medical associations of the District, expressed regret that up to that time no full record had been kept of the transactions of the Society or the history of the various epidemic diseases that had prevailed in the District, and suggested that thereafter the essays read before the Society, and its transactions, be published. October 28, 1868, he moved that a very interesting case just reported to the Society be sent to some journal for publication ; and the report was published in the *Richmond and Louisville Medical Journal*.[*]

At the same meeting the President of the Society (Dr. Thomas Miller) also spoke of the advantages of publishing the discussions in some medical journal, and the prospect of some such proposal being entertained at no very distant day. In his Presidential address, January 4, 1869, he formally recommended publication, and two days afterwards the subject was referred to a committee, consisting of Drs. J. H. Thompson, W. P. Johnston and Charles Allen, for consideration. March 17th, the committee reported that as far as practicable a full report should be kept of all dis-

[*] See Vol. VII, 1869, page 367 ; " Ovariotomy," by Dr. J. Harry Thompson ; with discussion.

cussions upon important subjects in the Society, and the Secretary should prepare reports for publication in some good medical journal; that a committee of three, called *Committee of Publication*, of which the Recording Secretary should be one, should be appointed annually by the Chair, to which all essays read before the Society should be referred, as it was proposed to establish in the District a Quarterly Medical and Surgical Journal, to be conducted by a corps of editors, all of whom should be members of the Society. The committee recommended that the transactions of the Society, essays, reports, etc., should be forwarded to the said journal for publication.

The chairman of the committee stated that the proposed journal would have four departments—medicine, surgery, obstetrics, and physiology and chemistry. The publishers had agreed to furnish a quarterly of 200 pages on tinted paper, with engravings when necessary, and bear the whole burden of expense and subscription list. The Society voted its approval of this scheme, as, indeed, might have been expected, since the expense was to be borne by another party.

It was some time before the promised journal material ized. The first number appeared as the *National Medical Journal*, April, 1870. Dr. C. C. Cox was the editor, Judd & Detweiler the publishers; it was a quarterly, of 128 pages. The Washington collaborators were Drs. S. L. Loomis, Noble Young, J. Harry Thompson, S. C. Busey, F. A. Ashford, T. B. Hood and J. K. Barnes, Surgeon General, U. S. Army. There were many other collaborators, resident in New York and elsewhere. Perhaps the venture would have been a success if the journal had not been launched on the stormy sea in which medical Washington rocked at that time and for some time thereafter. The first volume ended with the January number, 1871, and the second volume, beginning with the number for May, was under the editorial management of Drs. S. C. Busey and William Lee, and was published monthly, instead of quarterly. Publication entirely ceased with the February number, 1872.

Dr. Cox was never a member of the Medical Society. None of the proceedings of the Society, and apparently none of the papers read before it, appeared in the first volume of the journal. After the journal had passed into the editorial hands of Drs. Busey and Lee, both of whom were members of the Society, the latter took action toward publication. January 11, 1871, the Committee on Essays was instructed to arrange with some medical journal to publish a synopsis of the papers read and discussions thereon before the Society, and, February 8th, the committee reported, recommending that a copy of each paper read before the Society be filed with the Committee on Essays, to be placed in the archives of the Society; that pathological specimens should be accompanied by a written history, to go to the same committee; and that the committee should make a synopsis of such papers as it deemed worthy of publication, the synopsis and debate to be published. February 15th, this report was approved by the Society.

April 12th, Drs. Busey and Lee offered to publish the transactions in the *National Medical Journal*, and the Society ordered the publication. Much of the transactions from November, 1868, to December, 1870, including reports of cases, appeared in volume II of that journal.

While it is not a part of the present history to consider the reason for the change in editors of the journal, it would be interesting to those who recall those troublous times, were we to reprint the valedictory of Dr. Cox and the salutatory of Drs. Busey and Lee, both of which entirely failed to explain the reason why. The valedictory of

Busey and Lee, in February, 1872, is a six-line paragraph which states that the publishers insisted on publishing matter that did not meet the approval of the editors, and therefore they had withdrawn from the editorship. The publishers admitted this, and after stating that they had arranged for the appearance of the March and April numbers (which, however, never did appear), charged, and no doubt with truth, that the failure of the journal to succeed was largely due to the personal opposition to Dr. Cox. Thus ended the first medical journal published in the District of Columbia.

Nothing definite in the way of publication was now attempted until November, 1873, when Dr. Busey offered a resolution, which was adopted, that the Committee on Essays inquire into the expediency and expense of publishing a *Bulletin* of the debates of the Society, and report. November 19th, this committee reported that in its opinion it would be eminently proper and expedient for the Society to publish reports of its proceedings; such a course would enhance the usefulness of the Society, stimulate its members to present better papers and essays, and tend to improve the scientific character of the debates; and recommended a quarterly publication bearing the title, "Transactions of the Medical Society of the District of Columbia." The cost to be, pamphlet form, without cover, octavo, 48 lines solid to the page, 24 pages in each number, and 500 copies, $50 per quarter; which was $200 per year.*

The committee consisted of Drs. Benedict Thompson, A. F. A. King and Charles E. Hagner. The report was adopted and the committee proceeded with the work. The first quarter began April, 1874; the July, October and

---

* This was a high price as compared with prices now. The WASHINGTON MEDICAL ANNALS publishes a 48-line page octavo, bimonthly journal, 500 copies, *with covers*, and distributes it through the mails for about two-thirds the same sum, and with the advertising receipts deducted, the actual cost is only about half what it was in 1874.

January numbers, each 24 pages, appeared; the four numbers constituted the first volume, and brought the record up to October, 1874. The second volume began with April, 1875; the July and October numbers appeared together, and the January number ended with page 94. Volume III consisted of only three numbers, April, July and December, 1876, with a total of 72 pages. Volume IV began with May 24, 1876, and consisted of numbers for January, April, July and October, 1877, with a total of 94 pages. Then came volume V, with three numbers and a total of 73 pages, ending with July, 1878. The fourth volume introduced business matters, such as the election of new members and resolutions on the death of members. The last meeting reported, published in the *Transactions* was February 28, 1878.

As showing Dr. Busey's position on the question of publication, it may be added that in the discussion December 3, 1873, on the report of the committee, Dr. Busey said that "a journal would cost $1,200 per annum, and his experience had shown him that the profession here was not willing to raise that amount. Moreover, it was no easy position to be editor of a journal, even if the editor did not write a single line." From his salutatory while editor of the *National Med. Journal* we read that—

"The profession in this District owes it to itself to sustain a journal at the seat of government, and we appeal directly to it for that support which will insure success. Among our brethren here there are men of eminent abilities and of extensive experience, yet, comparatively, they are unknown to the country, a circumstance attributable to the absence of that medium of communication which we propose to supply."

In his Presidential address, December 18, 1895, he looked back over the events of nearly fifty years in the Society, and said:

"I believe, with the committee of 1873, that a society publication, preferably an annual volume of transactions, * * * would enhance the usefulness of the Society, stimulate its members to present better papers and essays and tend to improve the scientific character of its debates."

April 1, 1874, the committee reported that the *Bulletin* had been sent, not only to the members, but also to the American medical journals and to each medical society in the United States that published its own transactions. May 13th, the Society ordered that all papers and records of cases presented to or read before it should be sent to the Committee of Publication, and that members should not be allowed to publish elsewhere until after twelve months. This radical order was rescinded January 6, 1875.

September 1, 1875, the Society ordered that members who read papers should give a synopsis of the same to the Secretary, to be recorded on the minutes, and then be available for publication in the *Transactions* in case they were thought desirable by the Committee on Publication.

January 26, 1876, a committee was appointed to remodel the whole matter of publication of the transactions; it consisted of Drs. J. Ford Thompson, W. W. Johnston, W. H. Ross, R. Reyburn and Kleinschmidt. February 2d, the committee reported the following resolutions, which were adopted by the Society:

"That the *Transactions* be published quarterly, as heretofore; that the publication include original papers, reports of cases, autopsies or pathological specimens, read before the Society, and such parts of debates as would, in the judgment of the committee, if published, be of general interest to the profession at large, or tend to promote the advancement of medical science; that where papers were judged worthy by the committee, but were found to exceed the limits authorized by the Society, they might be pub-

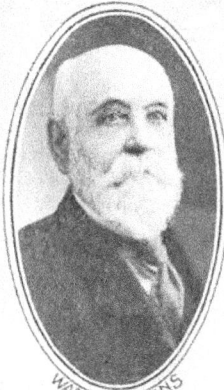

WARWICK EVANS

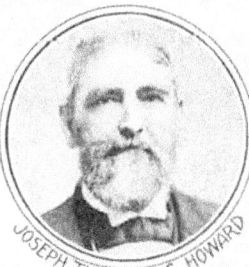

JOSEPH THEOPHILUS HOWARD

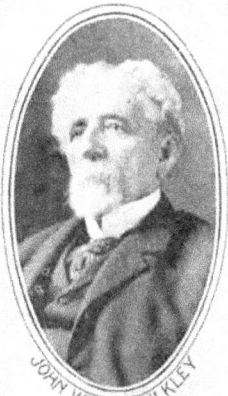

JOHN WELLS BULKLEY

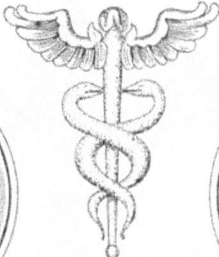

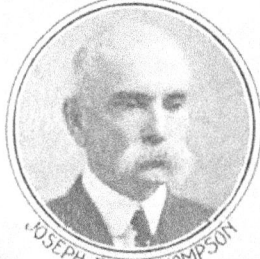

JOSEPH FORD THOMPSON

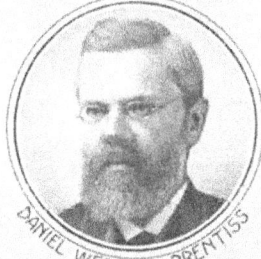

DANIEL WEBSTER PRENTISS

1864

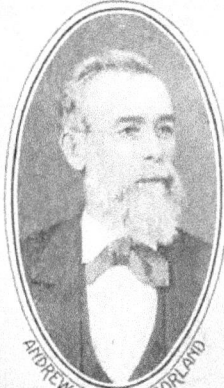

ANDREW JACKSON BORLAND

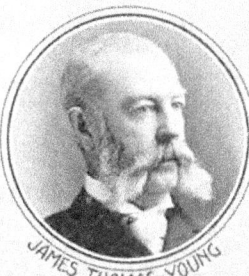

JAMES THOMAS YOUNG

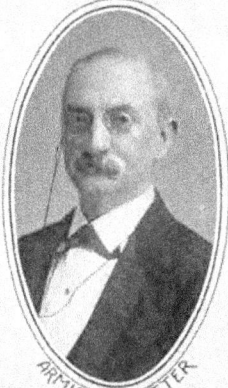

ARMISTEAD PETER

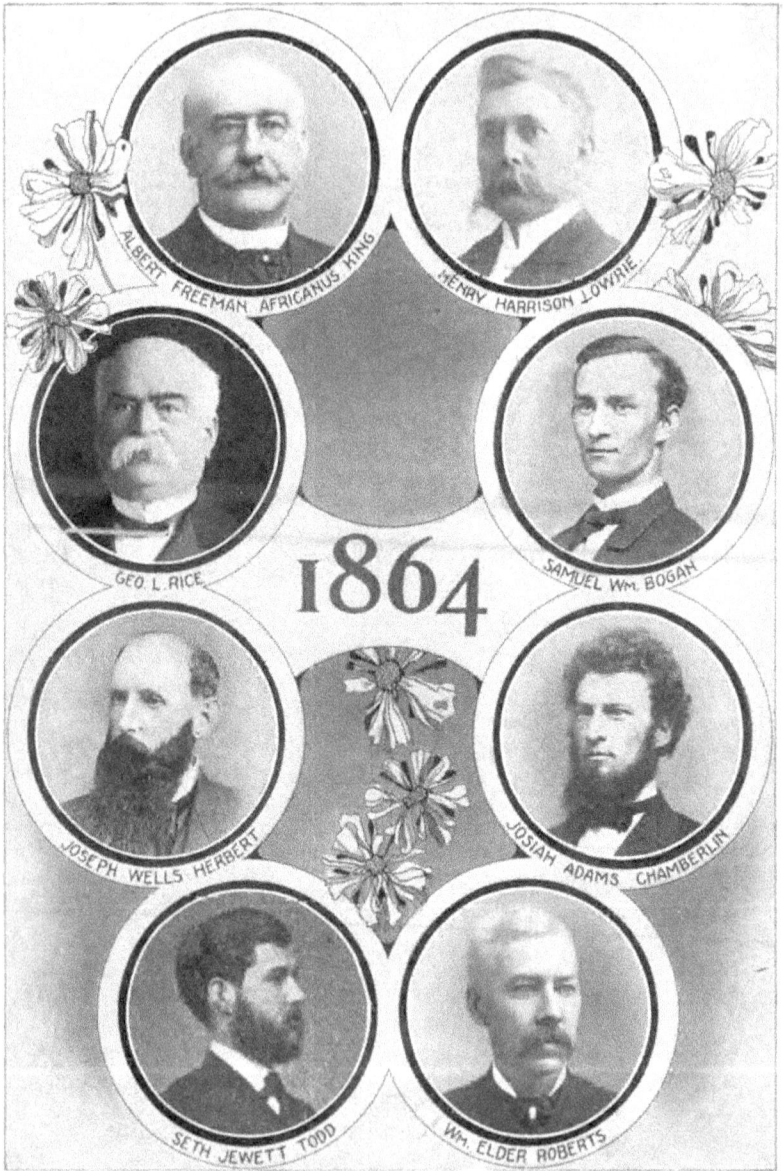

ALBERT FREEMAN AFRICANUS KING

HENRY HARRISON LOWRIE

GEO. L. RICE

SAMUEL WM. BOGAN

1864

JOSEPH WELLS HERBERT

JOSIAH ADAMS CHAMBERLIN

SETH JEWETT TODD

WM. ELDER ROBERTS

lished, provided the extra expense was defrayed by the author; that in the event of debates or papers being prolonged or diffuse, discretionary power be given to the committee to procure condensation of the same, either by the author or the committee, so that all matters of value and interest might be included and space might be economized; that the extra numbers should be disposed of, if called for, at the rate 20 cents per copy; provided that 50 copies were retained for preservation in the archives of the Society; that all matter submitted to the Society, likely to be used for publication, should be written on foolscap paper, with ink, and only on one side of the paper."

January 31, 1877, the Publication Committee, Drs. Wm. Lee, P. J. Murphy and Kleinschmidt, was authorized to commence each volume of the *Transactions* with the first month of the year, and, therefore, No. 3 of Volume III was dated December, 1876, and No. 1 of Volume IV, January, 1877—the numbers of Volume V to be issued during January, April, July and October of 1878. Also to insert, in addition to the matter published by resolution of the Society, such business matter as might be of general interest, including the organization and objects of committees, and especially resolutions passed and remarks made upon the deaths of members. Also to charge a nominal price of $1.00 a year to subscribers, said charge not to interfere, in any way, with proper exchanges, and its benefits to accrue to the Society. Also to receive advertisements.

February 21st, authority was given the committee to publish obituary notices and admissions of members.

April 11th and 18th, there was severe criticism on the work of the committee; more especially it was charged that remarks and discussions were not published as made. This brought up the whole subject of publication. Dr. J. Ford Thompson opposed further publication, except that inter-

esting papers might be published once a year. Dr. W. W.
Johnston favored publication because it had improved the
tone of debate. He held that it was the office of the
committee to condense debates, correct errors, eliminate
repetitions, &c. Many debates would have a bad appearance without such corrections. Dr. King maintained that
the *Transactions* were the outgrowth of a successful society.
Dr. J. E. Morgan opposed publication. Dr. Borrows favored
it. Dr. Reyburn favored publication; believed that the
transactions themselves would improve. Dr. Ashford
favored publication; believed that it had already improved
debate. Dr. Prentiss held that the Society owed it to the
profession to see that the valuable material in the Proceedings should be published. Publication gave greater
interest to the meetings, and reached members who were
not present at the meetings. He thought we ought to, and
some time would, have a regular medical journal in the
District. The *Transactions*, in the natural order of events,
would develop into such a journal. The Committee of
Publication should have the right to decline to publish
anything it deemed unsuitable.

May 16th, the committee made a report to the Society,
explaining and defending some things that had been criticised. It had been compelled to issue two numbers in
haste. The committee thought that if the publication
was to take rank with those of other societies, as an evidence of work done and an active interest in the medical
problems of the day, then the committee should be authorized to select for publication certain limited portions of
debates bearing directly and usefully on the subject under
discussion.

January 16, 1878, the committee that audited the report
of the Treasurer showed that the cost of publication of the
Transactions was increasing, and in the debate on the re-

port Dr. King stated that he considered the *Transactions* worth but little, because the material was not calculated to do much credit to the Society. He was, therefore, in favor of abridging the publication. Dr. A. Patze (Librarian) believed that the publication was gaining favor abroad, because of the number of requests for it received by him. At this point Dr. Toner moved to suspend the publication. Dr. Busey showed that some expenditures had been improperly charged to the *Transactions;* that, as a matter of fact, the cost had not really increased. He maintained that marked improvement had taken place in both the debates and the material offered to the Society. The publication had systematized debate, and statements therein were more accurate. The whole character of debate had been changed during the last few years. If we stopped publication the Society would retrogress. The publication should continue and should not be abridged. He rather favored an *annual.* As to the question of cost, the delinquent members should be made to pay up. Dr. W. H. Triplett said that to suspend publication would show poverty of both money and brains. The publication was educational in the highest degree, because it formulated thought and was the life and growth of medicine in the District. Dr. Toner thought that abroad the publication was not considered valuable.

At the close of the debate the Society ordered the publication continued, and appointed a committee to see if advertisements could be obtained to cut down expenses. Drs. Busey, Wm. Lee, P. J. Murphy, Kleinschmidt and W. H. Triplett constituted the committee.

February 20, 1878, a letter was written by Dr. Landon B. Edwards, editor and proprietor of the *Virginia Medical Monthly*, proposing to publish the transactions of the Society monthly, eight or nine pages a month, as prepared by the Secretary or Publishing Committee, on certain conditions. The letter was addressed to Dr. J. Ford Thompson, and was referred to a special committee. April 3d, the committee reported against the feasibility of the proposition, and the Society adopted the report.

October 16th, the Society ordered that publication be suspended. October 23d, a letter was received from Dr. Walter S. Wells, stating that he, with others, proposed to inaugurate a monthly medical magazine in Washington, with the title "National Medical Review," in which space would be given for reports such as had previously been published in the quarterly *Transactions*. The Society accepted the offer. November 20th, Dr. Busey offered a series of resolutions, of which the following was adopted: "That the resolution authorizing publication in the *National Medical Review* be rescinded." The other resolution, which provided for continuing the publication of the *Transactions* until the volume should be completed, failed to pass. The discussion was participated in by Drs. Triplett, E. M. Schaeffer, Kleinschmidt, A. F. A. King, W. W. Johnston, Reyburn, Noble Young, F. A. Ashford and J. Ford Thompson. As a matter of fact, the May number of the *Review* was the last published. July 7th, Dr. Wells wrote a letter to the Society, stating that although the journal had been sent to about 200 physicians, only 30 had paid subscription. Some portions of the work of the Society from February, 1878, to April, 1879, appeared in this journal.

October 6, 1880, there came an offer from Dr. Ralph Walsh, a member of the Society, to publish such parts of the Society transactions as he might judge to be of general interest, and the Society agreed to this. His journal was a quarterly—*Retrospect of American Medicine and Surgery*—published in Washington. Only a few articles from

Washington, however, appeared in this journal. Dr.
Walsh himself said in an editorial in his last issue, April,
1882 :

"Two years ago we were asked by the editor of the
New York Medical Journal why the Washington Medical
Society did not do more for medical literature. * * * At
an early meeting of the Medical Society of the District of
Columbia, we announced that in order to give the profession of Washington a voice, we had determined to depart
from the original plan of the *Retrospect* and create an original department, in which we would gratuitously publish
such portions of the Society's proceedings as in our judgment would be of general interest. To our great surprise,
the proposition met with little favor and some active opposition. * * * After debate, we were permitted to
publish papers, provided the authors did not wish to send
them to other journals, no part of the discussions being allowed publication. For about a year we patiently waited
an article, but nothing came."

January 17, 1883, the Society received a letter from the
Maryland Medical Journal, offering to publish the work
of the Medical Society in that journal. The proposition
was referred to the Committee on Publication, Drs. D. W.
Prentiss, A. F. A. King and T. E. McArdle, which reported February 7th, recommending the acceptance of the offer.
February 14th, the committee made a further report and the
report was adopted, that the material to be published
should be limited to original theories, or synopses of papers
containing such theories; original modes of practice;
cases testing modes of practice still *sub judice ;* cases, curious or rare ; new facts, experiments or discoveries appertaining to medicine or the allied sciences, and parts of
debates judged by the committee to be of general interest
to the profession or tending to promote the advancement
of medical science ; the publication to begin with January

1, 1883 ; the reports to be read to the Society before being published and opportunity given to members to revise remarks. The Society adopted the report and, May 9th, ordered that 150 copies of the printed reports should be bought quarterly.

The proceedings, accordingly, beginning with the meeting January 17, 1883, and ending with June 17, 1885, appeared in the *Maryland Medical Journal*, in volumes IX to XIII, 1882–1885. At first only the scientific work was printed ; afterwards, obituaries, &c. Some papers were published in full.

April 8, 1885, the Publication Committee was directed to take some action looking toward publishing the *Transactions* in some metropolitan journal of large circulation. September 30th, the committee reported in favor of the *Journal American Medical Association*, which offered to publish a judicious report about every two weeks and publish papers of merit in full and furnish reprints in neat pamphlet form at actual cost. The Society approved the action of the committee. January 4, 1886, the committee reported that the only condition of publication was that the material should be presented in proper form. The committee thought that the wide circulation that would be given the reports should be a stimulus to the members to do what they could to add to the interest of the proceedings. " Some papers presented showed careful preparation, and were promptly printed in the *Journal*, while other papers had not fulfilled the conditions."

The *Journal of the American Medical Association* published the proceedings, printing many of the papers in full, beginning with the meeting December 9, 1885, and ending with December 18, 1889, in Vols. VI to XV, 1886–1890, when publication of the proceedings ceased.

March 14, 1888, Dr. Lachlan Tyler suggested that the

Society was in a position to have its transactions published in pamphlet form and exchange with State societies. Dr. T. C. Smith, however, thought that such publication would cost too much, and the transactions were already being satisfactorily published in the *Journal American Medical Association.* Dr. Tyler then moved that the transactions be published in book form, and the Treasurer be authorized to pay for the same. Dr. A. F. A. King offered an amendment, that the Committee on Publication ascertain the cost of 500 reprints. Dr. Tyler accepted the amendment. Dr. Franzoni said that the Society's experience in publishing its transactions had been expensive and unsatisfactory; several times the treasury had been bankrupt. Dr. J. F. Hartigan thought that with $600 in the treasury, the Society was able to publish. The motion, however, was laid on the table.

June 6th, Dr. J. B. Hamilton called attention to the fact that the publication in the *Journal American Medical Association* was far behind, and wished the Committee on Publication to ask the editor to publish, as formerly, every two weeks. Dr. Busey replied that the journal was crowded, and was doing the best it could.

September 17, 1890, the Society requested the Committee on Publication to consider the propriety of publishing the transactions of the Society in some other journal than that of the American Medical Association. Dr. A. F. A. King was added temporarily to the committee. September 24th, the committee reported that the proposed change was not advisable.

November 19th, the Committee on Publication was instructed to take the best method for placing a paper read by Dr. D. S. Lamb on " School Hygiene" in the hands of the educationalists of the District. At the next meeting, however, November 26th, this action was rescinded.

April 6, 1892, the Society recommended that authors and essayists give their papers, or abstracts of the same, presented to the Society, to the *National Medical Review* for publication; and also ordered that the discussions on papers, etc., should also be given to the same journal. The *Review* began publication in March, 1892, under the editorship of Dr. Charles H. Stowell, a member of the Society. It was a monthly, 16 pages, double column. Much of the work of the Society was published in it, the discussions beginning with the November number, 1892. Volume V, 1896, contained only three numbers, a new arrangement of volumes being made; Vol. VI began with the June number, 1896, and the monthly pages were increased to 24. In October, 1897, Drs. George W. Johnston and T. E. McArdle became the owners and managers, in place of Stowell, and issued the November number. The journal was discontinued in 1901, the last number published being No. 1, Vol. XI, for June; the May number completing the Society transactions for 1900.

October 10, 1894, the editor of the *Virginia Medical Monthly* offered to publish the proceedings of the Society; and the editor of the *Maryland Medical Journal* had also the matter under consideration. The Society referred the subject to the Committee on Publication, which reported October 31st, recommending that the privilege of publication be continued to the *National Medical Review*, in consideration of Dr. Stowell's agreement to print promptly all discussions and abstracts of papers presented, when such abstracts were furnished by the authors. The Society adopted the report.

December 18, 1895, a committee was appointed to consider the advisability of publishing the transactions in some permanent form. Drs. W. W. Johnston, Kleinschmidt, S. S. Adams, J. H. Bryan and C. H. Stowell were the committee.

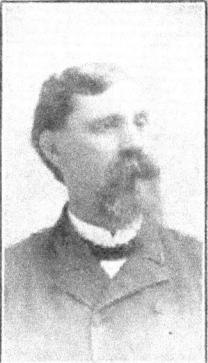

GEO. PHILIP FENWICK

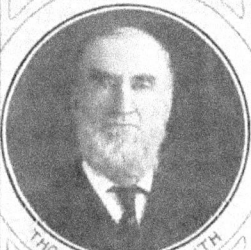

THOS. CROGGON SMITH

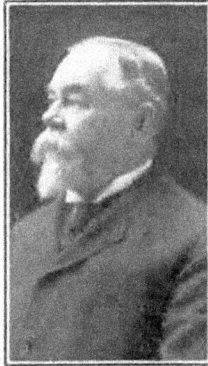

RALPH WALSH

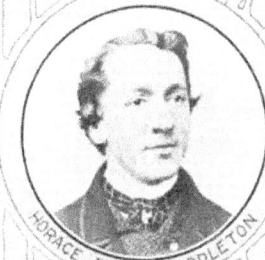

HORACE PECHIN MIDDLETON

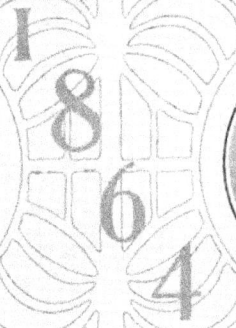

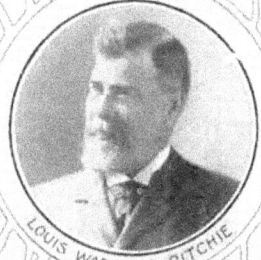

1864

LOUIS WARFIELD RITCHIE

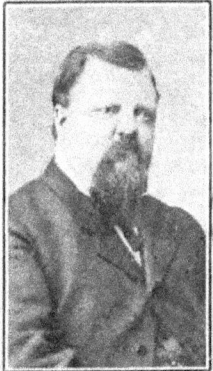

CHAS. MASON FORD

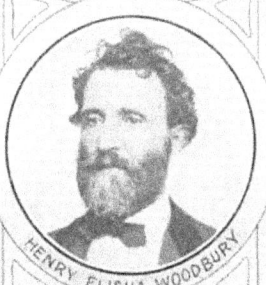

HENRY ELISHA WOODBURY

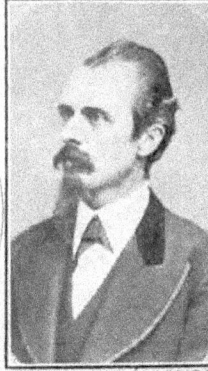

WM. HERBERT COMBS

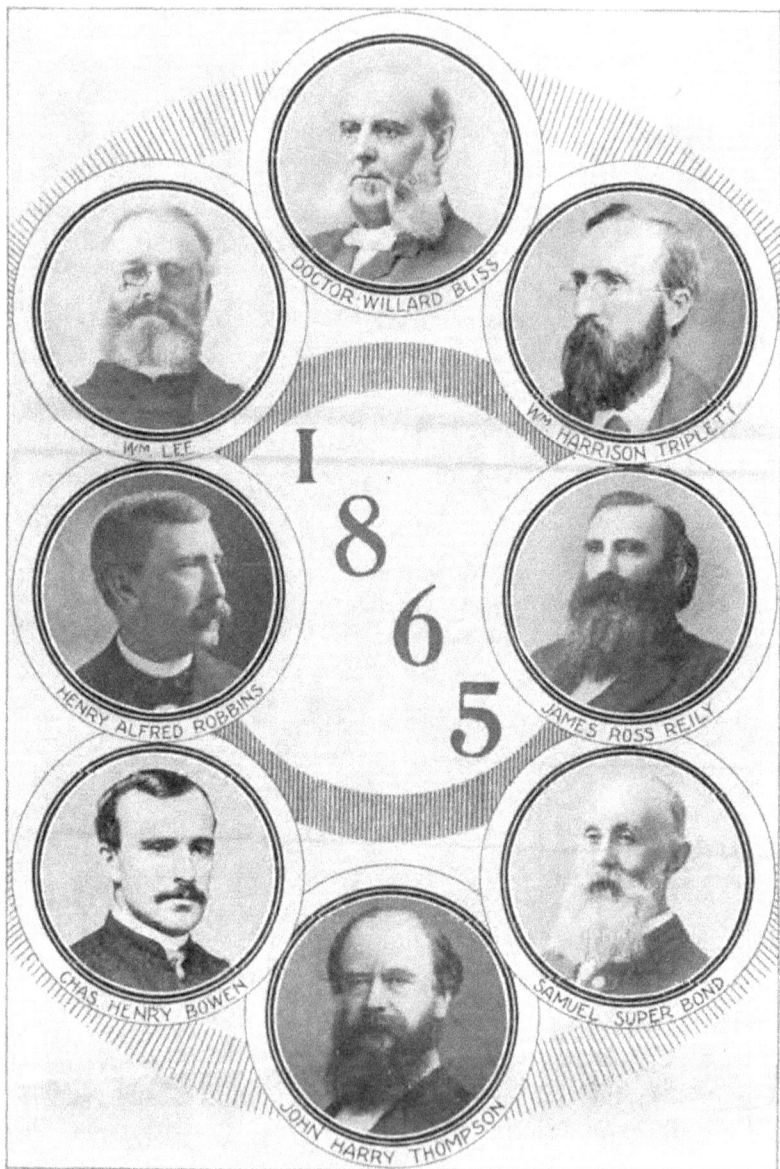

DOCTOR WILLARD BLISS

WM LEE

WM HARRISON TRIPLETT

1865

HENRY ALFRED ROBBINS

JAMES ROSS REILY

CHAS HENRY BOWEN

JOHN HARRY THOMPSON

SAMUEL SUPER BOND

The committee reported January 8, 1896, recommending an annual volume of transactions, to be published about
October 1st, and to include the Society work from the preceding October 1st to June 30th.   There should be a title
page, table of contents, list of officers and members, a condensed statement of matters of interest discussed and acted
on during the year, appertaining to legislation, public
health, &c.; papers, essays and discussions; and reports of
pathological specimens.   The editing to be done by a committee appointed by the President; this committee to have
full power to decide on the material for publication, and
exclude what was not thought worthy of preservation.   In
case of disagreement in the committee the President should
be the referee.

Readers of papers should furnish typewritten copies
for the use of the committee, but might publish their papers elsewhere, with the statement that they had been read
before the Society.   It was recommended to publish 500
copies at an annual cost of $800, with paper covers; each
member and member by invitation to receive a copy.   The
cost per page to be from $1.25 to $1.50; the volume not to
exceed 500 pages.   Illustrations, plates, prints in colors or
charts, at cost of author of paper.   After supplying the
members, the remaining copies to go to public medical
libraries, societies that publish their transactions and honorary members.

February 12th, after discussion, the report was laid on
the table.   February 19th, the Committee on Publication
was instructed to correspond with the *Journal of the American Medical Association*, the *Virginia Medical Monthly*,
the *New York Medical Journal*, and such other medical
journals as the committee might select, to ascertain the
conditions on which said journals would publish the transactions of the Society and furnish 500 reprints without
covers, paged in numerical order, with title page and index,
the index to be prepared by a committee of the Society.
March 18th, the Committee on Publication made a report,

6

and April 1st the report was discussed. The Society ordered that the transactions be published, and referred the subject to a special committee with instructions to present a method of publication. April 22d, the Society accepted the offer of the *National Medical Review;* a special assessment of one dollar per member was levied to pay for the journal, and an Editing Committee appointed with discretionary powers as to publication of papers and discussions; Drs. W. W. Johnston, G. M. Kober and J. D. Morgan were the committee.*

As a separate publication, but still a reprint from the *National Medical Review*, the *Transactions* of the Society from March to December, 1896, appeared as Vol. I, the paging being changed. The four succeeding volumes included, each, the Society work of the corresponding calendar year; the last was for the year 1900.

March 16, 1898, the Editing Committee reported that the contract for publication made with the *Review* would soon expire; that the managers of the journal had lost heavily; the cost of publishing the transactions of the Society was more than twice the sum the Society paid them for the work. They offered for $400 to continue publication and furnish 50 bound volumes of transactions, as before. The Society agreed to this proposition.†

February 21, 1900, the Society requested the Editing Committee to report on the advisability of continuing the publication of the *Transactions.* The committee reported March 21st,‡ and the Society ordered the publication continued in the same form, with the addition of the bound volumes.

April 17, 1901, the Editing Committee again made

---

* For this offer see *National Medical Review;* also *Transactions* of Society, 1896, I, p. 1.
† See *Transactions*, III, for 1898, p. 69; also *Review*, 1898–9, VIII, p. 187.
‡ See *Transactions*, V, 1900, p. 61.

report,* and on its recommendation, the Society work for 1901 was published as Vol. VI of the *Transactions.*

The Presidential address of Dr. D. S. Lamb, December 18, 1901, recommended that the Society publish its own journal. An editorial committee, Drs. D. S. Lamb, W. A. Wells and V. B. Jackson, was appointed to report on this proposition. The committee reported February 12, 1902, recommending the publication. The report was referred to the Executive Committee, which reported February 19th, recommending the publication, and the Society approved the recommendation.† The Editing Committee was authorized to proceed with the publication, keeping the expense within $600 for the year, and was also authorized to insert advertisements and solicit subscriptions.

February 18, 1903, the Editing Committee reported the results of the first year of publication ;‡ and February 17, 1904, the results of its second year.§ April 20th, some of the phases of publication were discussed by the Society,|| and May 4th, the Editing Committee made a report, which was adopted,¶ limiting the length of papers to ten pages, unless the authors would pay for the additional pages. October 19th, the committee reported that it had secured second-class rates at the post office.

The WASHINGTON MEDICAL ANNALS is the property and official organ of the Society; is a bimonthly, varying more or less in the number of pages of each issue, but making a total of between 400 and 600 pages yearly. Each issue comprises the papers read and specimens presented before the Society and discussions thereon; a brief statement of the proceedings of the Society; the editorial matter; and a medical miscellany, consisting of re-

---

* See *Transactions,* VI, 1901, p. 137.
† See ANNALS, I, 1902, pp. 79, 146.
‡ See ANNALS, 1903, II, p. 139.
§ ANNALS, 1904-5, III, p. 132.
‖ ANNALS, p. 241.
¶ ANNALS, p. 278.

ports of proceedings of other societies, of various medical institutions in Washington, of the Health Office of the District, etc.

Successive reports of the Editorial Committee have appeared in the ANNALS. The report January 1, 1908, for the year ending with the January number, shows a net cost of $1.13 per page, which covered all expenses incident to the publication. Since the publication began in 1902, the membership of the Society has increased from 285 to 429, about 50 per cent.

THE MEDICAL HALL.

It had long been in the minds of the members of the Society to have a building of its own. In course of time the members tired of going from one place of meeting to another. Apparently the first distinct movement toward such a building was made in the address of Dr. Toner, December 20, 1865. He wanted a medical library and museum for the use of the Society, and also a building in which the archives and other property of the Society might be permanently kept and meetings be held. He proposed a plan to raise $12,000 for the purpose. Drs. Liebermann, H. Lindsly, Toner and G. Tyler were appointed a committee to consider the question.

Nothing, however, was definitely done until nearly a year afterward, November 7, 1866, when Dr. W. P. Johnston submitted a plan for raising funds to buy a lot and erect a suitable building. The following resolution was adopted :

"*Resolved*, That a joint stock company be formed, composed only of members of the Society, with authority to raise by stock subscriptions a sum not less than $50,000 nor more than $75,000, for the purpose of erecting, under the auspices of the Medical Society, a commodious and fireproof building to be styled 'The Medical Hall of the District of Columbia.' "

At the same meeting, Dr. Toner, of the committee previously appointed, reported another plan for raising funds, by subscription and the issue of shares or scrip. His report was received and the committee discharged. November 14th, the committee provided for in Dr. Johnston's resolution was appointed: Drs. D. R. Hagner, from the first ward; W. P. Johnston, from the second; J. Ford Thompson, from the third; Harvey Lindsly, from the fourth; C. M. Ford, from the fifth; S. A. H. McKim, from the sixth; J. E. Morgan, from the seventh; Grafton Tyler and Louis Mackall, from Georgetown; and C. H. Nichols, from the County.

Promptly, November 21st, Dr. Johnston reported that $16,000 had already been subscribed by sixteen members, and December 5th, that the subscriptions amounted to $33,900. It was now desirable to have a legal opinion as to the purchase and holding of property by the subscribers, and Joseph H. Bradley, Esq., an eminent member of the Washington bar, was consulted. January 22, 1867, he gave a favorable opinion, and January 30th, a committee was appointed, consisting of the President, Dr. Liebermann, with Drs. Johnston, Joshua Riley, F. Howard and W. G. H. Newman, to which, February 6th, Dr. J. C. Hall was added, to buy a lot for the proposed building; they were to raise the funds by getting subscriptions, to be credited to the subscribers in stock, and propose plans for the building and make report to the Society; and, finally, to report proper regulations for the purchase and holding of stock, and other matters pertaining to the project.

February 13th, Dr. Johnston reported that a lot had

been bought at the southwest corner of Tenth and F Streets, N. W.; 75 feet on F Street and 74 feet on Tenth, for $25,000, $2,000 to be paid in cash, $10,000 in six months, and the remainder at stated periods to be determined. To help matters along, the Society, February 27th, transferred from its treasury $500 to the Treasurer of the "Medical Hall."

May 1st, the President of the Society was authorized to deliver to the Trustees of St. Joseph's Orphan Asylum, to which the property belonged, the necessary promissory notes, secured by deed of trust thereon, "purchased by the Society." June 19th, Dr. Riley resigned from the committee, and Dr. L. Mackall was appointed. The building already on the lot was rented at $100 a month, and the money was invested in six per cent. stock. July 24th, the Society ordered $300 more to be transferred to the Treasurer of the Medical Hall. August 21st, Dr. Hall resigned from the committee, and was succeeded by Dr. Toner. September 18th, the President was authorized to execute the necessary deed of trust to Messrs. A. Thomas Bradley and J. H. Bradley, Jr., to secure the payment of the scrip that had been issued in accordance with the action of the Society of January 30th.

October 2d, 9th and 23d, a committee was appointed to organize a course of lectures, to be delivered during the winter months, to help raise funds for the hall. The committee, however, failed to meet, and was discharged November 13th.

January 22, 1868, the Treasurer of the Hall Committee reported that up to January 1st, subscriptions had been received amounting to $3,286, rents to $760, and from the Medical Society, $800; total, $4,846, and he had given his bond for $5,000. There had been paid: for the purchase of the property, $3,200; interest on deferred notes, $788.91;

tax, $109.57 ; for stock bearing over 6 per cent. interest, $570 ; fees to notary, and stamps and recording deeds, $96.75 ; stationery, $40.28, and printing, $12 ; total, $4,826.76. The stock that had been bought was intended to meet any current demand that might be caused by the death or departure from the city of any subscriber. February 26th, $100 more was appropriated by the Society.

July 8th, the Hall Committee was authorized to erect a three-story building, and borrow the required amount, not exceeding $6,000, and pay the same with interest from the rents accruing from the building to be erected ; the building to be insured as it progressed ; $300 more was transferred from the Society to the Treasurer of the Hall. August 20th, ground was broken for the building.

January 6, 1869, the building being nearly completed, it was ordered that Dr. Johnston inaugurate the new hall by an address, and the medical profession of the District, with ladies, be invited to be present. January 20th, it was ordered that thereafter the officers of the Society should occupy seats on the platform ; also that the Treasurer of the Society should pay the current expenses on the property, including insurance, taxes, the purchase of furniture, fixtures, alterations, repairs and incidental expenses ; and that $150 be transferred to the Hall Committee, making $1,350 in all so transferred.

January 29th, the hall was inaugurated. Prayer was offered by Rev. Dr. Wm. Pinckney. Address by Dr. W. P. Johnston. The key of the building was given by Dr. Johnston to President Thomas Miller, who in turn gave it to Librarian Toner, who then also made an address. Addresses were also made by Drs. Liebermann, Tyler and A. F. A. King. The benediction was pronounced by Rev. Dr. G. W. Samson.

June 16th, Dr. Johnston stated to the Society that Mr.

A. T. Bradley, the attorney, had given an opinion that it would be necessary for each member of the Society to hold at least one share of stock in the Medical Hall. This was an unexpected complication.

The acoustic qualities of the hall were not the best, and November 3d, the Committee on Building was instructed to consult a "scientific" architect about the matter. Another more serious trouble, however, was now at hand. It had become evident that the Society was unable to raise the balance of funds necessary to complete the payments, and therefore could not hold the property. December 15th, the Society ordered that all its right, title and interest in the building should be transferred to three trustees for the benefit of the stockholders; the money interests of the Society and stockholders, respectively, to be ascertained by two members of the Society, one to report to the Society and the other to the stockholders, with power to select an arbitrator if the two were unable to agree. Dr. Antisell was appointed to represent the Society.

February 2, 1870, Dr. Liebermann, acting for the Society, presented the stockholders' bond in regard to the property, which was transferred, not to trustees, as had been proposed, but directly to the stockholders by their request. April 13, 1871, the Society was informed that all matters between it and the stockholders had been adjusted; and thus ended the first effort to secure a " Medical Hall."

ANOTHER MEDICAL BUILDING.

In his Presidential address of December, 1893, Dr. G. Wythe Cook recommended a medical building. March 7, 1894, he called the attention of the Society again to the matter, and a committee was appointed, consisting of Drs. Cook, Busey and J. D. Morgan, to consider it. The com-

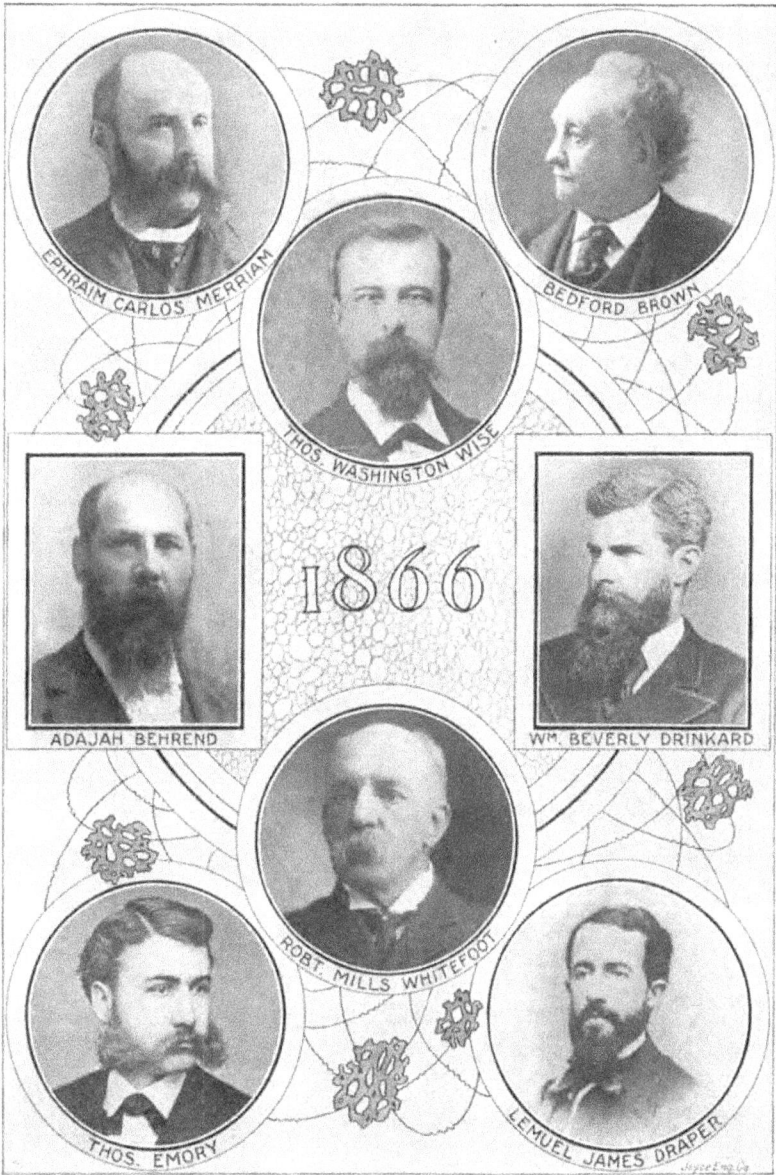

EPHRAIM CARLOS MERRIAM

BEDFORD BROWN

THOS. WASHINGTON WISE

1866

ADAJAH BEHREND

WM. BEVERLY DRINKARD

ROBT. MILLS WHITEFOOT

THOS. EMORY

LEMUEL JAMES DRAPER

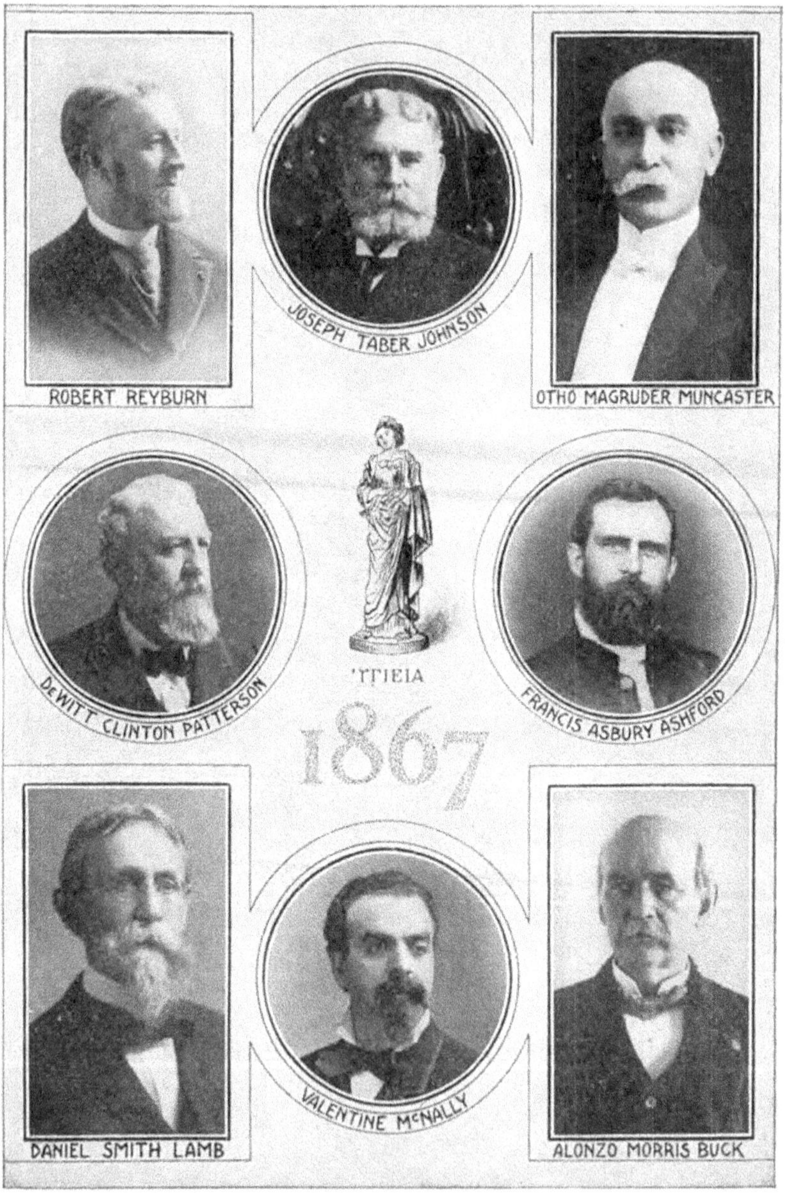

ROBERT REYBURN

JOSEPH TABER JOHNSON

OTHO MAGRUDER MUNCASTER

DeWITT CLINTON PATTERSON

'ΥΓΙΕΙΑ

1867

FRANCIS ASBURY ASHFORD

DANIEL SMITH LAMB

VALENTINE McNALLY

ALONZO MORRIS BUCK

mittee reported April 4th, recommending that some plan of organized and concerted effort be effected by which $30,000 or more could be raised or secured, to be held as a trust fund to be used only for procuring a permanent home and place of meeting.

The committee advised a joint stock company with a capital of $30,000, with 2,000 shares at $15.00 a share, payable in ten years, in annual installments of not less than $1.50, or in whole or in part at any period of the ten years, at the option of the holder, said shares to be issued only to members of the Society and such other persons as might be approved by a Committee of Finance to be appointed by the Society, and to bear interest, when paid in full, at the rate of two per cent. per annum. The shares to be irredeemable, except at the option of the Society, and not transferable, except with the consent of the Finance Committee, and sold only after the Society relinquished its option to purchase at their market value. In the event of the death of a holder of such shares, the Society would retain the option of purchase at such value as might be agreed upon, or otherwise the estate might dispose of them at its will and pleasure. Failure to pay the annual installment on each share, or to pay in full the par value in ten years from date of issue, should forfeit the said shares to the Society.

All shares purchased by the Society, or forfeited to it by delinquent holders, should be held by the Society on the same terms and conditions as applied to other shares, until such time as it might choose to cancel such stock, provided such cancellation was not prior to the accumulation of $30,000.

The duty of carrying into operation and the management of the project should devolve on a committee of finance, to consist of five members of the Society ; the committee should not be subject to change except by death or resignation. Vacancies to be filled by the Society in such manner as it might determine.

The report was ordered to be printed and distributed to members. April 25th it was adopted, and it was ordered that an attorney be employed to pass upon the legality of the project. A Finance Committee was appointed, May 2d—Drs. Busey, G. Wythe Cook, J. D. Morgan, W. W. Johnston and T. N. McLaughlin. October 31st, the committee reported that it had consulted W. E. Edmonston, of the Columbia Title Insurance Company, who had given an opinion that the Society could not legally carry out the project. The committee therefore asked authority to prepare a plan for voluntary contributions, and to ask Mr. Edmonston to draft a bill to be presented to Congress, giving the Society authority to raise funds. The report was adopted and authority given.

February 6, 1895, the Society recommended the efforts of the Building Committee. March 6th, however, the committee reported that the contributions to the building fund were wholly inadequate for the establishment of such a fund, and asked to be discharged. The record does not show what action, if any, was taken, but the matter was dropped.

PRIZE ESSAYS.

The first mention of a prize essay in which the Society took part was July 5, 1865, when Dr. Harvey Lindsly offered to give annually a prize for the best essay on some medical subject, the title to be selected by the Society. Drs. Antisell, Toner and Lovejoy were appointed a committee to see that essays were duly prepared for the consideration of the Society. December 6th, the committee reported, announcing a prize of $50 for the best essay on "Typho-malarial fever in the District and in the adjoining counties of Maryland and Virginia during the previous ten years." The essays were to be sent in by June 1, 1866, and the award to be made in July. January 17, 1866, a committee was appointed to carry out the wishes of the Society in regard to the award and, January 31st, the time was extended until October 1st. Time passed on until May, 1867, when Dr. Antisell reported that no essay had been received. Thus ended the first offer of a prize.

In his Presidential address, December 19, 1900, Dr. G. N. Acker recommended that a prize be offered yearly on some subject. The recommendation was referred to a committee consisting of Drs. A. F. A. King, T. N. McLaughlin and S. S. Adams. The matter went later to the Executive Committee, which made a favorable report, February 19, 1902. The report was adopted, and a printed circular of information was issued.* A number of essays were received and December 17th, following, the award was made.

The prize, $250, by private subscription, was given to Dr. F. P. Vale; his subject was " Concerning Shock, with a contribution to Pathology." Honorable mention was also made of the essay of Dr. J. B. Nichols, on "A study of acute leukemia and the etiology of leukemia." The judges were Drs. R. A. Marmion, U. S. Navy, W. C. Borden, U. S. Army, and H. D. Geddings, of the Public Health and Marine Hospital Service. The fund was raised mainly through the efforts of Dr. S. S. Adams; 25 members gave each $10.00.†

THE PHARMACISTS OF THE DISTRICT OF COLUMBIA.

The old grievance of physicians against druggists prescribing over the counter found its expression March 29, 1865, when the Society appointed a committee, consisting

---

* See Minutes, pp. 61, 155, and WASH. MED. ANNALS, 1902, I, p. 145.

† The subscribers were Drs. G. N. Acker, S. S. Adams, E. A. Balloch, J. H. Bryan, G. Wythe Cook, L. L. Friedrich, Franck Hyatt, H. L. E. Johnson, J. Taber Johnson, W. W. Johnston, A. F. A. King, G. M. Kober, T. N. McLaughlin, J. D. Morgan, W. G. Morgan, T. M. Murray, C. W. Richardson, S. O. Richey, T. C. Smith, Z. T. Sowers, W. M. Sprigg, I. S. Stone, W. H. Wilmer, J. T. Winter, W. C. Woodward.

of Drs. F. Howard, Joshua Riley, Johnson Eliot, J. E. Morgan and S. A. H. McKim, to report some proper means of preventing druggists from prescribing and practicing medicine. Apparently the committee never reported.

April 7, 1875, a letter was read from the National College of Pharmacy, inviting the coöperation of the Medical Society in a revision of certain formulae for so-called elegant preparations. The Society appointed a committee consisting of Drs. J. W. H. Lovejoy, Kleinschmidt, C. W. Franzoni, J. C. Riley and J. E. Morgan. The committee reported, April 14th, that it had met the Pharmacy Committee and the latter had submitted the following as the object of the conference:

"First. To secure with comparative certainty the furnishing to the patient of such medicines and in such doses as the physician wished to administer.

"Second. To secure uniformity in the vehicles employed in the administration of such medicines, and thus obviate the confusion which must arise so long as the preparations from different manufacturers are dispensed under similar names, and even those from one source often differ materially in color, taste, &c.

"Third. To do away with the necessity of taxing the public to the extent of a heavy profit for the manufacturers in addition to our own.

"Fourth. To recognize the fact that the compounding of medicines is the province of the apothecary; that by forcing him to sell the preparations of third parties, for the correctness of which he has to assume the responsibility without having control over them, thus reducing it to a mere matter of buying and selling, and incompetent parties are induced to engage in the same.

"We therefore propose to establish formulae for such of the elixirs, etc., as it may be desirable to retain, and a general formula for a simple elixir, to answer as a vehicle for most of the soluble salts.

"For this end we would ask your coöperation in selecting and determining such formulae and in using your best endeavors to bring about, as much as possible, a discontinuance of the use of the promiscuous preparations now offered by divers manufacturers."

After a full and free discussion, the following resolution was offered, and unanimously adopted:

"*Resolved*, That the respective committees report to their societies that the joint committee has agreed to recommend the establishment of uniform formulae for elixirs, etc., for use by the profession of the District of Columbia, and the appointment of a joint committee to carry out this object."

April 27th, the Society reappointed the same committee as a part of the joint committee agreed upon. October 20, 1877, the committee from the Society reported that the work had been completed, showed proofs of the printed matter and asked the formal endorsement of the Society, which was given. The title of the book was "Formulary for Non-official Preparations in General Use in the District of Columbia;" 48 pages.

In 1897 a bill was introduced into Congress to regulate the practice of pharmacy: Senate Bill 1330. The bill contained some features to which the Committee on Legislation of the Medical Society took exception, and April 7th, the Society directed the committee to oppose the passage of the bill.

May 20, 1903, a committee was appointed to confer with the Commissioners of Pharmacy with regard to formulating a new law concerning pharmacy and poisons.* The committee consisted of Drs. Z. T. Sowers, G. L. Magruder, R. Reyburn. T. A. Claytor and N. P. Barnes.

December 16th, Dr. M. G. Motter stated that a conference had been held by committees from the Medical Soci-

* See WASHINGTON MEDICAL ANNALS, 1903-4, II, pp. 307, 496.

ety, Homeopathic Medical Society, National College of Pharmacy, Retail Drug Clerks' Association, Medico-Legal Society, Registered Drug Clerks' Association and the Board of Pharmacy. The result was a bill which had been sent to the District Commissioners. March 2, 1904, the committee on the new pharmacy law reported to the Society that the bill agreed on had been introduced in Congress,* and November 8, 1905, the Society passed a resolution that it would coöperate with the District Commissioners in securing the passage of the bill.†

THE ANNIVERSARIES OF THE SOCIETY.

The question as to what time of the year should be celebrated as the anniversary of the formation of the Society was, perhaps, discussed from time to time, but the first record of the question being raised was when Dr. Toner made his anniversary address, September 26, 1866.‡ It will be remembered that this date was that of the preliminary meeting called in 1817 to consider the formation of the Society. At that meeting a resolution was adopted to the effect that it was "important and expedient to organize at once a society," etc., and apparently it was from this fact that Dr. Toner maintained that that date should be regarded as the true anniversary ; because, he argued that we celebrate the Fourth of July as Independence Day, although the resolution of the Continental Congress declaring the independence of the Colonies was not engrossed until July 19, and not signed until August 2, 1776.

September 26, 1867, what might be called a second An-

---

* House Bill 11967, introduced February 8th. See WASH. MED. ANNALS, 1904-5, III, pp. 134, 147.

† The bill passed and was approved May 7, 1906. See U. S. Statutes, 1905-6, part I, p. 175.

‡ "Anniversary address delivered before the Medical Society of the District of Columbia." Published in 1869, 80 pages.

niversary celebration took place. The meeting was held
at the Columbian Medical College ; there was an address by
Dr. W. P. Johnston, followed by a supper. Dr. Noble
Young, however, took exception to the date, September
26th, and wrote a letter to the Society, August 12, 1868,
when another celebration of September 26th was being
contemplated ; he maintained that the proper date was
that of the final organization of the Society, namely, January 5th, and that therefore the next celebration should be
January 5, 1869. The Society debated the question, September 2, 1868, and decided, by a vote of 9 to 4, that
January 5th was the proper date. Those who voted in the
affirmative were Drs. S. S. Bond, F. Howard, W. P. Johnston, A. F. A. King, C. H. Liebermann, G. R. Miller, J. E.
Morgan, C. M. Tree and Noble Young ; in the negative,
Drs. J. W. H. Lovejoy, Wm. Marbury, B. Thompson and
J. M. Toner. The attendance was too small to decide such
a matter. The Society accordingly celebrated January 5,
1869 ; the victor in the contest, Noble Young, made the
address, and those attending then adjourned to " Harvey's "
for supper.

As a matter of fact, however, January 5th was not always the date afterwards celebrated. It was January 26,
1870, when Dr. Lincoln made his address; Dr. Busey
made his, January 4, 1871 ; Dr. Louis Mackall, January 3,
1872, at Marini's Hall ; and January 9, 1873, at the same
place, Dr. Lovejoy officiated.*

Then the pendulum swung back to September 26th, for
September 26, 1873, the anniversary was held at Marini's,
and Dr. D. R. Hagner made the address ; September 26,
1874, at the same place, Dr. W. B. Drinkard was the orator. But the next year, 1875, the date was changed to

---

* Marini's Hall was previously the " Medical Hall."

November 23d ; the meeting was at the same place, and Dr. W. W. Johnston made the address.

It is well to note, going back for a moment, that January 6, 1851, Dr. Grafton Tyler was elected to deliver an annual address, and this must have been an anniversary address, because Dr. William Jones was President at that time, and the address was made January 5, 1852 ; and Dr. Tyler was elected to make the address again the next year, Dr. Jones still being President.

September 26, 1876, Dr. Antisell was the orator at Marini's Hall ; December 20, 1877, Dr. A. Y. P. Garnett, at Marini's ; December 28, 1878, Dr. A. F. A. King, at Talmadge Hall; November 26, 1879, Dr. Reyburn, at Gonzaga Hall; December 8, 1880, Dr. S. A. H. McKim, at the same place.*

With this date the anniversary celebrations ceased until February 16, 1894, when the 75th anniversary was celebrated. A full account of the events leading up to it, and the program as carried out, was published by the Society, under the title " Transactions and Proceedings of the 75th Anniversary of the Medical Society of the District of Columbia ;" 108 pages. The story is briefly as follows : April 5, 1893, Dr. C. H. Stowell called the attention of the Society to the fact that February 16, 1894, would be the 75th anniversary (*i. e.*, of the approval of the first charter). A committee was appointed to consider the propriety of celebrating it : Drs. Busey, Stowell and T. C. Smith. The committee reported favorably, and was enlarged by the addition of Drs. T. E. McArdle and S. S. Adams to prepare a program. This committee reported the program May 10th, and was again enlarged by adding Drs. G. C. Ober and A. A. Snyder to form a committee of arrangements.

---

* The titles of the anniversary essays up to 1878 were published in the *National Medical Review* for 1878-9, I, p. 64.

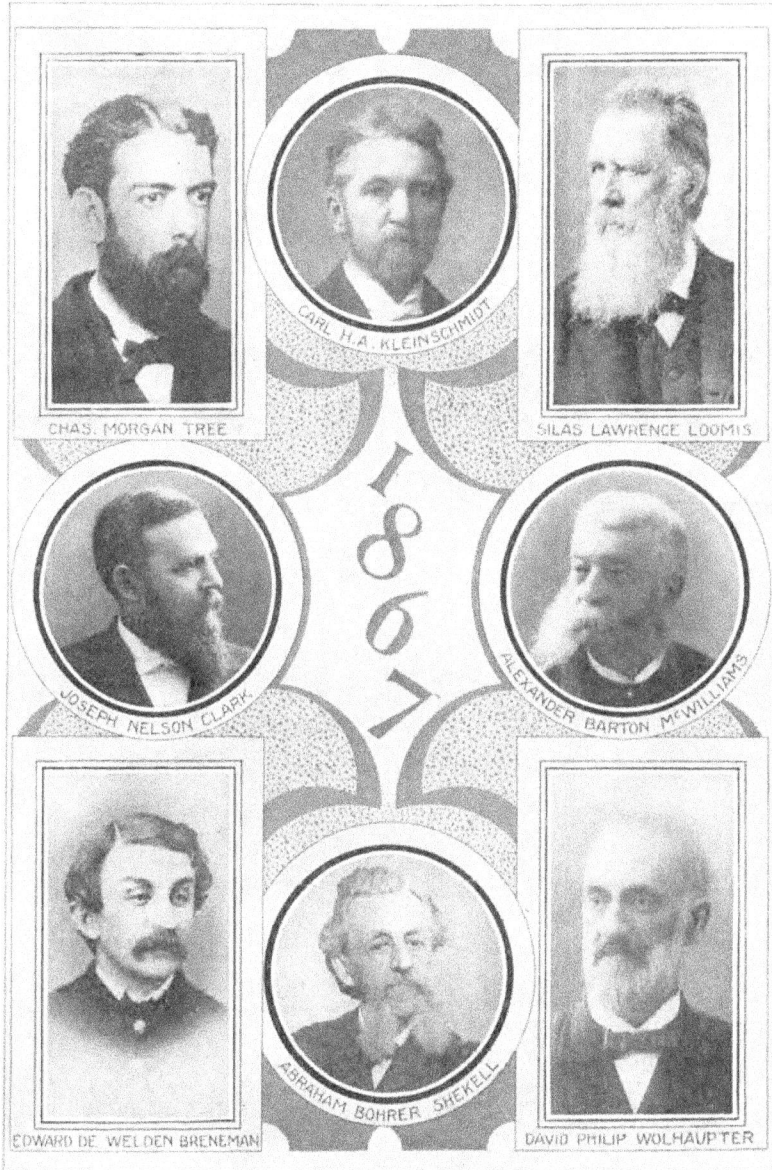

CHAS. MORGAN TREE

CARL H.A. KLEINSCHMIDT

SILAS LAWRENCE LOOMIS

JOSEPH NELSON CLARK

ALEXANDER BARTON McWILLIAMS

EDWARD DE WELDEN BRENEMAN

ABRAHAM BOHRER SHEKELL

DAVID PHILIP WOLHAUPTER

1867

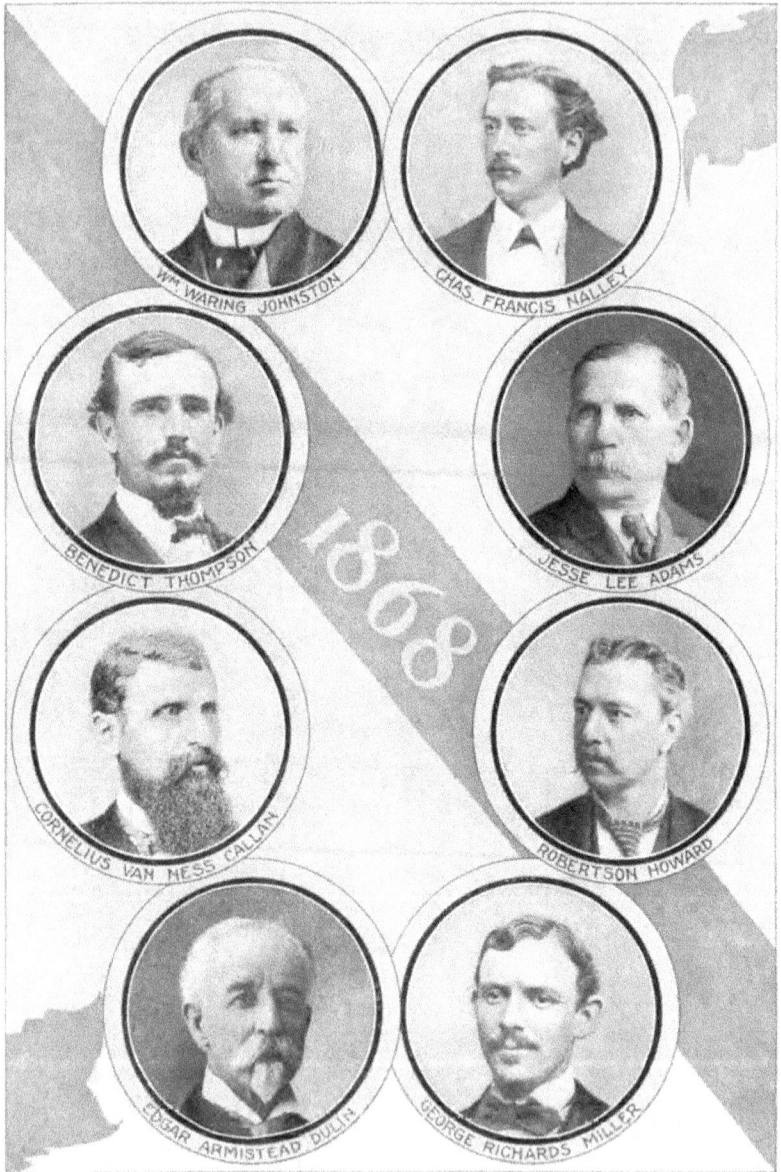

WM. WARING JOHNSTON   CHAS. FRANCIS NALLEY

BENEDICT THOMPSON   JESSE LEE ADAMS

CORNELIUS VAN NESS CALLAN   ROBERTSON HOWARD

EDGAR ARMISTEAD DULIN   GEORGE RICHARDS MILLER

1868

The committee reported details May 24th and again November 29th, and January 17 and February 7, 1894. The celebration was held February 16th, and on the 21st the Society adopted appropriate resolutions.

The program was opened with an address by Dr. Busey, who was President of the Society at the time ; Dr. W. W. Johnston followed with a "History of the Medical Society ;" Dr. J. Ford Thompson came next with a "History of the Hospitals of the District of Columbia ;" and Dr. T. C. Smith concluded with the "History of the Medical Colleges of the District of Columbia." The meeting then adjourned to The Arlington, where a banquet was served, with appropriate toasts.

PORTRAITS OF MEMBERS.

As early as 1866 the Society undertook to secure the portraits, or copies of them, of deceased members and, incidentally, of members still living. February 7th of that year, on motion of Dr. Toner, it was ordered that portraits of deceased members, to be hung up in the room of the Society, be requested from their families. April 4th, the portrait of Dr. B. S. Bohrer was received, and May 9th, that of one of the Worthingtons. December 9th, a committee was appointed—Drs. W. P. Johnston, F. Howard and A. F. A. King—to inquire into and report the best manner in which to frame these portraits. The committee reported, recommending a mounting costing $16.00 apiece. Of course, for only two portraits, this sum was not so large, but for a large number of portraits it would have been too much.

January 30, 1867, the committee was authorized to obtain the portraits of other deceased members, but at an expense as low as possible. April 24th, Dr. Thomas Miller

7

gave his photograph to the Society. The portrait of Dr. S. C. Smoot was received, but July 17th, Dr. Mackall reported that the photographer had lost it. Whether it was ever again found does not appear. February 19, 1873, the photograph of Dr. R. K. Stone was received. Dr. Stone had died the year before. June 7, 1882, the Secretary was requested to ascertain the names of all those members who, according to the rule adopted by the Society, might be requested to furnish their pictures for the Society rooms. There is no mention of any report in regard to the matter.

February 1, 1905, Dr. A. L. Stavely presented to the Society a photograph of Dr. Chas. Worthington, that had been made from an oil painting that was afterward burned in the " Knox" fire; the photograph was made by a granddaughter of Dr. Worthington, a Miss E. W. Trescott, of Washington.

The Historical Committee, February 7, 1906, sent out a circular letter to all living members, and to many persons not members, asking for photographs of members, both of those living and those deceased. It was the intention of the committee to assemble the photographs in albums as a permanent record, but it was afterward thought best to have them reproduced in half-tone for publication in the " History."

INVESTMENTS.

The charter of the Society limits its investments to what would bring an income of no more than $6,000 a year. As a matter of fact, it does not appear that it was ever contemplated by the Society as a body to do more than simply assess the members enough to pay the current expenses. At first a portion of the balance remaining from actual expenses was devoted to increasing the library; but this expenditure did not long continue. In 1866 the Society had some surplus, namely, $400, which was ordered to be invested in stock bearing dividends at 6 or 7 per cent. The Treasurer invested it in United States 7–30s, which, being at a premium, gave a return of $421, March 13, 1867, when the bonds were sold to help pay subsrcription to the "Medical Hall." The Society subscribed altogether $1,350 to this project.

July 14, 1892, the Treasurer was directed to deposit all moneys in the Washington Loan and Trust Company, which paid a small interest on deposits. April 1, 1896, he was instructed to invest $1,000 at five and a half per cent., with real estate security, with the American Security and Trust Company, of Washington. November 10, 1897, the period of investment having expired, it was ordered to be renewed.

THE SOCIETY AND MEDICAL HISTORY AND STATISTICS.

June 12, 1867, it was ordered, on motion of Dr. Toner, that a standing committee be appointed,

" To consist of one member from each ward, two from Georgetown and one from the county, to be known as the Committee on History and Statistics of the Medical Society of the District of Columbia, whose duty it shall be to collect and keep a record of all important facts, occurrences of interest to the medical profession and, particularly, to collect statistics of the frequency and prevalence of particular diseases, throughout the year, and of surgical operations and their results."

The committee was appointed March 24, 1869, and discharged May 12, 1869, apparently not having done anything.

January 25, 1871, the following resolution was adopted :

"That a committee be appointed at the first meeting in January (or as soon thereafter as practicable) to be called the Committee on the Medical Constitution of the District, to consist of six members; the committee to be divided into three sub-committees, respectively, on Meteorology, Endemics and Epidemics, and Medical Statistics, each sub-committee to submit a quarterly report to be embodied in the general report of the committee as a whole; the latter report to be laid before the Society at the first regular meeting in January, April, July and October. The committee to solicit information from individuals and organizations."

Drs. W. B. Drinkard, T. Antisell, B. F. Craig, W. W. Johnston, J. Ford Thompson and A. F. A. King were the committee. Apparently no report was ever made.

THE SOCIETY AND COLORED PHYSICIANS.

On the 9th of June, 1869, two colored physicians, Drs. C. B. Purvis and A. T. Augusta, were proposed for membership in the Society. At the next meeting, June 16th, they were reported as eligible. They failed, however, to receive the requisite number of votes to elect them. June 23d, another colored physician, Dr. A. W. Tucker, was proposed; on the 30th he was reported as eligible, but failed of election.

No further effort toward membership on the part of colored physicians was made till January 6, 1891, when Dr. J. F. Shadd was nominated. April 1st, the date of election, the vote was 16 to 37, a little less than one-third. No colored physician has since applied.

1869 TO 1872.

So many years, the life, indeed, of one generation, have passed away since the trouble of 1869 to 1872, that few of the present members of the Society have any recollection of it. The story, even now, is painful to tell, although the intense partisanship of that time has long since faded away.

The complete record of the trouble can be found in the minutes of the Society of those years, especially June 15, 1870; in Volumes XXI and XXIII, 1870 and 1872, *Transactions American Medical Association;* in the *Congressional Record* of 1869–70; in "Busey's Reminiscences," p. 245 *et seq.;* and in the *National Medical Journal*, 1870–1, Vol. I, pp. 168, 203, 214, 220 and 233.

Briefly told, the story is as follows: December 9, 1869, Senator Sumner offered the following resolution in the U. S. Senate:

"*Resolved,* That the Committee on the District of Columbia be directed to consider the expediency of repealing the charter of the Medical Society of the District of Columbia, and of such other legislation as may be necessary in order to secure for medical practitioners in the District of Columbia equal rights and opportunities, without distinction of color."

This resolution was discussed by Senators Sumner, Patterson and Norton, and was adopted. The discussion showed that the Society and Association were being confounded. Mr. Sumner stated that his object was to repeal the charter of the Society and then charter a new Society that should be founded on republican principles. He mentioned the rejection of colored physicians by the Society, and the difficulty they had in securing consultations.

December 29th, the Medical Society appointed a committee, consisting of all its officers and three other members, to represent the Society before Congress in a way deemed most expedient by said committee, having in view, especially, the action of the United States Senate. At the same meeting it was ordered that, as it was possible that the charter might be repealed, all moneys due the Society, all moneys in hand and all property should be delivered to Trustees, the money to be invested in the purchase of books for a medical library, and the other property to be held in trust. Drs. S. C. Busey, L. Mackall, J. M. Toner, J. W. H. Lovejoy and W. B. Drinkard were made the Trustees.

At the meeting January 12, 1870, Drs. Lovejoy, Toner and Liebermann were appointed a committee to draft a statement of facts, explaining the status of the Society with reference to the proposed action of Congress for the repeal of its charter. This committee made an appropriate report, which was adopted and ordered to be published.*

February 8th, Senator Sumner from the District Committee reported a bill (Senate Bill, No. 511) repealing the charter of the Society; it was read twice and ordered to be printed. February 16th, the Congressional Committee of the Society reported that the whole matter had been laid before the Senate Committee, and it was believed that Senators Patterson and Hamlin correctly understood it. March 2d, the Society appointed a committee—Drs. Wm. Marbury, C. M. Tree and T. Purrington—to take an inventory of its personal property, and the Treasurer was instructed to transfer to the trustees the property embraced in the deed of trust which had been executed under the resolution of January 12th.

March 4th, the repeal bill was called up in the Senate, but, after some debate, was passed over. It was again called up April 22d, and again passed over.

The trouble was taken to the American Medical Association, which met in Washington May 3 to 6, 1870. The majority of the local committee of arrangements made a report to the Association, which contained a list of members of the Medical Society entitled to sit as delegates;

---

* The report was an appeal to Congress. See Busey's "Reminiscences," p. 247.

there was also a minority report that objected to some names in the majority report and recommended others. Both reports were referred to the Committee on Ethics, of the Association; a majority of this committee reported favoring the report of the majority of the committee of arrangements, and the Association approved the same.

June 10th, the repealing bill was again called up in the U. S. Senate and again passed over. February 8, 1871, it was again called up and passed over. That night the Society appointed its President and two Vice Presidents a committee to look after the interests of the Society before Congress. February 15th, the committee reported that there was no likelihood of action being taken on the bill at that session of Congress.

Apparently the matter received no further notice from the Senate; but December 18th, a bill repealing the charter (House Bill, No. 733) was introduced into the House and referred to the Committee on the District of Columbia. The Society took notice of it January 24, 1872, appointing a committee, consisting of the President, Vice Presidents and Drs. Toner and Lovejoy, to protest against the repeal. The Committee of the House of Representatives, however, never reported.

At the meeting of the American Medical Association, at San Francisco, in 1871, Dr. Toner was the only accredited delegate from the District, and the question of the District's representation does not appear to have been raised. But at the meeting in Philadelphia, May 7 to 10, 1872, it came up and was decided favorably to the Medical Society.

September 29, 1886, Dr. Busey recalled how, in 1870, the Society, apprehending some danger of abrogation of its charter, had transferred to a board of trustees all its property, consisting of furniture, library and money on hand, to be held in trust for the Society. The furniture and library, however, had always remained in possession of the Society, and were continuously used. Several meetings of the Board were held, and Dr. Busey was elected chairman. No meetings had been held since 1871. In 1872 or 1873 Dr. Busey had made a report to the Society. Since that time he had been in possession of the money, but had forgotten all about the matter until June, 1886, and it was only September 29th that he had been able to find the record of the transactions. [He then read the minutes of the several meetings of the Board.]

The Society appointed a committee, consisting of the President, Secretary and Treasurer, to investigate the matter and report some way in which the trustees might be discharged from the trust. The committee reported October 27th, reciting the history of the matter from the beginning. The trustees had expended $5.75, leaving a balance of $195.25. The committee recommended that as the need for the trustees had passed and they wanted to be released, the Society release them and their representatives of all their obligations. The recommendation and report were adopted. But November 24th, Dr. Busey stated that the action of the Society had been pronounced by an attorney insufficient, and he offered a preamble and resolution [these are not given] providing for the reconveyance of the property in their hands to the Society. These were adopted by the Society.

April 9, 1890, the attention of the Society was called to the fact that Senator Dolph had introduced in the Senate a bill to repeal the charter of the Society. The Secretary of the Society was directed to ascertain the facts. April 16th he presented a copy of the bill, which read as follows:

"A bill to amend an act entitled 'An act to revive with amendments an act to incorporate the Medical Society of the District of Columbia, approved July 7, 1838:' *Be it*

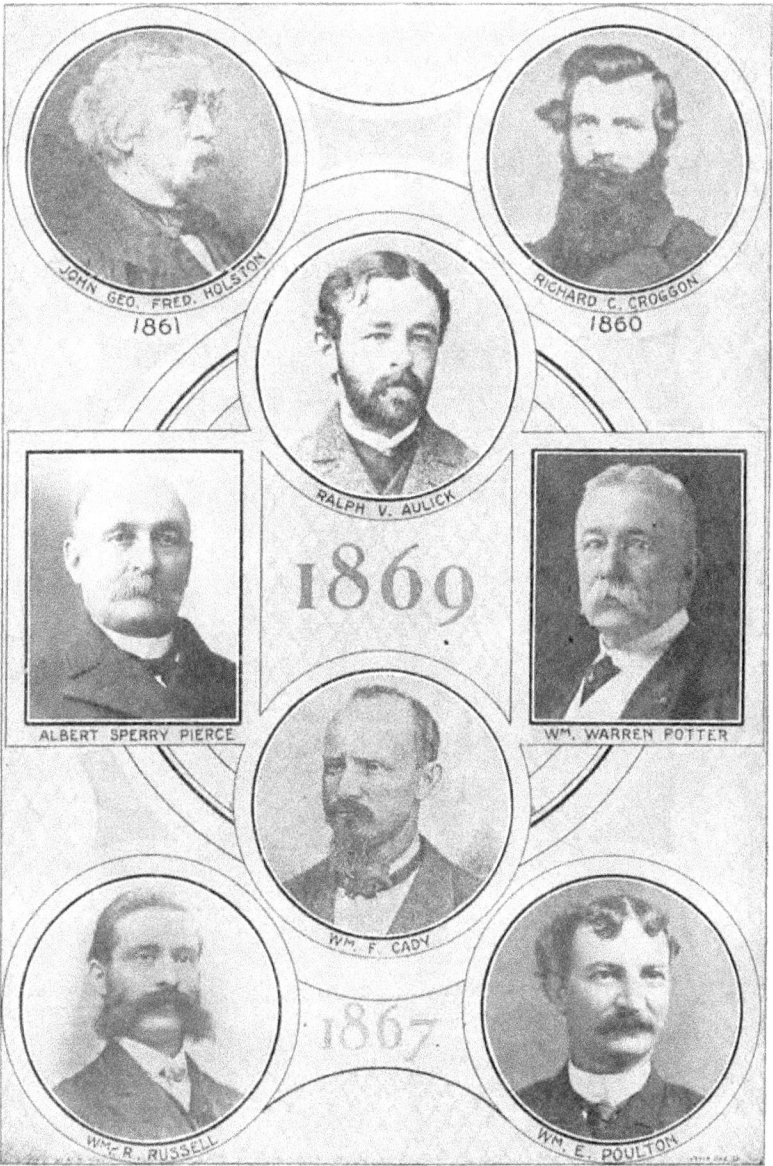

JOHN GEO. FRED. HOLSTON
1861

RICHARD C. CROGGON
1860

RALPH V. AULICK

1869

ALBERT SPERRY PIERCE

WM. WARREN POTTER

WM. F. CADY

1867

WM. R. RUSSELL

WM. E. POULTON

1871

JAMES FRENCH HARTIGAN

JOSHUA OTIS STANTON

CHAS. VERNON BOARMAN

WALTER CLARKE BRISCOE

HOWARD HINES BARKER

1872

JAMES KNOX POLK GLEESON

JAMES LITTLETON SUDDARTH

WALTER BOWIE TYLER

enacted by the Senate and House of Representatives of the United States of America in Congress assembled, That the act entitled 'An act to revive with amendments an act to incorporate the Medical Society of the District of Columbia, approved July 7, 1838,' be amended by striking out sections 3 and 5, the first eight lines, and first three words of the ninth line, counting from the top, of section 4, also the last seventeen lines of section 6, beginning with the words 10 'and provided also.' "

This bill was referred by the Society to the special committee on legislation.

The matter seems to have drifted along until April 12, 1892, when the Senate passed a resolution instructing the District Commissioners to inquire into and report whether the Medical Society admitted colored physicians to membership, or physicians who were or had been teachers in Howard University. After investigation, the Senate committee reported, July 22d, that the Society did " not admit to membership colored physicians, however reputable or well qualified they might be, and that as regards teachers in the medical school of Howard University, in some cases they were admitted and in others rejected."

This apparently disposed of the whole matter. No further action was taken.

THE SOCIETY AND THE HEALTH DEPARTMENT OF THE DISTRICT OF COLUMBIA.*

The necessity for a Health Officer or Board of Health to look after the sanitary needs of the District, was realized at an early date in the history of the District, but a number of years elapsed before such an officer or board was appointed. According to Dr. Toner,† it was mainly through

* This article was partly prepared by Dr. W. C. Woodward, from the records of the Health Department, D. C.

† Oration, p. 76.

the efforts of Dr. Henry Huntt, a member of the Society, that the Common Council and Board of Aldermen of Washington passed "An act to provide for the appointment of a Health Officer for the City of Washington," an Act approved by Mayor Samuel N. Smallwood, August 14, 1819. The text of this Act may be found, among a number of authorities, in the S. S. Adams Presidential address to the Society, December 17, 1902, entitled "Achievements of the conservators of the public health of the City of Washington during fifty years, 1819–1869."*

The first section of the Act provided that the Mayor, with the concurrence of the Board of Aldermen, should appoint a "discreet and prudent citizen, being a member of the Medical Society of the District of Columbia, to be Health Officer of the City of Washington." The Act then went on to recite the duties of this officer. By this Act, therefore, the Medical Society became directly interested in the office and the officer.

Four days after the approval, Dr. Henry Huntt was appointed Health Officer, and no doubt the influence of the Society was exerted, and effectually so, thereafter in shaping the sanitary legislation of the city.

For reasons which do not now appear the Common Council and Board of Aldermen passed a new law, that was approved by Mayor Smallwood, March 30, 1822, creating a "Board of Health," composed of one physician and one citizen not a physician, from each ward, and the physician attending the Washington Asylum. The first Board appointed (April 10, 1822) comprised, as physicians, Drs. Sim, Huntt, Sewall, Fred. May, Richmond Johnson, Hamilton and McWilliams—the last was the physician to the Washington Asylum. Dr. May was elected President, but declined, and Dr. Huntt was then elected and served

---

*Published as a Senate Document.

as such until 1833, when he resigned and Dr. Causin was elected President.

November 24, 1836, the Board of Health appointed a committee to memorialize Congress upon the subject of establishing an Insane Asylum and a National Hospital in Washington, and Drs. Young and Lindsly, who were members of the Board and also of the Society, were appointed by the Board a committee to present the matter to the Medical Society, and ask its concurrence and aid. Dr. Adams states* that the subject was presented to the Society, but was unceremoniously laid on the table, where it remained. The minutes of the Society for that period are not now in existence.

It may be mentioned here that the city of Georgetown had its own Board of Health, and by Sec. 10 of an Act of Congress, March 3, 1863, the "Levy Court" was given full power to make sanitary rules and regulations in the *county*, abate nuisances, &c. This court was composed of nine members, three from Washington, one from Georgetown and five from the County, appointed by the President of the United States and confirmed by the Senate.

As early as January 7, 1850, the Society appointed a committee, consisting of Drs. H. Lindsly, W. P. Johnston and J. C. Hall, to inquire into the expediency of establishing among the profession some system by which a more perfect registration of births and deaths might be effected. February 4th, the Society adopted a resolution approving the measure for procuring a registration of births which the Board of Health had adopted, and earnestly recommending the members of the Society to comply with the requirements of the same, so far as was compatible with professional confidence and a due regard to the feelings of patients.

---

* Ibid., p. 25.

In 1866 the Board of Health of Washington, because of the unsatisfactory results of its efforts to secure a complete registration of deaths, appointed a committee to consider the subject, and September 17th, the committee submitted a report, recommending that the Mayor be requested to recommend to the city Councils the adoption of an ordinance which the committee had prepared. The Board adopted the report. The proposed ordinance required the attending physician to sign the death certificate in each case of death, whereas previously he had simply been *requested* to do so; and certificates could also be signed by clergymen, members of the family of the deceased, and, indeed, by any respectable citizen. This action of the Board was communicated to the Medical Society, September 19th, and the Society passed an order requesting its members to oppose the passage of such a law. The law failed to pass, probably because of this opposition.

October 16, 1866, pursuant to a call, a few members of the Board of Health met, formed a temporary organization by calling Mr. M. G. Emery to the chair, and adjourned for one week, at the expiration of which time the Board was formally organized. November 9th, a resolution was adopted requiring physicians or midwives and certain other persons to report births to the Secretary of the Board of Health within a specified time, under a penalty of ten dollars. At the same meeting a resolution was adopted requiring all physicians, as well as undertakers, to keep on hand blank death certificates. The plan adopted by the Board for the registration of births does not appear to have given satisfactory results, for at the meeting of the Board November 19th, a request was made of the Boards of Aldermen and Common Council to enact into law the bill previously presented to the Board, referring principally to the ordinance enacted by the Board at its previous meeting.

April 29, 1868, the Medical Society appointed a committee, consisting of Drs. Lindsly, Tyler and D. R. Hagner, to apply to Congress for an act to establish a Commission of Health in the " District of Columbia."

The subject of reporting deaths seems to have been frequently before the Board of Health, because the minutes of the Board show that February 18, 1869, a resolution was introduced in regard to registration of deaths *before* burial. Up to that time such deaths had been registered by the superintendents of cemeteries after burial. The resolution was referred to a committee that reported one month later, but the nature of the report and the action of the Board thereon are not recorded. April 1st, the Undertakers' Protective Association protested that it was impossible for them to carry out the suggestions of the Board as to furnishing correct lists of burials, because some physicians refused to give the necessary information. Apparently the Board took no action on this. August 26th, the Board approved a draft of a new law for the registration of births, and instructed the Secretary to request of the Boards of Aldermen and Common Council their immediate action. By this bill the attending physician was made responsible for immediate report. What these legislative bodies did, however, does not appear.

At the meeting of the Board, October 21st, Mr. J. C. Willard moved that a committee be appointed to draft a bill to establish a Metropolitan Board of Health ; the motion was carried. Apparently, however, no bill was reported.

August 17, 1870, the committee of the Board on Burial Grounds and Registration was instructed to prepare a plan more effectually to secure a complete registration of births.

Apparently the Board of Health had no meeting between September 13th and October 4th. On the latter date the Board received an opinion from the Corporation Attorney relative to the powers of the Board. What the opin-

ion was is not stated.   A committee was appointed to call
on the Mayor and ascertain why the requests of the Board
had not been complied with.   This was the last meeting
of the Board of Health of the City of Washington.

By act of Congress, 1871, a Board of Health of the *District of Columbia* was created, and under this act a Board
was appointed, consisting of Dr. C. C. Cox, John Marbury,
John M. Langston, Dr. Tullio S. Verdi and H. A. Willard.   The Board organized at a meeting held April 13,
1871, by electing Dr. Cox President, Dr. Verdi Secretary,
and Mr. Willard Treasurer.   Dr. Verdi was subsequently
appointed Health Officer, and Mr. Willard having resigned,
Dr. D. W. Bliss was appointed in his place.   Dr. Cox,
however, was not a member of the Medical Society ; Dr.
Bliss was not in good standing in the Society, and Dr.
Verdi was a homeopathic practitioner.   April 26th, a committee, consisting of Drs. Antisell, Lincoln and Busey,
was appointed by the Medical Society to inquire into and
report upon the condition of the Health Department.
This committee was discharged May 3d, and a new one was
appointed—Drs. Lincoln, Miller and Marbury.   This committee also appears to have been unsatisfactory, for May
23d, Drs. Lovejoy, D.R.Hagner and Marbury were appointed to inquire into the constitution and action of the Board of
Health.   May 31st, the committee reported and was discharged.   Drs. Hagner, Lovejoy and Johnston were appointed a committee to have the report printed and sent to
all the medical journals and societies in the country.   The
memorial was as follows :

"*Memorial of the Medical Profession of the District of
Columbia to the Legislative Assembly :*
" The undersigned, regular practitioners of medicine in
the District of Columbia, respectfully represent to your
honorable bodies that the new code of laws adopted by

the Board of Health is of such a nature as to destroy, not only the privacy of the domestic household and the sacred relations existing between the physician and his patient, but is also a great act of injustice to the whole medical profession of the District.

"The law of Congress creating the Board of Health is as follows:

" 'SEC. 26. That there shall be appointed by the President of the United States, by and with the advice and consent of the Senate, a Board of Health for the said District, to consist of five persons, whose duty shall be to declare what shall be deemed nuisances injurious to the health, and to provide for the removal thereof; to make and enforce regulations to prevent domestic animals from running at large in the cities of Washington and Georgetown; to prevent the sale of unwholesome food in said cities, and to perform such other duties as shall be imposed upon said Board by the Legislative Assembly.'

" In reading this law it will be seen that the duties of this Board are: First, to declare what shall be deemed nuisances injurious to health, and to provide for their removal; Second, the prevention of domestic animals from running at large; and, Third, to prevent the sale of unwholesome food. These are all the duties assigned to said Board by Congress; no other powers can they assume, unless, as the law finally and emphatically states, ' To perform such other duties as shall be imposed upon said Board by the Legislative Assembly.'

"As no other duties have been imposed by the Legislative Assembly, your petitioners would most respectfully represent to your honorable bodies, that the powers as named by the Board, in the published code of laws, are not within their jurisdiction and militate most seriously against the interest and standing of the medical profession of this District, and are an infringement of the rights of every citizen. In regard to the final clause of the law of Congress, it is almost impossible for the Legislative Assembly to specify any other duties for the Board to perform, as already those assumed by it are so extensive and herculean in their character that it would take an army of assistants to execute them.

"The code of laws adopted by the Board of Health, of which Dr. C. C. Cox is chairman, declares that Tullio S. Verdi shall be the Health Officer and specifies certain duties that he had to perform, which none other than a medical man can discharge. Your petitioners respectfully represent that the said Verdi is not a regular practitioner of medicine, nor recognized as such by the American Medical Association, the representative body of the medical profession of the country; that no health officer of any city in the United States has ever yet been appointed who was not a regular practitioner of medicine, and therefore able to confer and advise with his medical brethren in regard to all hygienic rules that should be adopted for the safety and security of the public weal.

"The inspection of hospitals, all now under the control and management of regular practitioners, by the rules of this code is to be made by this Health Officer, and the existence of any infectious disease must be reported to him in twenty-four hours.

"The same section of the code, No. 46, also requires that every physician shall report to the sanitary superintendent or health officer every person having a contagious or infectious disease whom he has seen and prescribed for within forty-eight hours. It necessarily follows that the Board intends every case of measles, whooping-cough, mumps or scarlet fever occurring in the practice of a physician to be reported within forty-eight hours. It would be an onerous and almost impossible task, and the only result would be to keep the community in a constant state of alarm and anxiety, to frighten away all strangers from our midst, without any advantage to science or to the public.

"In the classification of diseases, scarlet fever, measles, yellow fever, typhoid and typhus fevers are considered infectious, actual contact being necessary for their propagation. Smallpox is considered by many both contagious and infectious, while venereal, itch and certain other skin diseases are purely contagious. According to the proposed law, the names and residences of all those suffering from

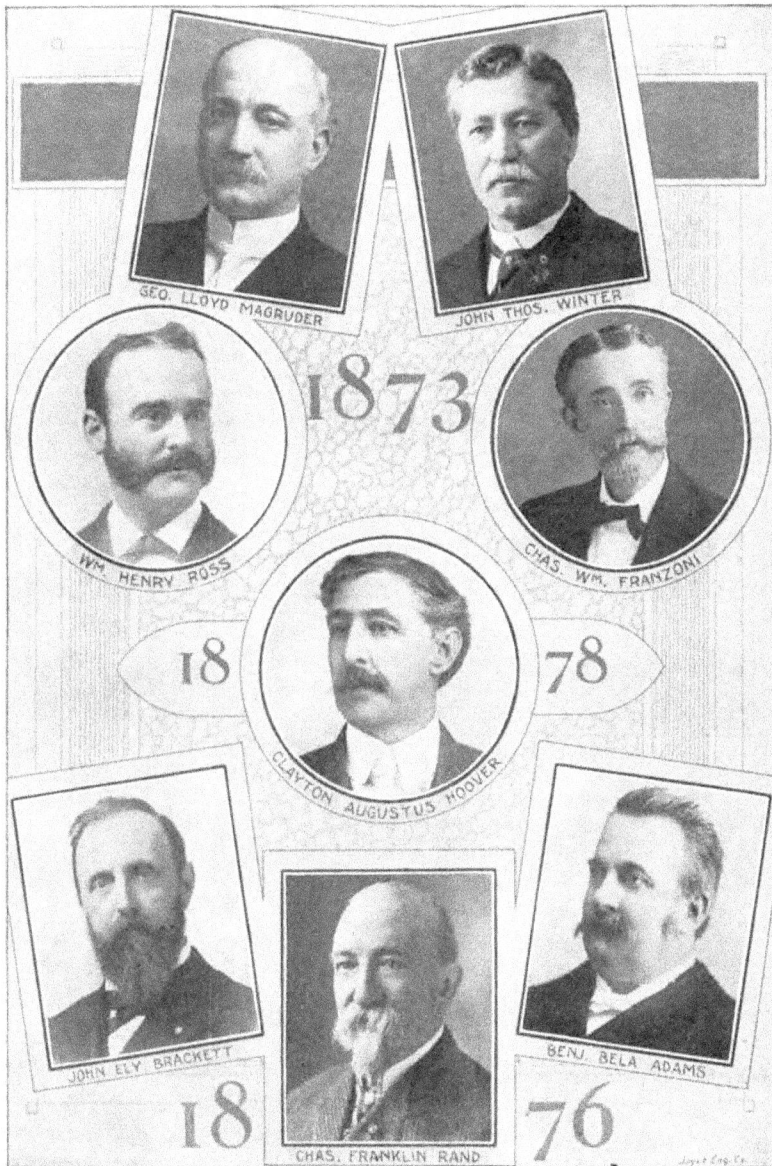

GEO. LLOYD MAGRUDER

JOHN THOS. WINTER

1873

WM. HENRY ROSS

CHAS. WM. FRANZONI

18

CLAYTON AUGUSTUS HOOVER

78

JOHN ELY BRACKETT

BENJ. BELA ADAMS

18

CHAS. FRANKLIN RAND

76

29

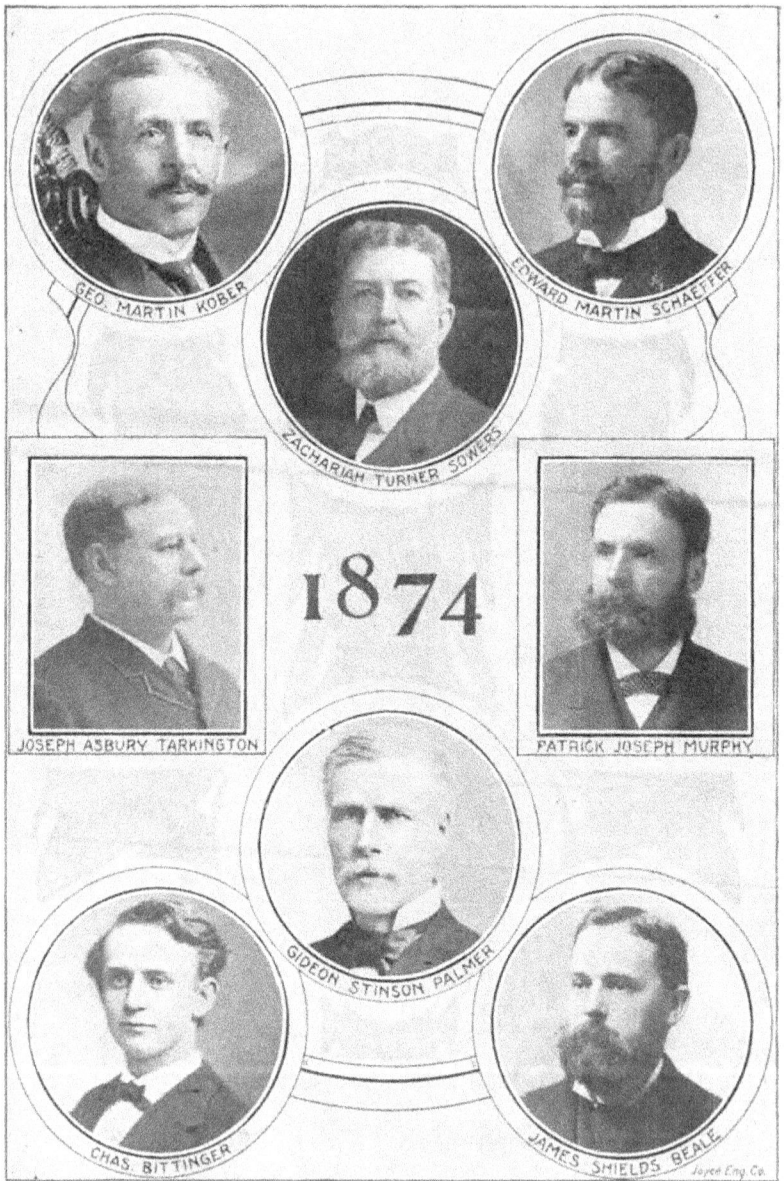

GEO. MARTIN KOBER

EDWARD MARTIN SCHAEFFER

ZACHARIAH TURNER SOWERS

1874

JOSEPH ASBURY TARKINGTON

PATRICK JOSEPH MURPHY

GIDEON STINSON PALMER

CHAS. BITTINGER

JAMES SHIELDS BEALE

Joyce Eng. Co.

these latter diseases are to be reported to the sanitary superintendent, or health officer, within forty-eight hours.

" In regard to hospitals, if this code is adopted the health officer will have the right to enter any hospital within the District, and require the physicians and surgeons in attendance to adopt his plans and ideas for ventilation and all other hygienic measures which in his judgment may seem best, however inconsistent they may be with the views of the medical men in charge.

" The regular medical profession of the District includes over 150 members; the homeopaths, hydropaths and herb doctors hardly a dozen in all. Of the class of men who compose the former we will leave your honorable bodies to judge, of the latter we will say nothing.

" It will also be seen that the Board of Health is to establish dispensaries, and appoint physicians to attend the poor, etc., all of whom are under the direction of the same health officer. If homeopaths are to hold all the offices they will doubtless discharge their duties to the entire satisfaction of the health officer, but how any regular practitioner of medicine can do so we are unable to understand. Such difficulties must arise in every instance where the regular physician and the homeopathic health officer come together, as their ideas of treatment of disease, of the remedies used, as well as the rules of hygiene, are as wide apart as the poles.

" In conclusion we respectfully request your honorable bodies not to subject the whole profession of the District, the representative of the regular medical practice of the country, to the control of one man who is irregular in practice and not recognized by the American Medical Association."

Signed by 78 members of the Society and Medical Association.

To this memorial the Board of Health made the following answer, July 1st.

"*Resolved*, That the memorialists and protestants misrepresent the Code of Health when they affirm that a provision exists therein requiring any physician to report

'all cases of contagious or infectious diseases' to the
Health Officer; that the Health Officer under said Code
has the right to enter any hospital and require the physicians in attendance to adopt his plans and ideas for 'ventilation or other hygienic measures;' or that any possible
conflict in regard to dispensaries and physicians to the
poor can possibly exist between 'the regular physician and
the homeopathic health officer,' no allusion being made
in the remotest degree, in any part of said Code, to such
'dispensaries' or 'physicians to the poor,' as every citizen
may know by reference to the printed message of the Governor, in which is enclosed the authorized draft of the
Code.

"*Resolved*, That the Board of Health has nothing whatever to do with the profession or occupation of any gentleman whom the Executive of the nation has thought
proper to designate as a member of the same; that it does
not concern them whether such member belongs to the
homeopathic or allopathic school of medicine; that no
principle of practice (which constitutes the difference between the two classes of practitioners) is involved in the
operations of the Board; and that, in their judgment, an
educated homeopathic physician is fully as competent to
judge of and direct the rules of hygiene as a graduate of
any other school of medicine.

"*Resolved*, That it is not true, as stated, that a homeopathic physician has never been recognized in the organization of any health department, as the sanitary history of
many cities of the country abundantly attests; that
the most prominent medical college in Europe, all of
whose professors are admitted by these very memorialists
and the profession at large, as 'regular' and 'in good
standing' includes, and has for years included in its faculty, a professor of homeopathy, thereby creating a direct
professional contact and intercourse between the two
branches of medical practice.

"*Resolved*, That Dr. Verdi, having received various
diplomas and certificates of merit, both from allopathic and
homeopathic institutions of credit, and holding, as he does,
a high position in this community for intelligence and

zeal in promoting the interests of the same, is entitled to our confidence, and is a suitable person, in our judgment, to hold a place in the Board of Health; that the Board regards the assault thus made upon Dr. Verdi as the offspring of personal malignity, of a reckless and disorganizing temper, and not as springing from any honest desire to conserve the public health or promote the welfare of the District.

"*Resolved*, That we call upon all citizens who have the good of the District at heart to frown down at once this attempt to subvert the purposes and aims of one of its most useful and self-sacrificing institutions; an attempt prompted only by prejudice and personal hostility."

The minutes of the Society do not record any further action in this matter. Apparently the Society and the Board were more or less in harmony thereafter, because no further reference to the Board appears on the minutes.

The Board of Health ceased to exist in 1878, when it was nominally replaced by a single-headed Department of Health. So far as the records of the Society show, the Society worked in harmony with the Health Officer, taking, however, but little active part in public affairs until February 7, 1894, when, on motion of Dr. G. Lloyd Magruder, the Society appointed a committee, consisting of Drs. Magruder, W. W. Johnston and C. M. Hammett, the last named being then Health Officer of the District, to investigate and report upon the prevalence and cause of typhoid fever in the District. The report of that Committee was submitted to the Society June 6th, and was subsequently printed as a public document, being probably the first report of the kind ever so printed. The action of the Society in the matter has exercised a marked influence on the entire subsequent work of the Health Department and on the relations between the Health Department and the Society. Nearly all the important legislation relating to public health in the District of Columbia has been approved by the Society, which has worked actively to promote its passage. The milk law of 1895 was in fact drafted by the Society. The influence of the Society was probably the moving cause leading to the establishment of the filtration plant, and determined the character of plant that should be constructed. Other matters, too, owe their present places on the statute books, to a large extent at least, to the stamp of approval that the Society placed upon them. Many of these are treated in other parts of this volume, to which reference should be made for further information concerning them.

It may be added that the change of Health Officer in 1894 was brought about through a request from one of the Commissioners of the District to members of the Society, though not the Society itself, to name some one for the office.

PRACTICAL ANATOMY.

February 3, 1869, a letter to the *Evening Star* from Dr. Adolph Patze, a member of the Society, was read. It related to a recent arrest for stealing a human body from a cemetery, and suggested the usual legal provisions for acquiring bodies for dissection purposes that avoid the necessity for such stealing.

In the discussion that followed Dr. Noble Young called attention to the difficulty of obtaining dissecting material, the opprobrium attached to the way in which it was usually obtained and the indisposition of members of Congress to legalize any method for procuring it. Dr. Liebermann also discussed the wrong and objectionable features of "resurrection," and referred to the laws in Europe governing such matters.

The letter was referred to a special committee, consisting of Drs. Young, Johnson Eliot, J. Ford Thompson, W. P.

Johnston and Wm. Marbury, these persons representing the two medical colleges, as well as the Society. May 19th, the committee, without making any report, was discharged.

May 10, 1876, the draft of a bill regulating dissecting material in this District, was presented to the Society; it originated with the Naval Medical Corps. The Society referred it to a committee—Drs. Busey, W. H. Triplett and J. F. Thompson. Nothing, apparently, was done by the committee, and it does not appear that the subject ever again came before the Society.

December 8th, the Society ordered that a petition should be presented to Congress in regard to the standing of medical officers of the Navy, to be signed by the President and Secretary of the Society, and have the seal of the Society attached.

In 1870 the Society placed itself on record in regard to the metric system, by instructing its delegates to the Pharmaceutical Convention—Drs. Antisell, Liebermann and B. F. Craig—to recommend the adoption of the metric system. May 12, 1880, however, when the question came up again, the Society decided against any such recommendation.

HOMEOPATHY.

When the bill creating the Washington Homeopathic Medical Society was introduced into Congress the matter was brought before the Medical Society of the District of Columbia. A committee was appointed to consider the bill, and was shortly afterward discharged, because, apparently, there was nothing for it to do. It seemed useless to oppose the bill, which passed and was approved April 22, 1870. Section 4 removed homeopathic practitioners from examination by the "Board of Examiners," as had been the law under the charter of the Medical Society, and gave the licensing power to the Washington Homeopathic Medical Society.

March 1, 1871, a committee of three was appointed by the Medical Society, to which the President of the Society was afterward added, to enquire into and report upon the exclusion of irregular practitioners from the position of examining surgeon in the U. S. Pension Bureau. It was stated that the homeopathic practitioners throughout the country were making an effort to secure such positions; that the Commissioner of Pensions, Dr. J. N. Van Aernam, who was a regular practitioner, had removed all irregulars from such positions; and that the homeopathic physicians had petitioned the President of the United States and the Secretary of the Interior, of which the Pension Bureau was a part, for the removal of the Commissioner of Pensions.

March 8th, the committee reported, and the report was adopted and ordered printed. The title was "Report of a Special Committee of the Medical Society of the District of Columbia upon the claims of homeopaths and other irregular practitioners for professional recognition in the medical service of the U. S. Government; and the charges brought against the U. S. Commissioner of Army and Navy Pensions, Washington, 1871."

It will suffice here to state the conclusions and recommendations of the committee:

"WHEREAS, The large majority of the present examining surgeons of the Pension Bureau have served in the medical corps of the volunteer forces during the late war; and whereas, none but regular physicians were admitted into that corps of the regular army and navy, and, therefore, none but regular physicians are provided with the medical experience requisite on examining boards; therefore

"*Resolved*, That this Society deems the action of the Hon. Commissioner of Pensions, in excluding irregular practitioners from the medical examining boards under that Bureau as made in the best interests of the public service, thereby leading to uniformity of action, increasing the efficiency of the Bureau and affording to the pensioners the benefit of the most skilled advice ; and it is earnestly hoped that the Government will not in this instance disregard the deliberate and expressed conviction of the whole legitimate medical profession of this country by appointing to medical position or office a class of men whose practice is not based on experience and observation, the only true groundwork of medical progress, but upon arbitrary dicta, not verified after nearly a century of trial, and which are wholly opposed to the ordinary exposition of the natural laws of physical science.

"*Resolved*, That a copy of the foregoing resolution be respectfully forwarded to the President of the United States and the Hon. Secretary of the Interior."

Within the past fifteen years, and especially concerning the District Medical Practice Act, the Society has worked satisfactorily with the Washington Homeopathic Medical Society of the District to secure legislation that would benefit the medical profession and advance the sanitary interests of the District.

WOMEN PHYSICIANS.

The first difficulty met with by women who desired to practice in this District was in obtaining a license to practice. Dr. Mary D. Spackman was the first to apply. Her application was addressed to the President of the Medical Society, March 14, 1872. The Society, April 10th, ordered that a copy of the charter be sent to her and that she be informed that under the charter she could not be granted a license. The letter was written by the Corresponding Secretary, William Lee, April 16th. June 17,

1874, it was reported to the Society that the Board of Examiners had likewise refused to grant a license to Dr. Mary A. Parsons.

This condition of things was, of course, too serious to go on indefinitely, and an effort was therefore made to have the charter of the Society amended in this particular. Congress was appealed to and amended the charter March 3d, 1875, changing the word "gentlemen" to "persons." March 17th following, Drs. Spackman and Parsons renewed their applications for license, and of course received them.

When women physicians first applied for membership in the Society there was opposition, and it was a long time before the first woman member, Dr. Parsons, was elected. December 29, 1876, Dr. Parsons applied, but April 4, 1877, the date of election, she received but 5 affirmative with 18 negative votes. She applied again January 7, 1878; at the election, April 3d, the report of the Censors was favorable, except that Dr. Busey dissented. She failed of election; the record does not show the number of ballots. January 6, 1879, she again applied, and April 2d, again failed of election; no details are given. In July, 1888, she again applied, and was elected October 3d; the vote was 17 affirmative, 2 negative.

July 6, 1891, Drs. Mary D. Spackman and Amelia Erbach applied. At the date of election, October 7th, Dr. Spackman was rejected, the vote being 15 to 14. Dr. Erbach was elected, the vote being 23 to 6.

After this date the only opposition to the admission of women as members was confined to a few votes, which did not prevent election. April 6, 1892, Drs. Ida J. Heiberger and Jeannette J. Sumner were elected; April 5, 1893, Dr. Mayne M. Pile; October 3, 1894, Drs. Anne A. Wilson, Anita N. McGee and Nancy D. Richards. In 1896, Drs. Sophie A. Nordhoff, Ada R. Thomas, Abbie C. Tyler,

DAVID HENRY HAZEN

PARKE GEORGE YOUNG

JAS. THOS. SOTHORON

HENRY A. DUNCANSON

1875

JOHN WALTER

SMITH TOWNSHEND

EDMUND A. ZEVELY

ARTHUR G. ADAMS

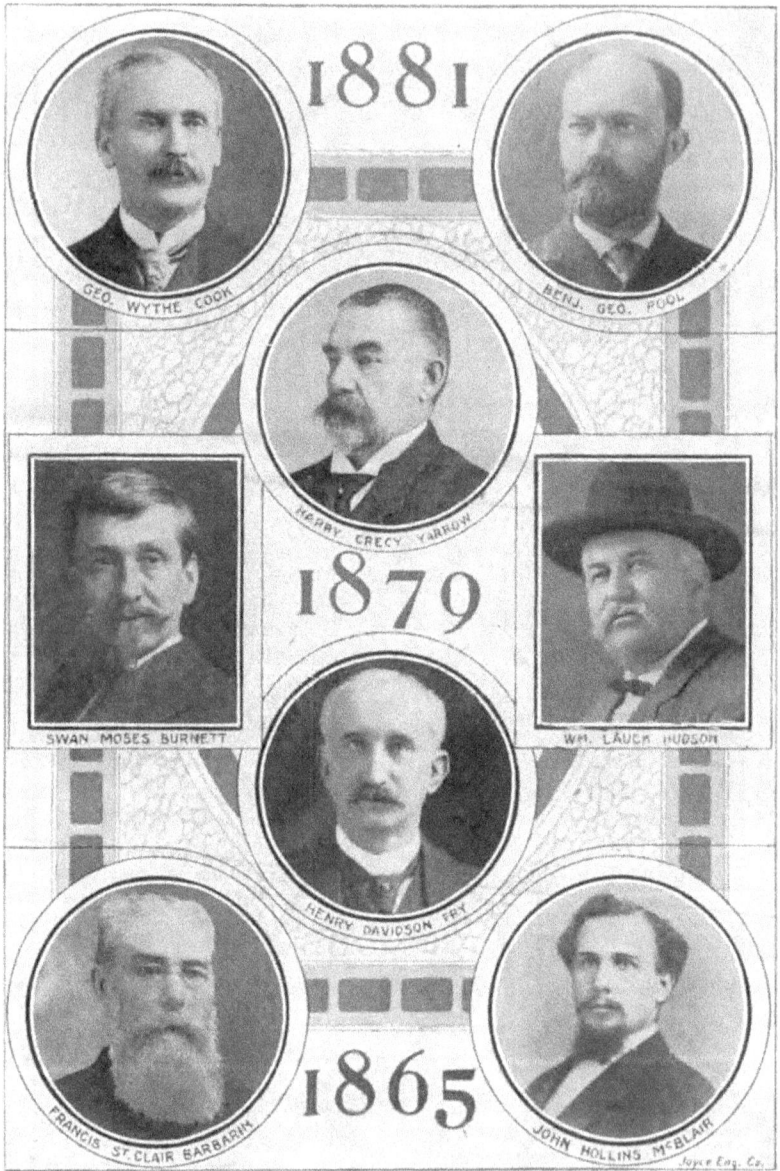

1881

GEO. WYTHE COOK

BENJ. GEO. POOL

HENRY CRECY YARROW

1879

SWAN MOSES BURNETT

WM. LAUCK HUDSON

HENRY DAVIDSON FRY

1865

FRANCIS ST. CLAIR BARBARIN

JOHN HOLLINS McBLAIR

Joyce Eng. Co.

Phoebe R. Norris, Susan J. Squire and Adeline E. Portman. In 1898, Dr. Isabel Haslup. In 1900, Drs. A. Frances Foye and Kathryn Lorigan. In 1901, Dr. E. B. Muncey. In 1902, Drs. M. Louise Strobel and Edith L. Maddren. In 1903, Dr. Laura M. Reville. In 1904, Drs. B. Rosalie Slaughter, B. A. Crush, L. Tayler-Jones, Mary Holmes and Anna Bartsch. In 1906, Dr. Emma L. Erving. In 1907, Dr. E. Corey Starr. In 1908, Dr. Mary O'Malley.

January 7, 1901, Dr. Mary Parsons was elected a Vice President of the Society. December 18, 1901, in expressing her thanks for the election, she stated that she had failed to do so at the time of election because she was so taken by surprise that she did not fully realize what it meant to her. But she had found this out week by week ever afterwards. It meant more to her than it could possibly mean to any man, and perhaps more than to any other woman. The year had been the happiest of her professional life.

CERTIFICATES OF ILLNESS.

December 4, 1872, Dr. Lovejoy called attention to the fact that he had been required in the case of an employee of a Government Department in Washington to state in the certificate of illness the name of the disease from which the patient suffered, otherwise the clerk would lose his pay for the period of absence. The subject was discussed, and finally the President and the two Vice Presidents were appointed a committee to lay the matter before the Attorney General of the United States for his opinion and decision. January 29, 1873, the committee, having no report to make, was discharged, and the matter was dropped.

November 10, 1886, Dr. T. C. Smith moved that the President appoint a committee of three to interview the Secretary of the Interior in regard to the order of General J. C. Black, the Commissioner of Pensions, that physicians should specify on sick certificates of clerks in the Pension Office the disease for which they were being treated. Dr. Smith had given a certificate to his patient and it was returned with the request that he specify the disease for which it was given. This he refused to do and it was again returned, with the information that unless the disease was specified the man would lose about $40 pay. Dr. Smith had again refused to accede to the request. Dr. T. E. McArdle seconded the motion, and stated that he had attended a clerk in a like position who was liable to lose $150 pay. Dr. Busey hoped that the question would not be pressed, as he thought that it was for the Medical Association of the District to consider all such questions, and moved as a substitute, that the President of the Society request the Medical Association to take up the matter.

January 31, 1894, the attention of the Society was called to the fact that a recent order of the Secretary of the Treasury appointed a member of the Marine Hospital Service to investigate all cases of illness reported to that office, even when they presented the certificate of a physician. This appeared like an insult to the profession of the District. A committee—Drs. T. E. McArdle, G. N. Acker and G. Wythe Cook—was appointed to inquire into the matter. The committee reported, February 7th, that after consulting the Supervising Surgeon General of the Marine Hospital Service it believed that there was no intention of infringing on the rights of the members of the Society. The report was adopted.

COMPENSATION TO THE OFFICERS OF THE SOCIETY.

The question of compensation to officers of the Society does not appear to have been raised for very many years; in fact, until 1865, when Dr. A. F. A. King began to keep a record of the proceedings, the work of the officers apparently was not onerous.   But Drs. King and Wm. Lee and afterwards Dr. Kleinschmidt gave much time and labor to the office of Recording Secretary, and while Dr. Kleinschmidt was serving, a resolution was offered, May 13, 1874, to pay him $200 a year; after discussion the resolution was withdrawn.   It was, however, the entering wedge, and January 4, 1875, the Society appropriated $50 to make him a "present."   January 27th, the committee charged with procuring the present reported that it had given the "check" to the Secretary.   Again, December 22d of the same year, the Society appropriated $75 to be given to that officer. January 6, 1879, it was ordered that $25 be paid quarterly, and the same amount was again ordered February 4, 1880.

In October, 1881, Dr. Kleinschmidt resigned as Recording Secretary, and October 19th Dr. J. Ford Thompson moved to cease paying any salary to the member holding that office.   The motion was adopted.   Dr. T. E. McArdle was elected to the office, and January 2, 1882, Dr. Thompson moved that the salary be restored, and it was done. From this time a salary was regularly paid each year. January 2, 1882, Dr. Patze was also given an honorarium of $100 in recognition of his long service as Librarian.

September 28, 1887, the Society ordered that the compensation of the Recording Secretary should be $200 a year.

January 7, 1889, it was ordered that the compensation of the Treasurer should be $50 a year.   January 4, 1897, the compensation was increased to $100, and to $200 January 6, 1908.

January 14, 1891, it was ordered that an appropriation of $25 should be given to the Corresponding Secretary for addressing postal cards.   The same was done again January 4, 1892.   In subsequent years this sum was included and paid as part of the bill annually rendered by the Corresponding Secretary.

February 6, 1895, the Society created the office of Assistant Recording Secretary, and ordered that the compensation should be $3 per meeting for active service.

In 1875, Dr. Busey was elected delegate to the International Medical Congress held in Philadelphia in September, 1876.

THE NATIONAL SURGICAL INSTITUTE OF THE DISTRICT OF COLUMBIA.

A bill was introduced in Congress in 1876, to charter a " National Surgical Institute of the District of Columbia." March 15th, the matter was brought to the attention of the Medical Society and a committee was appointed, consisting of Drs. W. H. Triplett, J. Ford Thompson, A. Y. P. Garnett, R. Reyburn and S. C. Busey, to oppose the bill. [The same committee was also instructed to oppose another bill which provided for an annual tax of $25 on physicians.] April 29th, Dr. Garnett stated that some members of Congress were disposed to report favorably on the bill, and the Society therefore ordered copies of the bill to be printed, to which a protest should be added, and the matter brought to the attention of the medical societies throughout the country, with a request for them to use their influence immediately to prevent the passage of the bill. The presidents of scientific and educational institutions in the District of Columbia were also asked to assist.

This Institute was to be a corporation, with a capital of $500,000—divided into shares of $100 each. Its objects were the treatment of surgical cases, the manufacture and sale of surgical instruments and appliances, the establishment of a college of surgery, the teaching of surgery in all its branches and the establishment of a surgical hospital.

The protest was as follows :

"*To the Honorable the Senate and House of Representatives of the United States in Congress assembled :* The undersigned, the officers and a committee of the Medical Society of the District of Columbia, in pursuance of instructions of said Society, respectfully protest against the passage of the bill entitled 'A Bill to incorporate the National Surgical Institute of the District of Columbia,' for the following reasons, to wit :

" 1. There are hospitals providing ample accommodations for the treatment of surgical diseases in successful operation in this District, in which all such diseases as are described in said bill are treated according to the most approved methods ; and if the persons named in said bill are possessed of any special skill, unusual dexterity, or extraordinary proficiency in the art and science of surgery, no protection is needed from the National Government to insure their success when brought in open competition with others pursuing the same profession.

" 2. If these gentlemen desire to practice their profession there is nothing to prevent their doing so in this, or any other locality ; but to establish a gigantic corporation of this description is simply using the Congress of the United States for an advertisement, and it would be a wrong upon the profession of medicine to confer special privileges upon any organization of men, or even by implication to acknowledge by an act of incorporation that any man or set of men can, or should claim as a vested right, any method of treatment or surgical appliance as his or their exclusive property, with the sole right of use and application.

" 3. Such an act of incorporation would be simply an instrumentality whereby certain men would become enriched at the expense of the health and lives of their unfortunate victims, and would be derogatory to the dignity of the medical profession, detrimental to the interests of the community at large and afford opportunity to charlatans and unprincipled persons to covertly conceal their blunders under the protecting aegis of an act of incorporation.

"4. Another provision of said bill authorizes the establishment of a 'school of surgery for teaching the science and practice of surgery in all its branches.' This, in other words, establishes a medical college for the instruction, alone, in one branch of medicine, with the full power to send forth its alumni as competent to practice that one branch, without a full, complete and necessary medical education, thus omitting entirely the usual safeguards and restrictions which have been found necessary to prevent unprincipled men from establishing 'bogus colleges' and selling diplomas to unqualified persons.

"5. In conclusion, may we not respectfully inquire if this may not be an effort to commit the Congress of the United States to the exercise of a doubtful power, in establishing an institution which purports to be local in its character, but which may eventually endeavor to extend the operation of its special privileges over the entire country, by virtue of the authority received from the General Government."

Signed by Drs. N. S. Lincoln, President; C. H. A. Kleinschmidt, Secretary; A. Y. P. Garnett, J. F. Thompson, R. Reyburn, W. H. Triplett and S. C. Busey, Committee.

The bill failed to pass.

October 11, 1876, a committee—Drs. A. Y. P. Garnett, S. C. Busey, J. W. H. Lovejoy, R. Reyburn and J. E. Morgan—was appointed, to confer with the Congressional Committee having in charge the framing of a new form of government for the District. January 7, 1878, Drs. J. Ford Thompson, Busey, Lovejoy, N. S. Lincoln, J. M. Toner, T. Antisell and Garnett were appointed a committee to watch over the interests of the profession in the District in the proposed bill.

February 7, 1877, the President of the Society called attention to the rule requiring officers to occupy seats on the platform; thereupon the Society rescinded the rule.

July 2d, Dr. Antisell favored uniting the Medical Society and Medical Association and asking Congress for a new charter, and moved the appointment of a committee to consider the matter. Dr. J. E. Morgan thought that such a movement would get the Society into difficulty with Congress and force persons on the Society whom it did not want. Dr. C. Boyle moved to lay the motion on the table, but as there was no quorum no action was taken.

July 10th, a special meeting was held to contradict in some authoritative way reports throughout the country that there was a severe epidemic in Washington—reports calculated to do harm to the business interests of the city. Drs. Garnett, Lovejoy, D. W. Prentiss, E. M. Schaeffer and Geo. McCoy were appointed a committee to prepare suitable resolutions. The committee reported resolutions, which were adopted, stating that the above-mentioned reports were false in every particular and that the health conditions of the city were even better than usual, and requesting the local press, as well as newspapers elsewhere, to contradict the reports.

COMPLIMENTARY ACTION OF THE SOCIETY TO CERTAIN MEMBERS.

March 13, 1878, Dr. Lovejoy called attention to the fact that some members of the Society had been practitioners for fifty years or more, and thought that the Society should take some appropriate action in regard thereto. A committee was appointed to take proper steps in that direction, and by vote of the Society the name of Dr. J. B. Blake was included, although he was not then a practitioner of medicine. Drs. Lovejoy, Toner and Mackall were the committee, which reported March 20th, as follows:

" WHEREAS, Harvey Lindsly, M. D. ; Jas. C. Hall, M. D. ; Joseph Borrows, M. D., and Noble Young, M. D., members of the Society, whose names appear in the act of incorporation reviving the charter of the Society, have now passed through fifty years of continuous practice of medicine in this District; and whereas, these gentlemen have during the whole of this long period retained the respect and esteem of their brethren in the profession and of the community at large, inspiring with each revolving year increasing confidence;

"Therefore *Resolved*, That this Society takes pleasure in calling the attention of its members to such notable examples of a career passed in the honorable and conscientious performance of the duties of life.

"*Resolved*, That the Society congratulate the above mentioned gentlemen upon the completion of half a century of usefulness in the profession and upon the honors and prosperity to which they have so deservedly attained.

"*Resolved*, That the Society trusts that there may be in reserve for them many more years of happiness and usefulness, and that when in the fulness of time the last claim of nature shall be made, they may each approach the inevitable hour ' like one who wraps the drapery of his couch about him and lies down to pleasant dreams.'

"WHEREAS, John B. Blake, M. D., a member of this Society, whose name appears in the act of incorporation reviving the charter of the Society, has now passed through more than fifty years from the date of his graduation in medicine; and whereas, Dr. Blake has throughout that long period continued his affiliation with the Society, though many years since it was his choice to retire from the active practice of medicine and engage in other pursuits in which he has obtained distinction and emolument;

"Therefore *Resolved*, That this Society congratulates him upon the completion of more than half a century of connection with the medical profession, and hopes that he may enjoy yet many years as happy and peaceful as his life heretofore has been prosperous and honorable.

"*Resolved*, That the eminent gentlemen named in the resolutions be requested at their earliest convenience to reduce to form and convey by letter their reminiscences and observations on interesting facts in medicine and of

SAMUEL SHUGERT ADAMS

STEPHEN OLIN RICHEY

THOS. EUGENE McARDLE

ETHELBERT CARROLL MORGAN

1880

HARRISON CROOK

FREDERICK C. VAN VLIET

THOS. HENRY TROTT

HENRY MARTEL NEWMAN

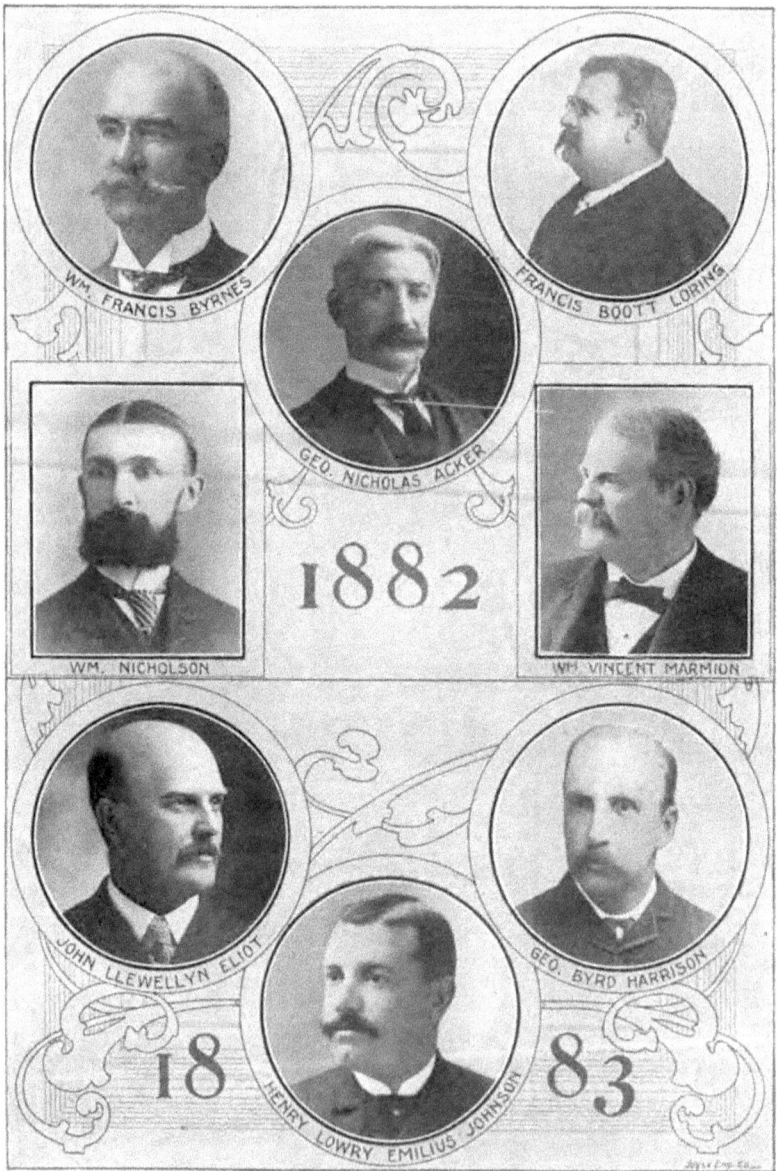

WM. FRANCIS BYRNES

FRANCIS BOOTT LORING

GEO. NICHOLAS ACKER

WM. NICHOLSON

1882

WM. VINCENT MARMION

JOHN LLEWELLYN ELIOT

GEO. BYRD HARRISON

18

HENRY LOWRY EMILIUS JOHNSON

83

34

noted persons and occurrences that may have interested them as practicing physicians at the Capital of our country, to be preserved as a legacy of the Society."

In reply, the following letters were received : Dr. Blake, March 23d, said that the resolutions were to him a mark of respect to which he had no claim, and were, therefore, the more highly prized. Dr. Hall said, March 22d, that the resolutions were an honor greater than any popular applause and purer than any material success. He stated that he had ever had the most friendly and pleasant relations with his fellow practitioners, and that no personal differences ever interrupted their professional intercourse. Dr. Lindsly, March 25th, said that the approbation and esteem of his professional brethren he considered the highest compliment to his character and conduct ; physicians were the best judges of other physicians' merits and deficiencies. He had never knowingly violated any rule of medical etiquette or done or said anything to injure a brother. He had the kindest feelings of friendship and respect for every member of the Society. He hoped for harmony among the medical brethren of the District.

September 18th, Dr. Toner offered a resolution in regard to Dr. Johnson Eliot, who was and had been ill for a long time. The illness was contracted in the discharge of his professional duties. The Society conveyed to him its sympathy and its gratification at the news that he was rapidly convalescing. To this Dr. Eliot replied, September 25th, that the action of the Society was quite unexpected but gratifying, and afforded him great consolation in his illness. His ambition had always been to merit the good wishes and esteem of his professional brethren.

December 13, 1896, the Society adopted the following resolution in regard to Dr. J. H. Mundell :

9

"WHEREAS, Dr. John Hodges Mundell, for many years a member in good standing in this Society, having attained the fiftieth year of his connection with the medical profession, during which period his upright, honorable conduct has won for him the esteem, respect and confidence of his associates; and the Medical Society desiring to manifest its appreciation of his many eminent qualifications, adopts the following resolution:

"*Resolved*, That the Medical Society extends to Dr. Mundell its warmest congratulations on the occasion of his half-century identification with the medical profession, during which time he has been deservedly honored by his professional brethren because of his high character as a gentleman and physician. He has been faithful to his obligations, has satisfactorily performed the duties imposed upon him by the Society, has earned and retained the good will and confidence of his associates and has lived a life worthy of emulation and commendation. The Society takes pleasure in calling the attention of the profession to the blameless life of our honored and honorable associate, and proffers him the kindest and heartiest wishes for a continuance for many years of his long and useful life and the hope that health and happiness may be his to the end."

April 6, 1898, the Society adopted the following resolution in regard to the fiftieth anniversary of the graduation of Dr. Busey in medicine :*

"WHEREAS, Samuel C. Busey, M. D., LL. D., President of this Society, will in a few days have passed through fifty years in the practice of medicine in this community, during which time he has faithfully served the Society as President, Censor, member of important committees and in many other ways, and is now the only practitioner among us who has been in practice so long a period; that he has always been prompt in maintaining the honor, dignity, rights and interests of the medical profession before Congress and the community; that his services in securing

---

* See *Trans.*, 1898, III, p. 79.

needed legislation for the protection of the public from ignorant and unlicensed practitioners, for the protection of
physicians before the courts of law, for the prevention of
contagious diseases, and in advocating other measures
which he has furthered by his industry and influence, will
ever be remembered. *Resolved*, That this Society takes
pleasure in calling the attention of its members to such a
notable example of a career passed in the honorable and
conscientious performance of the duties of life."

January 14, 1903, the Society formally endorsed a proposed memorial to Dr. Walter Reed, Surgeon, U. S. Army,
Chairman of the U. S. A. Yellow Fever Commission.
January 27, 1904, a committee, consisting of Drs. F. S.
Nash, G. Wythe Cook and A. F. A. King, was appointed
to confer with other similar committees upon the subject
of the memorial. May 11th, Drs. Cook, D. P. Hickling
and E. W. Reisinger were appointed a committee to collect
subscriptions. May 25th, the committee reported that it
had with other gentlemen incorporated, and had elected a
board of managers to collect funds; of this Board, Pres.
Gilman, of Johns Hopkins University, was President, and
Dr. Calvin DeWitt, U. S. Army, Secretary. January 16,
1907, Dr. Cook made a final report of the moneys collected,
and the Society appropriated $500 to the fund, to be added
to the collections made by the committee.* It may be
mentioned here that an address by Dr. W. C. Borden,
U. S. A., before the Society, October 3, 1906, was on the
subject "The Walter Reed U. S. Army General Hospital,
District of Columbia."

March 28, 1906, the Society adopted a complimentary
resolution to Dr. Louis Mackall, in view of the fact that he
had been a member of the Society over fifty years, had
been a graduate in medicine fifty-five years and was nearly

* See WASH. MED. ANNALS, 1907-8, VI, p. 52.

seventy-five years old. A committee—Drs. S. S. Adams,
D. S. Lamb and G. Wythe Cook—was appointed to arrange
for some further action by the Society. Pending the action
of the committee Dr. Mackall died and a memorial meeting was held.

January 16, 1907, the Society adopted a resolution con-
gratulating Dr. Wm. A. White, Superintendent of the
Government Hospital for the Insane, Washington, on the
vindication he had received from Congress in regard to his
administration of his office.

February 6th, the Society adopted a resolution congrat-
ulating Dr. Robert Reyburn on his attainment of a half
century in the practice of medicine. "Deserving and pos-
sessing, as he does, the respect, esteem and confidence of
the medical profession and the community, the Society
expresses its hearty good wishes, with the hope that Dr.
Reyburn's life of usefulness may be greatly prolonged."

February 20th, the Society decided to give an entertainment in honor of Dr. J. Ford Thompson, on the attainment
of his seventieth birthday and the fiftieth year of his professional life; and a committee, to consist of representatives
from the institutions with which Dr. Thompson was connected, was appointed to arrange the details of the entertainment, which was given March 2d, at "Rauscher's."*

March 20th, on recommendation of the Executive Committee, the Society passed a vote of thanks to Dr. G.
Lloyd Magruder "for his excellent work in seeking the
source of contamination of the milk supply in the District
of Columbia."

May 13, 1908, the Society congratulated Dr. G. M.
Kober on the distinction of having been invited by the
President of the United States to address the Conference of
Governors on "Public Sanitation."

---

* See ANNALS, VI, 1907, pp. 93 *et seq.*, and 167.

March 10, 1909, the Society congratulated Dr. J. T. Howard on his having practiced medicine fifty years and been a member of the Society forty-five years, and on his exemplary character as a practitioner; and expressed the hope that his useful and honorable life might be prolonged many years.

March 24th, resolutions were adopted in regard to Dr. Harvey W. Wiley, of the Department of Agriculture, and a member of the Society by invitation, setting forth that he was a man of sterling integrity, courage and persistent justice, an accomplished and skillful chemist; commending and endorsing his arduous and difficult work in protecting the American people from poisons, impurities and adulterations in their foods, drinks and medicinal remedies; and trusting that his humane efforts would be generously sustained by the Government, supported by the cordial sympathy of the profession and encouraged by the sincere appreciation of a grateful people.

February 5, 1879, a committee was appointed—Drs. A. Y. P. Garnett, S. C. Busey, J. M. Toner, J. Eliot, J. Ford Thompson and D. R. Hagner—to represent to Congress the injustice of imposing a license fee on physicians, and to do all in their power to prevent the enactment of the bill. December 17th, the committee was reappointed, and January 28, 1880, it reported that the matter had been dropped.

THE REGULATION OF THE PRACTICE OF MEDICINE IN THE DISTRICT OF COLUMBIA.

October 27, 1880, Dr. Ralph Walsh moved that a committee be appointed to frame a bill to regulate the practice of medicine in the District of Columbia and report to the Society. The discussion on the motion showed that the Society preferred to leave the matter to a general convention of the profession.

March 12, 1886, a petition was presented to the Society urging the passage of a bill by Congress to regulate the practice of medicine in the District. It was laid on the table. [No details are given.]

January 29, 1890, the attention of the Society was called to the fact that a bill had been introduced in the Senate by Senator Ingalls to regulate the practice of medicine in the District. The Society instructed the Board of Examiners to procure a copy of the bill, ascertain its author, examine into its merits, and report. February 5th, the Board reported that the bill had been introduced in the Senate January 30th, and the author of the bill was Dr. J. M. Carroll. The Board also stated its objections to the bill. The subject was discussed and decision postponed. February 19th, the report of the Board was adopted and a committee appointed, consisting of Drs. R. T. Edes, J. M. Toner, G. N. Acker, G. Wythe Cook and J. B. Hamilton, to secure the passage of a law to regulate the practice of medicine in the District; that, if practicable, such a law should be an amendment to the charter of the Society, granting it the power to regulate the practice. The committee reported March 5th, a majority and minority report; two distinct bills. The question was whether to have a new bill or one that simply amended the charter; the Society voted for a new bill, which also would amend the charter. Amendments were made and the bill as amended adopted by the Society, March 19th. [The details of the bill are not given.]

May 28th, the Secretary stated that the subcommittee of the Senate had reported to the Senate the bill originally prepared by Dr. Carroll, with a few alterations. The matter was referred by the Society to the Special Committee on Legislation. June 4th, the Society instructed this committee to ask that the bill be recommitted so that the representatives of the Society might be heard. July 7th, Dr. Edes reported that the committee had failed to have the Senate bill recommitted, but had presented the bill adopted by the Society to the House Committee on the District.

December 3d, Dr. Edes reported that he had addressed a letter to the House Committee on the District, pointing out the differences between the Senate and Society bills. December 10th, a letter was received from Dr. Carroll in regard to his bill and referred to the Committee on Legislation.

January 4, 1892, the Society directed the Board of Examiners to prepare a bill to regulate the practice of medicine in the District, to confer with the Homeopathic Medical Society in regard to it, and, after ratification by this Society, present the bill to Congress and urge its passage. January 20th, the Board reported, and after some discussion the report was adopted by the Society and the Board instructed anew to present it to Congress and urge its passage. [See page 19 *et seq.* of the minutes for text of bill.] February 3d, the Society reconsidered the bill and amended it.

December 14th, the Board reported that a Senate bill to regulate the practice of medicine had passed two readings, and December 21st, that the bill had passed the Senate. (What the text of this bill was does not appear.) January 25, 1893, the Committee on Legislation reported that the " Society's" bill had been introduced into the House of Representatives.

April 25, 1894, a letter was received from the Chairman of the Committee on Legislation of the Washington Homeopathic Medical Society, desiring to meet a like committee of this Society to consider the necessity for legislation to regulate the practice of medicine in the District ; the letter was referred to the special Committee on Legislation. Dr.

Busey says, "Annual Addresses," page 46, "that the joint committee failed to agree, and the *Society* committee on the bill to regulate the practice of medicine in the District reported a bill to the Society, May 23d." The Society ordered the bill printed [see the minutes for the bill]. June 20th, the bill was debated and amended, and as amended, adopted.* A committee was appointed to present the bill to Congress—Drs. Busey, W. W. Johnston, G. Wythe Cook, R. Reyburn, Z. T. Sowers, W. C. Woodward and J. S. McLain. [House Bill 7661, introduced by Mr. McMillin, July 7, 1894.]

October 31st, the Committee on Legislation recommended some changes in the proposed Medical Practice Act; the changes were adopted by the Society and were embodied in a new bill [House Bill No. 8133, introduced in the House, December 10th, by Mr. Heard].

December 17th, a bill [House Bill 8229] was introduced by Mr. Blair, giving to the Physio-Medical School of Medicine the same rights, etc., in the District as other schools of medicine. It failed to pass.

January 23, 1895, Senate Bill 2645 was introduced by Senator Teller, and January 31st, Senate Bill 2685 by Senator Harris, to regulate the practice of medicine in the District. February 13th, letters written by President Busey, one to the Chairman of the Senate Committee on the District, one to the Commissioners of the District and a third to the Committee of the Washington Homeopathic Medical Society, all three letters objecting to the bills then before the Senate, were read, and approved by this Society.

December 4th, another bill, Senate Bill 325, was introduced by Senator Harris. This was a new Congress and,

---

* See the Minutes, p. 225, for bill as amended; also Busey's Annual Address of December 18, 1895, p. 33.

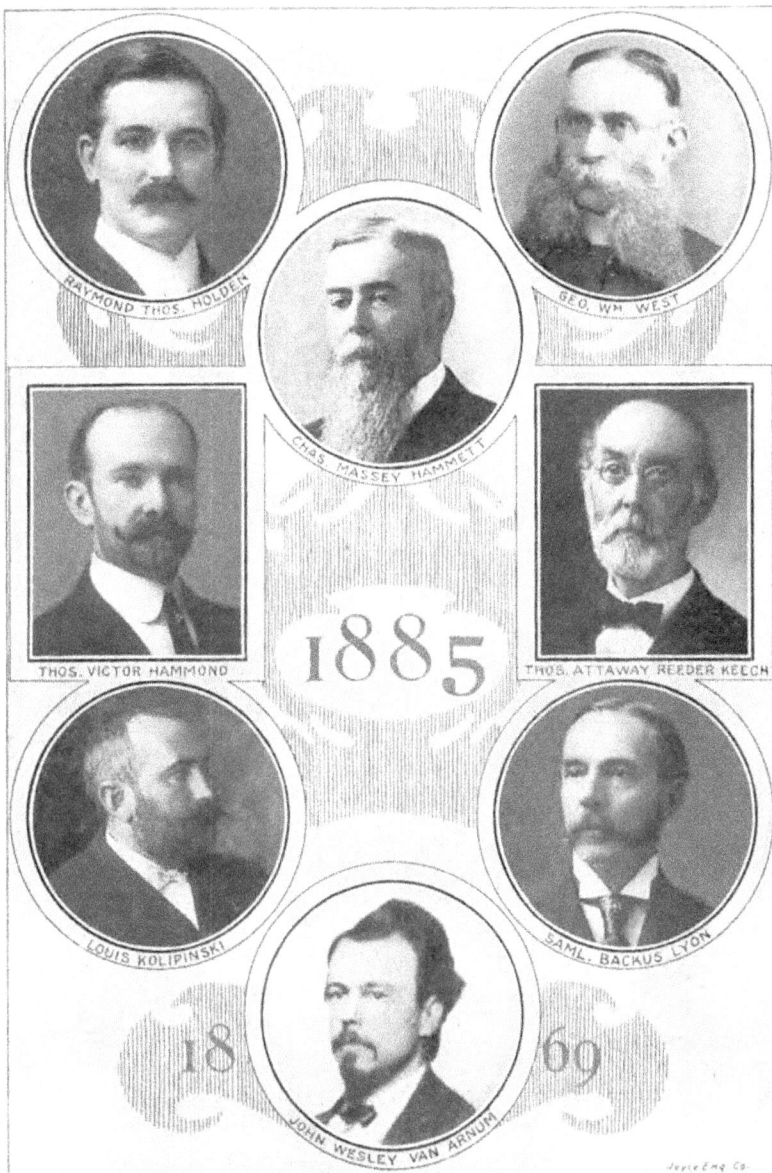

RAYMOND THOS. HOLDEN

GEO. WM. WEST

CHAS. MASSEY HAMMETT

THOS. VICTOR HAMMOND

1885

THOS. ATTAWAY REEDER KEECH

LOUIS KOLIPINSKI

SAML. BACKUS LYON

18 69

JOHN WESLEY VAN ARNUM

Joyce Eng. Co.

35

JOHN HODGES MUNDELL

18

JOHN BROWN HAMILTON

THOS. TAYLOR

84

1886

MILLARD FILLMORE THOMPSON

DANL. PERCY HICKLING

THOS. MORRIS MURRAY
1888

ISADORE S. L. BERMANN

ROBT. THAXTER EDES
1888

18   87

Jones Eng. Co.

188

therefore, a new bill. April 22, 1896, the Society adopted a
" memorial" recommending House Bill 5731, and the memorial was sent to Congress and printed as Document 228,
Fifty-fourth Congress, First Session. It was signed by
representatives from both the Medical Society and the
Homeopathic Medical Society.

May 13th, the Committee on Legislation reported that
an amendment had been introduced in the Senate exempt-
ing from the action of the proposed bill matriculates who
had matriculated prior to January 1, 1896. The Society
considered that the amendment was detrimental to the best
interests of the community, and a blemish to an otherwise
good measure that had been already endorsed by the Society.
The Corresponding Secretary was instructed to notify the
Senate committee of the Society's action. The amendment failed to pass.

The bill passed, approved June 3, 1896, and was published as Public Document No. 174.*

February 24, 1904, the Society was informed that a bill
had been introduced in the Senate [No. 4346] permitting
physicians who had practiced ten years or more in any
State of the United States to practice in this District without examination, provided they furnished certificates of
good moral character from the State Board of Health of
the State in which they had been practicing.† The Executive Committee was instructed to oppose the bill. It
failed to pass.

May 9, 1906, the Society adopted a resolution to accompany a memorial to Congress protesting against the passage
of a bill to regulate the practice of osteopathy and to license

---

* For interesting reading in connection with this bill, see Busey's address, December
18, 1895, published both separately and as a part of his "Annual Addresses;" also his
" Souvenir," p. 342 *et seq.*, and p. 372 ; also *National Medical Review*, 1896-7, VI, p. 4 ; also
Trans. of the Medical Society, 1896, I, p. 4.

† See ANNALS, 1904-5, III, p. 133.

osteopathic physicians in this District.   February 20, 1907, the Society was informed that the bill had been defeated in the House of Representatives.

Section 8, of the Act of June 3, 1896, was amended January 19, 1905, by Congress, authorizing the Medical Supervisors of the District to license without examination physicians from outside the District who should fulfill certain conditions.*

MALARIA IN THE DISTRICT OF COLUMBIA.

November 2, 1881, Dr. Harvey Lindsly stated that there was much talk about the prevalence of malaria in Washington.   While traveling during the summer through the North and East he met gentlemen from all parts of the country, who took it for granted that malaria prevailed at the Capital to an alarming extent.   Every newspaper that he read was full of the subject, and much blame, he thought, must rest on our own newspapers, and more especially on the correspondents of outside papers having offices here. He thought it would be wise for our citizens to take cognizance of this matter, and the medical profession should take the lead.   Many, especially the older members, remembered well how persons talked about the old canal. He had lived on its very banks for eighteen years, and no member of his family, consisting of nine or ten persons, had ever suffered from fever and ague.   Indeed, there were very few cases in the neighborhood.   When he afterwards moved to the corner of Fourth and C Streets, he and some of his family were attacked by intermittent fever.   But a committee of wise men from the Smithsonian, with Professor Henry at its head, pronounced the canal deadly and pernicious.   As for the pestilential atmosphere of the

---

* See ANNALS, 1905-6, IV, p. 78.

White House, history proved the opposite. When he first came here John Quincy Adams was President ; Dr. Lindsly doubted if any President during these fifty years was ever unable to attend to business or ever suffered from malaria. Only four Presidents had died in Washington, two from violence, one from pneumonia and one from exposure to the sun's rays and imprudence in diet. The majority of the Presidents lived here the whole year round and none of them were ever sick. Malaria was not more prevalent in the White House or its vicinity or even on the "Island"* near the river, than in any other part of the city. He offered the following resolution :

" WHEREAS, The impression so general throughout the country of the unprecedented prevalence of malaria in Washington is likely to prove a serious injury to the material interests of the city, and this impression, if not wholly unfounded, is at least grossly exaggerated ; therefore, *Resolved*, That a committee of five be appointed, in connection with the Health Officer, to investigate this whole subject and report to the Society at its earliest convenience."

Dr. J. E. Morgan seconded the resolution and approved Dr. Lindsly's course. Dr. Morgan had had a similar experience ; they knew these reports to be false. There was no more malaria in Washington than in any other city similarly situated. If a person had the toothache, got drunk or suffered from a boil, all were attributed to malaria. The thing had been going on for years, and something must be done to stop it. Last year one of the outside papers stated that half the population of south Washington was down with fever, which had assumed a continued form. Dr. Morgan consulted the physicians of that sec-

* The name " Island" was applied to that part of south Washington between the canal and river.

tion and found that not a single case of malaria existed. Lately he saw in the *Baltimore Sun* that one physician had thirty cases of typhoid fever in the immediate vicinity of the White House. There were not thirty families in that neighborhood. Last year the Commissioners became alarmed, and one of them spoke to Dr. Morgan about the terrible amount of sickness. Dr. Morgan at that time pronounced the statement false, and would now have the Secretary read some statistics emanating from the Board of Health proving his assertion concerning the healthfulness of Washington. Whilst we were a perfect graveyard, according to the outside papers, these figures showed us to be the healthiest people in the United States. But there was something behind all this. It was the anxiety of speculators to make money. There had been filed two different claims to the " flats."* These men conceived that they had a bonanza, a regular Golconda. Every part of this reclaimed land would be worth many dollars. The obstruction of the Washington channel had been brought about, not by God but by man. This was clearly demonstrated by the Citizens' Committee.

Dr. Noble Young said that it was time that the medical profession informed the public. Dr. Lindsly had referred to the canal, and Dr. Young would corroborate Dr. Lindsly's statements. Dr. Young had lived for thirty years on its banks and knew whereof he spoke. Despite the hue and cry which resulted in its closure, Dr. Young asserted that there never was a case of fever caused by the canal. The water was clear and limpid, with a beautiful sandy bottom; many times as a boy he had bathed in it. It was a means of draining the whole city ; sections which before had been marshy, by its means became dry and healthful. There

---

* The " Flats" was the stretch of river bottom adjoining the north shore, that was covered with only a foot or two of water.

was a great stir made at one time because it had been resolved to clean it. It was declared that a pestilence would prevail. But on the contrary, all that was found was a species of black sand. Of course, when it was neglected and every dead dog and cat was thrown into it, things were materially altered. He averred, on his professional reputation, that the several squares in his immediate neighborhood were as healthful as any other place in the United States. He never knew of a case of malaria originating there. The White House was notoriously healthful. Garfield's physicians expressly stated that he did not have malaria. This cry had nearly ruined the eastern section of the city, and nothing of any respectability was ever built there. It was with the greatest difficulty that we succeeded in getting the Insane Asylum in its present location. Speculation was at the bottom of all these reports. Men with property in the northwest section wanted a new President's house to be built there. Others wanted "Kidwell's Bottoms"* reclaimed for their benefit. Major Hoxie had a plan. And so on. But as long as the causeway of the Long Bridge existed, so long would we have emanations from the filth there collected.

Dr. J. M. Toner bore testimony to the widespread rumors concerning the unhealthfulness of Washington. During the summer he had heard this asserted by men who did not seem to fear contradiction. Dr. Toner silenced the doctors by telling them that speculators were at the bottom of the reports. The trouble had been in our thinking it due to our material interests not to say anything about the matter. He now proposed that we ask the National Board of Health to investigate the affair and make report. We would be considered apologists, and our action would not have as much weight as that of the National Board of

---

* "Kidwell's Bottoms," part of the "flats" above mentioned; a Mr. Kidwell claimed it.

Health.   If we could with propriety ask it to do this, Dr. Toner thought the Society should do so.

Dr. W. W. Johnston was glad that Dr. Lindsly had initiated the subject.   Individually we had been contending against these rumors, but collectively we had done nothing. It would take ten years to correct these reports.   We should not cast all the blame on the newspapers.   Most of it rested on us as physicians.   We should be careful in our diagnoses and we should not certify to deaths from malaria when the patients died of typhoid fever.   (He here read statistics from the Health Officer showing that if the death certificates were correct, malaria did prevail to an undue extent.)   We had no specific for typhoid, we had one for malaria.   Was it possible that seventy-eight persons had died from these fevers?   What was the explanation? Deaths certified to from malaria when the patients really died from typhoid.   If malarial fevers were as fatal here as typhoid no wonder persons were afraid to come here. According to statistics, Washington stood first in deaths from malaria ; from typhoid it had the third place.   The error arose from non-recognition of mild cases of typhoid. He would be glad if we could unite on some means of correcting the returns.

Dr. S. Townshend (Health Officer) thought with Dr. Johnston that physicians were much to blame.   Whenever we were in doubt about a diagnosis we said " malaria." [He read some data to prove the comparative freedom of Washington from zymotic diseases.]

Dr. W. H. Taylor wanted to know if it would mend matters if we increased our death rate from typhoid.

Dr. J. T. Sothoron testified to the prevalence of typhoid fever over malarial fevers in his section.

Dr. E. M. Schaeffer wanted the matter carefully studied, and not trust the reputation of the city to outsiders until we had considered that New Orleans and Baltimore had suffered at the hands of the National Board of Health.

Dr. P. J. Murphy said that the Health Officer was the proper person to take cognizance of this affair, and protested against calling in the National Board of Health.

The resolutions were adopted, and the committee—Drs. Lindsly, Noble Young, J. E. Morgan, D. W. Prentiss, W. W. Johnston and S. Townshend—was appointed.

November 16th, the committee reported as follows:

" The committee believes and reports that the statements so generally published are entirely unfounded ; that Washington now, as heretofore, is unquestionably as healthful as the most favored cities in this country or Europe ; and that, instead of deteriorating, it has been much improved in its general sanitary condition during the last few years, as compared with its state ten or fifteen years since. There has been a gradual but decided diminution in the extent and intensity of diseases of a malarial nature, owing, no doubt, to improved drainage, better paved streets, the filling in of low lands, and other improvements which are constantly being made by our present efficient government. Malarial diseases are almost wholly confined to those portions of the city immediately bordering on the Potomac river and its tributaries, the Eastern Branch and Rock Creek.

" A large portion of the so-called malarial diseases are not in our opinion due to malarial influences, but to other causes, which exist to an equal or greater extent in large cities, such as sewerage, the use of unwholesome food, overcrowding and bad ventilation among the poorer classes. The form of malarial diseases most commonly met with is simple intermittent fever, which is the least serious and most curable form. Death from well defined, uncomplicated malarial diseases is a rare event in our city. A careful comparison of the death rate of Washington with that of other principal cities of the United States shows conclusively that it does not exceed the average, notwithstanding the very large proportion of colored persons, one-third of the whole, whose death rate is generally almost or quite double that of the whites. The proportion of the colored race is greater in Washington than in any city north or west of us, and when the proper deduction of the death rate on this account is made it will show a sanitary condition not surpassed anywhere. It is proper to remark here that the records of the Health Department of Washington are believed to be absolutely correct as to the number of deaths annually occurring among us.

"The total number of deaths in the District of Columbia for the year ending June 30, 1881, was 4,136, of which number 2,206 were white persons and 1,931 colored, showing a death rate of 18.18 per 1,000 per annum for the whites, 31.27 for the colored, and 22.60 for the whole population. The mean annual death rate from September 1, 1874, to June 30, 1881, was, white, 19.27; colored, 37.67; total, 25.30.

"We believe, too, that the unfavorable reports so industriously circulated of the unhealthful condition of the President's house are equally unfounded. This has been the residence of all the Presidents for eighty-one years, and during all of that time, with the exception of Presidents Harrison and Taylor, who died after short illnesses from acute diseases, in no way dependent on climatic influences, the chief magistrates, although generally men of advanced age, have enjoyed excellent health and been able to attend to their official duties with scarcely a day's interruption—a most remarkable exemption and proof enough of itself of the favorable condition both of the White House and the city. We may add, too, in confirmation of this view, that all the former Presidents spent the whole year here, except a very short visit to their respective homes, the practice of living for a part of the summer in the suburbs having been first adopted by Mr. Buchanan; and when the present anomalous condition of the Potomac flats opposite the city shall have been remedied, which in their present state are at least a menace for the future, we know of nothing likely to prevent Washington from being hereafter, as heretofore, one of the most healthful as it is one of the most beautiful cities in our country."

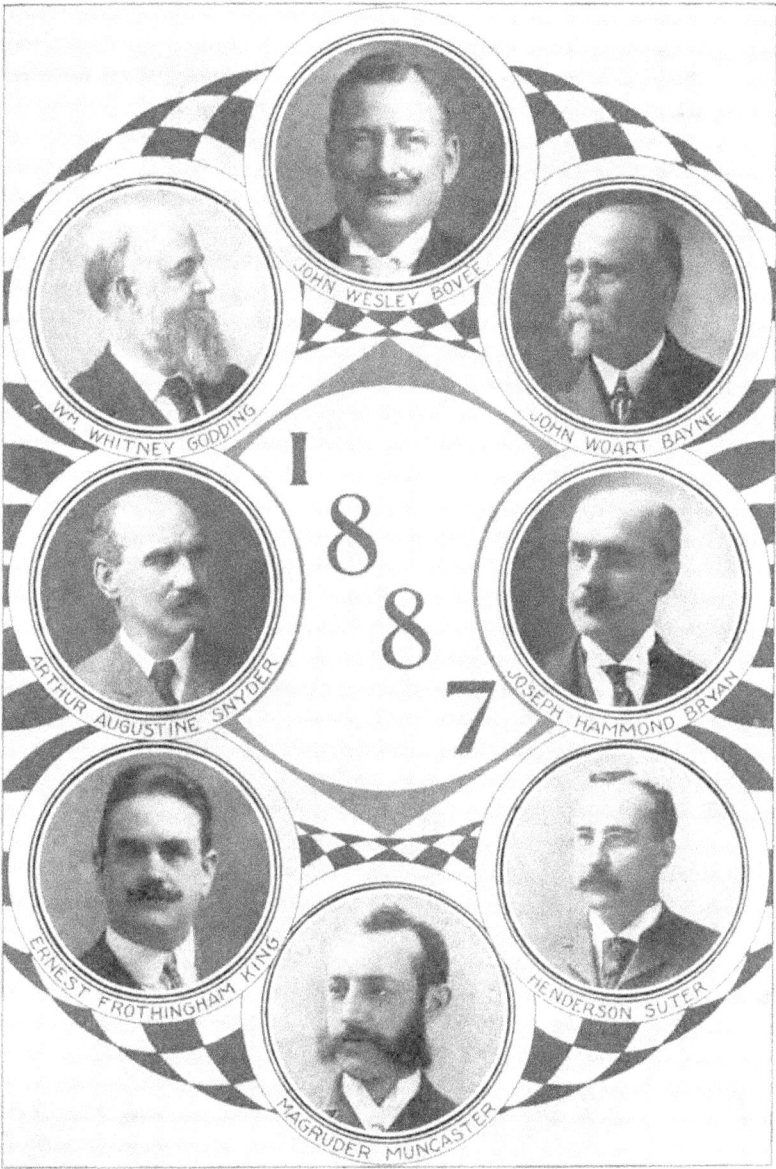

JOHN WESLEY BOVEE

WM WHITNEY GODDING

JOHN WOART BAYNE

ARTHUR AUGUSTINE SNYDER

1887

JOSEPH HAMMOND BRYAN

ERNEST FROTHINGHAM KING

MAGRUDER MUNCASTER

HENDERSON SUTER

37

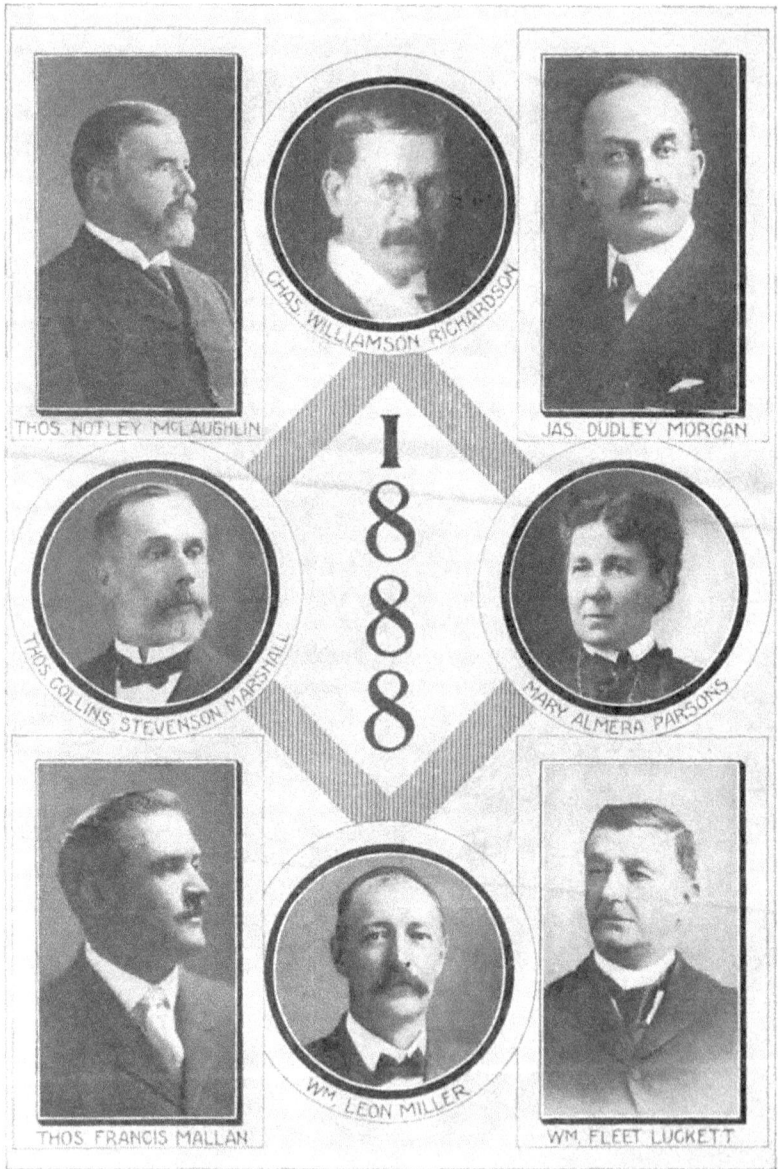

THOS. NOTLEY McLAUGHLIN
CHAS. WILLIAMSON RICHARDSON
JAS. DUDLEY MORGAN
THOS. COLLINS STEVENSON MARSHALL
1888
MARY ALMERA PARSONS
THOS. FRANCIS MALLAN
WM. LEON MILLER
WM. FLEET LUCKETT

The Society adopted the report.

May 18, 1898, the Committee on Public Health made a report concerning malaria in the District, more especially as it affected the school children.* The fever was most prevalent in the country east of the Anacostia River and, next to this, along the Potomac side.

NURSES.

In Washington the nurses, or "sick" nurses, as they were so often called, were rather an indifferent lot until the "training school" began to give them an adequate preparatory education. In course of time a number of such schools were opened, usually in connection with the hospitals. Finally, the question of a Directory for nurses was considered and, November 15, 1882, the Society appointed a committee—Drs. W. W. Johnston, S. M. Burnett and T. E. McArdle—to confer with the Washington Training School for Nurses as to the advisability of establishing such a Directory. November 22d, the committee reported the details of the conferences that had been held and what had been agreed on, and recommended the following resolution, which the Society adopted:

"*Resolved*, That the Medical Society of the District of Columbia learns with pleasure of the proposal of the Washington Training School for Nurses to establish a Nurses' Directory, and the Society promises the object its most hearty coöperation, and, as a pledge of its official sanction, directs the President of the Medical Society to appoint three members who shall compose a committee to join with the Training School in the establishment and management of said Directory."

The same committee was reappointed.

---

* See *Trans. Med. Society*, III, for 1898, p. 116, and *National Med. Review*, 1898-9, VIII, p. 322.

10

November 4, 1891, the committee from the Society reported that the matron had resigned in September and the nurses had become scattered. The committee recommended a change in the financial conduct of the Directory, a classification of the nurses and regulation of their charges, and made suggestions as to the methods to be adopted by the profession and the public in securing a nurse or nurses. After discussion, the committee was instructed to report further details. December 2d, the committee reported that it had had a conference with the nurses, and submitted a plan of reorganization which, with some alterations, had been accepted.

Owing to the number of training schools and the lack of support from the nurses themselves, the Washington Directory for Nurses was abandoned and the property turned over to the Washington Training School for Nurses, now the Capital Training School for Nurses. The Committee of the Society has been annually appointed, but for a long time has been ignored by the Training School.

February 15, 1882, the Society appointed a committee to lay before Congress the advisability of erecting a fireproof building for the Army Medical Museum. Drs. Lovejoy, W. G. Palmer and D. C. Patterson were the committee. January 7, 1884, the same committee was reappointed for the same purpose.

THE ABATTOIR.

A bill [House Bill 5634, 1882] providing for an abattoir in the District of Columbia was referred by the Committee of the House of Representatives to the Medical Society for its opinion as to what sanitary benefit would accrue to the city, and was referred, April 26, 1882, by the Society, to a committee consisting of Drs. T. E. McArdle, T. Antisell and D. W. Prentiss. The committee reported May 10th, recommending an abattoir, to be built east of and not less than a mile from the city limits, and suggested a location across the Eastern Branch; also that legislation be enacted to prevent the crowding around the abattoir of rendering houses, blood-boiling or fertilizing establishments and other manufactures from "waste residues"; and that the local government should define the conditions under which the establishment should be conducted, especially adopting smoke-consuming methods. The benefits to the city were stated to be: skilled inspection of the cattle; the best methods of slaughtering; the best methods of preparing the meats for food; the probabilities of the place being kept clean, and the riddance of the nuisance of private slaughter houses.

The report was adopted by the Society and the committee instructed to send it to the House District Committee. In due time the abattoir was built.

REMINISCENCES.

On the 21st of March, 1883, Dr. Borrows gave some reminiscences of the early physicians of the District of Columbia. He said that his heart was with the Society, and he had offered to appear that evening that he might perhaps amuse and instruct by the recollections of a very busy professional life of fifty-five years. His connection with the profession commenced about the year 1822, when he was admitted into the Freshman class of Columbian College. Shortly afterward he became identified with Drs. Thos. Sewall, J. M. Staughton and Alex. McWilliams, who were professors in the classical department and at the same time gave lectures in medicine—Sewall on anatomy, Staughton on materia medica and McWilliams on botany.

Borrows was persuaded to study medicine, that he might add to his general knowledge. As his studies went on he found that his taste for it increased, and it did not require much persuasion to urge him on to graduation.

Among his earlier recollections was Chas. Worthington, who practiced in Georgetown; a man venerable in appearance and a high Christian gentleman, though not a bigot. This was exemplified by his not objecting to the playing of cards by the students of his son Nicholas, who was professor of materia medica. This son also was a man of character and refinement, the pink of politeness, bashful and modest as a girl. He never married. Dr. Sewall, the professor of anatomy, was a New England man, who came to Washington under a cloud, having robbed the grave of a near relative in his devotion to the study of medicine. Hingham's loss was Washington's gain, for Sewall became celebrated not only in this country but in Europe by his work on phrenology.

Dr. Thos. Henderson had all the pomp of a professor, and had he commenced early in life to give lectures in a large school he would have become prominent. His lectures were well written and well delivered. The same could be said of Dr. Fred. May, who was professor of midwifery. He had the faculty of amusing at one moment and bringing tears the next. Whenever he spoke of uterine hemorrhage he always enlisted the sympathies of his hearers, for it was known that his wife had died from that cause. He was most courteous and refined in manner. Dr. E. Cutbush, the professor of chemistry, was a high-toned gentleman. He had been an officer in the navy, but retired to private life upon the election of Jackson as President. Dr. R. Randall, another professor of chemistry, was a gentleman of elevated character. In his anxiety to distinguish himself he accepted the position of Governor of

Liberia, and in that perilous climate lost his life. Dr. James M. Staughton, who delivered the address at the first opening of the medical department of Columbian College, was a clergyman in appearance ; fifty-one years ago he was the attendant of the most fashionable persons in Washington. His son was to Dr. Borrows as a brother. Dr. Staughton became professor of surgery, in Cincinnati, and died there, leaving many friends.

Dr. Borrows' fellow students were Harvey Lindsly and Noble Young ; two others had since died—Jones in New Orleans and Collins in Virginia, of yellow fever. The latter was a member of the legislature, and had been auditor, succeeding Dr. Tully Wise. Dr. Peregrine Warfield was a stout, blunt man of great medical acquirements, and well known as a surgeon. Dr. B. H. Bohrer was a man of great personal address, with accomplished manners and most acceptable as a companion. Dr. Thos. Sim, of the West End, died of cholera in 1832. He had great success as an accoucheur and told many stories of his wonderful performances. There were several others in that section, amongst them Drs. Elzey and N. P. Causin ; the latter prominent as a politician, etc., and ended his life whilst returning from the races by falling into an ice house where the Patent Office now stands. Poor old Dr. Munding was one of the most charitable doctors, who never become rich. He attended the poorest patients without hope of compensation. Dr. J. Lovell was the Surgeon General, U. S. Army, and was identified with the Phrenological Society. Dr. Henry Huntt was a dandy. He drove a fine horse and was followed by two dogs. He had more tact than any other doctor whom Borrows ever knew. He was equally good in medicine, surgery and obstetrics. He had been in the army during the war of 1812, and after settling in Washington moved immediately into the fashionable practice, and he fully deserved it. Though somewhat abrupt in manner, he was still agreeable, and ever maintained his own dignity and the responsibility of the profession. He was President of the Board of Health when we were prosecuting Williams, the oculist, for obtaining money under false pretenses. It was proven that the Medical Society had forfeited its charter by not meeting sufficiently often.

Dr. Causin came from Maryland, and was appointed judge, retaining the office till his death. Dr. Fred Dawes was a man of great medical acquirements, who was more easily influenced by the solicitations of his friends than by the ethics of the profession. He died poor. Dr. George May was a man whom Borrows ever esteemed; his character was always that of a gentleman; his personal appearance was good. His knowledge of the three branches of the profession was greater than that of any other man of Borrows' acquaintance. Dr. Thomas Scott was of a retiring disposition and not so prominent as some of those mentioned. He took families by the year, some as low as $10, obstetrics included. He was a very stout man. He came from one of the lower counties. Dr. Richmond Johnson was not as much identified with the profession as with the Surgeon General's Office. He was a person of fine address and acquirements. Dr. Magruder commenced the practice of medicine in 1832, the year of the cholera. The first cases of that disease were treated in the old medical college on E Street, near Tenth. This not being found large enough, Stone's building on the Avenue was occupied; afterwards the cholera hospital was on M Street between First and Second. The attending physicians were Magruder, B. and T. Miller, Davis, Warren and Borrows. The first case of cholera was reported by Dr. Alex. Davis. The Board of Health increased the number of physicians in each ward from two to five, making thirty in all.

Dr. James H. Blake was Mayor of Washington in 1812–14. He had a very extensive practice, and had associated with him Dr. Wm. Jones, afterwards postmaster for three terms. Dr. C. F. Wilstach was more of an apothecary than physician, and had a place of business on Pennsylvania Avenue between Ninth and Tenth Streets. Dr. James Ewell was a very corpulent man; he wore a ruffled shirt and was dandified in his manner. His brother Thomas built the house in which General Sickles lived when he shot Key. These brothers were rivals for professional fame. One was the author of the "Medical Companion," the other of the "Family Physician," both popular works in medicine. The charges then for bleeding and pulling teeth were 50 cents, for attendance $1 and for obstetrical services $10.

Dr. Flodoardo Howard said that he remembered Dr. Semmes very well; as an apothecary he had put up many of the doctor's prescriptions. He would start out in the morning on a bob-tailed horse and visit from twenty to thirty families during the day. His prescription for each was generally the same, calomel and Dover's powder. It was true that the majority of his patients suffered from malarial troubles. Another favorite prescription was equal parts of laudanum, compound spirit of lavender and Hoffman's anodyne. He was an exceedingly successful accoucheur. Dr. William B. Magruder distinguished himself in the treatment of cholera, and this reputation gave him a great start in practice. After becoming Mayor and dabbling in politics he lost a great deal of business. He was exceedingly popular, but had the bad habit of not collecting his fees, and died poor. A more disinterested physician than Dr. Richmond Johnson never lived. He was the accoucheur in the first ward for a long time, and this gave him great popularity. He was exceedingly kind to the poor, and after his work for the day was over at the Sur-

geon General's Office he frequently visited from fifteen to
twenty poor patients. He was an accomplished physician
and an exceedingly devoted Christian.

Dr. Johnson Eliot said that there was one subject connected with the old doctors which should be a matter of
pride to the profession : that was the first use anywhere, by
Dr. Alex. McWilliams, of adhesive straps in extension. In
1822 Dr. McWilliams applied adhesive straps in the Washington Asylum ; he sent an exemplification of the process,
with a large doll, to the French Academy, and received in
return a very complimentary letter, which, as a young man,
Eliot read.   Drs. Borrows, Hall and May had written letters corroborating the statement.   Dr. Gross, however, said
that in 1834 a pupil of his suggested it, and in 1841 some-
body else claimed it ; but in 1828 Eliot spread the adhesive
straps and assisted McWilliams to apply them.

Dr. W. H. Taylor said that a Dr. Minor, of New York,
came to Washington in 1855, claiming that he had devised
the plan of using adhesive straps to make extension.   Dr.
Taylor hunted up the old apparatus which had been used
at the Infirmary for a number of years and showed it to
Minor, whereupon the latter returned to New York a wiser
but a sadder man.

Dr. Borrows recollected that McWilliams had used adhesive straps for extension in 1827.

October 15, 1884, a committee was appointed, consisting
of the President, Dr. A. Y. P. Garnett and Drs. J. W. H.
Lovejoy, C. W. Franzoni, J. Ford Thompson, D. R. Hagner, J. F. Hartigan, E. M. Schaeffer, T. C. Smith, W. W.
Johnston and W. G. Palmer, to consider the propriety or
necessity of revising the charter, and go to Congress and
urge such changes as the Society might think advisable.
Apparently nothing further was done.

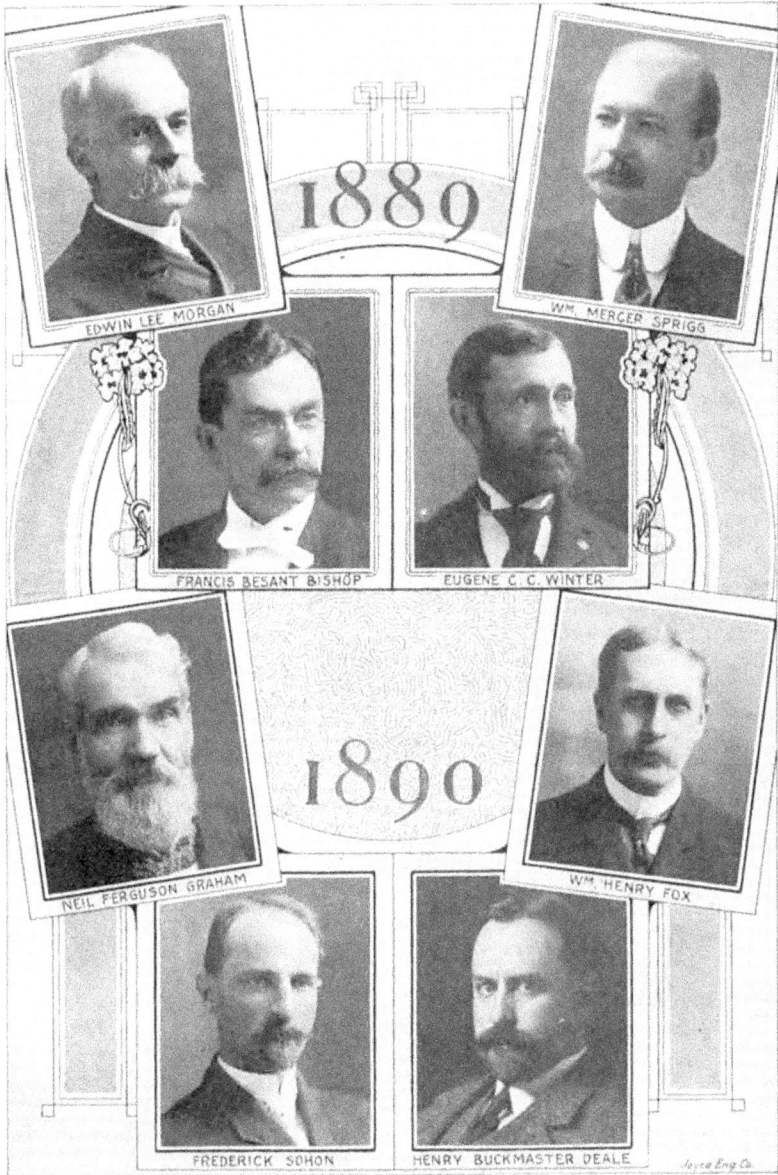

1889

1890

EDWIN LEE MORGAN

WM. MERCER SPRIGG

FRANCIS BESANT BISHOP

EUGENE C. C. WINTER

NEIL FERGUSON GRAHAM

WM. HENRY FOX

FREDERICK SOHON

HENRY BUCKMASTER DEALE

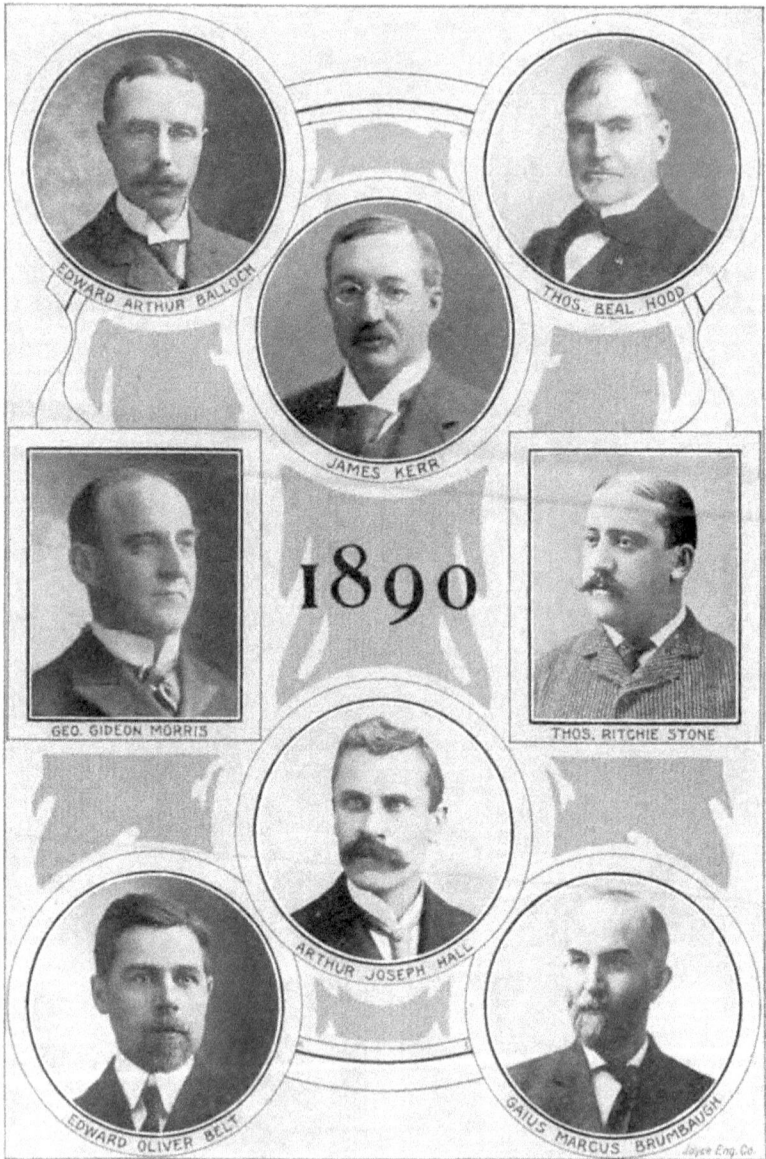

EDWARD ARTHUR BALLOCH

THOS. BEAL HOOD

JAMES KERR

1890

GEO. GIDEON MORRIS

THOS. RITCHIE STONE

ARTHUR JOSEPH HALL

EDWARD OLIVER BELT

GAIUS MARCUS BRUMBAUGH

Joyce Eng. Co.

September 22, 1886, a letter was received from the South Carolina Medical School, stating that its buildings had been injured by the earthquake and asking for assistance. The Society appropriated $100.

THE SOCIETY AND THE WATER SUPPLY OF THE DISTRICT OF COLUMBIA ; AND TYPHOID FEVER.*

The records of the Medical Society show that it has been ever alert in matters pertaining to public health, and the more or less voluminous reports of the various committees that have been appointed from time to time to investigate and study health problems attest its vigilance in this respect. Perhaps more attention has been given to a careful inquiry into the purity and potability of the water supply than to any other one subject. It is not necessary here to go into the history of the public water supply of Washington. It will be sufficient to say that it is derived from the Potomac River. The aqueduct "was so far completed in 1859 that the water from the receiving reservoir was available and turned into the mains. This supply was independent of the Potomac and was furnished by the watershed of Little Falls Branch. * * * The conduit was completed and water supplied from the Potomac, December 5, 1863, and since that date the system has been in successful operation."

In the spring of 1885, owing to the offensive odor present in the water, it was alleged that the water supply of the city was in some way contaminated, and in order to determine, if possible, so vital a matter, the Society appointed a committee, May 27th, to investigate and report upon the character of the water in the reservoirs and as supplied to the dwellings in Washington. After careful consideration of "several chemical analyses of the Potomac water,

* This article was prepared by Dr. G. Wythe Cook.

made by competent chemists, who have recently examined our water supply," the committee reported, June 10th, " that the water is a healthy and potable one," and, further, "there is no epidemic of intestinal or febroid disease in Washington at present; the experience of the medical profession has been that during the existence of this condition of the water the health of the community has been generally good." The committee, while believing that Potomac River water, which is our main supply, is one of the purest, cautioned against its contamination by allowing "minor feeders or additional streams to commingle with it. It is the opinion of the committee that the offensive odor lately prevalent in the water has been due to the decomposition of various aquatic forms of vegetable and animal life in the reservoir and pipes. * * * As a remedy, frequent and thorough flushings of the pipes" was recommended. The committee stated that "many of the evils now complained of might be prevented or remedied by proper filtration and aeration of the water on a complete scale by the authorities." The report is an admirable one, and shows close observation and careful thought. The committee consisted of Drs. E. M. Schaeffer, Thomas Antisell, J. Ford Thompson, Louis Mackall, Jr., and D. W. Prentiss.

The next year, April 14, 1886, Dr. W. W. Johnston, remarking upon the muddiness of the water supply, said that Captain Symonds, of the Engineer Corps, in charge of the water works, had made an elaborate report to the War Department recommending the filtration of the Potomac River water before its delivery into the water pipes. Upon Dr. Johnston's motion, Captain Symonds was invited to address the Society upon " The Filtration of the Water Supply," which he did, April 21st.*

---

* See *Jour. Amer. Med. Asso.*, Aug. 21, 1886, p. 219.

So far as the writer knows, the first published reference to the probability that the Potomac River water might be contaminated by pathogenic germs is found in an address entitled " A Contribution to the Etiology of Typhoid Fever," by Dr. G. M. Kober, of this Society, delivered in Berlin in 1890 at the Tenth International Medical Congress. In this address he considered an epidemic of typhoid fever prevailing at Cumberland, Md., as being the probable cause of the same disease in the City of Washington, by reason of the fact that the drainage from Cumberland falls into the Potomac River, from which stream Washington receives its water supply.

February 5, 1894, Dr. Charles Smart, U. S. A., in an address before the Sanitary League delivered at the Columbian University in this city, emphatically declared that the high death-rate in Washington from typhoid fever was attributable to polluted Potomac River water. Dr. G. L. Magruder, who was present, called in question the correctness of Dr. Smart's statement; and the views of some others, subsequently published in the *Evening Star*, coincided with Dr. Magruder's. At the next meeting of the Medical Society, February 7th, Dr. Magruder brought to the attention of the Society the statement of Dr. Smart, and upon his motion he and Drs. W. W. Johnston and C. M. Hammett (Health Officer) were appointed a committee to investigate the causes of the prevalence of and high death-rate from typhoid fever in the District of Columbia. June 6th, this committee, after much labor and painstaking, presented its report, together with numerous maps and diagrams and the following recommendations, which, after consideration by the Medical Society, were unanimously adopted:

" 1. The immediate abandonment of all wells within the city limits, exception only to be made in case of the absence of the Potomac supply, and where the wells, after repeated chemical and bacteriological examinations, have been found to be free from all possible sources of danger ; but even these to be abandoned as rapidly as possible.

" 2. Purification of the sewerage system already existing by replacing as rapidly as possible all damaged or defective drains.

" 3. The introduction of new sewers in advance of other improvements in parts of the city not now supplied with drainage, and the extension of the system as far outside of the city limits as the rapidly growing population demands, so as to prevent soil contamination.

" 4. The adoption of some system by which the lower sections of the city can be more completely drained, and the risks arising from the backing up of tidewater and sewage prevented.

" 5. The final and safe disposal of the sewage.

" 6. To make all existing privies, vaults or other receptacles of human excreta watertight, and by rigid inspection and penalties to prevent the danger from leakage and overflow.

" 7. The early completion of the plans recommended by Colonel Elliott, in charge of the Washington Aqueduct, and now in course of execution, which have in view the sedimentation of the Potomac water, and ultimately the completion of works for filtration, the only proper method of purification.

" 8. The suppression of all privies and the enforcing of the law to make sewer connections.

" 9. Careful inspection of all dairies in the District from which our milk supply is drawn, and the enactment of a law by which no milk shall be sold in the District without a permit from the Health Office. The inspection shall cover an examination of the dairies, of all possible sources of infection, including the water supply.

" 10. The urging upon the members of the profession of a careful collation of all facts bearing upon the mode of infection in each case and the advantage of reporting such facts to the Society, and the propagation of the doctrine that immediate disinfection of the stools is the first duty of the physician as guardian of the health of the community."

Immediately after the adoption of this report the Medical Society received an invitation, through Commissioner George Truesdell, from the Committee of the House of Representatives on the District of Columbia, to attend its meeting, and June 14th, through its committee, composed of Drs. S. C. Busey, W. W. Johnston, G. L. Magruder, C. H. A. Kleinschmidt, G. Wythe Cook, S. S. Adams and D. W. Prentiss, presented the report to the Committee of the House, which, after two hearings, ordered it to be printed as a public document.

October 24th, Dr. John S. Billings read by request before the Society a paper entitled "Filtration Methods of Water Supply and Sewage Disposal in Some Large European Cities," in which the distinct statement was made that "the securing of an abundant and pure water supply appears to be the most urgent need of Washington at the present time," and that, "Sedimentation alone will not give us satisfactory results, and rapid filtration through steel cylinders, with or without the addition of alum or other chemicals, while quite as costly as the simple sand filtration, does not give an equal guaranty of the purity of the water."

January 30, 1895, Prof. W. P. Mason, of Troy, New York, delivered, by invitation, an address before the Medical Society on the subject of the water supply of cities, in which he emphasized the necessity of sedimentation and the superiority of sand filtration over all other known methods.

The report of the Committee of the Medical Society on Public Health, January 26, 1896, says, "The agitation of the subject of the purification of the Potomac water is forced upon us, as physicians, by every recent addition to our knowledge of the subject," and declares that sand filtration is the "most convenient and effective method for the purification of drinking water," and "must be adopted ultimately for the water supply of Washington." At the same meeting the following, among other resolutions relating to sanitation, was unanimously adopted : "That the general water supply should be purified by sedimentation and filtration (the first being necessary at certain times and the second at all times) before it is admitted to the mains."

October 26, 1898, Dr. Robert Reyburn read before the Society a paper on the pollution of the Potomac River at Piedmont, West Virginia, and Cumberland, Maryland. This paper was based on his personal investigations and observations of the discharge of the filthy waste water from factories at the above named places into the Potomac River.*

Owing to the sometime repulsive character of the water as it appeared in the glass and in the bath tub, there was a universal demand for its improvement, and the cry went up from all sections of the city for a clean, wholesome water. The Commissioners, the Board of Trade, the Business Men's Association, various independent organizations, the newspapers and, indeed, the unanimous sentiment was for a purified water supply, and Congress was disposed to provide the means for it when the best way to secure it was pointed out. Accordingly in the Act making appropriations for the District of Columbia, approved March 3, 1899, is contained the following clause :

"For additional amount to enable the proper officer of the Government having charge of the Washington Aqueduct and water supply to the City of Washington to make an investigation of the feasibility and propriety of filtering the water supply of Washington, and to submit to Congress a full and detailed report thereon, and to meet all necessary expenses of said investigation, five thousand dollars, to be immediately available."

* See *Trans. Med. Society* for 1898, p. 153; *Nat. Med. Review*, 1898, VIII, p. 421.

Upon Col. A. M. Miller, Corps of Engineers, U. S. A., "in charge of the Washington Aqueduct and of the increase of the water supply of the City of Washington," devolved the duty of the investigation of the feasibility and propriety of filtering the water supply of the City of Washington. After a careful and painstaking investigation Colonel Miller rendered an elaborate report, dated March 28, 1900. He considered the source of the water supply, the character of the water-shed, the first introduction of Potomac water through the aqueduct, the various reservoirs and the pumping station. He detailed the methods of filtration and described the experimental filters used. The slow sand filter "consisted of a cylindrical white-pine tank, eleven feet in diameter," in which were placed the filtering materials, with the necessary pipes, valves, meter, etc., to admit the raw water, control its velocity through the filter or rate of filtration, and dispose of the filtered water.

The mechanical filter used in experiments was erected by the New York Filter Manufacturing Company, and combined all the recent improvements in this method.

"It consists of a cylindrical steel tank, set up vertically and divided by a horizontal diaphragm into two compartments, the lower compartment serving as a preliminary sedimentation basin, and receiving the raw water and coagulant. The influent is so arranged that a centrifugal motion is given to the water on entering. From this lower compartment the water passes to the second or upper compartment, in which is situated the filtering device.

"The filtering device consists of a cylindrical steel vessel, smaller in diameter than the outer cylinder, resting on the horizontal diaphragm. In the bottom of this interior vessel are placed, set in cement, the strainers, which collect the filtered water and pass it to a main drain, whence it is passed through a regulator to the effluent of the filter.

"The object of the investigation was to ascertain whether

the Potomac water, as delivered to the consumer at Washington at present, could be rendered by filtration, with either method, acceptable in appearance and hygienically fit for a domestic supply.

"An acceptable appearance of the water requires the removal of the turbidity to an extent which will render the water unobjectionable. Hygienic requirements are satisfied by the reduction of the number of bacteria to an acceptable quantity."

Under the direction of Colonel Miller frequent chemical and bacteriological examinations of the raw and filtered water were made by skilled analysts.

The committee—Drs. S. C. Busey, G. Wythe Cook, G. M. Kober, Z. T. Sowers and W. C. Woodward—appointed by the Medical Society of the District of Columbia, March 7, 1900, "to inquire into the relative merits of natural or slow sand filtration and mechanical filtration in their relation to the public water supply of this District," by the courtesy of Gen. John M. Wilson, Chief of Engineers, U. S. A., visited the experimental plant established by Colonel Miller and found the filters as described above. The mechanical filter was the *very best that could be made*, while the slow sand filter was necessarily merely in miniature of what it would be when in practical use. The product of the mechanical filter was a beautiful and clear water; that of the slow sand filter was not quite so transparent, but sufficiently so to suit reasonable requirements. The bacterial results were in favor of the slow sand filter. Colonel Miller believed that the bacterial efficiency of the mechanical filter was sufficient for safety, and as he desired to furnish the most attractive looking water, he recommended the mechanical method of filtration. The committee was considerably perturbed at this outcome of Colonel Miller's investigations. It was confronted by this report

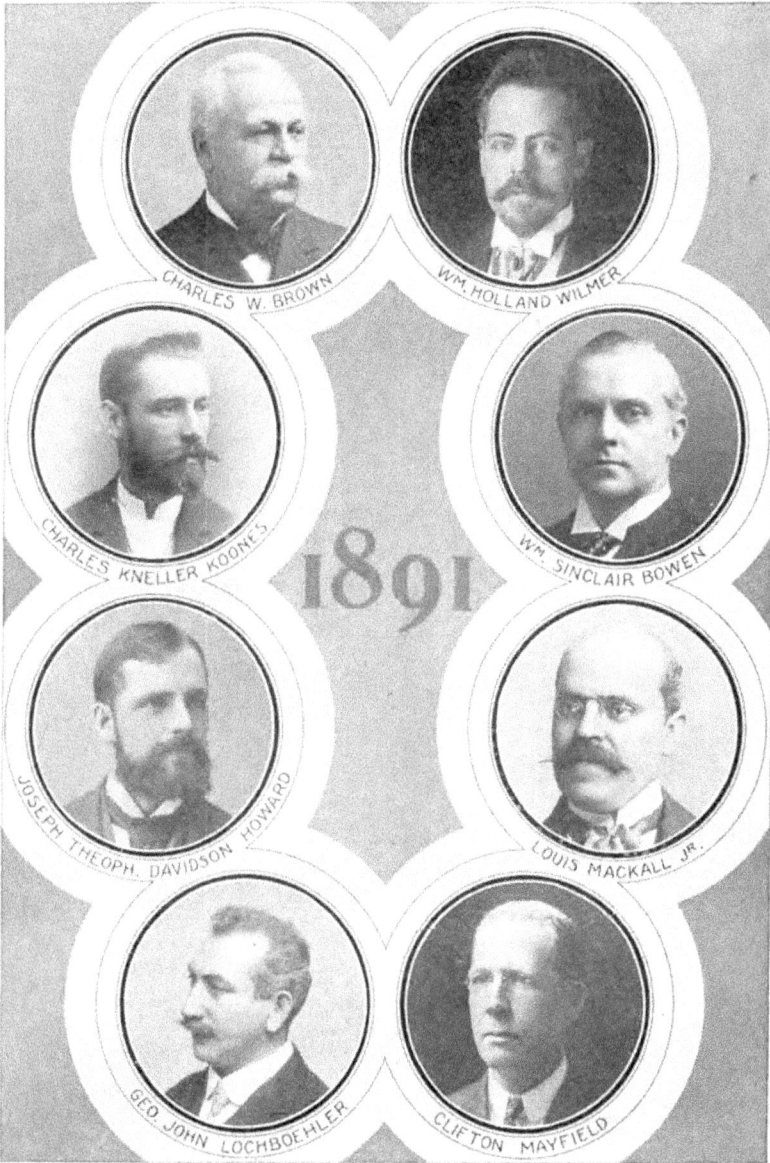

CHARLES W. BROWN

WM. HOLLAND WILMER

CHARLES KNELLER KOONES

WM. SINCLAIR BOWEN

1891

JOSEPH THEOPH. DAVIDSON HOWARD

LOUIS MACKALL, JR.

GEO. JOHN LOCHBOEHLER

CLIFTON MAYFIELD

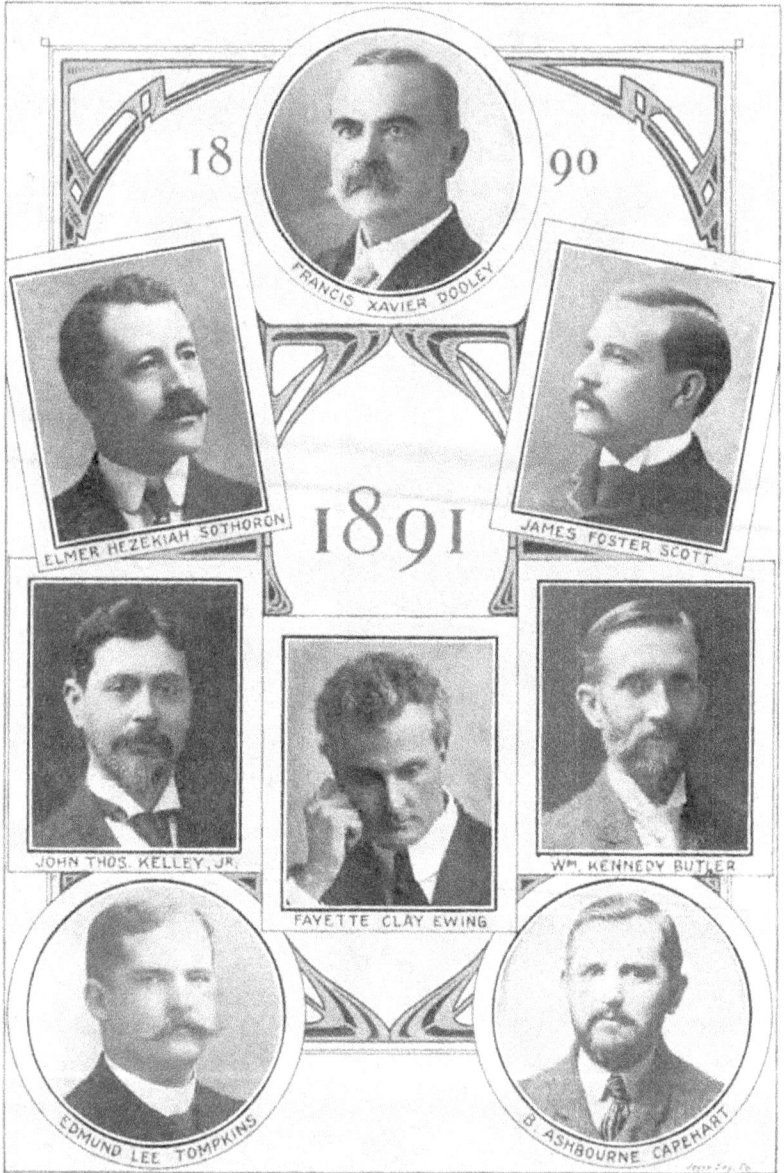

18 90

FRANCIS XAVIER DOOLEY

ELMER HEZEKIAH SOTHORON

1891

JAMES FOSTER SCOTT

JOHN THOS. KELLEY, JR.

FAYETTE CLAY EWING

WM. KENNEDY BUTLER

EDMUND LEE TOMPKINS

B. ASHBOURNE CAPEHART

42

from the War Department to the United States Senate, recommending the mechanical method of filtration, while it had strongly urged the natural or slow sand method, as the main contention of the Medical Society was for the greatest bacterial efficiency, and that no chemical or other agent be added to the water before or during the process of filtration. There was no means of knowing how the Senate Committee might view the matter, but it was certain they desired the best method; so that Dr. Busey, though in feeble health, with his accustomed energy and pertinacity, with the committee of the Medical Society, proceeded to analyze the report of Colonel Miller, and laid the results before the Society, December 5th, "earnestly and unhesitatingly recommending the prompt installation of the natural sand filters." This recommendation was unanimously adopted by the Society, December 7th, and a copy of the report was transmitted to Hon. James McMillan, chairman Committee on the District of Columbia, U. S. Senate, and was printed as Senate Document No. 27, Fifty-sixth Congress, Second Session.

February 19, 1901, Mr. McMillan, from the Committee on the District of Columbia, submitted a report on the relative merits of the mechanical and the slow sand systems of filtration for the water supply of the District of Columbia, in which he says:

"After a very long and careful investigation the report from the War Department, known as Colonel Miller's report, took the ground that the water supply of the District of Columbia contained suspended clay in such fine particles as to make it practically impossible to use the slow sand system of filtration, and he, therefore, recommended the adoption of the rapid, or mechanical, system of filtration.

"This report was sharply attacked by the Medical Society of the District of Columbia, and, following the lead of the Medical Society, by the Board of Trade and the Busi-

11

ness Men's Association. It was argued by these bodies that the use of alum as a coagulant was in itself objectionable, and that the mechanical process was inferior to the slow sand system as a means of removing those forms of pollution that are the cause of typhoid fever.

"An inquiry conducted by this committee in New York City on January 4, 1901, was attended by men who have made for themselves the highest reputation in the matter of the construction and operation of filters for public water supplies. No large filter plant, either in existence or projected, was unrepresented at that meeting. The plants at Lawrence, Mass.; Albany, N. Y.; East Providence, R. I.; Norfolk, Va.; Elmira, N. Y., were among those as to which direct testimony was given; and the projects at Philadelphia, Pittsburg, Louisville, Cincinnati, Paterson and New Orleans were discussed by men who had served or were then serving upon the boards of experts for those cities. No such representative gathering of filtration experts ever before took place in this country. It is true that the discussion of the subject of the filtration of public water supplies held at the meeting of the American Association of Civil Engineers in London, England, in July, 1900, brought together a larger representation of foreign experts; but the leaders of the discussion in London were also present in New York, and at the latter gathering the American problem had its fullest discussion.

"The result of this discussion established the fact that the slow sand filter, wherever it had been put into operation, had produced uniformly good results, both in clearing the water from turbidity and also in removing bacteria."

At that inquiry Dr. W. C. Woodward, in behalf of natural, slow sand filtration, conducted the examination of the experts in a masterful and efficient manner, and the examination of the mechanical method was managed by Colonel Miller. The report of the Committee of the Medical Society, known as Senate Document No. 27, was made the basis for exceptions to Colonel Miller's recommendation.

Subsequent to the inquiry held by the Senate Committee

in New York City, and after the House of Representatives had passed a bill appropriating $200,000 for filtration purposes, without defining any method, Dr. G. L. Magruder succeeded in obtaining a hearing for the Medical Society before the subcommittee of the House of Representatives on Appropriations. At that hearing there were present Drs. D. S. Lamb, W. W. Johnston, G. Wythe Cook, Wm. C. Woodward, G. L. Magruder and D. P. Hickling, of the Committee on Legislation, and Drs. G. M. Kober, Wm. C. Woodward and G. Wythe Cook, of the Committee on Filtration. Arguments were presented by Drs. G. M. Kober, W. W. Johnston, D. P. Hickling and Wm. C. Woodward.

Fortunately, after the inquiry was held in New York City, the Senate Committee asked for a professional report from Mr. Rudolph Herring, Mr. George W. Fuller and Mr. Allen Hazen. These able and experienced experts, after a thorough review and consideration of all the conditions, made the following report:

"In consideration of the full evidence we recommend the construction of a complete system of slow or sand filters, with such auxiliary works as may be necessary for preliminary sedimentation, and the use of a coagulant for a part of the time. There is no reason to believe that the use of this coagulant will in any degree affect the wholesomeness of the water."

Upon the lines of this recommendation the authorization of the construction of the filtration plant was based. How much credit may be due the Medical Society for the accomplishment of slow sand filtration may be found in the fact that the report of its committee was the stumbling block of the mechanical filters.

November 8, 1905, the Medical Society resolved to cooperate with the Commissioners of the District of Columbia in the endeavor to secure the passage of a bill to prevent the pollution of the Potomac River; and to assist in the public movement to consider the "Pollution of the Potomac River" and the "Methods to Secure a Pure Water Supply for the District of Columbia."

The Civic Center of Washington having invited the Medical Society of the District of Columbia to be present at its meeting, December 11, 1905, the Society in accepting the invitation appointed Dr. G. Wythe Cook to speak for it on that occasion. The subject of his address was: "Historical Account of the Installation of Slow Sand Filtration of the Potomac River Water for the City of Washington." From that address a large part of this article is taken. The subject of pure water was still a live one, and Dr. T. N. McLaughlin, in his Presidential address before the Society, December 13, 1905, spoke on the subject of "The Pollution of the Potomac River." This address was illustrated with numerous lantern slides. At this meeting the President was directed to appoint a committee "to enquire into the efficiency of the filtration plant and make such recommendations as appeared necessary." This committee, composed of Drs. G. M. Kober, G. Wythe Cook, D. Percy Hickling, Z. T. Sowers and W. C. Woodward, made a careful enquiry and reported to the Society, January 31, 1906, recommending the installation of water meters as a means of checking waste of water; "Removal of all sediment from the receiving reservoirs which has accumulated for years," and "That the Society suspend judgment with reference to the advisability or inadvisability, from a sanitary standpoint, of adding a coagulant to our water supply for the purpose of purifying it."

It will thus be seen that the Medical Society was continually alert and energetic in its endeavors to secure a pure and abundant water supply for the District of Columbia. It is but fair to say that the records of the Society show that Dr. G. Lloyd Magruder was especially vigilant in regard to proposed legislation respecting filtration and reporting his information to the Society.*

AN INEBRIATE ASYLUM IN THE DISTRICT OF COLUMBIA.

December 1, 1886, Dr. W. W. Godding, Superintendent of the Government Hospital for the Insane of the District of Columbia, read a paper on the "Problem of the Inebriate." The discussion brought out the fact that a bill had passed the Senate and was pending in the House of Representatives providing for the treatment of inebriates in the Government Hospital for the Insane. To this proposition Dr. Godding objected. The Society appointed a committee, consisting of Drs. Godding, N. S. Lincoln and J. M. Toner, to consider the question of the best treatment of the inebriate. The committee reported, December 22d.†

February 2, 1887, Dr. Toner, from the committee, reported a copy of a bill which the committee had prepared and introduced in Congress, providing for an inebriate asylum. The bill, however, failed to pass, and there is as yet (1909) no asylum for inebriates in the District of Columbia.

LICENTIATES OF THE SOCIETY.

October 26, 1887, the Society ordered that licentiates should be notified of its meetings by postal card. January 14, 1891, the question was raised as to the advisability of continuing this privilege, and a committee was appointed to inquire into the matter, consisting of Drs. H. L. E.

---

* See also *Trans. Med. Society*, 1898, III, pp. 35-64, and 1900, V, p. 47; *Nat. Med. Review*, 1898-9, VIII, pp. 87-92, 139-152; 1900-1, X, p. 103, and 1901, VI, p. 54; WASH. MED. ANNALS, 1903-4, II, p. 56, and 1905-6, IV, p. 362.

† The report and copy of the bill that had passed the Senate were printed in the *Journal American Medical Association*, 1887, VIII, p. 49, *et seq.*

Johnson, T. C. Smith, C. H. A. Kleinschmidt, T. E. Mc-
Ardle and S. S. Adams. The committee reported ad-
versely, February 4th. The matter went over till the
11th, when, after a full and free discussion, the whole subject was tabled. It was brought up again, July 6th; the
report of the committee was adopted and it was ordered
that only those persons should be permitted to attend the
meetings who were provided for in the Constitution of the
Society.

June 5, 1889, the Society donated $100 to the sufferers
by the flood at Johnstown, Pa.

CONTAGIOUS DISEASES OTHER THAN SMALLPOX IN THE DISTRICT OF COLUMBIA.

June 12, 1889, a committee, consisting of Drs. J. B.
Hamilton, T. E. McArdle and B. G. Pool, was appointed
to ascertain if there were any laws in the District of Columbia for preventing the spread of scarlet fever, measles
and diphtheria. October 2d, the committee made a
lengthy report stating that there was a law, approved July
19, 1872, and entitled "An Act for the prevention of diseases in the District of Columbia," authorizing the Board
of Health, in its judgment, to make regulations for the
removal or prevention of epidemic and infectious or contagious diseases. Another act of Congress, April 24, 1880,
legalized the regulations then in force for the control of
smallpox, but said nothing about other infectious or contagious diseases, and did not legalize the Act of 1872,
thereby leaving the Health Officer powerless in regard to
the control of such other diseases. The committee recommended an amendment to the Act of 1880, making the
regulations in regard to smallpox applicable to measles,

diphtheria and scarlet fever. The report was much discussed, *pro* and *con;* finally, the Society ordered that the recommendation be printed and sent to the members, after which the subject would be further considered.

October 9th, the committee made a supplemental report, which was ordered to be printed and sent to the members in place of the preceding one. October 30th, the committee offered a third form of bill, and this was much discussed; there was still much opposition to any action being taken. Drs. S. C. Busey, R. Reyburn and T. C. Smith offered amendments. The Society ordered that a copy of all proposed amendments be printed and sent to the members. November 6th, the subject was again fully discussed. November 13th, the amendments offered by Drs. Busey, Smith and Reyburn were voted on, but failed to pass. The bill proposed by the committee was then rejected by a vote of 12 to 11. November 20th, an effort was made to reconsider, but the Society ordered the subject postponed. December 4th, a motion to reconsider was passed and December 11th was appointed as the date for discussion. On that date Dr. G. Wythe Cook offered a new bill which, after some amendments, was adopted, and a "Committee on Legislation," composed of Dr. Busey, chairman, and Drs. Hamilton, S. Townshend, W. W. Johnston and Ralph Walsh, was appointed to take it to Congress.

March 12, 1890, Dr. Busey reported that the bill had been introduced in both the Senate and House of Representatives; April 23d, that it had passed the Senate and was then in the House, where he anticipated that there would be much opposition. The bill, however, passed, and was approved, December 20th (see Statutes U. S., 1890–1, Chap. 251).

March 15, 1896, the Society was informed that a bill

(House Bill 9023) had been introduced in the House of Representatives "To prevent the spread of contagious diseases in the District of Columbia." The bill passed, and was approved March 3, 1897 (see Statutes U. S., 1896–7, Chap. 383).

November 8, 1899, the Society empowered its Committee on Legislation to draft a law to make householders responsible for reporting contagious diseases. Apparently the committee made no report to the Society.

February 11, 1903, the Executive Committee reported to the Society a copy of a bill providing for the reporting of the minor contagious diseases to the Health Officer, who had asked for the opinion of the Medical Society on the subject. The Committee was authorized by the Society to take such steps as it saw fit. March 11th, the committee reported that the bill had been favorably acted upon by the Senate Committee but that there the consideration had stopped.

June 27, 1904, the Executive Committee reported that there was then pending in Congress a bill (Senate Bill 3786, House Bill 10,955) for the further prevention of communicable diseases. The committee was instructed by the Society to favor this legislation. [The bills expired by limitation with the session of Congress.]

Congress passed a bill, approved February 9, 1907, entitled "An Act for the prevention of scarlet fever, diphtheria, measles, whooping cough, chicken pox, epidemic cerebro-spinal meningitis and typhoid fever in the District of Columbia" (see U. S. Statutes, 1906–7, p. 889). March 13th, a letter was received by the Society from the Health Officer, transmitting a copy of the regulations proposed under the act and asking an expression of opinion. The letter was referred to the Executive Committee, which reported, March 20th, recommending that the proposed reg-

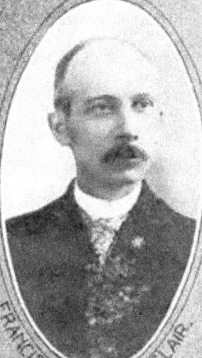

FRANCIS ALPHONSO ST.CLAIR.

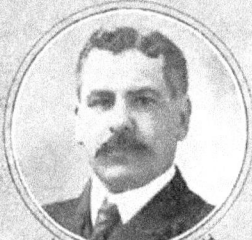

JOHN EDGAR WALSH

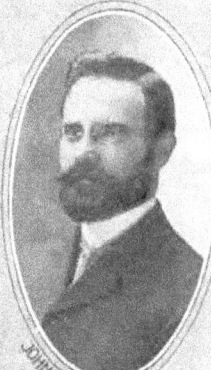

JOHNSON ELIOT JR.

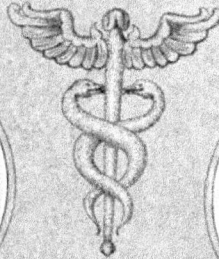

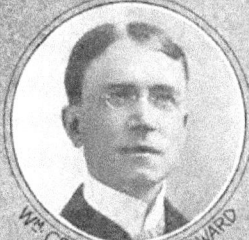

W.M CREIGHTON WOODWARD

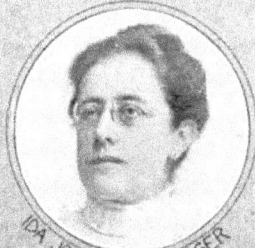

IDA JOHANNA HEIBERGER

1892

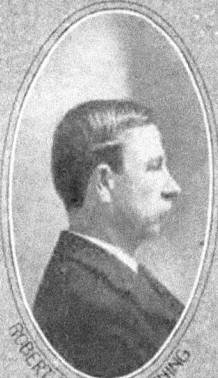

ROBERT EDMOND HENNING

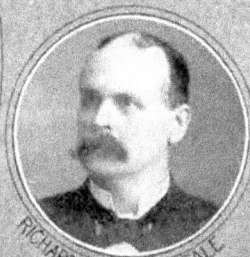

RICHARD ALOYSIUS NEALE

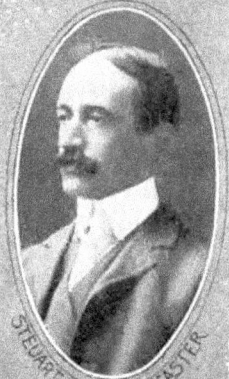

STEUART BROWN MUNCASTER

43

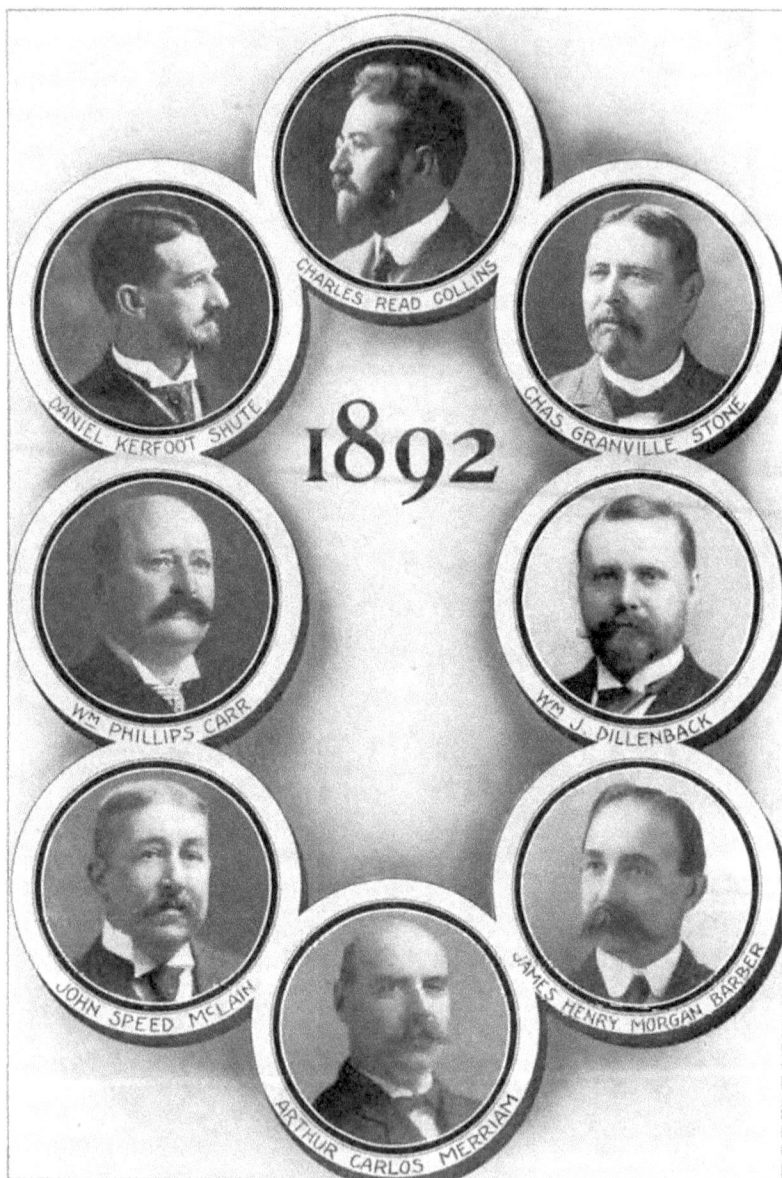

CHARLES READ COLLINS

DANIEL KERFOOT SHUTE

CHAS GRANVILLE STONE

1892

WM PHILLIPS CARR

WM J. DILLENBACK

JOHN SPEED McLAIN

JAMES HENRY MORGAN BARBER

ARTHUR CARLOS MERRIAM

ulations be endorsed by the Society, and the report was adopted.

December 18th, the Committee on Public Health made an elaborate report on these diseases, which was discussed, January 15 and 29, 1908.*

July 7, 1890, the Society ordered that thenceforward, immediately after the stated meeting in January, 500 copies of the list of members should be printed.

THE TESTIMONY OF PHYSICIANS IN COURT.

December 16, 1891, the retiring President, Dr. D. W. Prentiss, suggested that something should be done to protect the physician in giving testimony in court. March 2, 1892, Dr. Busey presented to the Society a form of bill relating thereto, which had been prepared by Dr. Z. T. Sowers.

March 16th, a committee, consisting of Drs. Lovejoy, Reyburn, A. F. A. King, Franzoni and G. Wythe Cook, was appointed to consider all the suggestions made by Dr. Prentiss. The committee reported, November 16th, and the report was discussed on the 23d. The bill recommended by the committee was amended to read as follows, and the Board of Examiners was instructed to put it in proper form and present it to Congress:

"An Act defining as privileged evidence in courts of law or equity a confidential communication of patients to their physicians.

"*Be it enacted by the Senate and House of Representatives in Congress assembled:* No physician authorized to practice medicine or surgery in the District of Columbia shall be allowed to disclose any information, which he may have acquired in attending any patient in a professional

*See ANNALS, VI, p. 496, and VII, p. 28.

character, and which information was necessary to enable him to prescribe for such patient as a physician or to do any act for him as a surgeon."

January 23, 1895, a second bill, drawn by Dr. Busey, was adopted by the Society and referred to the Committee on Legislation, with instructions to urge its passage by Congress:

"*Be it enacted by the Senate and House of Representatives of the United States in Congress assembled:* That in the courts of the District of Columbia no physician or surgeon shall be permitted, without the consent of the person affected, to disclose any information which he shall have acquired in attending a patient in a professional capacity and which was necessary to enable him to act in that capacity, whether such information shall have been obtained from the patient or from his family, or from the person or persons in charge of him : *Provided*, That this Act shall not apply to evidence in criminal cases where the accused is charged with causing the death of, or inflicting injuries upon a human being and the disclosures shall be required in the interests of public justice."

The bill (House Bill 2647) was passed and became a law May 26, 1896, without the signature of the President of the United States.*

THE ECLECTIC MEDICAL SOCIETY OF THE DISTRICT OF
COLUMBIA.

April 6, 1892, the Medical Society was informed that a bill to incorporate the Eclectic Medical Society of the District of Columbia had been reported to the Senate by the Committee on the District. This bill passed, and was approved February 18, 1893.

---

* Public Document No. 156. See Busey's " Souvenir," pp. 376 and 363, for his letter to the Commissioners in regard to this bill. See also *Nat. Med. Review*, 1896-7, VI, p. 9, which is a complete statement; also *Trans. Med. Society*, 1896, I, p. 9.

THE ICE TRUST.

April 5, 1893, the Society adopted the following:

"WHEREAS, The companies engaged in the business of supplying ice to the citizens of the District of Columbia have announced through the local press the formation of a combination of the several companies, in which they have agreed to suspend the delivery of ice on the Sabbath day to the retail consumers during the months of June, July, August and September; therefore be it

"*Resolved*, That a committee of five, of which the President and Recording Secretary shall be members, be appointed to consider what action, if any, this Society should take in relation thereto."

The committee consisted of the President, Dr. G. Wythe Cook; Secretary, Dr. S. S. Adams; and Drs. S. C. Busey, G. L. Magruder and L. Eliot. April 12th, the committee reported, taking the ground that the proposed suspension of delivery of ice on Sundays during the summer months would not only be an inconvenience to householders but detrimental to health, would add to the sufferings of the sick and to the morbidity and mortality of the city. The report was adopted. The Society also adopted the following:

"*Resolved*, That the Medical Society of the District of Columbia, in this effort to secure the continuous daily delivery of ice to the retail consumers during the heated months of the year, invites the support and coöperation of the Commissioners of the District of Columbia, the Health Officer, the local press, the Sanitary League and all other organizations and persons interested in the matter."

The Society ordered that 1,000 copies of the report should be printed and copies sent to the Attorney General of the United States, the District Attorney, the Commissioners of

the District, the Health Officer, the local press, the officers
of the Sanitary League, the presidents of the several ice
companies and the members of the Society.

THE FEEDING OF INFANTS.

June 7, 1893, the Secretary of the Society reported that
the Sanitary League of the District wanted information in
regard to the proper "feeding" of infants. A committee,
consisting of Drs. T. E. McArdle, S. S. Adams and J. D.
Morgan, was appointed to consider the matter. June 14th,
the committee reported* rules which applied especially to
the clothing and feeding of infants during the summer
months, and as they were for the benefit of the poor, the
simplest language possible was used. No reference was
made to pasteurizing milk, because it was impossible to
formulate such a rule in language that would be intelligi-
ble to the parents for whom the rules were made. The
committee said nothing about contagious diseases, because
the Health Officer issued regulations on that subject. The
report was adopted.

February 21, 1894, Dr. W. W. Johnston was requested
to ascertain the cost of a safe. Apparently nothing was
done about it. November 6, 1901, Drs. Johnston, G. L.
Magruder and E. L. Morgan were appointed a committee
on the same subject. January 6, 1902, the committee reported that it had found a safe that would answer the needs
of the Society. The committee was directed to buy it.

THE MEDICAL COLLEGE ACT.

March 7, 1894, the Society received from the Commissioners of the District of Columbia a copy of a bill to reg-

---

* See the report in full on page 128 of the minutes.

ulate medical colleges in the District.* The Society referred it to Drs. Lovejoy, A. F. A. King, H. H. Barker and D. S. Lamb, as representing the four medical schools in the District. March 21st, two reports were made, a majority report by Drs. Lovejoy, King and Lamb; a minority report by Dr. Barker.

Majority report: "WHEREAS, The Revised Statutes of the United States, known as the 'General Incorporation Act,' permits 'Any three or more persons of full age, citizens of the United States, a majority of whom shall be residents of the District, who desire to associate themselves for benevolent, charitable, educational, literary, musical, scientific, religious or missionary purposes, including societies for mutual improvement, or for the promotion of the arts, may make, sign and acknowledge before any officer authorized to take acknowledgment of deeds in the District, and file in the office of the Recorder of Deeds, to be recorded by him, a certificate in writing in which shall be stated, first, the name or title by which such society shall be known in law; second, the term for which it is organized; third, the particular business and objects of the society; fourth, the number of its trustees, directors or managers for the first year of its existence; and, fifth, whereas, the said Act does not seem to require the person so desiring to form an incorporation to produce evidence of proper qualifications and of the possession of the proper facilities for the carrying out of the objects proposed by them; and whereas, the science and art of medicine constitute a branch of knowledge of peculiar importance to the community, and there is no other occupation so necessary to the preservation of the health and well being of the people; therefore

"*Resolved*, first, that we hold it to be a matter of the utmost importance that the laws should throw around the study of medicine all the safeguards that are possible; that

---

* Senate Bill 1652; introduced into the Senate, February 19, 1894, and referred to the Committee on the District. Referred by this committee to the District Commissioners, and by these to the Medical Society, for such recommendations as it might wish to make.

our lawmakers should require that the persons professing to teach this science and art should themselves have acquired the ability to teach, by study, by practice and by experience, and should offer to their students the proper facilities to learn this important branch of knowledge and should protect a confiding and easily deceived public from the charlatanry and imposture of ignorant and selfish pretenders. *Resolved*, second, that we heartily endorse the apparent object of the bill, which seems to prevent the organization of medical colleges that may be incompetent to properly educate their students. *Resolved*, third, that we cannot endorse the method proposed by the bill of carrying out this object, which seems to be to empower the Honorable Commissioners of the District of Columbia to grant permits to such proposed colleges, under specific conditions. *Resolved*, fourth, that we recommend that the bill should provide that no medical college shall be incorporated without a special act of Congress. *Resolved*, fifth, that this Society has no knowledge of the source whence the proposed bill proceeded."*

This report was adopted by the Society. The minority report was as follows:

"I fully endorse and concur in the motives which have actuated the majority in their report, which are indicated in their preambles and first resolution, but I cannot view the present bill in the light in which it is viewed by them. I do not concur in the second resolution, for I fail to see anything in the bill which proposes to prevent the organization of incompetent medical colleges. The bill recognizes the fact that there are now or may be medical colleges in the District of Columbia incorporated by special act of Congress, but both creatures of Congress. It then declares that it shall be unlawful for those colleges incorporated in the latter manner to begin or continue business, except under certain restrictions, which are not imposed upon colleges incorporated in the former manner. This is class

* Dr. Busey in his " Souvenir," p. 375, states that the bill originated with the Homoeopathic Medical Society.

legislation, and being therefore unconstitutional cannot be commended, nor could its provisions be enforced if it were adopted. If the bill provided that all medical colleges should furnish evidence that they are fully equipped both by the character and fitness of their faculty and the sufficiency of their appliances, the above objections to the bill might have less force. But who are to decide upon the sufficiency of such evidence? the District Commissioners, composed of two lawyers and one engineer; certainly not such persons as would be considered experts upon medical colleges.

" The third resolution of the majority recognizes this fact and expresses our disapproval of such provisions of the bill as confer such powers upon the Commissioners. The adoption of this, the third resolution, by this Society will be a virtual condemnation of the entire bill, for if it is stripped of these provisions there is nothing left to it. The fourth resolution is open to the same objection urged against the original bill: that it contemplates class legislation and therefore cannot and will not be adopted by Congress. If Congress desires to prevent the future incorporation of medical colleges under the General Incorporation Act, it must strike out of that act the word "educational," or repeal the act.

" The fifth resolution seems to be in the nature of an apology to some one. If the Society must apologize for approving the bill it had better not approve it. I would therefore recommend that the bill be returned to the Commissioners, with the statement that in the opinion of the Society it does not throw proper safeguards around the method of medical education in the District of Columbia; and that the Commissioners be requested to urge in lieu of this bill the passage of the Medical Practice Act, with such provisions therein as will compel candidates for graduation in medicine to submit to an examination by the Board of Medical Examiners to be created by that act, before obtaining their diplomas. In conclusion I would urge upon the Society the impropriety of weakening whatever influence it may have with Congress by attempting to wet-nurse this sickly foundling. Rather let it reserve all its forces for a well-directed, systematic and persistent effort to secure the passage of the Medical Practice Act."

The bill passed both houses of Congress, and was approved May 4, 1896. [See Public Document 99. See also Busey's "Souvenir," page 375, where he says, "the act will prevent the multiplication of the class of bogus medical schools which have turned loose upon a credulous public so many ignorant frauds and venal charlatans. It is the beginning of the end of mills than grind out diplomas at so much per square inch of parchment."]

TUBERCULOSIS.

March 7, 1894, the attention of the Society was called to steps that were being taken in different cities to check the spread of tuberculosis. A committee, composed of Drs. C. H. Stowell, J. H. Bryan and E. A. Balloch, was appointed to examine into the question, and recommend what measures, if any, should be taken by the Society to stop the ravages of tuberculosis in the District of Columbia. May 9th, the committee made a report recommending that a committee be appointed to prepare a circular of instructions, to be popularly distributed, and setting forth the danger of communicating the disease by one person to another and how such communication might be prevented; that hospital authorities should be urged to set apart certain wards for consumptives, or, better, that special hospitals be built; that physicians should be requested to instruct their patients in regard to the disinfection of sputa, and that rooms occupied by consumptives should be disinfected; and that the Society should take steps toward the enactment of a law that would secure the purity of milk offered for sale in the District. An amendment was offered by Dr. T. E. McArdle requesting the Health Officer of the

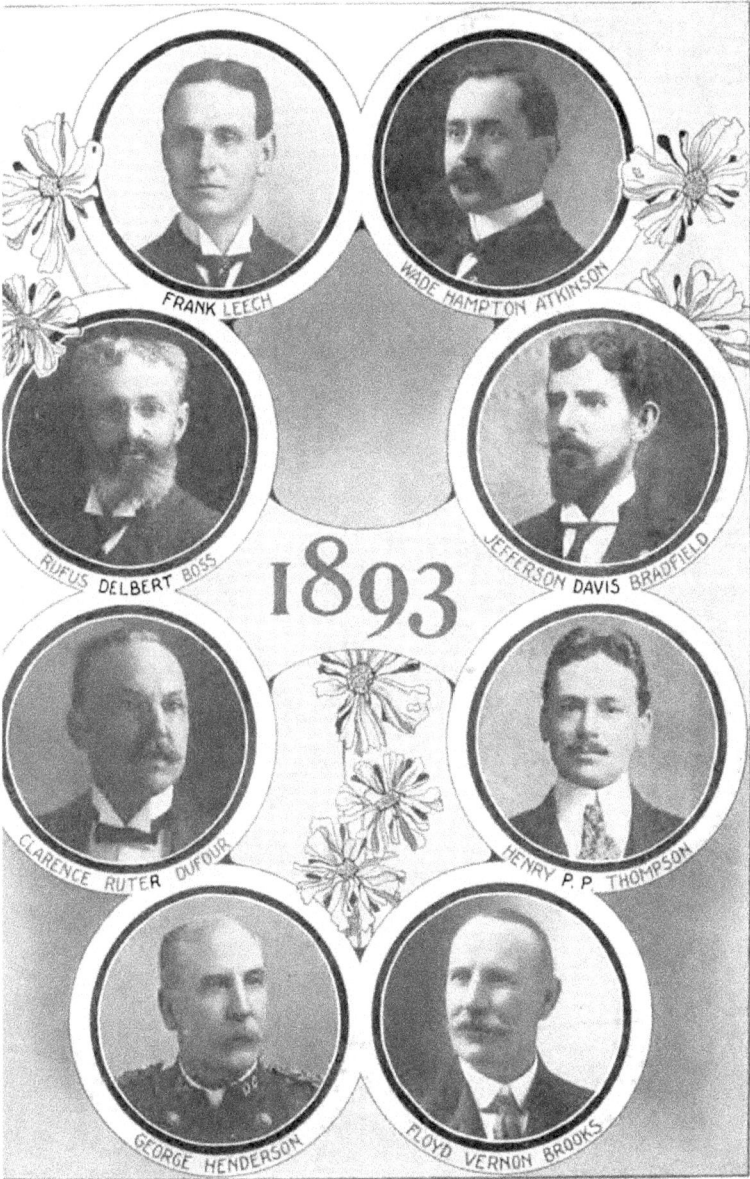

FRANK LEECH

WADE HAMPTON ATKINSON

RUFUS DELBERT BOSS

JEFFERSON DAVIS BRADFIELD

1893

CLARENCE RUTER DUFOUR

HENRY P. P. THOMPSON

GEORGE HENDERSON

FLOYD VERNON BROOKS

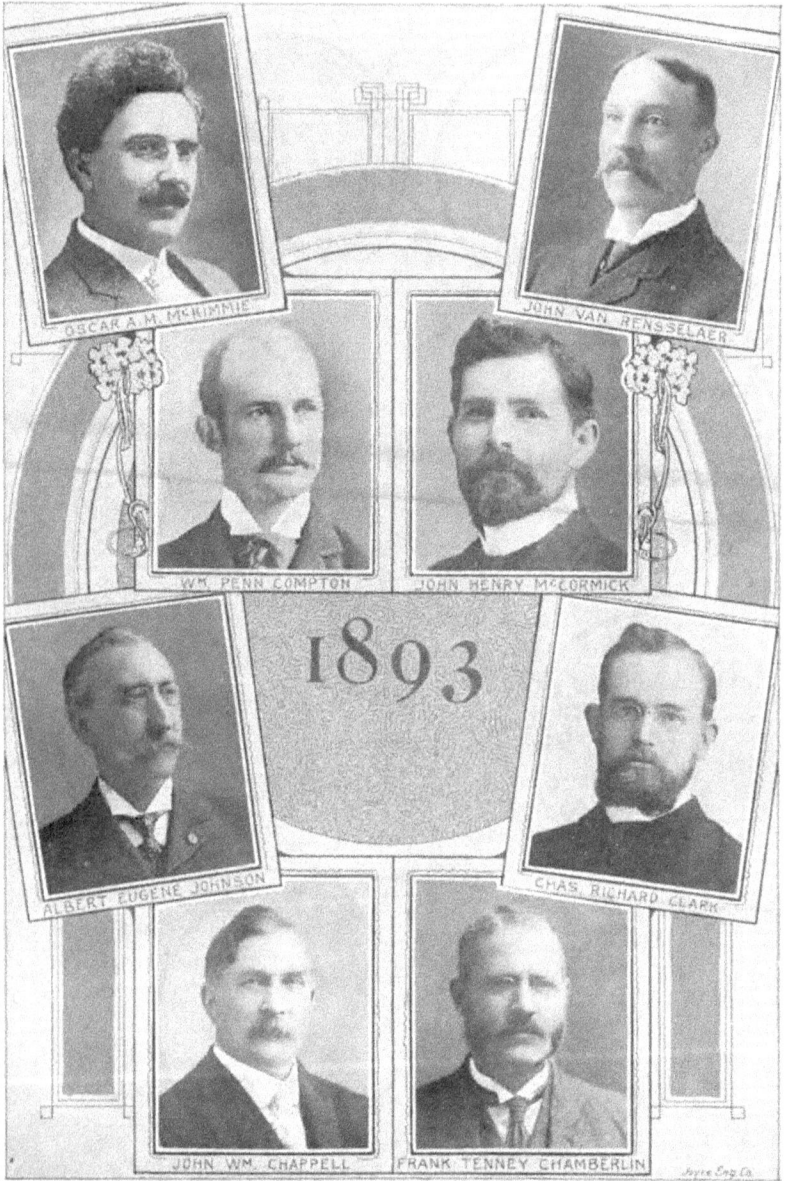

OSCAR A. M. McKIMMIE

JOHN VAN RENSSELAER

WM. PENN COMPTON

JOHN HENRY McCORMICK

1893

ALBERT EUGENE JOHNSON

CHAS. RICHARD CLARK

JOHN WM. CHAPPELL

FRANK TENNEY CHAMBERLIN

46

District to formulate such regulations as would assure the freedom of vaccine virus from tuberculous infection. May 16th, the report was exhaustively considered; June 6th, was further considered, and adopted, as also the amendment offered by Dr. McArdle.*

February 17, 1904, a letter from the Health Officer of the District in regard to physicians notifying that officer of cases of pulmonary tuberculosis coming under their care, was received by the Society, asking its opinion. The letter was referred to the Executive Committee, which, September 21st, reported unfavorably, but recommended that the Health Officer issue a circular of instructions in regard to the prophylaxis of the disease. The report was adopted by the Society November 30th. It may be mentioned here that October 26th there was a symposium on tuberculosis before the Society, in which Drs. W. C. Woodward, D. P. Hickling, A. F. A. King, W. P. Carr, General G. M. Sternberg, Frederick Sohon, S. S. Adams and T. A. Claytor took part.†

January 1, 1906, the Society endorsed the project of the District Commissioners for the erection of a hospital for consumptives.

March 7th, the Executive Committee made a report upon the registration of tuberculosis in the District of Columbia, and March 21st a committee—Drs. J. B. Nichols, S. Ruffin and J. D. Thomas—was appointed to prepare a bill for the legal supervision of tuberculosis in the District. The committee reported two bills, of which one entitled *B* was adopted by the Society, and the committee was instructed, March 28th, to take steps to secure its enactment by Congress.

---

* See *National Medical Review*, 1894-5, III, p. 60.
† See ANNALS, III, 1904-5, p. 145.

THE SOCIETY AND THE MILK SUPPLY OF THE DISTRICT OF COLUMBIA.*

The first record of any effort to control the milk supply of the District of Columbia was contained in an ordinance promulgated May 15, 1871, by the Board of Health created by the Act of February 21, 1871, reorganizing the government of the District. Repeated efforts were made by the District authorities between that date and 1894 to improve the conditions of the production and sale of milk, without accomplishing much of value. While preparing the report on typhoid fever in 1894 Dr. G. Lloyd Magruder had frequent conferences with the District Commissioners. The influence of milk as one of the most prominent causes of typhoid fever and the often-urged necessity for its careful supervision were promptly recognized. These facts so impressed the Committee on Typhoid Fever that the following recommendation was inserted in its report :

"Careful inspection of all dairies in the district from which our milk supply is drawn and the enactment of a law by which no milk shall be sold in the District without a permit from the Health Officer. The inspection should cover an examination at the dairies of all possible sources of infection, including the water supply."

At Dr. Magruder's suggestion the District Commissioners sought the aid of the Medical Society to secure the much-needed legislation along the lines above indicated. In compliance with this suggestion, June 6, 1894, the Society received a communication from the Commissioners enclosing the draft of a bill to regulate the milk supply and to secure pure milk. In this communication the Society was asked to perfect the bill.

---

* This article was partly prepared by Dr. G. Lloyd Magruder.

The Society appointed Drs. Kleinschmidt, S. S. Adams and Woodward a committee to consider the bill and return it, amended, to the Commissioners.* The committee reported June 13th.

February 6, 1895, the Committee on Legislation reported that the bill had been so much altered in the Senate Committee that it was worse than none, and the Legislative Committee had entered a protest. The Society approved the protest. The House bill (8231), as endorsed by the Society and Commissioners, passed the House of Representatives. February 27th, the Society was informed that the bill was in conference. It passed and was approved, March 2d.†

The influence of the Society was a most potent factor in securing this legislation, which required the inspection of the dairy farms and a permit from the Health Officer before milk could be shipped to this city. This made Washington one of the first cities in the United States to require such a permit. It appears justifiable to claim that this law has largely contributed towards saving many lives of children under one year old. In 1894, previous to the passage of the law, the death rate was 5.70 per 1,000 of the entire population; in 1905, ten years afterwards, the death rate was 3.52 per 1,000.

October 20, 1897, Dr. S. S. Adams presented a plan for the establishment of a milk laboratory, and a committee—Drs. Kober, E. A. de Schweinitz and Adams—was appointed, to have a general supervision over the same and report from time to time to the Society. January 12, 1898, the committee made an elaborate report.‡ March 1, 1899, it made a report for the previous year.§

* See Minutes, page 194. *National Med. Rev.*, 1894-5, III, p. 85.

† See Busey's "Annual Addresses," pp. 41 and 65; Minutes of Society, pp. 52-70.

‡ See Minutes of the Society, pp, 10-17; *Trans. Med. Society*, 1898, III, p. 64; *Nat. Med. Review*, 1898-9, VIII, p. 152.

§ See *Trans. Med. Society*, 1899, IV, p. 36; *Nat. Med. Review*, 1898-9, VIII, p. 483.

January 7, 1901, a bill (Senate Bill 4804) was introduced in Congress, regulating the production and sale of milk in the District of Columbia. There was also a report (Report 1665) from the Senate District Committee, June 5, 1900. March 5, 1902, the Society endorsed the Senate bill (1686, House 11,005) for the regulation, production, etc., and instructed the Executive Committee of the Society to try to secure its passage.

April 29, 1903, the Committee on Laboratory (Walker-Gordon Laboratory) recommended a Milk Commission like those in New York City and other cities, with the object of securing careful daily inspection of milk delivered in the city, by competent veterinarians appointed for the purpose. The Society endorsed the plan.* May 20th, the commission was appointed—Drs. Adams, de Schweinitz, McCormick, Sprigg and Woodward.

July 7th, the commission reported that it had organized and incorporated, that all dairymen would have an equal chance before the commission, and that scientific experts would be employed to make the necessary examination of the milk supply. October 7th, the commission made another report.†

March 30, 1904, House Bill 14,473, supplementary to an act to regulate the sale of milk in the District, was presented to the Society and referred to the Executive Committee.

July 4th, the Milk Commission reported again and for the last time.‡

April 24, 1895, the Society was informed that Dr. Busey had dedicated his " Personal Reminiscences" to the Society, and members could procure copies with the author's compliments by calling at his residence.

---

*ANNALS, 1903-4, II, p. 267.
† See ANNALS, 1903-4, II, pp. 251 and 490.
‡ See ANNALS, III, 1904-5, p. 280.

VIVISECTION.

A bill, popularly known as the anti-vivisection bill (Senate Bill 1552, for the further prevention of cruelty to animals in the District of Columbia), was introduced in the U. S. Senate, and January 22, 1896, this fact was reported to the Society and the Committee on Legislation was instructed to oppose the bill. April 22d, the Society adopted a "memorial" against the bill.* May 26th, the Senate Committee on the District reported the bill with amendments (Report No. 1049, Calendar No. 1144).

October 7th, the Society adopted the following resolutions :

"The Medical Society of the District of Columbia hereby invites the bureaus, departments, schools of medicine and scientific societies hereafter named to unite with it in the organization of a commission to be constituted of one representative from each of such bureaus, departments, schools of medicine and scientific societies, which shall be known as the 'Joint Commission on Vivisection,' charged with the duty of investigating the practice of animal experimentation in this District and representation of the constituent organizations before Congress in such manner as said commission may determine.

" 2d. That this invitation be extended to the Bureaus of Medicine and Surgery of the Army, Navy and Marine Hospital Service and Animal Industry, the Medical Departments of the Columbian, Georgetown, Howard and National Universities, and to the Chemical, Biological, Anthropological, Entomological and Philosophical Societies of the District of Columbia.

" 3d. That the expense of the Joint Commission shall be defrayed in equal proportion by each bureau, department, school and society represented in said Joint Commission.

* This memorial is printed in Senate Report No. 1049, Calendar No. 1144, p. 128 ; also in the *National Medical Review*, 1896-7, I, p. 14 ; also in *Trans. Med. Society*, 1896, I, p. 14.

"4th. The Corresponding Secretary is requested to transmit a copy of the preamble and resolutions to each of the bureaus, departments, schools and societies named and request their concurrence and the name and address of their representatives."

The resolutions were adopted. Dr. S. C. Busey was appointed to represent the Medical Society.

February 3, 1897, Dr. Busey stated that a movement had been made to have the medical societies of the several States organize committees to meet in Washington once a year to look after matters of interest to physicians and the passage of such bills as the American Medical Association might approve. February 17th, the Society decided to coöperate with this movement.

May 13th, the Senate Committee on the District reported favorably an anti-vivisection bill (1063); the bill was similar to 1552 of the previous session.

The attention of the Society was next called to the matter December 6, 1899, when it was informed that a new bill on the subject (Senate, 34) had been introduced and referred.

February 21, 1900, Dr. W. C. Woodward reported to the Society an analysis of the arguments on vivisection ; the Society approved the same, and ordered that a copy be sent to the Senate Committee on the District.*

[The subject has not since been brought to the attention of the Society. Anti-vivisection bills have continued to be introduced in Congress, but none have passed. The work of the Joint Commission itself may be summarized as follows :

[The Commission met November 23 and December 18, 1896, and January 23, 1897. Dr. Busey was elected Chairman, Dr. D. S. Lamb, Secretary, and Dr. G. M. Sternberg,

---

* See Senate Document 337 ; a hearing before the Committee, February 21, 1900.

Treasurer. The members of the commission were : Drs. S. C. Busey, representing the Medical Society ; Walter Reed, the U. S. Army ; D. V. Salmon, the Bureau of Animal Industry ; E. A. de Schweinitz, Medical Department Columbian University ; C. W. Stiles, Georgetown University ; R. Reyburn and D. S. Lamb, Howard University ; W. M. Sprigg, National University ; H. N. Stokes, the Chemical Society ; G. M. Sternberg, the Biological Society ; Frank Baker, the Anthropological Society. The Navy and Marine Hospital Service were not then represented. Later Dr. M. J. Rosenau, of the Marine Hospital Service, was added.

[Drs. Sternberg, Salmon and Stiles were appointed a committee to prepare an appropriate reply to the Senate report. General Sternberg offered to admit to the Army Medical Laboratory any one interested in seeing the work done there.*

[At the meeting, March 30th, General Sternberg was directed to prepare a letter to the Senate District Committee asking that before any legislation was enacted there should be an investigation of the charges of cruelty. Dr. Busey was directed to try to interest the Amer. Med. Assn. and induce it to appoint a committee to assist in opposing the bill. He stated that the State Medical Societies of New York and Ohio had each resolved to appoint a committee to attend during the session of Congress and influence legislation in medical matters.

[At the meeting, May 18th, Dr. Busey stated that the Congress of American Physicians and Surgeons at its recent meeting had appointed a committee to take suitable action. Drs. Salmon, Sternberg and Baker were appointed a committee to prepare a protest against bill 1063.†

[At the meeting, November 12, 1898, Dr. Busey stated that the American Humane Society would meet in Washington in December and would consider the regulation of vivisection in the District. The Commission directed the Secretary to call the attention of the prominent medical and scientific journals of the country to the meeting of the

---

* See Document 31 to accompany Report 1049, Senate Bill 1552.

† See Document 104, Senate, January 31, 1898.

American Humane Society and request that editorial notice be taken of the danger that the influence likely to be exerted at that meeting might cause the vivisection bill pending in the Senate to be called up and passed.

[January 9, 1902, the Commission had another meeting; Dr. Busey having died, Dr. G. N. Acker represented the Medical Society; Drs. W. W. Johnston and G. M. Kober were also added to the Commission, and Dr. Kober was elected Chairman. The meeting was called because another anti-vivisection bill had been introduced into the Senate and it was desirable to secure a hearing. Accordingly a letter asking such a hearing was prepared and sent to the Senate Committee.

[No further meetings have been held.—D. S. LAMB.]

May 6, 1896, the Society contributed $100 to the fund for the " Pasteur" monument.

THE EYES OF SCHOOL CHILDREN.

June 3, 1896, the Society appointed a committee to report upon the advisability of a systematic examination of the eyes of school children in the District; Drs. C. R. Dufour, E. O. Belt and I. Bermann were the committee. June 10th, the committee reported that it believed the welfare of the school children required such examination, and the matter should be brought to the attention of the trustees of the schools. The committee found that a large majority of the children suffered from lack of visual acuity, but did not know it. An examination made yearly would reveal all ocular troubles and give the opportunity to have them corrected. The committee was recommended by the Society to wait upon the trustees and urge the adoption of such regulations as would secure such examination; the committee to coöperate with the trustees.

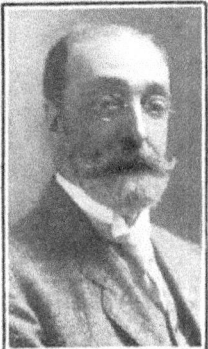

CHAS. VOLNEY PETTEYS

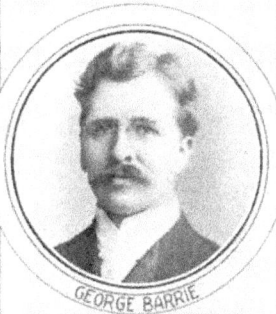

GEORGE BARRIE

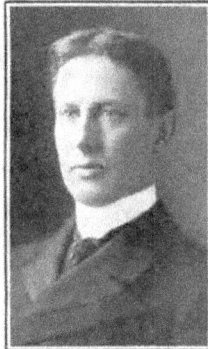

STERLING RUFFIN

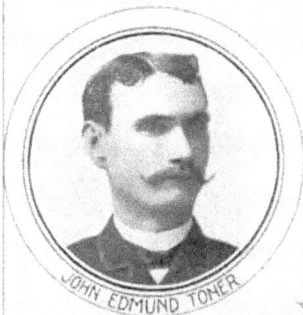

JOHN EDMUND TONER

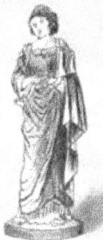

ΥΓΙΕΙΑ

1894

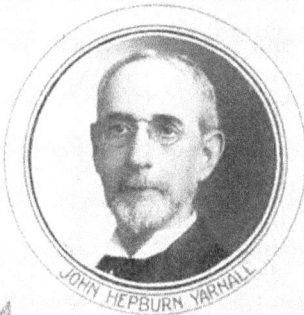

JOHN HEPBURN YARNALL

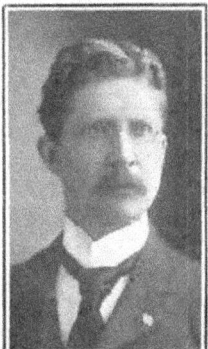

WM. LITTLETON ROBINS

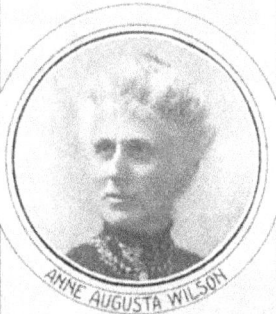

ANNE AUGUSTA WILSON

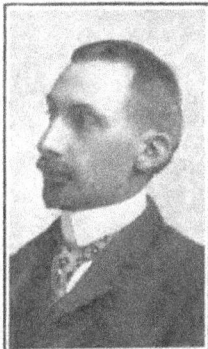

PRESLEY CRAIG HUNT

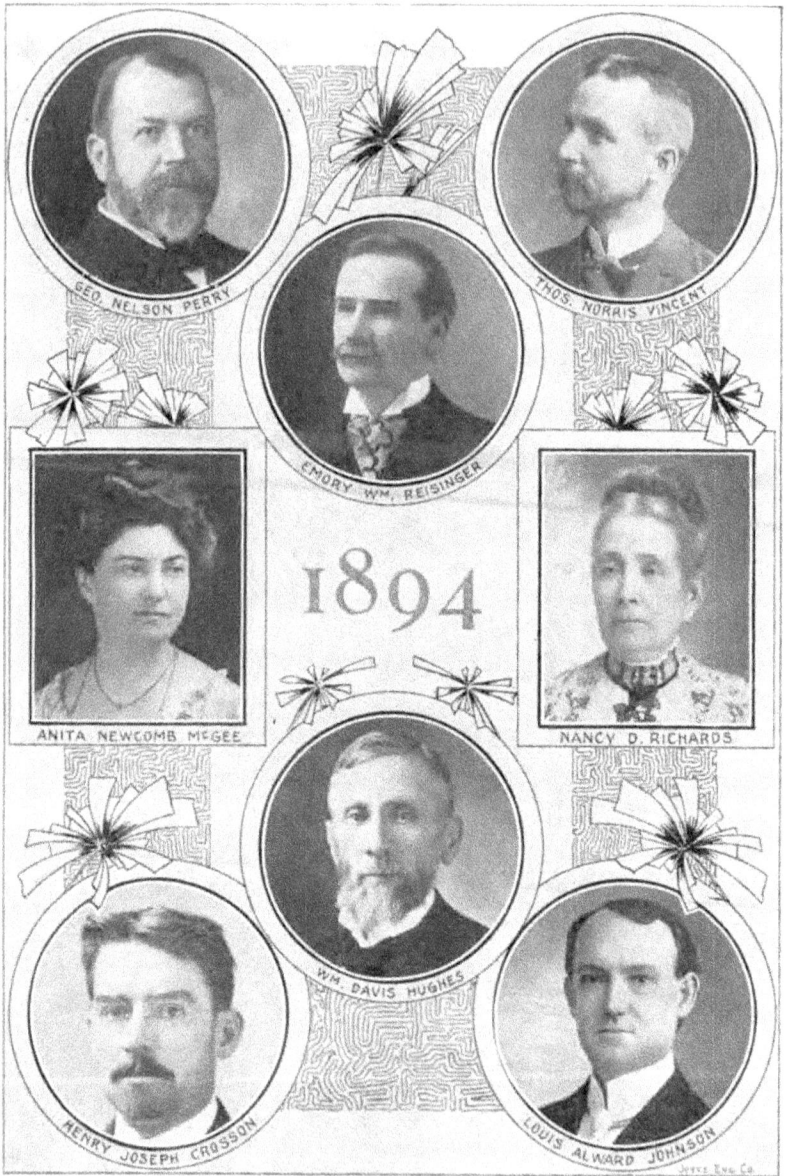

GEO. NELSON PERRY

THOS. NORRIS VINCENT

EMORY WM. REISINGER

1894

ANITA NEWCOMB McGEE

NANCY D. RICHARDS

WM. DAVIS HUGHES

HENRY JOSEPH CROSSON

LOUIS ALWARD JOHNSON

48

PURE FOOD AND DRUGS IN THE DISTRICT OF COLUMBIA.

January 4, 1897, the Committee on Legislation presented to the Society a bill (House Bill 9842), which had passed the House of Representatives, in regard to the adulteration of food and drugs. The Society approved the bill and instructed the committee to urge its passage in the Senate.

February 9, 1898, Drs. G. N. Acker and L. W. Glazebrook were appointed by the Society delegates to the Pure Food Congress, and Drs. G. M. Kober and G. Wythe Cook members of the Advisory Committee of the Congress.

November 8th, five delegates were appointed by the Society to the next succeeding Food Congress, namely, Drs. Z. T. Sowers, W. W. Johnston, C. H. A. Kleinschmidt, G. L. Magruder and G. M. Kober.*

April 18, 1900, the Society adopted resolutions to the effect that the interests of medical science required the establishment of a Bureau of Materia Medica in order to institute disinterested investigation into the character and value of new drugs. The Society recommended to the Decennial Committee of 1900 on the revision of the Pharmacopœia the creation of such a bureau under its authority.

January 14, 1903, the Executive Committee of the Society made a report to the Society† which stated that a bill had been passed by the House of Representatives that prejudiced the results of all the work that the Society had done toward securing purity of food and drugs, including milk, in this District. The committee asked that the Society endorse a protest that it had made against the pas-

---

* December 18, 1899, a bill was introduced in the House (House Bill 4618) to establish a Food Bureau in the Agricultural Department. January 3, 1900, a bill (Senate Bill 2050) was introduced into the Senate; January 8, another (Senate Bill 2222); March 5th, still another (Senate Bill 3618), and December 18th, still another (Senate Bill 5262). In the House a report was made (Report No. 1426).

† See WASH. MED. ANNALS, 1903-4, II, p. 54.

sage of the bill. The Society approved the action of the committee.

January 27, 1904, the Executive Committee reported that there were two bills (Senate, 198, and House, 6295,) pending, the object of which was to prevent the adulteration of food, drugs, etc., but that the House bill was objectionable. The Society instructed the committee to favor the Senate bill.

March 14, 1906, the Society approved Senate Bill 88, Pure Food and Drugs. The bill passed June 30th.* October 3d, the Executive Committee was instructed to consider what effect, if any, the so-called Pure Food and Drugs Act would have on the practice of medicine in this District. It does not appear that the committee made any report.

THE OPIUM HABIT.

January 20, 1897, a letter was read to the Society stating that a committee of The Medical and Surgical Society of the District of Columbia had investigated the extent of the opium habit in Washington and had made a report. A copy of this report was transmitted to the Medical Society and was referred by it to its Committee on Legislation; this committee forwarded the report to Congress, by which it was printed as Senate Document 74 and introduced into the Senate, January 21st, and referred to the District Committee. The report was considered in connection with House Bill No. 10,038 (Senate Bill 3575), regulating the sale of poisons. The House bill having passed, the Society, April 7th, ordered a memorial favoring the bill.†

March 30, 1898, the Society became a constituent member of the Washington Academy of Sciences, and Drs. D. S. Lamb, G. M. Kober and S. M. Burnett were appointed

* See Statutes, U. S., 1905–6, chap. 3915.
† See Senate Document 15, 1897.

a committee to make nominations of members of the Society to membership in the Academy.

April 20, 1898, a joint meeting of the Washington Anthropological Society and Medical Society was held at the room of the latter, at which the subject of "Treatment and Education of the Deaf" was discussed. Papers were read by Drs. Frank Baker, R. Reyburn, E. M. Gallaudet and D. S. Lamb.

May 4th, the Committee on Public Health was requested to investigate and report on the plumbing regulations of the District, with regard to the use of lead pipes in the water-supply service, and to especially consider the question of the danger of lead poisoning.

May 11th, the Society requested the delegates from the District of Columbia to the American Medical Association to coöperate with the other delegates in organizing a Committee on National Legislation.

April 26, 1899, there was another joint meeting of the Washington Anthropological Society and Medical Society at the room of the latter. The subject was "The Effects of Modern Firearms in War." Papers were read by Dr. G. M. Kober and three medical officers of the U. S. Army—Drs. L. A. La Garde, W. C. Borden and E. L. Munson.

May 3, 1899, a letter was received from M. P. Key, suggesting that the Society make a study of the subject of longevity in connection with the announced World's Fair in Paris, 1900. A committee was appointed by the Society, consisting of Drs. Z. T. Sowers, W. W. Johnston and G. M. Kober, to consider the matter and report. May 31st, the committee made a partial report, which was accepted.* The complete report was published in *Trans. Med. Society*, V, 1900, page 1.

---

*Nat. Med. Rev., 1899–1900, IX, pp. 365, 647.

THE SOCIETY AND THE HEALTH OF SCHOOL CHILDREN.

October 4, 1899, the Committee on Public Health made a report in regard to the health of children in the public schools of the District of Columbia. On the 11th, the Society appointed a committee of 76 members, auxiliary to the Committee on Public Health, to assist in the investigation into the health of these children.* Some objection was made to the published report, and March 10, 1900, the Committee on Public Health made another report,† and June 13th still another report.

CODIFICATION OF THE LAWS OF THE DISTRICT OF COLUMBIA.

December 13, 1899, the Committee on Legislation reported that December 11th a letter had been sent to A. S. Worthington, Esq., the Chairman of the Committee of the Bar Association on the District Code,‡ protesting against some proposed changes in the code.

February 28, 1900, the Committee on Legislation reported to the Society that it had collected certain laws relating to the health of the District, and submitted them to the Bar Association with the understanding that they would be included in the code.

May 16th, the Society ordered that a protest be sent to the U. S. Senate against the amendments to Senate Bill 3812, which amended the law in regard to the testimony of physicians ; also against section 1636 of the code which repealed the charter of the Society and the act regulating

---

* See *Trans. Med. Society*, IV, 1899, p. 135, for report of committee.

† See *Trans. Med. Society*, V, 1900, p. 43, and *Nat. Med. Rev.*, 1900-1, X, pp. 99 and 431.

‡ See Senate Bill 5530, Fifty-fifth Congress ; Minutes of Society, pp. 345-9 ; *Trans. Society*, 1899, IV, pp. 212-4 ; *Nat. Med. Review*, 1899-1900, IX, p. 596.

the practice of medicine in the District of Columbia, and all health and sanitary regulations.*

October 3d, letters were read in regard to the proposed code, stating that it repealed the Medical College Act and other matters of interest to the medical profession. The letters were referred to the Committee on Legislation.†

December 12th, the Committee on Legislation submitted the correspondence, including the letters of Dr. G. Wythe Cook of December 7th, as chairman of the committee, to Ashley M. Gould, Esq., of the Bar Association, relating to Senate Bill 3812, and December 8th, and Gould's reply of this date.‡

March 13, 1901, the Society was notified that the " Code bill" had passed Congress and had become a law.

March 24, 1900, the District Commissioners referred Senate Bill 3424, Fifty-sixth Congress, First Session, to the Society, for remark. The bill was entitled " For the regulation of scientific experiments upon human beings in the District of Columbia," and had been introduced into the Senate March 2d. March 28th, the matter came before the Society and was referred to the Committee on Legislation. The committee reported, April 4th ; the report was approved by the Society and ordered to be forwarded to the Commissioners. It took the ground that the bill was unnecessary and, if enacted, would be harmful.§ The bill failed to pass.

April 11, 1900, the Society directed the Committee on Public Health to inquire into the subject of hydrophobia and make report. The committee made a report, June 13th, recommending that all dogs appearing on the streets

---

* See *Trans. Society*, 1900,V, p. 94 ; *National Medical Review*, 1900-1, X, p. 270.
† *National Medical Review*, 1899–1900, IX, p. 495.
‡ See Public Document 159.
§ See *Trans.*, V, 1900, p. 65 ; *Nat. Med. Review*, X, 1900-1, p. 201.

and highways be required to be muzzled; that owners be held liable for damage done by their dogs; that the pound-master take up and destroy all dogs not so muzzled, etc. The report and recommendations were adopted and the committee directed to send copies to the District Commissioners, to the Senate Committee on the District of Columbia, to the public press and the Marine Hospital Service.*

October 3d, a letter was read from the National Association for the Study of Epilepsy, asking the Society to appoint a committee to ascertain the number and condition of epileptics under public' care in the District of Columbia. The letter was referred to the Committee on Public Health.

The same evening a letter was read from the Committee on Revision of the Pharmacopœia of 1900, requesting the Society to recommend what substances and preparations should be dropped from or added to its new Pharmacopœia. The Society appointed a committee, consisting of Drs. F. P. Morgan, G. J. Lochboehler, W. M. Sprigg, J. E. Brackett and S. E. Lewis, to consider the matter. November 7th, the committee reported a list of substances recommended to be dropped, and the report was accepted November 14th.†

January 23, 1901, the Society appointed Dr. H. L. E. Johnson a delegate to the Pan American Congress.

SPITTING IN PUBLIC.

May 29, 1901, the Committee on Public Health reported to the Society the following resolution: " Spitting upon paved sidewalks creates a nuisance dangerous to health,

---

* See Bull. 25, 1900, Dept. Agriculture ; *Trans. Med. Society*, V, 1900, p. 135; *Nat. Med. Review*, 1900-1, X, p. 431.

† See *Trans. Med. Society*, V, 1900, p. 201.

and should be forbidden by law." The resolution was adopted.

March 18, 1903, the same committee reported the following resolutions, which were adopted by the Society:

"*Resolved*, That the Committee on Public Health is hereby authorized to use the best efforts to obtain the enactment of the law which should prohibit the spitting upon the sidewalks by persons in the District. *Resolved*, That the Medical Society of the District endorse the proposed action of the Honorable Commissioners of the District in promulgating a public regulation which shall prohibit the spitting upon the sidewalks by persons of the District."

MEDICAL INSPECTION OF SCHOOLS IN THE DISTRICT OF COLUMBIA.

June 5, 1901, Dr. D. S. Lamb read a paper on "The Medical Inspection of Schools," which was referred to the Committee on Public Health, with instructions to prepare a plan of inspection. The committee reported, December 4th,* and its report was referred to the Committee on Legislation. This committee, however, had already considered the report and promptly made thereon its own report,† and recommendations, which were adopted by the Society, and the Committee on Legislation was instructed, January 6, 1902,‡ to forward a copy of the report to the District Commissioners, Board of Education, D. C., and to Congress, and use all proper efforts to secure legislation providing for such inspection. January 14, 1903, the Executive Committee reported§ that it had communicated with the Committee on Appropriations of the House of Repre-

---

* See *Trans. Med. Society*, VI, 1901, p. 304.
† *Trans.*, VI, 1901, p. 315.
‡ WASH. MED. ANNALS, 1902, I, p. 79.
§ WASH. MED. ANNALS, 1903-4, II, p. 54.

sentatives, urging the establishment of such inspection under the supervision of the Health Department. An appropriation was made, taking effect July 1, 1903.

PSYCHO–PHYSICAL LABORATORY.

October 30, 1901, the Society adopted a resolution favoring the establishment of a psycho-physical laboratory·in Washington, in the Department of the Interior, for the study of the physiology and psychology of man, with the view of applying the resulting knowledge to the problems of sociology and jurisprudence. The resolution further stated that the scientific study of criminals of the pauper degenerate classes in an institution would tend to settle many vexed questions as to their proper management and control; that such study could emanate only from a laboratory fitted with instruments of precision. The study of precocity and defective mental conditions in children would be of great service in determining the best methods for their rearing and education. February 3, 1904, a letter was read from Dr. Arthur McDonald, asking the further coöperation of the Society in securing the passage of the bill to establish the laboratory. The letter was referred to the Executive Committee.

THE INSANE OF THE DISTRICT OF COLUMBIA.

December 4, 1901, the Society instructed the Committee on Legislation to take action towards securing the enactment of a law providing for the detention of alleged lunatics pending formal adjudication of the question of lunacy, when such lunatics were believed to be dangerous and their environment militated against recovery; also the appointment of trustees to take charge of the property of persons incompetent from the drug habit.

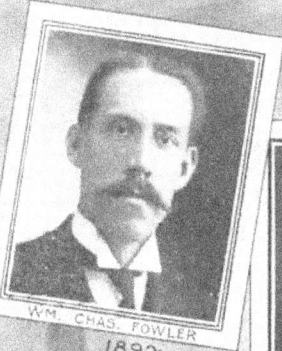

WM. CHAS. FOWLER
1892

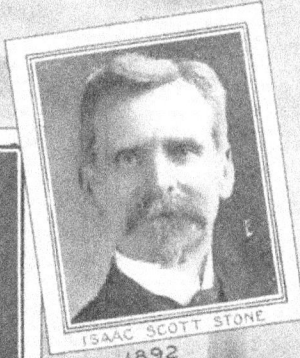

WILFRED MASON BARTON
1895

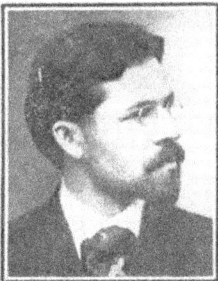

ISAAC SCOTT STONE
1892

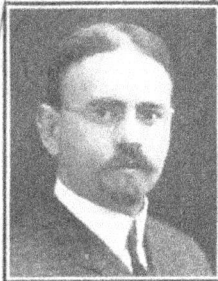

JOHN ALBERTSON STOUTENBURGH
1894

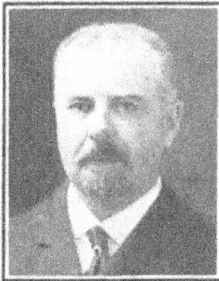

JOHN RYDER WELLINGTON
1894

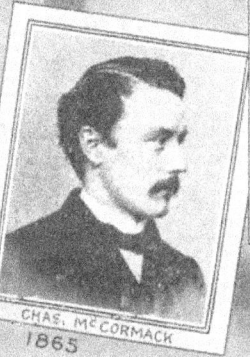

CHAS. McCORMACK
1865

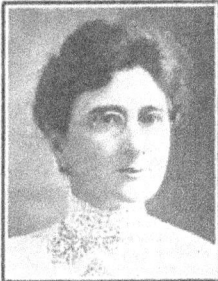

PHOEBE RUSSELL NORRIS
1896

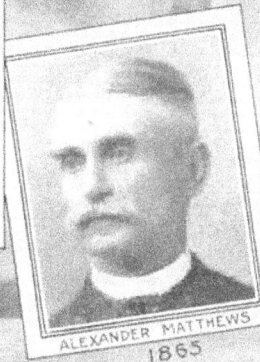

ALEXANDER MATTHEWS
1865

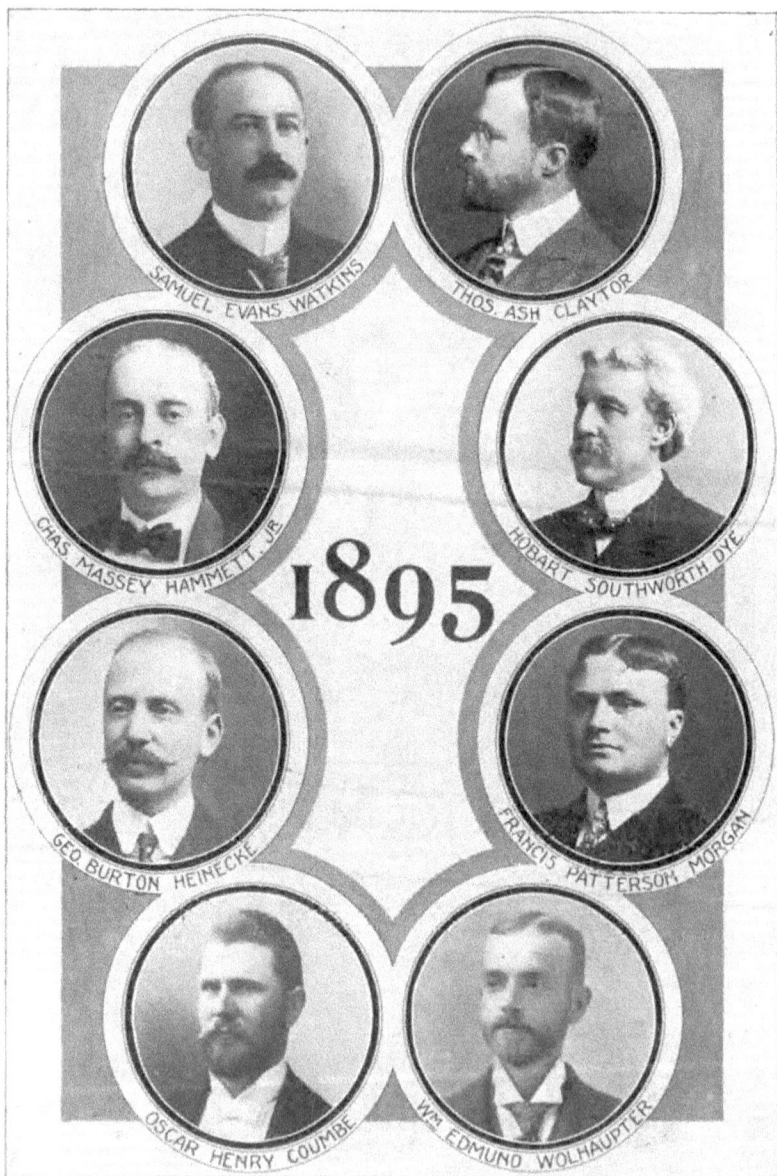

SAMUEL EVANS WATKINS

THOS. ASH CLAYTOR

CHAS. MASSEY HAMMETT, JR.

HOBART SOUTHWORTH DYE

1895

GEO. BURTON HEINECKE

FRANCIS PATTERSON MORGAN

OSCAR HENRY COUMBE

WM. EDMUND WOLHAUPTER

50

January 27, 1904, the Executive Committee reported two bills (Senate 2880, House 8692) for the apprehension and detention of the insane, and stated that the bills should be amended. The Society instructed the committee to try to secure the desired amendments.

January 17, 1906, a letter from the Secretary of the Interior was read, asking the coöperation of the Society in his efforts to secure the passage of a bill amending the laws regulating commitments of the insane. The letter was referred to the Executive Committee.

THE EXECUTIVE COMMITTEE OF THE SOCIETY.

An Executive Committee was provided for by the Society, January 8, 1902, to replace the Committee on Legislation. Its duties were—

" To keep informed in all matters concerning the interests of the medical profession generally and of the Society and its members in particular ; to consider such resolutions as may be referred to it by the Society ; to suggest improvements in the conduct of the business of the Society; to consider and report upon matters requiring legislative action ; to represent the Society before Congress and the Commissioners of the District of Columbia, and to report its operations to the Society from time to time, as occasion may require, together with such recommendations as it may deem proper."

The committee went promptly to work, and until 1908 gave its attention to many matters that were referred to it by the Society. Subcommittees were formed, to which subjects for inquiry were referred. The committee communicated at intervals with the committees of the U. S. Senate and House of Representatives in regard to legislation, especially with the Committees on Appropriations

13

and the District of Columbia; also with the Commissioners of the District and with officers of the executive departments of the U. S. Government. From time to time members of the committee attended "hearings" before the bodies and persons indicated, for the purpose of securing or opposing legislation. Altogether, the Executive Committee has done much and excellent work, the extent and scope of which are almost unknown to the members of the Society other than those who have been members of the committee.

The most important subjects considered by the committee have been as follows:

1902—February 19th—Recommended the Society to authorize a prize essay and rules in regard thereto.

Recommended the publication of a journal of the Society and some conditions therefor.

In regard to the proposed municipal hospital.

March 5th—In regard to the condemnation of insanitary buildings.

The production and sale of milk and cream in the District of Columbia.

That the initiation fee for membership should be reduced to $5.00.

Recommended approval of certain recommendations of the Auditing Committee.

That one Wednesday evening in the month should be devoted to pathological specimens.

That meetings should begin promptly at 8 o'clock.

That papers should be discussed the same evening that they are read.

Protesting against a certain bill in Congress (Senate 190) to prevent cruelty to animals in the District of Columbia.

Against a bill (Senate 3068) to regulate scientific experiments on human beings in the District of Columbia.

March 22d—Urged appropriation to complete filter plant.

April 2d—In regard to the proposed consolidation of the medical work of the government of the District of Columbia.

April 16th—Report on bill to regulate sale of serums, etc., in the District of Columbia.

May 8th—Medical inspection of schools.

June 11th—In regard to Maryland physicians practicing in the District of Columbia.

November 11th—In regard to the filtration plant.

November 19th—Report on certain legislation authorizing appointment of guardians for property of persons addicted to use of opium, etc.

In regard to promotion of anatomical science.

1903—January 14th—Report in regard to manufacture and sale of adulterated food and drugs.

January 13th—In regard to medical inspection of schools.

In regard to a certain prize essay.

January 29th—In regard to accessibility of records of births and deaths in the Health Department, D. C.

January 30th—In regard to the filtration plant; mechanical filtration.

Medical inspection of schools.

February 1st and 18th—Report on the minor contagious diseases.

In regard to a complimentary dinner to Charles Moore.

March 11th—In regard to inspection of food in the District of Columbia.

In regard to commitment of lunatics in the District of Columbia.

March 18th—In regard to having a reference library in the Public Library, D. C.

November 4th—Proposed change in counting votes in the Society.

November 18th—The Milk Commission.

1904—January 27th—In regard to the adulteration, mis-branding and imitation of foods, beverages, candies, drugs and condiments in the District of Columbia.

In regard to the abatement of nuisances in the District of Columbia.

Apprehension and detention of insane persons in the District of Columbia.

Condemnation of insanitary buildings in the District of Columbia.

In regard to the commission to examine into the sanitary condition of the U. S. Government Departments.

The prevention of communicable diseases in the District of Columbia.

In regard to physicians to the poor.

February 24th—In regard to the registration of physicians in the District of Columbia.

In regard to the issuance of patents covering operations on the human body or methods to be employed in operations.

March 6th—Legislation on tuberculosis in the District of Columbia.

1905—November 8th—To control the pollution of the Potomac water.

In regard to the pharmacy and poison law.

1906—January 10th—Endorsing the efforts of the Commissioners of the District of Columbia to secure an appropriation for erection of hospital for consumptives.

Recommending that the proper representatives of the Society join the Association of State Medical Journals.

January 17th—Recommending that the Society meet at the Columbian University.

In regard to preliminary steps toward preventing pollution of interstate streams.

March 16th—Legislation in regard to the insane of the District of Columbia.

May 9th—Memorial protesting against passage of bill to regulate practice of osteopathy in the District of Columbia.

December 5th—Report of action of committee on osteopathic bill.

1907—January 7th—In regard to the reclamation of the Anacostia flats.

In regard to the American Medical Union.

January 23d—In regard to regulation of production and sale of milk in District of Columbia.

February 20th—In regard to the osteopathic bill.

March 20th—Thanking Dr. G. L. Magruder for his work in regard to the milk supply in the District of Columbia.

In regard to the spread of communicable diseases in the District of Columbia.

May 22d—In regard to the proposed building of a place for meetings of the Washington Academy of Sciences, etc.

November 20th—In regard to transferring legislative matters from the Medical Society to the Medical Association of the District.

December 4th—Ditto.

1908—May 13th—In regard to the proposed weekly periodical of the Washington Academy of Sciences.

February 26, 1902, the Committee on Public Health made a report recommending that the laws of the District in regard to poisons be amended so as to include methyl alcohol and all substances known to contain it, in the list of poisons.* The committee also recommended that a printed copy of a paper read before the Society by Dr. S. M. Burnett, on the same subject, be sent to the Commissioners of the District and the District Committees of Congress. The Executive Committee of the Society was

---

* See Report of the Health Officer, 1900, p. 74.

requested to make an effort to secure appropriate legislation.

March 5th, the Society authorized the Executive Committee to endorse a bill (Senate Bill 3244) creating a commission for the condemnation of unsanitary buildings, etc., and to take such action as might be necessary to secure the legislation. January 27, 1904, the committee reported that two bills in relation to this subject were before the Senate (2131 and 3155, House 6289 and 9293). The committee was instructed to favor the better legislation.

April 2, 1902, the Executive Committee made a report favoring the consolidation of all the medical work of the District Government under one officer, namely, the Health Officer.* The committee was authorized to take appropriate action.

April 16th, the Executive Committee made a report recommending a bill to regulate the sale of viruses and serums in the District of Columbia. The Society endorsed the recommendation and authorized the committee to take appropriate action.†

May 14th, a committee of Maryland physicians—Drs. Griffith, Taylor and Perry—appeared before the Society, asking its aid in obtaining legislation that would secure reciprocity in medical practice between Maryland and the District. The matter was referred to the Executive Committee.

June 4th, by invitation of Dr. A. B. Richardson, Superintendent of the Government Hospital for the Insane, D. C., many members of the Society visited the hospital and were entertained by the hospital staff. A paper on " The treatment of acute insanity" was read by Dr. Richardson, and

---

* See WASH. MED. ANNALS, 1902, I, p. 269.
† See WASH. MED. ANNALS, 1902, I, p. 274.

an inspection made of the hospital by the members of the Society.

January 14, 1903, the Society endorsed the proposition that a medical man should be appointed upon the Isthmian Canal Commission.

ASSOCIATION OF STATE MEDICAL JOURNALS.

March 9, 1904, a letter was read to the Society from Dr. J. O. Bullitt, Secretary of the Kentucky State Medical Association, asking the appointment of a delegate to a meeting to be held at Atlantic City to organize an association of State medical journals. The letter was referred to the Editorial Committee, which reported March 30th, recommending that the delegate be appointed as requested. Accordingly, Dr. D. S. Lamb was appointed, with Dr. W. A. Wells as alternate.

May 24, 1905, Dr. G. M. Kober was appointed delegate to the Association of State Medical Journals.

January 10, 1906, the Society authorized those who should be the proper representatives of the Society, namely, the members of the Editorial Committee, to join the Association of State Medical Journals.

November 16, 1904, Drs. G. M. Kober, H. L. E. Johnson and N. P. Barnes were appointed delegates to the Pan-American Medical Congress, to meet at Panama.

November 22, 1905, Dr. G. Wythe Cook was appointed to represent the Society at the meeting of the Civic Center, Washington, D. C.

November 29th, a joint meeting of the Anthropological Society and Medical Society was held at the room of the latter. The subject "Diseases among the Indians" was discussed by Dr. A. Hrdlicka, of the U. S. National Museum.*

REVIEWERS.

December 13, 1905, Dr. McLaughlin, in his Presidential address, recommended that "a number of the younger members should be selected to review the progress made during the year in the different specialties and in general medicine," and appointed a member and a subject for each month of 1906 during the session of the Society, the reviewer to alternate with the monthly essayist. The custom of appointing reviewers then inaugurated has since then been followed each year by the retiring President.

January 17, 1906, the Society requested the Commissioners of the District to take steps to bring about a meeting of the Supervising Surgeon General of the U. S. P. H. and M. H. S. and the chief of the Bureau of Hydro-economics of the Geological Survey, to consider the subject of the pollution of interstate streams.

March 7th, the Executive Committee made a report recommending the establishment of a public crematorium as a means of limiting the spread of contagious diseases. Also recommending Senate Bill 3644, relating to police surgeons. The Society adopted both recommendations. The committee opposed the incorporation by Congress (Senate Bill 3603) of the American Institute for Drug Proving, unless the bill should state that it was in the interest solely of the Homeopathic school. The Society endorsed the position of the committee. The committee also reported favorably House Bill 4462, regulating child labor. Also House Bill 8997, regulating the practice of pharmacy; Senate Bill 47, creating a board for the condemnation of unsanitary buildings; and Senate Bill 2475, in regard to

* See WASH. MED. ANNALS, 1905, IV, p. 372.

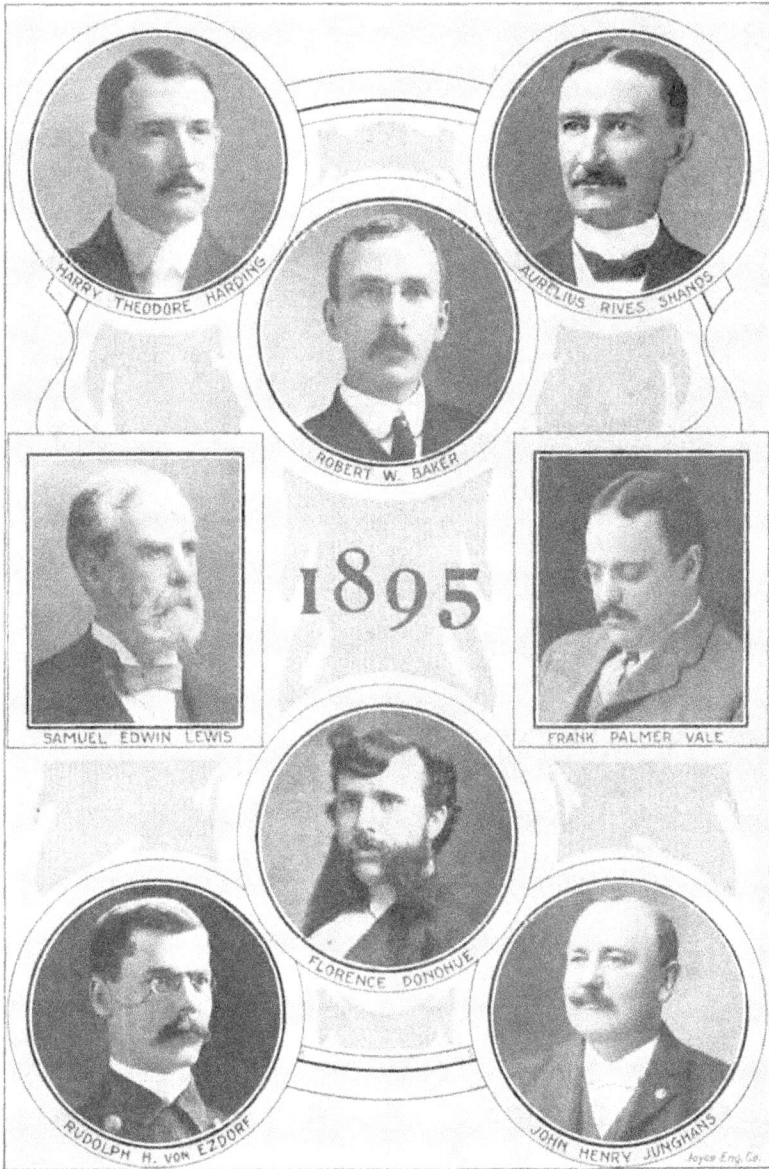

HARRY THEODORE HARDING

AURELIUS RIVES SHANDS

ROBERT W. BAKER

1895

SAMUEL EDWIN LEWIS

FRANK PALMER VALE

FLORENCE DONOHUE

RUDOLPH H. VON EZDORF

JOHN HENRY JUNGHANS

Joyce Eng. Co.

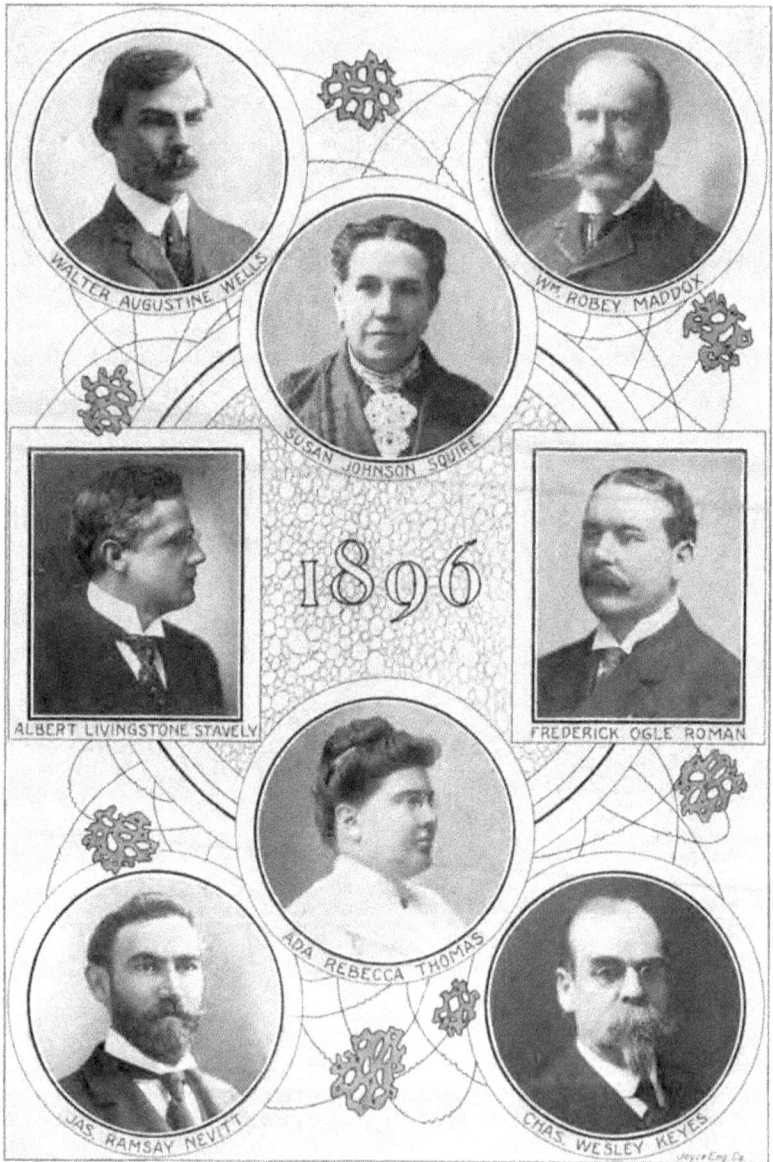

WALTER AUGUSTINE WELLS

WM. ROBEY MADDOX

SUSAN JOHNSON SQUIRE

1896

ALBERT LIVINGSTONE STAVELY

FREDERICK OGLE ROMAN

ADA REBECCA THOMAS

JAS. RAMSAY NEVITT

CHAS. WESLEY KEYES

Joyce Eng. Co.

the public schools of the District, recommending the'continuation of medical inspection and the appointment of visiting school nurses. All of which were approved by the Society.

March 14th, the Society approved the bill for the improvement of the Anacostia flats; Senate Bill 4506, for the registration of births; and the regulation by the Health Officer of the sanitary condition of barber shops. Also House Bill 15,918, regulating the manufacture and sale of patent and proprietary remedies, and Senate Bill 4830, for the registration of deaths and removal of dead bodies.

April 11th, the Society appointed a committee—Drs. Sowers, S. S. Adams, Hickling, Nichols and S. Ruffin—to coöperate with a corresponding committee of the Homeopathic Medical Society in regard to the common interests of the medical profession.

The same date, the Executive Committee reported to the Society, objecting to House Bill 16,955, to regulate the practice of osteopathy in the District of Columbia, and approved Senate Bill 5118, favoring legislation toward preventing scarlet fever, etc.

May 9th, the Society adopted a memorial to Congress, opposing the bill regarding osteopathy.

May 23d, a letter was read from the Red Cross Association, asking donations of books and instruments for San Francisco physicians who had lost books and instruments in the San Francisco earthquake and fire. The Society authorized the Librarian to receive and transmit such donations.*

October 3d, a letter was read from Hon. Wm. H. De-Lacey, Judge of the Juvenile Court of the District, asking the coöperation of the medical profession in certain aspects

* See ANNALS, V, p. 427.

of the work of that Court.   The letter was referred to the
Executive Committee.

December 5th, the Executive Committee was instructed
to appear before the Committee on Legislation of the
Amer. Med. Association and oppose the " Osteopathy" bill.
The Executive Committee was also directed to aid in securing the establishment of a bacteriological laboratory for
the Health Department of the District.

January 7, 1907, the Executive Committee was instructed to coöperate with the Commissioners of the District of
Columbia in securing the passage of a bill before Congress
for the reclamation of the Anacostia flats ; also to oppose
the bill in Congress to incorporate the "American Medical
Union."

March 27th, the Executive Committee was instructed to
consider a letter received in regard to the desirability of a
home for the Washington Academy of Sciences and the
affiliated societies.   May 22d, the committee reported, endorsing the project as advisable, and stating that the Society
would require a room large enough to accommodate 500
persons, and a small room for its library, safe, etc., and
would be willing to pay about $200 per year as rent ; and
pledged the coöperation of the Society in the effort to provide the desired building.   The report was adopted.

THE MEDICAL ASSOCIATION.

April 10th and 24th, a committee, consisting of Drs.
Acker, W. F. R. Phillips, L. Mackall, J. D. Morgan and
J. W. Chappell, was appointed to meet a similar committee .
of the Medical Association, D. C., to consider the relations
of the Medical Society and Medical Association.   May
15th, the committee reported, recommending that the constitution of the Medical Association be so amended as to

provide for the consideration of all matters relative to questions of legislation on medical subjects both general and local; and that the Medical Association be so constituted as to make it sufficiently a scientific body to have it conform to the requirements of the American Medical Association. The report was adopted and the committee continued.

November 20th, the Executive Committee recommended that the legislative matters in its hands be transferred to the corresponding committee of the Medical Association of the District. December 4th, a resolution was adopted by the Society providing that the Executive Committee should suspend consideration of any legislative matters then pending before Congress until otherwise instructed by the Society.

April 15, 1908, the Society was entertained at St. Elizabeth Hospital for the Insane, D. C., by invitation of the Superintendent, Dr. Wm. A. White.

May 13th, the Executive Committee reported favorably on a proposition of the Washington Academy of Sciences to publish a weekly periodical; and the Society adopted the report.

January 4, 1909, a letter was read from Dr. W. A. White, Superintendent Government Hospital for the Insane, inviting the members of the Society to attend meetings of the staff of that hospital, at which papers would be read upon psychiatry, etc. The Society accepted the invitation and ordered that the notice of the meetings should appear on the program cards of the Society.

January 27th, the Executive Committee recommended that the Society approve the Medical Practice Act then before Congress. The Society gave its approval.

February 10th, the Editorial Committee was authorized

to publish the dates of meetings of the medical societies of the District.

April 21st, Dr. Biscoe requested a ruling from the President as to the right of members to smoke during the meetings of the Society. The President ruled that smoking was out of order, basing his decision on the long established custom of the Society.

April 28th, a letter was received from the Secretary of the Washington Academy of Sciences setting forth a proposition to coöperate with the George Washington Memorial Association in efforts to erect a memorial building to George Washington, the building to provide meeting places for the Academy of Sciences and its affiliated societies, and asking the Medical Society to appoint a committee to consider the matter jointly with one from the Academy. Drs. I. S. Stone, McLaughlin and Shute were appointed.

May 5th, the following were appointed delegates to the Pharmacopœial Convention: Drs. Motter, Chappell and Prentiss.

MEMBERSHIP.

MEMBERSHIP.

HONORARY MEMBERS OF THE SOCIETY.

ELECTED IN 1819.

WILLIAM BEANS, Upper Marlboro, Md.,   Died Oct. 12, 1823.
JOHANN HEINRICH CHAUSEPIÉ, Hamburg, Germany. Died.
JAMES MANN, Asst. Surg., U. S. A.,   Died Nov. 7, 1832.
SAMUEL LATHAM MITCHILL, New York City,   Died Sept. 7, 1831.
JOHN SPENCE, Dumfries, Va.,   Died May 18, 1829.

1820

NATHANIEL CHAPMAN, Philadelphia, Pa.,   Died July 1, 1853.
JOSHUA FISHER, Beverley, Mass.,   Died March 21, 1833.
JOHN McCLELLAN, Greencastle, Pa.,   Died 1836.
WILLIAM N. MERCER, New Orleans, La.,   Died.

1821

PARKER CLEAVELAND, Brunswick, Me.,   Died Oct. 15, 1858.
DANIEL CONEY, Augusta, Me.,   Died Jan. 21, 1842.
THOMAS TICKELL HEWSON, Philadelphia, Pa., Died Feb. 17, 1848.
JAMES JACKSON, Boston, Mass.,   Died Aug. 27, 1867.
PHILIP SYNG PHYSICK, Philadelphia, Pa.,   Died Dec. 15, 1837.
NATHANIEL POTTER, Baltimore, Md.,   Died July 2, 1843.
JOHN COLLINS WARREN, Boston, Mass.,   Died May 4, 1856.
BENJAMIN WATERHOUSE, Boston, Mass.,   Died Oct. 2, 1846.

1823

JOSEPH PARRISH, Philadelphia, Pa.,   Died March 18, 1840.

1839

LEWIS FIELDS LINN, St. Louis, Mo.,   Died Oct. 3, 1843.
LUTHER RILEY, Pennsylvania,   Died.
WILLIAM TAYLOR, Manlius, N. Y.,   Died Sept. 16, 1865.

1866

JOSEPH K.* BARNES, Surg. Gen., U. S. A.,   Died April 5, 1883.

1874

WILLIAM MAXWELL WOOD, Surg. Gen., U. S. N.,   Died March 1, 1880.
JOSEPH JANVIER WOODWARD, Surg., U. S. A.,   Died Aug. 17, 1884.

1875

JOHN SHAW BILLINGS, Surgeon, U. S. A.,   New York City.
CHARLES HENRY CRANE, Surg. Gen., U. S. A.,   Died Oct. 10, 1883.
GEORGE ALEXANDER OTIS, Surg., U. S. A.,   Died Feb. 23, 1881.

1892

†THOMAS ANTISELL, Washington, D. C.,   Died June 14, 1893.

1895

THOMAS ALMOND ASHBY, Baltimore, Md.
†BEDFORD BROWN, Alexandria, Va.,   Died Sept. 13, 1897.
LANDON CARTER GRAY, New York City,   Died May 8, 1900.
WILLIAM OSLER, Baltimore, Md.,   Now Oxford, Engl'd.
W. H. PALMER, Providence, R. I.
THEOPHILUS PARVIN, Philadelphia, Pa.,   Died Jan. 29, 1898.
MOSES WADLEIGH RUSSELL, Concord, N. H.,   Died April 18, 1896.
FREDERICK CHEEVER SHATTUCK, Boston, Mass.
GEORGE MILLER STERNBERG, Surg. Gen., U.S.A., Washington, D. C.
JAMES RUFUS TRYON, Surg. Gen., U. S. N.
WALTER WYMAN, Sup. Surg. Gen., U. S. M. H. S., Washington, D. C.

1896

ROBERT FLETCHER, Army Med. Library,   Washington, D. C.

1900

ABRAHAM JACOBI, New York City.

1905

WILLIAM WILLIAMS KEEN, Philadelphia, Pa.
JOHN HERR MUSSER, Philadelphia, Pa.

---

* General Barnes used the letter " K " to distinguish himself from another Dr. Joseph Barnes.

† See name also among active members.

SOFIE AMELIE NORDHOFF JUNG

CHAS. CLAGETT MARBURY

JOHN HITZ METZEROTT

ABBIE CUTLER TYLER

1896

RANDOLPH BRYAN CARMICHAEL

LOUISA MILLER BLAKE

18

ANTHONY HEGER

95

WM. FRANCIS WALTER

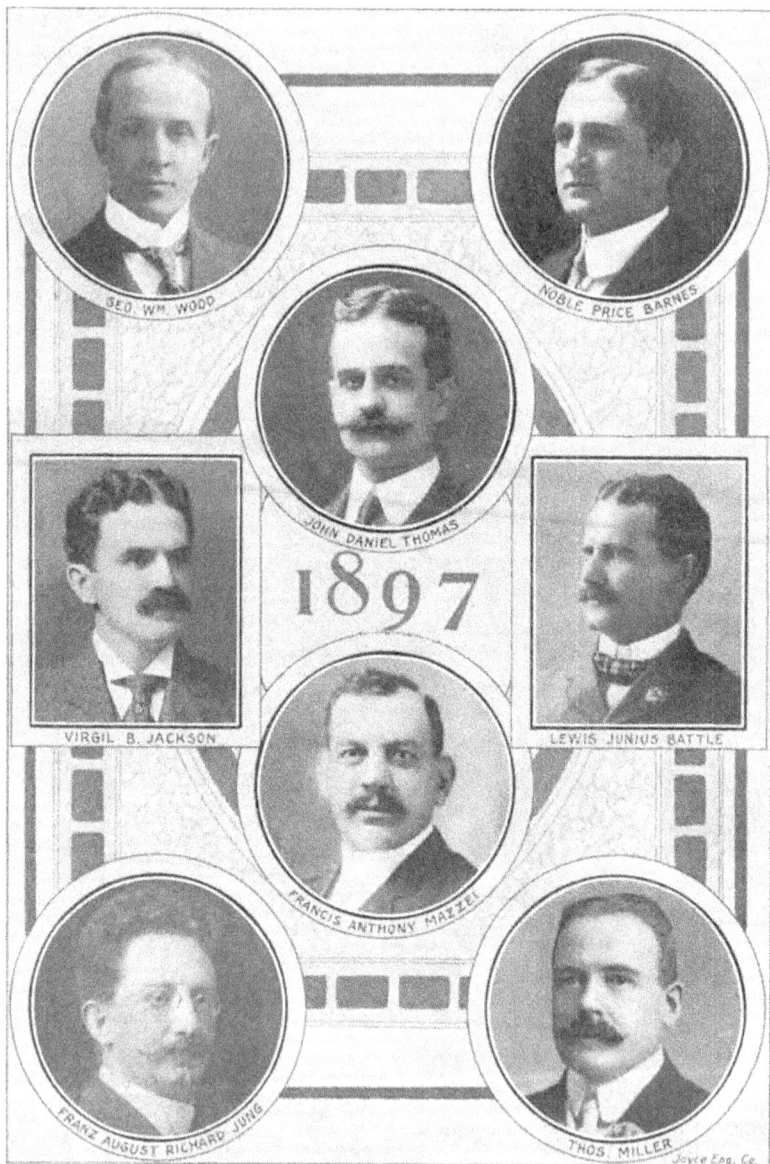

GEO. WM. WOOD

NOBLE PRICE BARNES

JOHN DANIEL THOMAS

1897

VIRGIL B. JACKSON

LEWIS JUNIUS BATTLE

FRANCIS ANTHONY MAZZEI

FRANZ AUGUST RICHARD JUNG

THOS. MILLER

Joyce Eng. Co.

54

ACTIVE MEMBERS OF THE SOCIETY.

The names of the active members of the Society have been arranged in the order in which they were elected to membership, so far as the dates could be ascertained. January 5, 1870, the constitution was amended to the effect that thereafter a member *elect* should become an *actual* member on signing the constitution and by-laws. As more than one hundred members since 1838 have not signed the constitution at all, and some signed many years after election, the only equitable arrangement prior to 1870 seems to be according to the date of election.

The records in many cases are defective, and in such cases the date of election can only be approximate; some persons were nominated to membership, but there is no date at all of their election although they paid their assessments and were recognized as members. There are many mistakes and contradictions in the records, such as inevitably occur to some extent in all records, especially those which have been kept by different officers, having different degrees of accuracy in their methods. It is believed, however, that in the main the following records of elections are correct; certainly very much valuable time has been spent in the effort to make them so.

May 10, 1889, the attention of the Society was called to the fact that some members had never signed the constitution, and a committee was appointed, consisting of Drs. Toner, T. C. Smith and Franzoni, to "ascertain and report the names and number of such physicians, the status and seniority, if any, of such membership, how such defect or lapsed membership may be determined and corrected, and how the seniority of such incomplete or lapsed membership

14

may be adjusted with fairness and justice to the seniority of complete membership. The committee shall also determine and prepare, on or before the first Monday in January, 1894, a full and complete roster, arranged according to seniority of membership, of every living resident member; to each must be affixed the date and place of birth, the date of graduation in medicine, with name of *alma mater*, together with all scientific degrees and institution, with date of such decoration."

June 7th, the committee reported the names of members who had failed to sign the constitution, and recommended that opportunity should be given to them to sign and in that way preserve their seniority. The report and recommendation were adopted.

In addition to the records named in the Preface as having been consulted in preparing the general history, the following have also been consulted for personal histories:

Dictionary of American Biography; by F. S. Drake; Boston, 1872.

History of the Medical Department, U. S. Army, 1775 to 1873; by H. E. Brown; Washington, 1873.

Medical Register and Directory of the United States; by S. W. Butler; Philadelphia, 1874.

Physicians and Surgeons of the United States; by W. B. Atkinson; Philadelphia, 1878 and 1880.

Alphabetical list of Battles and Roster of Regimental Surgeons; N. S. Strait; Washington, 1882.

Polk's Medical Directory; nine editions, 1886 to date.

Appleton's Cyclopedia of American Biographies; New York, 1887-9; 6 volumes.

Army and Navy Register; T. H. S. Hamersly; New York, 1888.

Biography of Eminent American Physicians and Surgeons; by R. F. Stone; Indianapolis, 1894.

Physicians and Surgeons of America; by I. A. Watson; Concord, N. H., 1896.

List of Officers of Army of United States, 1779 to 1900; by W. H. Powell; New York, 1900.

Howard University Medical Department; by D. S. Lamb; Washington, 1900.

History of the City of Washington; by the *Washington Post*, 1903.

Notable Americans; Twentieth Century Biographical Dictionary; by Johnston and Brown; Boston, 1904; 10 volumes.

American Men of Science; by J. M. Cattell; New York, 1906.

The War of the Rebellion; 106 volumes.

Who's Who in America; four editions.

Georgetown University in the District of Columbia; New York, 1907.

University of Maryland; New York and Chicago, 1907; 2 volumes.

American Biographical Directory; Washington, 1908.

In order to save space some abbreviations have been used in the sketches, all of which probably are self-explanatory; but lest some should not be so, it may be stated that the letters A. M. A. mean the American Medical Association; U. S. A., the United States Army; U. S. N., the United States Navy; U. S. P. H. and M. H. S., the United States Public Health and Marine Hospital Service; C. S. A., Confederate States Army; M. C. F., Maryland, Med. and Chirurgical Faculty of Maryland; N. G., National Guard; G. A. R., Grand Army of the Republic; A. A. A. S., American Association for the Advancement of Science.

Names of Colleges and Universities are briefly stated; thus, Georgetown is Georgetown College or University, D. C. Where an institution has been known by several names, that by which it has been longest and best known has been adopted in the sketches ; thus, the present Medical Dept. of George Washington University was at first known as the Med. Dept. of Columbian College ; in 1847 this was changed to "National" Medical College, with the provision, however, that the relation to Columbian College should continue.   In 1873 the Columbian College became Columbian University.   In 1894 the name "National" was dropped.   In fact, there was at the time another college in Washington known by the name of the Med. Dept. of the National University.   In 1904 "Columbian" was changed to "George Washington" University.   In these sketches the institution is known as Columbian.

No mention is made in the individual sketches of membership or of offices held in the Medical Society (except only in a few instances) because, as a matter of course, the mere fact of the presence of the name indicates such membership ; and there are lists of officers in the Appendix.

Authorship.—An examination of the Index Catalogue of the Surgeon General's Library will show that altogether the members of this Society have published some books, large and small, and very many papers in the medical periodicals.   The list is so extensive that, while at first it was the intention to publish under the name of each member the titles of all his literary productions, it was found that the publication would require much more space than could possibly be given thereto.   As it would be invidious to publish for one and not another, it was decided to simply state the fact that such lists can be found under the respective names in the said Index Catalogue, to which the inquirer is therefore referred.   The titles of the more important works, as books, have been mentioned under the members' names.

As originally prepared, the following sketches were

rather full; a revision was necessary and was made, but it was evident that even with this revision they would occupy more space than could legitimately be given to them. Accordingly a second revision was made, reducing them to statements of the facts of little more than the medical life of the individual. The sketches begin with a synopsis of the birth of the individual, his degrees and whence derived, and prominent military or civil positions held. Where biographical sketches had been previously published the references thereto are given, so that the inquirer can consult them.

SEPTEMBER 26, 1817

1. CHARLES WORTHINGTON—Born Oct. 8, 1759, "Summer Hill," Anne Arundel Co., Md. M. B., 1782, Univ. Penna. One of the founders of the Med. and Chirurg. Faculty of Maryland ; an incorporator of the Medical Society, D. C., under its first charter. Father of Dr. N. W. Worthington, *infra*. Died Sept. 10, 1836. [His grandfather, John Worthington, was the first of the family in America.] Studied medicine with Dr. James Murray, of Annapolis, Md. Was Surgeon to four barges, "Maryland flotilla," captured in Chesapeake Bay, 1782. Removed to Georgetown, Md., in 1783 ; lived on "Quality Hill," corner of Prospect and Fayette Streets. One of the founders of St. John's Church, Georgetown, the second Episcopal Church in the District of Columbia. Dressed in the old style, hair *en queue*, knee breeches, long stockings, shoe buckles. Drove a coach and four. The first President of the Medical Society. He and Dr. Frederick May were the most influential medical men of the time in the District. At the time of the battle of Bladensburg and the burning of Washington some wounded British officers were brought to Worthington's house. He "so won the hearts of the English by his hospitality and skillful care that one of the officers presented him with a gold snuffbox." Married Miss Elizabeth Booth, of Jamestown, Va. See Trans. Med. Soc., 75th Anniv., p. 30; Busey's Reminiscences, p. 122; Minutes Med. Society, Feb. 1, 1904; WASH. MED. ANNALS, 1905-6, IV, p. 71; Cordell, Med. Annals of Maryland, 1903, p. 632.

2. JAMES HEIGHE BLAKE—Born June 11, 1768, Calvert Co., Md. Graduated, 1789, at American Med. Society, Philadelphia; *not* M. D. Was an incorporator of the Med. Society, D. C., under the first charter; Medical Supervisor of Hospitals, Washington, in 1814; Mayor of Washington, 1813-17. Father of Dr. J. B. Blake, *infra*. Died July 26, 1819. [Son of

Joseph and Mary Heighe Blake; descendant of a family of lower Maryland planters, who came to the colony soon after its first settlement.] Removed to Georgetown soon after 1789. Built a house S. W. corner Gay and Congress Streets, and began to practice. In 1800 removed to Colchester, Va.; was chosen a member of the Legislature. In 1809 resumed practice in Washington, and was also appointed Collector of Internal Revenue, D. C. Largely through his efforts the charter of Washington was changed, and he became Mayor in June, 1813; was re-elected annually till 1818. In 1818–19 was Register of Wills, D. C. Married in 1789. See Busey's Reminiscences, p. 125.

3. HENRY HUNTT—Born in Maryland, 1782. Licentiate of Med. and Chirurg. Faculty, Maryland; Honorary M. D., 1824, Univ. Md. An incorporator of the Medical Society under both charters; Hospital Surgeon, U. S. Army, 1814-15. The first Health Officer of Washington, afterward President of Board of Health, 1822-33. Consulting physician, Central Cholera Hospital, 1832; one of the founders of the Med. Association, D. C.; member Washington Med. Society; delegate to Amer. Pharm. Convention, 1819; established a Dispensary in Washington, Oct. 20, 1819. Died Sept. 21, 1838. Author of "Observations on a change of climate in pulmonary consumption," etc., Washington, 1834; "A visit to the Red Sulphur Springs of Virginia," etc., Washington, 1838, Boston, 1839, Philadelphia, 1853. See Brown's History, p. 270; Powell's History, p. 107; Busey's Reminiscences, p. 133; Medical Examiner, Philadelphia, 1838, p. 363.

4. THOMAS HENDERSON—Born Jan. 6, 1789, Dumfries, Va. M. D., 1809, Univ. Penna. An incorporator of the Society under the first charter; Assist. Surgeon, U. S. Army. Died Aug. 11, 1854, at his son-in-law's, Gen. F. H. Smith, Commandant Va. Mil. Institute, Lexington, Va. [Son of Alexander Henderson, of Dumfries, prominent as a friend of the colonies in the war of the American Revolution; brother of Gen. Archibald Henderson, many years Commandant, U. S. Marine Corps.] Began practice in Warrenton, Va. In 1816 removed to Georgetown, D. C., and in 1826 to Washington. In 1824-33 was Prof. Theory and Practice of Medicine, Columbian Med. College, Washington. In 1833 was appointed Asst. Surg., U. S. A. Served on various medical boards for examination of candidates for admission to army medical staff. On the basis of his recommendations the Medical Corps was reorganized in 1834. It is believed that the establishment of the Naval School at Annapolis was partly due to his letters to the Secretary of the Navy in 1845. He was largely instrumental in the rebuilding of Christ Church, Georgetown, and in building Trinity Church, Washington. In his house were held the conferences that led to the establishment of the Theological Seminary,

Alexandria, Va. Author of "Epitome of the physiology, general anatomy and pathology of Bichat," Philadelphia, 1829; "Hints on the medical examination of recruits for the Army," etc., Philadelphia, 1840, 1856. See Brown's History, p. 292; Powell's History, p. 369; Busey's Reminiscences, p. 135.

5. WILLIAM JONES—Born April 12, 1790, Rockville, Md. Undergraduate, Univ. Penna., 1812. Licentiate, Med. and Chirurg. Faculty, Maryland; *not* M. D. Was an incorporator of the Society under both charters. Hospital Surgeon's Mate, U. S. Army, 1813-15. One of the founders of the Med. Association, D. C., and President, 1850-8. Postmaster of Washington, 1829-39, 1841-5, 1858-61. Died June 25, 1867. One of the founders of Washington Med. Institute and Med. Association, D. C. Educated in Breckenridge's classical school, "Harewood" (now part of Soldiers' Home Park), and his Academy at Rockville. Studied medicine with Dr. Tyler, of Frederick, Md. After taking one course of lectures at Univ. Penna. he entered the U. S. Army. Assistant to Dr. J. H. Blake, *supra*, in the military hospital near U. S. Arsenal, Washington. At the close of the war of 1812 he formed a partnership with Dr. Blake, and when the latter died, fell heir to his practice. Member of the noted "Jackson Central Committee" that antagonized President John Quincy Adams. Member of Washington Med. Institute, National Institute and Patholog. Society, Washington. See Brown's History; Powell's History; Minutes of Med. Society, June 26, 1867; Trans. A. M. A., 1868, XIX, p. 433; Busey's Reminiscences, p. 127; Biograph. Sketch, by J. B. Blake, 1867; Cordell's Med. Annals of Maryland, 1903, p. 461.

6. THOMAS SIM—Born 1770, Frederick Co., Md. Son of Dr. Joseph Sim. Removed to Washington about 1810. M. B., 1820; M. D., 1823, Univ. Penna. An incorporator of the Society under its first charter. Married Harriet Love, of Langley, Va. In 1813 (June 26) delivered a eulogy on Dr. Benj. Rush, one of the signers of the Declaration of Independence and sometime Physician-General of the Continental Army. Died of epidemic cholera, Sept. 13, 1832, while President of the Society. See Busey's Reminiscences, p. 138.

7. ALEXANDER McWILLIAMS—Born in 1775, St. Mary's Co., Md. Undergraduate Med. Dept. Univ. Penna.; Honorary M. D., 1841, Columbian. Incorporator of the Society under both charters; Asst. Surgeon, U. S. Navy, 1802-5; President of Med. Association, D. C., 1847-50. Father of Dr. Alexander McWilliams, *infra*. Died March 31, 1850. [Was of Scotch descent. The first of the family who came to this country. Escaped from threatened arrest for treason on account of political connection with the party of the Pretender.] Served in the Tripolitan War; was present at the burning of the "Philadelphia." On his return voyage was taken ill with a continued fever and was left at Gibraltar for several weeks. Returned home on the frigate "Constitution," and was then stationed at the Navy Yard, Washington. Soon afterward resigned from the Navy and commenced private practice, locating near the Navy Yard, which was in the most thickly populated part of the city. It is said that Dr. Frederick May expressed to him regret that he should commence the practice of medicine in this city, because there was no more business than May could conveniently attend to. He gave attention to the natural sciences, especially botany, to the neglect of his professional work. Sometime Professor of Botany in Columbian Med. College. Published "Flora of the District of Columbia." Member of Botanic Club that published in 1830 "Prodromus of the Flora Columbiana." Built a conservatory and aviary and made a large collection of minerals. Invented a ship gauge that was approved by a board of naval officers ; some of his models were destroyed in the Patent Office fire. Was the first physician in this country to use adhesive plaster for extension in fracture. Consulting physician to Eastern Cholera Hospital, 1832; physician to Washington Asylum, 1815-50. Member Med Institute, National Institute and Patholog. Society of Washington. See Minutes Med. Society, April 1, 1850; Busey's Reminiscences, p. 132 ; Therap. Gaz., Sept. 15, 1894.

8. ROBERT FRENCH—Born in 1787,* D. C. M. D., 1809, Univ. Penna. Practiced medicine for a while in Georgetown. Incorporator of the Society under the first charter; Asst. Surgeon, U. S. Army and Asst. Surgeon, U. S. Navy, 1820-35. Died. Aug. 13, 1835. See Brown's History, p. 290; Powell's History, p. 319.

9. SAMUEL CABELL HORSLEY--Born in 1798,† Amherst Co., Va. Probably not M. D. Incorporator of the Society under the first charter ; Asst. Surgeon and Surgeon U. S. Navy, 1809-14. Died Sept. 8, 1821 or 1828, at Portsmouth, Va. Educated at Washington College, now Washington and Lee Univ., Va., 1804-6. Was on Perry's flagship at Battle of Lake Erie, escaping with Perry in an open boat when the ship went down. Married Mary Ann Banning-Denny, of Talbot Co., Md. See Hamersly's Register.

10. JAMES T. JOHNSON—M. D. Incorporator of the Society under the first charter. Nothing more known of him.

11. J. PONTE COULANT McMAHON—M. D. Surgeon's Mate, 3d U. S. Inf.; Post Surgeon; Asst. Surgeon and Surgeon, U. S. Army, resigning Oct. 30, 1834. Died April 14, 1837, at New Orleans, La. See Brown's History, pp. 281-290; Powell's History, p. 473.

*Probably Maryland ; the District was not created until 1790.
† So stated in the catalogue, 1885, but evidently a mistake ; probably 1778.

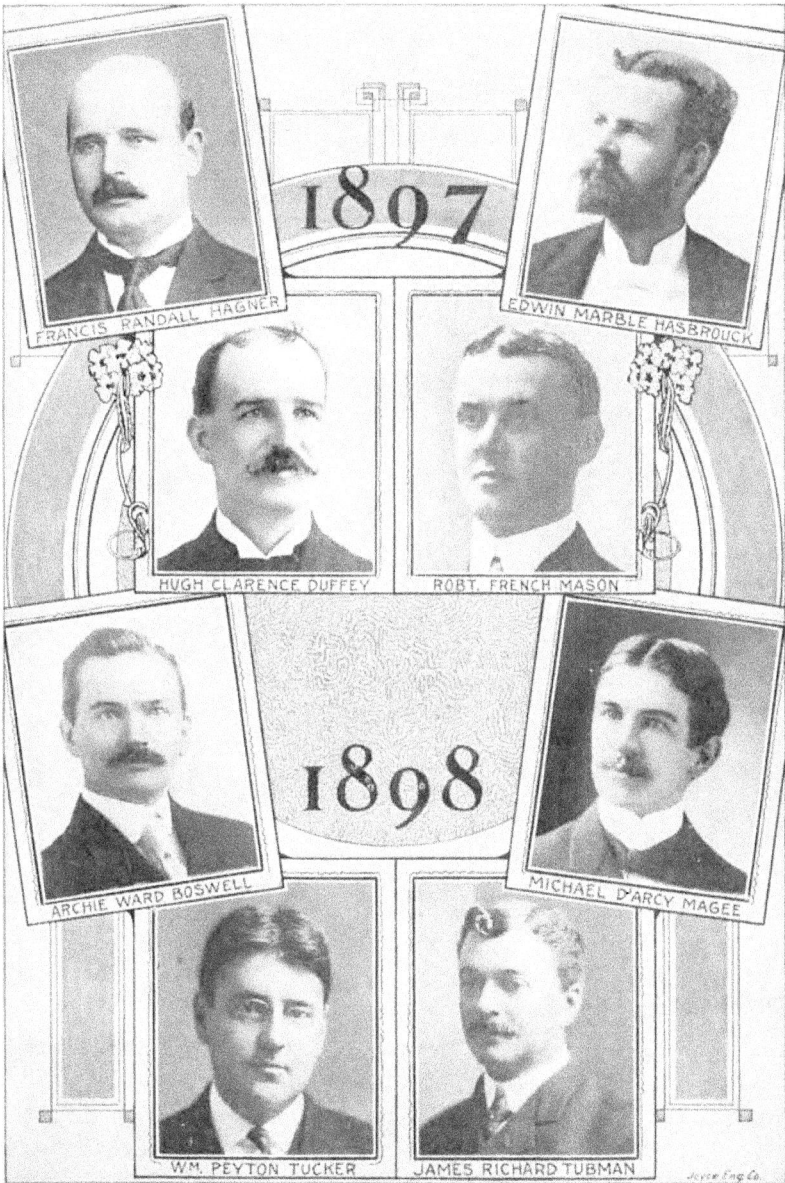

1897

FRANCIS RANDALL HAGNER

EDWIN MARBLE HASBROUCK

HUGH CLARENCE DUFFEY

ROBT. FRENCH MASON

1898

ARCHIE WARD BOSWELL

MICHAEL D'ARCY MAGEE

WM. PEYTON TUCKER

JAMES RICHARD TUBMAN

Joyce Eng. Co.

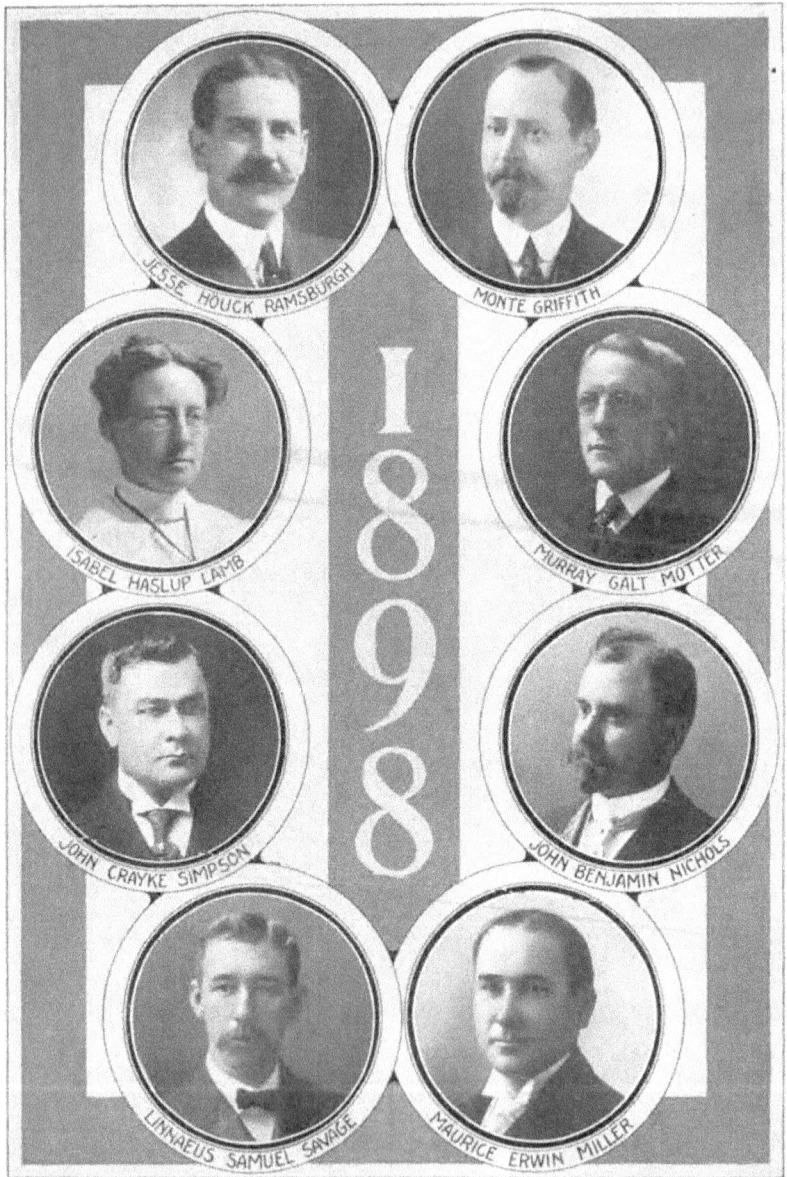

JESSE HOUCK RAMSBURGH

MONTE GRIFFITH

ISABEL HASLUP LAMB

MURRAY GALT MOTTER

JOHN CRAYKE SIMPSON

JOHN BENJAMIN NICHOLS

LINNAEUS SAMUEL SAVAGE

MAURICE ERWIN MILLER

1898

56

12. PEREGRINE WARFIELD—Born Feb. 8, 1779, Anne Arundel Co., Md. [Son of Dr. C. A. and Eliza Warfield; he was one of the founders of the Med. and Chirurg. Faculty of Maryland.] Licentiate, 1817, Med. and Chirurg. Faculty; practiced a few years at Liberty, Md.; married Harriet, daughter of Dr. Francis Sappington, of Liberty. In the political riots in Baltimore, 1812, was wounded while defending the Federalist Press of Hon. C. A. C. Hanson. Removed to Georgetown, D. C. Incorporator of Medical Society under both charters. Died at Georgetown, July 24, 1856. See Minutes Med. Society, Aug. 5, 1856; Busey's Reminiscences, p. 129; Cordell's Med. Annals Maryland, 1903, p. 609.

13. GEORGE CLARKE (spelled both with and without the terminal "e"). Born in Essex Co., Va. M. D., 1810, Univ. Penna. Incorporator of the Society under the first charter. Died, Oct. 5 or 10, 1822, Essex Co., Va., where he had gone on a professional visit.

14. BENJAMIN SCHENKMYER BOHRER—Born April 6, 1788, D. C.* M. D., 1810, Univ. Penna. Incorporator of the Society under the first charter. Sometime President of Board of Health, Georgetown. Died Aug. 19, 1862, of paralysis. Educated at private academy. Studied medicine with Dr. Chas. Worthington, *supra*. Practiced awhile in Georgetown, D. C. Removed to Cincinnati, Ohio, in 1822; appointed Prof. Materia Medica, Ohio Med. College. Served several sessions, then returned to Georgetown. Member Med. Assn., D. C.; delegate, 1851, to Amer. Med. Assn. Visitor to Govt. Hosp. Insane, D. C. Married twice— first, Eliza, daughter of Nathan and Jane Luffborough; afterwards, Mrs. Maria (Taylor) Forrest. Was the originator of the project to establish an insane asylum in this District. See Minutes Med. Society, Aug. 20, 1862; Trans. A. M. A., 1880, XXXI, p. 1018; Busey's Reminiscences, p. 129.

15. JOHN HARRISON—Born in Prince George Co., Md. Probably not M. D. Incorporator of the Society under the first charter; Surgeon's Mate, U. S. Navy. Died March 4, 1825. [His father emigrated from England and became a successful planter in Maryland, where he married a Miss Contee.] Studied medicine with Dr. John Tyler, of Frederick, Md. Was many years Surgeon at Washington Navy Yard. Married Elizabeth, daughter of John and Catherine (Gibson) Hoffman, of Frederick. A son, John Hoffman Harrison, became an eminent physician.

16. NICHOLAS WILLIAM WORTHINGTON—Born 1789, D. C.* M. D., 1815, Univ. Penna. Incorporator of the Society under both charters. Son of Dr. Charles Worthington, *supra*. Retired from practice because

---

*Probably Maryland; see note to No. 8.

of feeble health, and removed to Brentwood, near Washington. Died July 24 or 30, 1849. See Minutes Med. Society, July 31, 1849; Busey's Reminiscences, p. 121.

17. JOHN THOMAS SHAAFF—Born 1763, Frederick Co., Md. Probably not M. D.; Licentiate Med. and Chirurg. Faculty, Md. Incorporator of the Medical Society under the first charter. Died April 28, 1819. One of the founders of the Med. and Chirurg. Faculty; its Treasurer, 1799-1801; member of "Governor's Council" of Maryland, 1798-1800. Said to have been an alumnus of Univ. of Edinburgh, Scotland. Married Mary Sydebotham, of Bladensburg, Md. June 29, 1807, a public meeting was held at Annapolis, to denounce the attack of the British Frigate "Leopard" upon the U. S. Ship "Chesapeake," on June 22d off Norfolk, and to "support such measures as should be adopted by the Government." Dr. Shaaff was one of a committee of twelve, including the Governor of the State, "to carry out the resolutions." See Cordell's Med. Annals of Maryland, 1903, p. 564.

18. FREDERICK MAY—Born Nov. 16, 1773, Boston, Mass. M. B., 1795; M. D., 1811, Harvard. Incorporator of the Society under both charters; President Med. Assn., D. C., 1833-46. Father of Dr. John Frederick May and brother of Dr. Geo. W. May, *infra.* Died Jan. 23, 1847. Came to Washington in 1795. Physician to the Eastern Cholera Hospital in 1832; member of National Institute, Patholog. Society of Washington, and first Board of Health, Washington. In 1823, on the establishment of the Med. Dept. Columbian College, Washington, he was appointed Professor of Obstetrics. See Minutes Med. Society, Jan. 25, 1847, published in Boston Med. and Surg. Jour., 1847, XXXVI, p. 249; also Drake's Dict. Amer. Biog., 1872, p. 611; Busey's Reminiscences, p. 124.

19. JOEL TRUMBULL GUSTINE—M. D. Incorporator of the Society under the first charter. Died.

20. ELISHA HARRISON—Born in 1762, Cecil Co., Md. Probably not M. D. Surgeon's Mate, Maryland line, War of the Revolution; member Society of Cincinnati; one of the founders of the Med. and Chirurg. Faculty, Maryland. Incorporator of the Society under the first charter. Died Aug. 24, 1819. See Cordell's Med. Annals of Maryland, 1903, p. 430.

21. GEORGE WASHINGTON MAY—Born in 1789, Boston, Mass. A. M., 1810; M. D., 1813, Harvard. Incorporator of the Society under both charters. Brother of Dr. Frederick May, *supra.* Died in 1845. One of the founders of the Med. Assn., D. C.; member Washington Med. Society and Patholog. Society. See Busey's Reminiscences, p. 205.

22. ARNOLD ELZEY—Born in 1756, Somerset Co., Md. A. M., 1775, Princeton ; M. D. (?) Garrison Surgeon's Mate and Post Hospital Surgeon, U. S. Army, 1814-18. Died June 6, 1818. Of English descent. One of the founders of Med. and Chirurg. Faculty of Maryland. Physician to President Madison. See Brown's History, pp. 271, 282 ; Powell's History, pp. 108, 301 ; Cordell's Med. Annals of Maryland, 1903, p. 391.

23. RICHARD WEIGHTMAN—Born about 1792, Alexandria, D. C. M. D., 1817, Univ. Maryland. Incorporator of the Society under the first charter. Post Surgeon and Asst. Surg., U. S. A. Died Oct. 30, 1841, at Fort Marion, Fla. [His father was from Whitehaven, England ; on his mother's side he came of the Chew family, Maryland ; Gen. Robert C. Weightman, sometime Mayor of Washington, was his brother.] Educated in Alexandria, and at Union College, Schenectady, N. Y. When the British entered Washington, in 1814, Weightman was captured and imprisoned. Studied medicine with Drs. J. H. Blake and Wm. Jones, *supra*. Practiced in Washington until appointed Asst. Surgeon in the Army, was then ordered to Florida and was on duty at St. Augustine, Fla., until his death, which was caused by a wound and exposure. Buried at Weightman's Bluff, opposite Jacksonville. He never married. See Brown's History, pp. 283, 290 ; Powell's History, p. 661.

24. EDMUND BRICE ADDISON—Born Oct. 5, 1794, at Oxon Hill, Prince George Co., Md. Educated at St. John's College ; studied medicine with Dr. George Clarke, *supra*, and Dr. Philip Syng Dorsey, Philadelphia. M. D., 1815, Univ. Penna. Practiced in Baltimore, at Upper Marlboro, Reistertown and Owings Mills, Md., till he retired, in 1849, and removed to Alexandria, Va. ; thence to Washington, in 1877, where he died Feb. 14, 1878. Was completely blind from cataract for fifteen years. See Cordell's Med. Annals of Maryland, 1903, p. 298.

25. ELISHA CULLEN DICK—Born in 1750 or 1752, Chester Co., Pa. M. B., 1782, Univ. Penna. Resided in Alexandria, D. C.; was Mayor and Health Officer of Alexandria. Attended Gen. George Washington in his last illness. Colonel of Cavalry. Died Sept. 22, 1825. He came of a distinguished Colonial family of Pennsylvania. Studied medicine with Drs. Benj. Rush and Wm. Shippen, Philadelphia, Pa.; began practice in Alexandria in 1782. He seems to have adopted the name Cullen after graduation. One of the founders and for some years Worshipful Master of the first lodge of Masonry in Alexandria, chartered in 1783, and which became Alexandria Lodge in 1788, with Gen. George Washington as Worshipful Master. After the retirement of General Washington, in 1789, Dr. Dick was re-elected and served for some years. He conducted the Masonic ceremonies at the laying of the corner stone of

the District of Columbia, April 15, 1791, at Jones Point, at the mouth of
Hunting Creek, below Alexandria, and when the corner stone of the
Capitol at Washington was laid, in 1793, he marched arm-in-arm with
Washington and took part with the latter in the ceremonies. He also
conducted the Masonic services at the funeral and burial of General
Washington, and presided at the Lodge of Sorrow. He was one of the
two consulting physicians and the first to arrive in the last sickness of
General Washington, and remained with the illustrious patient during
the last hours of his life, striving with his colleagues, Drs. Craik and
Brown, to save the life of the "first citizen of the Republic." "The his-
toric events with which he was so prominently associated directly connect
the Medical Society of the District and the profession of medicine with
several of the most noteworthy and conspicuous occurrences in the foundation and early history of the District. Before going from Alexandria
to Jones' Point he invoked the blessing that the stone to be laid might
'remain an immovable monument of the wisdom and unanimity of North
America,' and after the return of the Commissioners and others to Alexandria, he offered the following sentiment : 'Brethren and Gentlemen :
May jealousy, that green-eyed monster, be buried deep beneath the work
which we have this day completed, never to rise again within the Federal
District.'" See Trans. Med. Society, Virginia, 1885, XVI, p. 267 ; Busey's Reminiscences, p. 144.

26. WILLIAM ARNOLD—M. D. Resided in Alexandria, D. C.
Died.

27. THOMAS SEMMES—Born Aug. 13, 1779, Prince George Co.,
Md. M. D., 1801, Univ. Penna. . Died July 31, 1833, in Alexandria, D.
C. Studied medicine with Dr. E. C. Dick, *supra*. After graduation
spent some time in Europe, after which he practiced in Alexandria. See
Williams' Amer. Med. Biog., 1845, p. 513.

28. GUSTAVUS ALEXANDER BROWN—Born about 1790, Alexan-
dria, D. C. A. B., 1806, Princeton; M. D., 1815, Univ. Penna. Resided
in Alexandria until 1825, when he removed to Smithland, Ky., and practiced there until he was killed, in 1835, in a private encounter. Son of
Dr. Wm. Brown, of Alexandria, who was Physician General during the
War of the American Revolution, and of Catherine Scott, of Scotch descent. Unmarried. See Jour. A. M. A., I, 1883, p. 602.

ELECTED IN 1818

29. RICHARD RANDALL—Born May 13, 1796, Annapolis, Md. M.
D., 1818, Univ. Penna. Surgeon's Mate, Surg., 4th U. S. Inf., Post
Surg. and Asst. Surg., U. S. A., 1818-1821; practiced in Washington,
1821-1828, when he was appointed by the Amer. Colonization Society,

Governor of Liberia.   Died at Monrovia, Liberia, April 19, 1829.   Son of
John and Deborah Knapp Randall.   Educated at St. John's College, An-
napolis, Md.; studied medicine with Dr. John Ridgely, of Annapolis.
In 1827 was appointed Prof. Chemistry, Med. Dept. Columbian College,
D. C.   See Brown's History, p. 290 ; Powell's History, pp. 283, 545.

PROBABLY 1819

30. WILLIAM THORNTON—Born May 27, 1761, Tortola Island,
West Indies.   M. D., 1784, Edinburgh.   Architect of U. S. Capitol.   Died
March 27, 1828.   After graduation he continued his medical studies in
Paris, and travelled extensively through Europe ; then came to the United
States.   Married in 1790 and returned to Tortola.   Returned to Washington in 1793.   The same year published his "Elements of Written
Language ;" and afterwards published many papers on other subjects,
including medicine, astronomy, philosophy, finance, government and art.
Was associated with Fitch in the early experiments in running boats by
steam.   Invented a number of patents ; was in charge of patents from
the passage of the act of Congress, 1802, till his death ; and during the
war of 1814 was the means of preserving the records of the Patent Office
from destruction by the British.   Was the first architect of the Capitol,
as also its designer.   Was first Lieutenant, then Captain, in the war of
1812-14.   In 1794 was appointed by President Washington one of the
three Commissioners of the District of Columbia.   Designed and built
many buildings in the District of Columbia and elsewhere.   See Appleton's Biog., 1889, VI, p. 104 ; Hist. U. S. Capitol, Washington, 1900, p. 81.

31. NATHANIEL POPE CAUSIN—Born, 1781, in Maryland.   M. D.,
1805, Univ. Penna.   Licentiate, Med. and Chirurg. Faculty, Maryland.
Incorporator of the Society under the second charter.   President of Board
of Health, Washington, 1833-36.   Judge of Orphan's Court, D. C., 1838-
49.   Died Nov. 14, 1849.   Practiced for thirteen years at Port Tobacco,
Md. ; in 1818 removed to Washington, where he practiced until 1838.
Was Attending Physician to the Dispensary, 1819 ; Consulting Physician,
Central Cholera Hospital, 1832 ; one of the founders of Med. Assn., D. C.;
member of National Institute, Washington Med. Society and Pathological
Society.   See Busey's Reminiscences, p. 175 ; Cordell's Med. Annals of
Maryland, 1903, p. 345.

32. EDWARD CUTBUSH—Born in 1772, Philadelphia, Pa.   M. D.,
1794, Univ. Penna.   Surg., U. S. N., 1799-1829.   Died June 23, 1843, Geneva, N. Y.   Studied medicine with Dr. Benj. Rush.   Seven years a physician at Pennsylvania Hospital, Philadelphia.   In 1794 was Surgeon General in Washington's expedition against the insurgents in Pennsylvania.
Resigned, 1829, from the Navy and removed to Geneva ; appointed Prof.

Chemistry in Geneva Med. School, and Dean of Med. Faculty. Honorary member of Philadelphia Med. and Chem. Society, of Linnaean Society of Philadelphia, of Amer. Med. Society (?); corresponding member New Orleans Med. Society; member Med. Society of Ontario County, N. Y.; corresponding member Yale Natural History Society; member Natural History Society of Geneva College; corresponding member National Institute, Washington ; sometime President Columbian Institute at Washington, revived by the National Institute.   Oct. 21, 1824, married Sarah Reese, daughter of James Twanley, of Philadelphia.   Author of "Observations on the means of preserving the health of soldiers and sailors," Philadelphia, 1808.   See Williams' Amer. Med. Biog., 1845, p. 118.

1820

83. BAILEY WASHINGTON—Born May 12, 1787, Westmoreland Co., Va. M. D., 1810, Univ. Penna. Surg., U. S. Navy, 1813. Died Aug. 4, 1854. Son of Lawrence Washington ; nephew of George Washington. During the War of 1812, was Surgeon on the "Enterprise" when she captured the "Boxer." On Lake Ontario, at a later date, was selected as Fleet Surgeon, although a junior officer ; afterwards served as Fleet Surgeon in the Mediterranean, and closed his active service during the Mexican War. At the time of his death was Visiting Surgeon of the Navy Yard and Marine Barracks, Washington. Member Med. Assn., D. C. Author of "Observations on yellow fever." See Jour. A. M. A., Feb. 27, 1897, p. 431 ; Chicago Med. Recorder, May, 1897, p. 364.

34. THOMAS SEWALL—Born April 16, 1786, Augusta, Me. M. D., 1812, Harvard. Incorporator of the Society under the second charter. Died April 10, 1845. Son of Thomas and Priscilla (Cony) Sewall. Removed to Washington about 1820. Was appointed Prof. Anatomy, Med. Dept. Columbian College, 1821; served till 1839, when he was transferred to the Chair of Practice, in which he continued till his death. One of the founders of Columbian College in 1821 ; Consulting Physician, Central Cholera Hospital, 1832 ; one of the founders of Washington Infirmary, 1844 ; one of the founders of Med. Assn., D. C.; member National Institute, Washington Med. Society ; President of Patholog. Society, 1843 ; member Board of Health, 1819. One of the first opponents of phrenology, against which he wrote "The errors of phrenology exposed." He also wrote, shortly after Beaumont's work on digestion, "The Enquirer ; pathology of drunkenness," 1841, which was translated into German, and was "possibly the first monograph on the post mortem appearance of the gastric mucosa in alcoholics." Married, Nov. 28, 1813, Mary Choate, sister of Rufus Choate. See Appleton's Biog., 1889, V, p. 469 ; Minutes Med. Society, April, 1, 1845 ; Med. Examiner, Philadelphia, 1845, I, p. 291.

35. CHARLES BEALE HAMILTON—Born 1792. M. D. (?) Entered the Navy as Assistant Surgeon, April 2, 1811; was made Surgeon, April 15, 1814; served under Commodore Waring during the entire war with Great Britain. Resigned from the Navy, April 12, 1826, and went into private practice. Preferred agricultural pursuits, and, except that he continued to practice within a limited circle, he lived on a farm a few miles from Washington. Died April 24, 1851. See National Intelligencer, April 26, 1851.

1822

36. ELIJAH RICHARDSON CRAVEN—Born Feb. 3, 1796, Morrisville, N. J. A. B., 1815, Princeton; M. D., 1819, Univ. Penna. Died Dec. 4, 1823, from hemorrhage caused by being thrown from his horse. Son of John Craven. Studied medicine with Dr. P. S. Dorsey, Philadelphia, Pa. After graduation, practiced in Washington. Sometime Prof. Botany, Columbian College, D. C.

37. JOSEPH LOVELL—Born Dec. 22, 1788, Boston, Mass. M. D., 1811, Harvard. Surgeon, 9th U. S. Infantry, 1812-14; served on Niagara frontier; Hospital Surgeon, 1814-18; Surgeon General, U. S. A., 1818-36. Died Oct. 17, 1836, of pneumonia. One of the founders and a counsellor of the Med. Assn., D. C. "Army and Navy surgeons were actively instrumental in the organization of the two medical societies in the District of Columbia; and the profession of the District owes to two army surgeons the inception, organization and successful defence of a society established in 1833 to define and prescribe the rules and regulations of ethical intercourse and relations of medical gentlemen and of the profession with the public at large." Furnished a transcript of the rules and regulations of a similar society in Boston as a guide to its formation. Member of National Institute. Married E. Mansfield, Sept., 1817. See Drake's Amer. Biog., 1872, p. 565; Brown's History, pp. 268, 282, 286; Powell's History, pp. 59, 80, 121, 441; Busey's Reminiscences, p. 204.

38. CHARLES FREDERICK WILSTACH—Born Sept. 3, 1794, Philadelphia, Pa. M. D., 1820, Univ. Penna. Died July 1, 1860, at Lafayette, Ind. [Son of Chas. Wilstach, from Germany, and Hannah Lubrech, from Hesse Darmstadt.] Had a good classical education; spent several years in a drug store; studied medicine with Dr. P. S. Dorsey, of Philadelphia. Served one year as House Surgeon, Philadelphia Almshouse. Removed to Harper's Ferry, where he practiced two years; thence to Washington, where he practiced medicine and also kept a drug store. In 1830 removed to Cincinnati, Ohio, and in 1838 to Lafayette, Ind. Married in 1821 Hannah W. Ustick.

1823

39. JAMES MARTIN STAUGHTON—Born in 1800, Bordentown, N. J. Son of Rev. Dr. Wm. and Maria Henson Staughton. A. B., 1818; M. D., 1821, Univ. Penna.; A. M., 1821, Princeton. Resident student, Philadelphia Almshouse. Practiced medicine in Washington; helped to organize Med. Dept. Columbian College; was appointed Prof. Chemistry and Geology ; afterwards Surgery. Spent two years in Europe. Said to have been the first physician to operate successfully in Washington for stone in the bladder. Removed to Cincinnati, and was appointed Prof. of Surgery in Med. College of Ohio ; was also connected with the Commercial Hospital and Ohio Lunatic Asylum. One of the founders of Ohio Med. Lyceum; co-editor Western Med. Gazette. Died Aug. 7, 1833. See West. Med. Gazette, 1833, I, p. 271.

40. JAMES SAMUEL GUNNELL—Born March, 1788, Fairfax Co., Va. M. D., 1820, Univ. Penna. Was Lieutenant, 1812, Virginia Light Horse. Incorporator of the Society under the second charter. Died in 1852. See Busey's Reminiscences, p. 167.

1826

41. JOHN B. BLAKE—Born Aug. 12, 1800, Colchester, Va. Son of Dr. J. H. Blake, *supra*. M. D., 1824, Univ. Maryland. Incorporator of the Society under the second charter. Died Oct. 26, 1881. Sometime Commissioner of Public Buildings and Grounds, D. C. ; President National Metropolitan Bank. Practiced medicine only a short time. Had a son, Dr. Ebenezer Tucker Blake. Author of " Biographical sketch of the late Dr. Wm. Jones," Washington, 1867. See Minutes of Med. Society, Oct. 26, 1881 ; Busey's Reminiscences, p. 141.

42. THOMAS CLAGETT SCOTT—Born Dec. 4, 1784, Prince George Co., Md. M. D., 1812, Univ. Penna. Died of congestive chill at Washington, Sept. 7, 1837. Son of Judson and Martha Ellen Clagett Scott, both from early settlers of Maryland. Educated at Charlotte Hall, Md.; studied medicine under Dr. Wm. Beans, of Upper Marlboro, Md. Attended Univ. Penna., 1804-5. In 1806 became a licentiate Med. and Chirurg. Faculty of Maryland. The same year married Miss Ann H. Boone, daughter of Francis and Mary Sansbury Boone, whose ancestors came to America with Lord Baltimore. Began to practice medicine in Montgomery Co., Md. In 1809 removed to Loudoun Co., Va.; in 1813 to Frederick Co., Md., and attended lectures at the Univ. Maryland. In 1823 removed to Washington and associated himself with Dr. N. P. Causin, *supra*. Was physician to the penitentiary, Washington. One of the founders Med. Assn., D. C. See Cordell's Med. Annals of Maryland, 1903, p. 562.

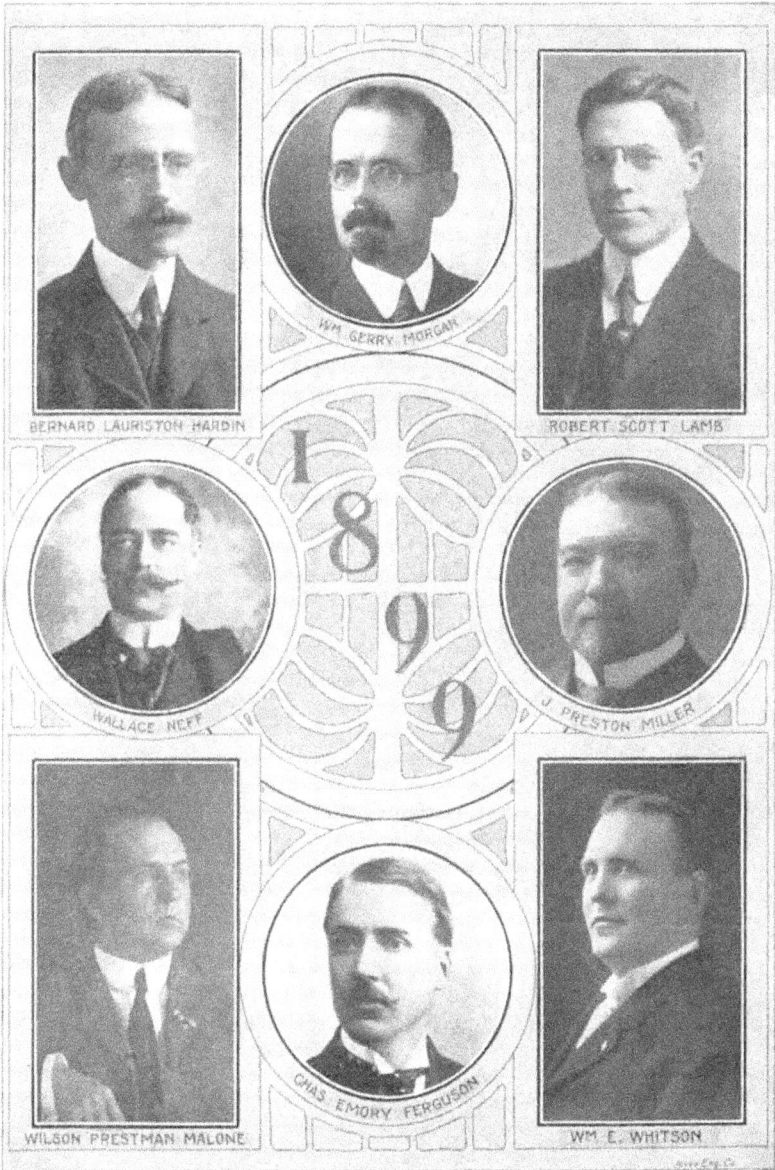

BERNARD LAURISTON HARDIN

WM GERRY MORGAN

ROBERT SCOTT LAMB

1899

WALLACE NEFF

J. PRESTON MILLER

WILSON PRESTMAN MALONE

CHAS EMORY FERGUSON

WM E. WHITSON

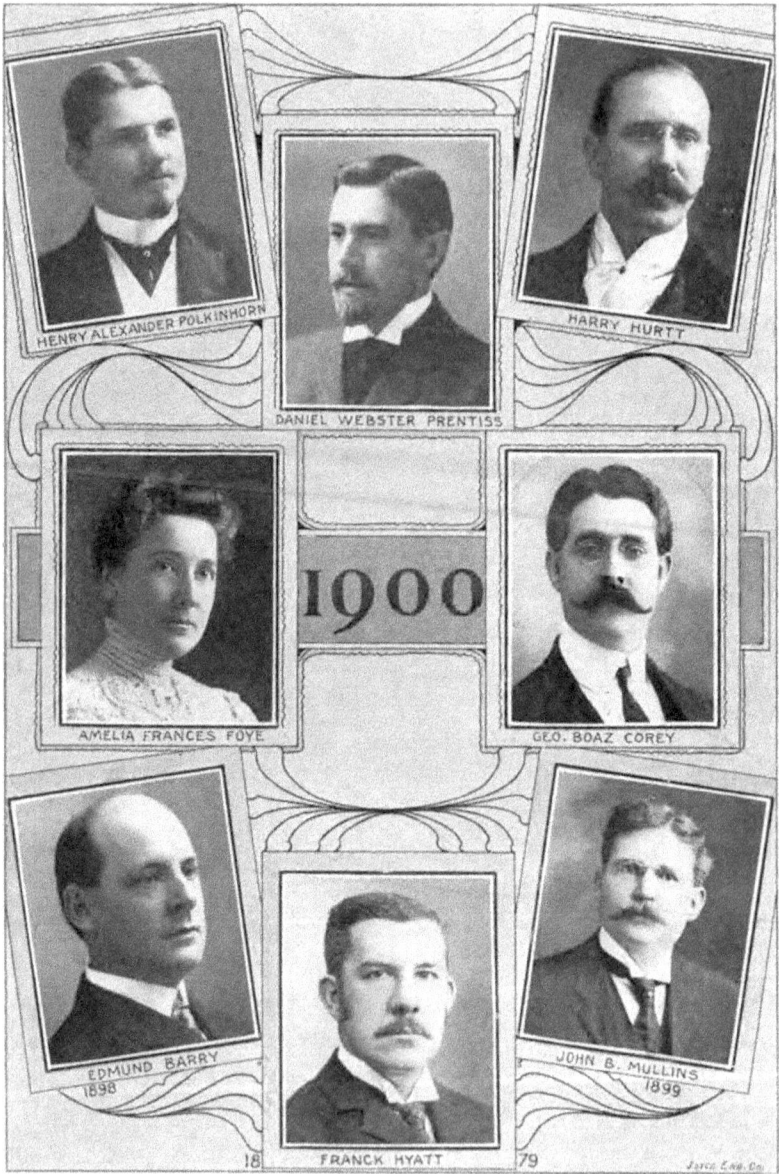

HENRY ALEXANDER POLKINHORN

DANIEL WEBSTER PRENTISS

HARRY HURTT

AMELIA FRANCES FOYE

1900

GEO. BOAZ COREY

EDMUND BARRY
1898

FRANCK HYATT

JOHN B. MULLINS
1899

18   79

Joyce Eng. Co.

58

43. JOSHUA RILEY—Born Jan. 19, 1800, Baltimore, Md. M. D., 1824, Univ. Maryland. Father of Dr. J. C. Riley, *infra*. Incorporator of the Society under second charter. President Med. Assn., D. C., 1858-68. Died Feb. 11, 1875. Came to Georgetown, D. C., when 18 years old; sometime clerk in a drug store. Studied medicine with Dr. George Clarke, *supra*. After graduation, practiced in Georgetown. Was Prof. Materia Medica, Med. Dept. Columbian College, 1844-9; one of the founders of the Washington Infirmary; member of Board of Aldermen, Georgetown, and of Council of Territorial Government, D. C.; President of Potomac Fire Insurance Co. "He taught physicians how to collect accounts for services from a certain class of delinquent clients by taking their notes for the amount, and renewing them annually thereafter, with the addition of the interest accrued, until it was paid either by the drawer or his estate." See Minutes Med. Society, Feb. 13, 1875; Trans. A. M. A., 1875, XXVI, p. 453; Busey's Reminiscences, p. 159.

1830

44. ORLANDO FAIRFAX—Born Feb. 14, 1806, Alexandria, D. C. M. D., 1829, Univ. Penna. Son of Thomas, the ninth Lord Fairfax. Resided in Alexandria; removed in 1861 to Richmond, Va., where he died, Jan. 11, 1882. See Busey's Reminiscences, p. 147.

1834

45. RICHMOND JOHNSON—Born 1791, Annapolis, Md. Not M. D. Surgeon's Mate, U. S. N., 1812-14. Incorporator of the Society under the second charter. Died March 12, 1874. Came to Washington in 1800; educated at Washington Institute. Grand nephew of Thomas Johnson, the first Governor of Maryland. Studied medicine with Dr. Fred. May, *supra*. After the close of the war of 1812-14, practiced in Washington. Sometime chief clerk in office of Surgeon General, U. S. A. One of the founders of Med. Assn., D. C. Consulting Physician to Western Cholera Hospital, 1832. See Minutes of Med. Society, March 14, 1874; Trans. A. M. A., 1874, XXV, p. 526; Busey's Reminiscences, p. 152.

46. HARVEY LINDSLY—Born Jan. 11, 1804, Morris Co., N. J. A. M., 1820, Princeton; M. D., 1828, Columbian. Father of Dr. W. Lindsly, *infra*. Incorporator of the Society under second charter. President of Board of Health, Washington, 1836-46. President Amer. Med. Assn., 1859. Died April 28, 1889. Of English descent. Educated at academy in Somerset Co., N. J. Honorary member Rhode Island Med. Society, Historical Society of New Jersey, etc. Prof. Obstetrics, 1839-45, and Practice of Medicine, 1845-6, Med. Dept. Columbian College, Washington. Member Amer. Colonization Society over 30 years,

15

and Chairman of its Executive Committee. President, 1878, of Washington Alumni of Princeton College. One of the founders of Washington Infirmary, Patholog. Society, Med. Assn., D. C.; member of National Institute. "During a period of discontent the Standing Committee of the Medical Association of the District, which had been instructed to investigate prevalent insinuations and charges of violations of ethical methods and proprieties, concluded its report with a resolution recommending the members to 'bury all past grievances in oblivion, and for the future to observe the Golden Rule.' Dr. Lindsly moved to strike out the words 'Golden Rule' and insert 'Rules and By-laws of this Association,' which was carried." In 1859, "in his address of welcome to the American Medical Association, then assembled in this city, after giving expression to his regret that the city was so barren of all that would interest the votaries of medical science, he added, in words that read like the inspiration of prophecy, 'The day is not far distant when, by the liberality of a great people, our public buildings, our literary and scientific institutions, our national parks and botanic gardens will be worthy of the grand metropolis of a nation which, perhaps within the next half century, will be the most populous, powerful and wealthy in Christendom.' He lived long enough afterward to realize the fullness of his prophecy." Author of "Origin and introduction into medical practice of ardent spirits," Washington, 1835. See Atkinson's Phys. and Surg., 1878, p. 119; Minutes Med. Society, April 29, 1889; Lamb's History, p. 111; Busey's Reminiscences, pp. 109, 155.

1835

47. THOMAS MILLER—Born Feb. 18, 1806, Port Royal, Va. M. D., 1829, Univ. Penna. Father of Dr. G. R. Miller, *infra*. Incorporator of the Society under the second charter. President Board of Health, Washington, 1846-55; President Med. Assn., D. C., 1873. Died Sept. 20, 1873. Son of Major Miller, who came to Washington in 1816. Educated at Washington Seminary; studied medicine with Dr. Henry Huntt, *supra*. After graduation, practiced in Washington. In 1830 he and six other physicians formed the Washington Med. Institute, for the instruction of students; in 1832 he began to teach practical anatomy; the same year was physician to the Central Cholera Hospital. One of the founders of the Med. Assn., D. C., 1833. From 1839 to 1859 was Prof. Anatomy, Med. Dept. Columbian College; first President of Patholog. Society of Washington; attending Surgeon, Washington Infirmary; member Board of Aldermen; consulting physician to Providence Hospital and Children's Hospital. Originated the movement to establish and enforce a system of registration of births and deaths in Washington; active in securing the establishment of the Government Hospital for the Insane. Married,

in 1833, the daughter of Gen. Walter Jones. See Minutes of Med. Society, Sept. 22, 1873, and Sept. 30, 1874; Trans. A. M. A., 1874, XXV, p. 523; Busey's Reminiscences, p. 169.

JULY, 1838

48. JOSEPH BORROWS—Born Jan. 20, 1807, D. C. A. B., 1825 (?); M. D., 1828, Columbian. Incorporator of the Society under second charter. President Med. Assn., D. C., 1884-5. Died May 30, 1889. See Minutes of Med. Society, June 1, 1889; Busey's Reminiscences, p. 142.

49. ALEXANDER McDONALD DAVIS—Born 1807, D. C. M. D., 1828, Columbian. Incorporator of the Society under second charter. Died May 29, 1872. Studied medicine with Dr. Wm. Jones, *supra*. After graduation, practiced only a few years. Was President of the City Council; member of Board of Aldermen; Health Officer. Physician in 1833 in the Cholera Hospital. See Minutes Med. Society, May 29, 1872.

50. NOBLE YOUNG—Born June 26, 1808, Baltimore, Md. M. D., 1828, Columbian. Incorporator of the Society under second charter. President Med. Assn., D. C., 1868-70. A. M., 1876, Georgetown. Died April 11, 1883, at Sacketts Harbor, N. Y. Of Scotch-Irish descent. Educated at Washington Seminary. After graduation in medicine, practiced in Washington; member of Amer. Med. Association, ex-Vice President; Prof. Principles and Practice of Medicine for twenty-five years, Georgetown Med. School; one of the four who organized the school. For many years was physician to U. S. Penitentiary, Washington. Married, May 6, 1836. Delivered the address at the laying of the corner stone of College Physicians and Surgeons, Wilmington, N. C., 1871. See Minutes of Med. Society, April 13, 1883; Jour. A. M. A., 1883, I, p. 520; Atkinson's Phys. and Surg., 1878, p. 537; Busey's Reminiscences, p. 162; Georgetown Univ., II, p. 73.

51. BENJAMIN KING—Born Aug. 24, 1797, Calvert Co., Md. M. D., 1818, Univ. Maryland. Incorporator of the Society under second charter. Surgeon's Mate, 7th U. S. Inf.; Asst. Surg., U. S. A.; retired, Nov. 9, 1863. Removed, 1870, to Weston, Md., where he died June 24, 1888. Served with his regiment in Georgia to June, 1821; at Baton Rouge, La., to November, 1822; at Augusta, Ga., to March, 1823; at Military Academy, West Point, to Aug. 19, 1823; at Fort McHenry to October, 1825; shipwrecked in November on Body's Island, S. C., while *en route* to Charleston; at Charleston, Savannah, Forts McHenry and Severn and in Washington to November, 1832; Philadelphia to February, 1833; in Surgeon General's Office, Washington, till Oct. 16, 1840;

in the Seminole War, Florida, to July, 1842 ; at Fort Severn, Md., to September, 1845 ; at Frankford Arsenal, Philadelphia, to September, 1849 ; at Carlisle Barracks, Pa., to Feb. 10, 1851 ; at Soldiers' Home, Washington, to Nov. 26, 1864. See Brown's History, pp. 285, 291 ; Powell's History, p. 414.

52. JAMES CROWDHILL HALL—Born Jan. 10, 1805, Alexandria, D. C. A. B., 1823, Jefferson College, Cannonsburg, Penna.; M. D., 1827, Univ. Penna. Incorporator of the Society under second charter. Died suddenly June 7, 1880. While he was an infant his father died ; in 1810 his mother remarried. He studied medicine with Dr. Thomas Henderson, *supra*. After graduation was Resident Physician one year at Blockley Hospital, Philadelphia, Pa. 1830-9, Prof. Surgery, Med. Dept. Columbian College, Washington. Member Med. Assn., D. C. ; Washington Med. Society ; National Institute. Vice President Patholog. Society. Conducted a private course in practical anatomy at Washington Med. Institute. Gave large bequests to Washington City Orphan Asylum and Children's Hospital. " Family physician of every President of the United States from Jackson to Lincoln. For many years attended the family of every Justice of the Supreme Court ; through many administrations the family of every Cabinet Officer ; and for a long series of years every foreign legation residing in Washington, and every prominent Senator and member of the House of Representatives, the heads of departments and many honored citizens." See Minutes of Med. Society, June 8, 1880, and April 6, 1881 ; Boston Med. and Surg. Jour., 1880, CII, p. 621 ; Trans. A. M. A., 1881, XXXII, p. 506 ; Busey's Reminiscences, pp. 147, 166.

53. HENRY FORD CONDICT—Born 1804, Littleton, N. J. A. M., 1822, Princeton ; M. D., 1830, Columbian. Incorporator of the Society under second charter. Removed, about 1875, to Montgomery Co., Md. Dropped from membership, 1877. Died Oct. 31, 1893. Attended school at Littleton. For some time after graduation he prepared students for college. Practiced medicine in Washington, at first in partnership with Dr. N. P. Causin, *supra*, whose daughter he married. Author of "The Plague of Athens," a translation from Thucydides. See Busey's Reminiscences, p. 143.

54. WILLIAM B. MAGRUDER—Born Feb. 11, 1810, Baltimore, Md. M. D., 1831, Univ. Maryland. Incorporator of the Society under second charter. Mayor of Washington, 1856-8. Died May 30, 1869, from an obscure disease of the stomach. Son of James A. and Millicent Magruder. Studied medicine with Dr. B. S. Bohrer, *supra*. " Practiced in Georgetown until the summer of 1832, when, the cholera epidemic having

driven away the physicians resident in that part of Washington known
as the First Ward, he was called by the citizens to take charge of a
cholera hospital, and was the only active physician in that section during
the epidemic." Sometime member of the City Council, and also Alderman. Married twice. See Minutes of Med. Society, May 31, 1869;
Trans. A. M. A., XXIII, 1872, p. 577; Busey's Reminiscences, p. 168.

55. FREDERICK DAWES—M. D. Born Jan. 26, 1778, in Huntingdon, England. Died Feb. 10, 1852, after an illness of nineteen months.
Was first an apothecary at Wisbeach, Lincolnshire, England. Studied
medicine with Sir Astley Cooper; practiced at Wisbeach. Served as Surgeon on Russian man-of-war. Returned to Wisbeach and then, in 1819,
emigrated to the United States, and came to Washington. After a few
years, bought a farm at and removed to Shelby, Ill. Later removed to a
farm in Westmoreland Co., Va. In 1839 returned to Washington. One
of the founders of the Med. Association, D. C., member of Pathological
Society, Washington. Married, about 1797, Miss Ward, of Wisbeach;
in 1819, Charlotte M. Taylor, of Montgomery Co., Md. See Busey's
Reminiscences, p. 143 ; Minutes of Med. Society, Feb. 11, 1852.

JULY 1, 1839

56. JOHN MOYLAN THOMAS—Born Sept. 26, 1805, Anne Arundel
Co., Md. M. D., 1826, Univ. Maryland. Died Oct. 16, 1853. Son of
Philip S. Thomas. Educated at St. Mary's College, Baltimore, Md.
Practiced a few years at his native place, then removed to Washington;
member Amer. Med. Association ; sometime Prof. Physiology, Med.
Dept. Columbian College, Washington. July 25, 1829, married Miss
Sarah Brooks Lee Ringgold, daughter of Frank Ringgold, sometime
Marshal, D. C. See Minutes of Med. Society, Oct. 17, 1853 ; Trans. A.
M. A., 1880, XXXI, p. 1088.

57. JAMES B. C. THORNTON, M. D.—Born 1809. Died Jan. 15,
1839, at Snickersville, Va. Practiced medicine some time at Occoquan,
Va. [According to Dr. Toner, he was a member of the National Institute which, however, was not founded till 1840.]

PROBABLY JULY 1, 1839

58. JOHN FREDERICK MAY—Son of Dr. Frederick May, *supra*.
Born May 19, 1812, D. C. A. B., 1831; M. D., 1834, Columbian. Re-
moved to Nashville, Tenn., 1858. Returned to D. C., 1880. Father of
Dr. William May, *infra*. Died May 2, 1891. Soon after graduation in
medicine he went to Europe and spent over a year in the hospitals of
London and Paris. Licentiate, M. C. F., Maryland, 1837. In 1839 be-

came Prof. Anatomy and Physiology, Med. Dept. Columbian College, Washington; in 1841, Prof. Surgery; resigned in 1858. Was also Prof. Surgery, 1837-9, in Univ. Maryland; member National Institute; Med. Association, D. C.; Pathological Society, Washington; Amer. Med. Association. In 1858 became Prof. Surgery in Shelby Med. College, Nashville, Tenn., and continued there till 1861. Sometime Surgeon to Washington Infirmary. About 1865 removed to New York City. Returned to Washington in 1880. In 1884 became member of consulting staff Garfield Hospital; President for five years. See Minutes Med. Society, May 4, 1891; Stone's Biog., 1894, p. 319; Jour. A. M. A., 1891, XVII, p. 121; Busey's Reminiscences, p. 158; Cordell's Med. Annals of Maryland, 1903, p. 492.

PROBABLY JANUARY 6, 1840

59. SAMUEL FORRY—[Forry was nominated July 1, 1839; there is no record of his election, but he was recognized as a member.] Born June 23, 1811, Berlin, Pa. M. D., 1832, Jefferson. Licentiate, M. C. F., Maryland, 1836; Asst. Surg. and Surg., U. S. A.; editor N. Y. Journal Med. and Collateral Sciences, 1843-4. Died Nov. 8, 1844. Studied medicine with Dr. Fahnestock. While Surgeon, U. S. A., in the campaign in Florida, he made many interesting observations on the climate. Afterwards compiled from these observations and others made by surgeons at different military posts, under the direction of Dr. Lawson, Surgeon General of the Army, "The Meteorological Register" and "Statistical report on the sickness and mortality in the army," both of which were published as the official reports of the medical department of the army. The numerous facts contained in these works, with others which he collected, were afterwards used in the preparation of his work on the "Climate of the United States, and its endemic influence." This work obtained for him a high and well-deserved reputation, both in his native country and among scientific men in Europe. The Boylston prize, of Harvard University, for 1844, for the best essay on the protective power of vaccinia, was awarded to him, and appeared in the New York Journal for September, 1844. In such high estimation was he held by the physicians of the city of New York that they raised a subscription for a monument to his memory, to be erected in Greenwood Cemetery, where he is buried. See Drake's Dict. Amer. Biog., 1872, p. 234; Appleton's Biog., 1887, II, p. 506; Trans. A. M. A., 1850, III, p. 440; Brown's History, p. 292; Powell's History, p. 314.

1840

60. JOSHUA A. RITCHIE—[The catalogue of 1885 states that Ritchie was elected in 1840, but on what foundation the statement is made is unknown. His name appears on the minutes for the first time in January,

1858. The first record of dues paid by him was Nov. 7, 1865.] Born
July 1, 1815, D. C. M. D., 1839, Jefferson ; A. B., 1835; A. M., 1840 (?)
Father of Dr. L. W. Ritchie, *infra*. Dropped from membership, 1875.
Died Nov. 2, 1887. See Minutes of Med. Society, Nov. 2, 1887; Busey's
Reminiscences, p. 160.

PROBABLY JANUARY 11, 1841

61. JOHN MACKALL ROBERTS—[There is no record of any meet-
ing between Jan. 11, 1841, and Jan. 5, 1842 ; Roberts attended the latter.]
Born June 11, 1815, D. C. M. D., 1836, Jefferson. Father of Dr. W. E.
Roberts, *infra*. Died Sept. 11, 1865. Son of Charles and Ann Loker
Roberts, St. Mary's Co., Md. Educated in Washington schools. Studied
medicine with Dr. Thomas Sewall, *supra*. Practiced in Washington.
Member Med. Assn., D. C. Director of Bank of the Metropolis and
Franklin Insurance Co., Washington. Married Oct. 18, 1838, Matilda
Campbell Elder, daughter of Wm. and Matilda Stamp Elder, of Charles
Co., Md. See Minutes Med. Society, Sept. 12, 1865 ; Trans. A. M. A.,
1872, XXIII, p. 576.

JANUARY 5, 1842

62. WILLIAM PATRICK JOHNSTON—Born June 11, 1811, Savannah, Ga. A. B., 1833, Yale ; M. D., 1836, Univ. Penna. Father of Drs.
W. W. and G. W. Johnston, *infra*. President of Board of Health, Washington, 1856-8. Died of chronic disease of the heart, Oct. 24, 1876. Son
of Col. James and Ann Marion Johnston ; grandson of Dr. Andrew Johnston, M. D., Univ. Edinburgh. Educated at Round Hill School, Northampton, Mass., of which George Bancroft was then the head. Studied
medicine with Prof. Wm. Horner, of Philadelphia, Pa. Served in drug
store of Samuel Griffith, Philadelphia, and one year as Resident Physician, Blockley Hospital, Philadelphia. In 1837 was Physician to Philadelphia Dispensary. In Europe, 1837-40, partly in travel, partly attending the Paris hospitals. Began to practice medicine in Philadelphia, but
after marrying, in 1840, Miss Hooe, of Alexandria, D. C., he settled in
Washington. In 1842 became Prof. Surgery, Med. Dept. Columbian College ; 1845, Prof. Obstetrics and Diseases Women and Children. Resigned in 1871. Aided in establishing the Washington Infirmary. Sometime President of Medical Faculty, Columbian College. One of the
founders Pathological Society of Washington. Member Med. Assn.,
D. C. ; Amer. Med. Assn., Vice President in 1866. Aided in formation
of Clin. Path. Society of Washington. Member Consulting Board Providence Hospital ; sometime Clinical Lecturer there. One of the founders
of Children's Hospital ; sometime President of Medical Board. During
the period that Confederate soldiers were confined in the Old Capitol

Prison in Washington, he obtained permission for Dr. J. C. Hall, *supra*. Mr. F. B. McGuire and himself to visit the prisoners, and for a long time he administered to their urgent and material wants. Was the first physician in Washington to devote special attention to the diseases of women. See Minutes Med. Society, Oct. 25, 1876; Trans. A. M. A., 1878, XXIX, p. 686; Atkinson's Phys. and Surg., 1878, p. 705; Busey's Reminiscences, p. 178; and "In Memoriam Board of Directors Children's Hospital, Washington, 1876."

63. BENJAMIN F. PERRY—Born in Maryland. M. D., 1829, Univ. Maryland. Removed to Hillsville, Va., about 1870. Died March 21, 1898, Carroll Co., Va.

PROBABLY JANUARY 5, 1842

64. EDWARD FLORENS RIVINUS. [Rivinus and Perry (No. 63) were both nominated Jan. 6, 1840; there is no record of the election of Rivinus, but apparently he was recognized as a member.] Born Jan. 1, 1802, Düben, Saxony. M. D., 1830, Univ. Penna. Died Feb. 14, 1873, at Hyeres, France. Author of "Catalogue of the Medical Library of Philadelphia Almshouse," Philadelphia, 1831. See Larrey (D. J.), "Observations on wounds," Philadelphia, 1832.

JULY 5, 1842

65. FLODOARDO HOWARD—Born March 11, 1814, Stafford Co., Va. M. D., 1841, Columbian; Phar. D., 1872, Georgetown. President Med. Assn., D. C., 1873-5. Father of Dr. Robertson Howard, *infra*. Died January, 1888, at Rockville, Md. Educated at Brookville Academy, Brookville, Md. For some years conducted a pharmacy. Studied medicine with Dr. Henry Howard. Practiced medicine in Washington; member Amer. Med. Association. Was one of the four who organized the Georgetown Med. School, and was Prof. Obstetrics and Diseases of Women until 1876, except for 1857-63, when he resided in Brookville. Consulting Physician to Providence Hospital and Women's Christian Home; Attending Physician St. Ann's Infant Asylum, Washington. Married, June 11, 1833, Lydia M., daughter of Samuel Robertson, of Maryland. See Atkinson's Phys. and Surgeons, 1878, p. 34; Minutes Med. Society, Jan. 18, 1888; Busey's Reminiscences, p. 152; Georgetown Univ., II, p. 71.

66. WILLIAM W. HOXTON—Born in District of Columbia. M. D., 1834, Univ. Penna. Asst. Surg., U. S. A., resigning Sept. 30, 1841. Died Aug. 23, 1855. See Brown's History, p. 292.

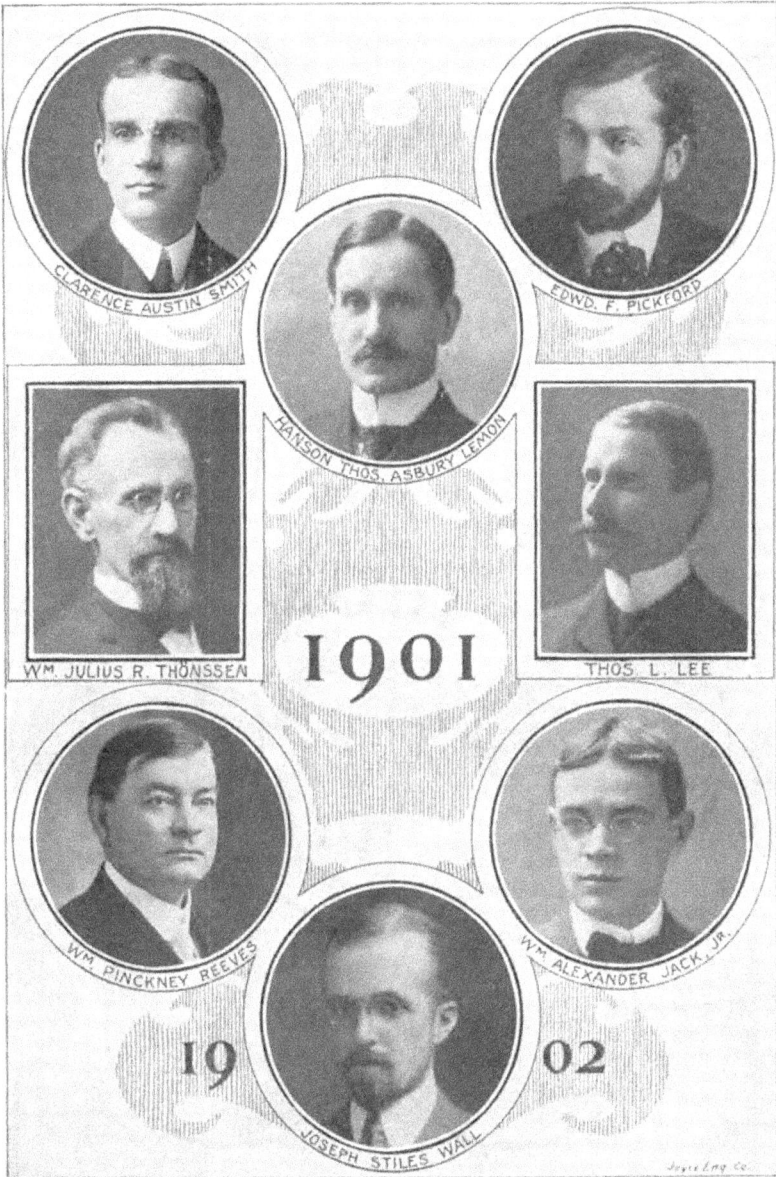

CLARENCE AUSTIN SMITH

EDWD. F. PICKFORD

HANSON THOS. ASBURY LEMON

WM. JULIUS R. THONSSEN

1901

THOS. L. LEE

WM. PINCKNEY REEVES

WM. ALEXANDER JACK, JR.

19

02

JOSEPH STILES WALL

Joyce Eng Co.

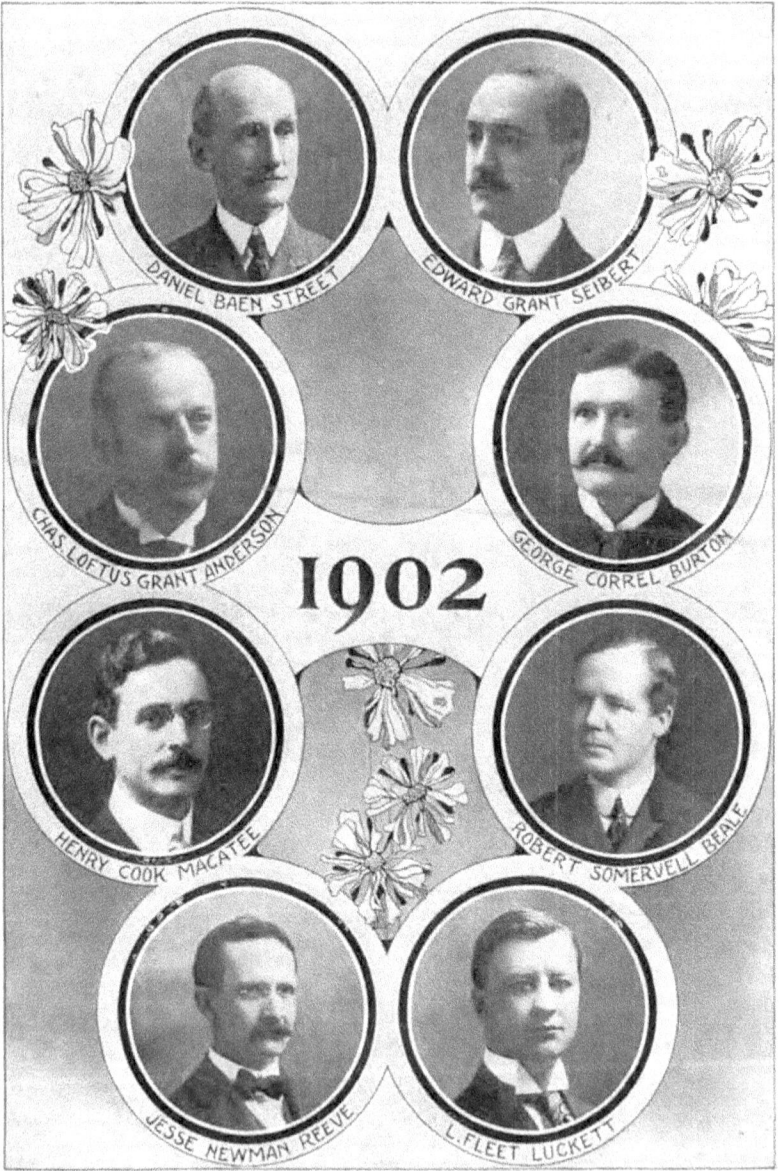

DANIEL BAEN STREET

EDWARD GRANT SEIBERT

CHAS. LOFTUS GRANT ANDERSON

GEORGE CORREL BURTON

1902

HENRY COOK MACATEE

ROBERT SOMERVELL BEALE

JESSE NEWMAN REEVE

L. FLEET LUCKETT

1842

67. WILLIAM HOLMES VAN BUREN. [There is no record of Van Buren's election, but he was recognized as a member.] Born April 5, 1819, Philadelphia, Pa. A. M., 1866, LL. D., 1878, Yale; M. D., 1840, Univ. Penna.; appointed Asst. Surg., U. S. A., June 15, 1840; resigned Dec. 31, 1845. Removed to New York City; died March 25, 1883. He came of a family of physicians. [Great-great-grandson of Dr. Johannes Van Buren (a pupil of Boerhaave); graduate of Univ. Leyden; emigrated to New York in 1700; physician to the N. Y. City Almshouse. Great-grandson of Dr. Beekman Van Buren and grandson of Dr. Abraham Van Buren.] Educated in Philadelphia and at Yale College. Spent eighteen months at Charité Hospital, Paris. While in U. S. Army, served in Florida, on Canadian frontier and in the Surgeon General's Office, Washington. In 1845 became Prosector to Chair of Surgery, Med. Dept. University City of New York; in 1852, Prof. Anatomy. Was Consulting Surgeon to St. Vincent's Hospital and to Charity Hospital, Blackwell's Island; Prof. Surgery, Bellevue Hospital Med. College; in 1859, elected Vice President N. Y. Acad. Medicine; in 1861 was active in forming the U. S. Sanitary Commission. Was offered the place of Surgeon General, U. S. A.; declined in favor of Dr. W. A. Hammond. In 1842 married a daughter of Dr. Valentine Mott, of N. Y. City. Author of "Lectures upon diseases of the rectum," New York, 1870, 1878, 1881, "Inflammation," in Ashhurst's Surgery, 1881; translated Morel's "Compendium of human histology," 1861; "Contributions to practical surgery," Philadelphia, 1865, etc. See Brown's History, p. 293; Powell's History, p. 642; Boston Med. and Surg. Jour., 1883, CVIII, p. 332; N. Y. Med. Jour., 1883, XXXVII, p. 393; Appleton's Biog., 1887, VI, p. 234.

JANUARY 9, 1843

68. JOHNSON ELIOT—Born Aug. 24, 1815, D. C. Father of Drs. J. L. and Johnson Eliot, Jr., *infra*. M. D., 1842, Columbian. Hon. A. M., 1869, and Phar. D., 1872, Georgetown. President Med. Assn., D. C., 1880–1. Died Dec. 30, 1883. Descendant of Sir John Eliot, of Devonshire, England, and of colonial settlers of Massachusetts and Maryland; grandnephew of President Andrew Eliot, of Harvard College. Educated at McLeod Seminary, Washington. Sometime clerk in Dr. Chas. McCormack's drug store, Washington. Studied medicine with Dr. Thomas Sewall, *supra*. Sometime steward in Washington Naval Hospital. After graduating in medicine was appointed Demonstrator of Anatomy, Columbian Med. College. One of the four who founded the Georgetown Med. School; Prof. Anatomy, 1849; Materia Medica and Physiology, 1854, In 1861, he became Prof. Surgery and so continued till 1876; for twenty years was Dean of the Faculty. Served on Surgical Staff of Providence Hospital, Columbia Hospital for Women, and Children's Hospital. Member of Pathological Society of Washington, National Institute and Amer. Med. Assn. Vice President Alumni Association, Georgetown University. Consulting Surgeon to Central Dispensary ; for some years Physician to Smallpox Hospital ; Surgeon to Metropolitan Police ; Consulting Surgeon St. Ann's Infant Asylum. After the second battle of Bull Run (1862), when a call for volunteer surgeons was made, he went to the front, taking with him the necessary appliances, and while in attendance on the sick and wounded was taken prisoner, but was soon released, and walked from Chantilly to Washington. Among those on whom he operated was Corporal James Tanner. Married Nov. 30, 1850, Mary John, daughter of John Llewellin, of St. Mary's Co., Md. See Minutes of Med. Society, Dec. 31, 1883; Atkinson's Phys. and Surg., 1878, p. 85 ; Maryland Med. Jour., 1883-4, X, p. 671 ; Med. and Surg. Reporter, 1884, L, p. 64 ; Jour. A. M. A., 1884, II, p. 79 ; Busey's Reminiscences, p. 187 ; Georgetown University, II, p. 65.

JANUARY 3, 1844

69. ANTHONY HOLMEAD, JR.—Born 1822, District of Columbia. M. D., 1841, Columbian. Died Oct. 26, 1855. See Minutes of Med. Society, Oct. 27, 1855.

JULY 1, 1844

70. JAMES HYMAN CAUSTEN, JR.—Born July, 1818, Baltimore, Md. M. D., 1842, Columbian. Died Oct. 3 or 5, 1856. [Eldest son of J. H. Causten, U. S. Consul to Ecuador ; his mother was the daughter of Thomas Meyer, of Baltimore.] Attended St. Mary's College, Baltimore, in 1830, and Georgetown College in 1835. After graduation in medicine, went abroad with Dr. R. K. Stone, *infra*. Retired early from practice of medicine to engage in translation of documents. Married, April 9, 1850, Miss Anna Payne, adopted daughter of "Dolly Madison." Author of "Claims against France," Washington, 1871.

71. SAMUEL CLEMENT SMOOT—Born Feb. 3, 1818, District of Columbia. A. B., 1835, A. M., 1838, Columbian; M. D., 1838, Jefferson. Acting Asst. Surg., U. S. N., Oct. 5, 1861, to Jan. 27, 1862, when he resigned ; sometime President Board of Health, Washington. Died Sept. 29, 1866. His ancestors were among the early settlers of Maryland. He studied medicine with Dr. Thomas Sewall, *supra*. Practiced some time at Jackson, Miss.; in 1839 returned to Washington. In 1856 was elected Secretary to Board of Trustees of Columbian College ; was Demonstrator of Anatomy in Med. Dept.; member of Med. Association, D. C. See Minutes Med. Society, Oct. 1, 1866; Trans. A. M. A., 1867, XVIII, p. 340.

72. CHARLES H. LIEBERMANN—Born Sept. 15, 1813, Riga, Russia. A. B., 1836, Dorpat; M. D., 1838, Univ. Berlin. Died March 27, 1886. His father was a military surgeon ; his mother was one of the Radetzkeys of German and Polish history. Studied medicine first at Wilna, then at Dorpat, finally at Berlin ; was private pupil of Prof. Dieffenbach. After graduation, visited hospitals in the principal capitals of Europe. In 1840, came to United States, and began to practice in Washington. For over twenty years was the leading oculist of Washington. Member Med. Association, D. C.; National Institute; one of the founders of Georgetown Med. School ; Prof. Surgery, 1849–53 and 1857–61 ; member of Pathological Society; Amer. Med. Association ; Physician to Convent of Visitation ; Consulting Physician Georgetown College and Convent ; Consulting Surgeon Providence Hospital ; Member of Board of Managers Children's Hospital. In 1841 married Miss Betzold, of Alexandria, D. C. See Minutes Med. Society, March 29, 1886 ; Jour. A. M. A., 1886, VII, p. 222 ; Busey's Reminiscences, p. 153 ; Georgetown Univ., II, p. 72.

73. THOMAS E. W. FEINOUR or FERNIOUR, M. D.—[There was a Dr. T. Feinour in Baltimore in 1874. There was also a Thos. E. W Feinour, clerk at Police Headquarters, D. C., in 1869.]

PROBABLY JULY 1, 1844

74. JAMES GRIFFITH COOMBE—[Coombe attended the meeting Jan. 6, 1845, and subsequent meetings, and was recognized as a member.] Born Jan. 1, 1812, D. C. M. D., 1835, Univ. Maryland. Died Feb. 4, 1883.

JANUARY 6, 1845

75. THOMAS BAKER JOHNSON FRYE—Born 1820, District of Columbia. A. M. and M. D., 1840, Columbian. Removed to Alexandria, Va. Died May 31, 1889, in Washington, D. C., of cancer of tongue.

76. JOSEPH F. MUNDING, M. D.--[Munding attended a special meeting April 11, 1845 ; he is not afterwards mentioned in the minutes but the Catalogue of 1885 records him as having been a member.] Born in 1808. Member of Pathological Society of Washington. Died March 3, 1852.

JULY 7, 1845

77. CORNELIUS BOYLE—Born Nov. 12, 1817, District of Columbia. Father of Dr. C. B. Boyle, *infra*. M. D., 1844, Columbian. Provost Marshal General, Army of Northern Virginia (Confederate). Died March 11, 1878. [Son of John Boyle, an Irish patriot, who came from Londonderry, Ireland, about May 1, 1801—was for nearly thirty years

Chief Clerk, Navy Department, Washington—and Catherine Annie Burke, daughter of Richard Burke, of Baltimore Co., Md.] Educated at the academy of John McLeod, Washington. For some time was in the drug business. After graduating in medicine, practiced in Washington. One of his patients was Senator Sumner, of Massachusetts, after the *Brooks* assault in 1856; another was Brooks himself. At the outbreak of the Civil War Dr. Boyle "went South." Was sometime Major in the command of Stonewall Jackson; afterwards Provost Marshal General, Army of Northern Virginia, from May, 1862, to April, 1865. Then took passage for Mexico, but was wrecked off Cape Hatteras; in Mexico he was in a banking house. Later he bought and managed the Fauquier White Sulphur Springs, Va. About 1869 returned to Washington and resumed practice. Member Med. Association, D. C.; Amer. Med. Association; Pathological Society and National Institute, Washington. Married in 1852, Fannie R., daughter of Wm. Greene, of Fredericksburg, Va.; afterwards Cherry Bethune, daughter of Gen. Joseph N. and Frances Grinley Bethune, of Georgia. See Minutes Med. Society, March 12, 1878; Trans. A. M. A., 1878, XXIX, p. 618; Atkinson's Phys. and Surgeons, 1878, p. 381.

JANUARY 19, 1846

78. CHARLES HARTWELL CRAGIN—Born Sept. 7, 1817, Alsted, N. H. A. B., 1837; A. M., 1840, Amherst; M. D., 1844, Columbian. Died April 1, 1887. Son of Isaiah and Hannah H. Cragin. Attended school at New Ipswich, N. H., and afterwards the Academy of Groton, Mass. Taught school at Richmond, Va., in 1837 and 1838, and at Fitchburg, Mass., during part of the years 1838 to 1840. While teaching school at Fitchburg, studied medicine with Dr. J. A. Marshall. Removed to Washington in 1840 and continued his studies with Dr. Thomas Sewall, *supra*, teaching school while attending lectures. Practiced medicine in Washington in 1844 and 1845, and afterwards in Georgetown, except during 1849 and 1850, when he resided in Sacramento, Cal., being one of the "Forty-niners" who went to California when the memorable gold discovery was made; the journey occupied six months and, with the exception of the trip across the Isthmus of Panama, was made in sailing vessels. Retired from practice in 1865 because of ill health. Member of Board of Common Council, Georgetown; for several years Police Commissioner, D. C.; member of School Board; Postmaster of Georgetown; Secretary and Treasurer Columbia Hospital, Washington. Married, Oct. 2, 1845, Mary, daughter of Samuel and Mary A. F. McKenney, of Georgetown; April 16, 1857, her sister, Henrietta F. McKenney. See Minutes of Med. Society, April 13, 1887.

79. JAMES F. T. [or J.] McCLE[A]RY—Born Jan. 24, 1820, District of Columbia. M. D., 1842, Columbian. Surgeon, C. S. A. Died Feb. 16, 1871. His parents were natives of Maryland, where he himself was educated. Soon after graduation in medicine he accompanied Robert Dale Owen in an exploring expedition through the Western States. Returned to Washington; practiced medicine here a short time, then practiced in Loudoun Co., Va. During the Civil War served as medical officer, C. S. A. In July, 1865, embarked for South America; for three years was Surgeon on a vessel bound for China. Returned to Washington and resumed practice. Member of Med. Association, D. C. See Minutes Med. Society, Feb. 22, 1871; Trans. A. M. A., 1872, XXIII, p. 581.

JULY 6, 1846

80. GRAFTON TYLER—Born Nov. 21, 1811, "La Grange," Prince George Co., Md. M. D., 1833, Univ. Maryland. Licentiate M. C. F., Maryland, 1839. Father of Dr. W. B. Tyler, *infra*. President of Board of Health, Georgetown. Died Aug. 26, 1884. Descended from a family of Tylers that came from England and settled on the Patuxent River, Maryland, in 1660. Son of Grafton and Ann H. Plummer Tyler. Educated at Carnochan's and McVean's school, Georgetown. Studied medicine with Dr. Richard Duckett, of Maryland, with whom he formed a partnership after graduation. In 1845 removed to Georgetown, D. C. In 1846 became Prof. Practice of Medicine, Columbian Med. School, and a few years later, Prof. Clinical Medicine, Washington Infirmary; resigned both in 1859; member of first Board of Visitors of Government Hospital for Insane, D. C.; President of Board of Council of Georgetown; member Med. and Chirurg. Faculty, Maryland; Med. Association, D. C.; Amer. Med. Association, Vice President in 1855; Consulting Physician to Providence Hospital and President of the Board for its opening; incorporator and director of Children's Hospital. Married, January, 1836, Mary M., daughter of Walter Bowie, Esq., Prince George Co., Md. Author of "Medicine as a science and an art," Washington, 1852. See Minutes Med. Society, Aug. 27, 1884; Maryland Med. Jour., 1884, XI, p. 379; Atkinson's Phys. and Surgeons, 1878, p. 238; Busey's Reminiscences, p. 161; Jour. A. M. A., 1884, III, p. 307; Cordell's Med. Annals of Maryland, 1903, p. 601.

JANUARY 3, 1848

81. JAMES ETHELBERT MORGAN—Born Sept. 25, 1822, St. Mary's Co., Md. M. D., 1845, Columbian; Actg. Asst. Surg., U. S. A.; President Med. Assn., D. C., 1879-80. Father of Drs. E. C. and J. D. Morgan, *infra*. Died June 2, 1889. [His ancestors belonged to the families of Morgan, of Monmouthshire, and Cecil, of Kent, England. They were adherents of the cause of Charles I and Roman Catholics, and were therefore glad to seek an asylum in the Catholic colony of Maryland.] Educated at St. John's College, Md. After graduation in medicine practiced in Washington. In 1848 was appointed Demonstrator of Anatomy, Columbian Med. College; also Asst. to Prof. Anatomy. In 1852 Prof. Physiology, Georgetown Med. College; afterwards of Med. Jurisprudence. In 1858 Prof. Materia Medica and Therapeutics, which he held until 1876. Physician and Surgeon to Washington Asylum and Smallpox Hospitals. In 1862 had charge of Soldiers' Rest, under the control of U. S. Sanitary Commission; also 1862-5 Surgeon to the Quartermaster's Hospital. Member of Board of Health many years. He and Dr. R. K. Stone, *infra*, investigated the mysterious "National Hotel Disease." Member Amer. Med. Assn. and of its Judicial Council. For many years had charge of the medical staff of the District Militia. At the outbreak of the Civil War he organized the 4th D. C. Vols., and at first was its Colonel, but resigned and was made its Surgeon. Member of Board of Trustees of Public Schools. In 1850 was elected an alderman, but soon retired. In June, 1854, married Nora, daughter of Wm. Dudley Digges, of Maryland, a descendant of Gov. Edward Digges, of Virginia, and of the Carroll family, of Maryland. See Minutes of Med. Society, June 3, 1889; Atkinson's Phys. and Surgeons, 1878, p. 116; N. Y. Med. Jour., 1889, XLIX, p. 635; Med. Record, N. Y., 1889, XXXV, p. 692; Busey's Reminiscences, p. 196; Georgetown University, II, p. 76.

82. HAMILTON PLEASANTS HOWARD—Born 1820, Brookville, Md. M. D., 1841, Univ. Va. Removed from the District about July 3, 1848. Died Dec. 29, 1863. Was President Board of Health, Washington, 1855-6. Surgeon and Medical Purveyor, C. S. A.

83. ALFRED HOWLAND LEE—Born April 19, 1819, Ridgfield, Conn. M. D., 1839, Jefferson. Dropped from membership 1891. Died Oct. 24, 1903.

84. WILLIAM McKENDREE TUCKER—[Tucker was first nominated in January, 1839.] Born 1821, D. C. A. B., 1840; M. D., 1844, Columbian. Died Jan. 31, 1890, of consumption. Removed for burial to Ballston, N. Y.

85. PHILANDER GOULD—Born in Maine. M. D., 1845, Columbian. Nothing more known of him.

86. ROBERT KING STONE—Born in 1822, D. C. A. B., 1842, Princeton. M. D., 1845, Univ. Penna.; 1849, Univ. Louisville; 1851, Univ. City of New York. Father of Dr. T. R. Stone, *infra*. Was physician to President Abraham Lincoln. President Board of Health of Washington, 1858-61. Died April 23, 1872, in Philadelphia, Pa. His ancestors were among the earlier settlers of Washington. He studied medicine with Dr. Thos. Miller, *supra*, and assisted the latter in the dissecting room. After graduation in medicine he attended clinics at the hospitals of London, Edinburgh, Paris and Vienna, paying special attention to diseases of the eye and ear; was a private pupil of Desmarres. Returned to Washington in 1847 and began practice. In 1848 became Adjunct Prof. Anatomy and Physiology, Columbian Med. College; afterwards, Prof. Anatomy, Physiology and Microscopic Anatomy; later became Prof. Ophthalmic and Aural Surgery. In consequence of a fracture of the thigh he gave up outdoor practice. Member Pathological Society, Washington. In 1849 married the daughter of Thomas Ritchie, who founded the Richmond Enquirer in 1804, and Washington Union in 1845. See Minutes Med. Society, April 24, 1872; Trans. A. M. A., 1873, XXIV, p. 338; Busey's Reminiscences, pp. 54 and 56.

PROBABLY JANUARY 3, 1848

87. SAMUEL ELLICOTT TYSON—[Tyson was nominated Jan. 4, 1847. There was no meeting of the Society in July, 1847, and he was, therefore, most probably elected at the next January meeting.] Born Nov. 16, 1809, in Maryland. M. D., 1832, Washington Med. Coll., Baltimore. Licentiate M. C. F., Maryland, 1832. Died March 29, 1883. Grandson of Elisha Tyson, the philanthropist. Studied medicine with Dr. Wm. Handy, of Baltimore, Md. After graduation, he served some time in a hospital in Philadelphia, Pa. After practicing medicine awhile in Washington his health failed and he engaged in pharmacy. See Busey's Reminiscences, p. 162; Cordell's Med. Annals, Maryland, 1903, p. 602.

JULY 3. 1848

88. GEORGE McCAULEY DOVE—Born Oct. 5, 1817, District of Columbia. M. D., 1839, Univ. Penna. Licentiate M. C. F., Maryland, 1841. Acting Asst. Surg., U. S. A.; Surgeon to Baltimore Battalion, in Mexican War, 1846; Secretary and afterwards President Board of Health, D. C. Died Jan. 30, 1874. Son of Marmaduke and Margaret Dove. Studied medicine with Dr. Kearney, U. S. Navy. After graduation, practiced in Washington. For many years Physician to Washington Asylum; also Attending Physician Providence Hospital, and in 1849 of Smallpox Hospital. For a long time Prof. Practice of Medicine, Columbian Med. College; also sometime Demonstrator and Adjunct Prof. Anatomy, Georgetown Med. School. During the Civil War was in charge of a military hospital. See Minutes Med. Society, Jan. 31, 1874; Trans. A. M. A., 1874, XXV, p. 525; Cordell's Med. Annals of Maryland, 1903, p. 381.

89. JOSEPH WALSH—Born Oct. 28, 1806, Dublin, Ireland. M. D., 1843, Columbian. Sometime apothecary in Washington. Acting Asst. Surg., U. S. A. Father of Dr. J. K. Walsh, *infra*. Died of pneumonia,

Nov. 9, 1879. Son of Joseph and Margaret Corrigan Walsh, of Dublin.
Educated at the Jesuit College, Dublin. Graduated in pharmacy, 1828,
at Apothecaries' Hall, Dublin. Travelled much, over the world; finally
settled in Washington. Served some time in U. S. Marine Barracks and
studied medicine. After graduation, was contract physician at Marine
Barracks, and also practiced among the citizens. Sometime physician to
the poor. Member Med. Association, D. C.; Amer. Med. Association.
Married, Sept. 7, 1843, Elizabeth, daughter of Wm. and Malinda Tench
Smith, of Washington. See Minutes Med. Society, Nov. 10, 1879;
Trans. A. M. A., 1880, XXXI, p. 1096.

90. JOSEPH B. EDELIN, M. D.—Born in Maryland. Acting Asst.
Surg., U. S. A. Died May 18, 1876.

91. JOHN IGNATIUS DYER—Born May 17, 1827, District of Columbia. M. D., Columbian, 1847. Dropped from membership, 1866. Removed to St. Marys Co., Md. Returned to Washington, 1876; appointed
Visiting Physician Washington Asylum, also Physician St. Vincent's Orphan Asylum. Died May 9, 1903.

92. ISAAC STREIGHT LAUCK—[Lauck's name appears only once
in the minutes of the Society, namely, May 18, 1864, the day after he
died. The 1885 list dates his election in 1848, but on what authority
does not appear.] Born March 11, 1820, Martinsburg, Va. M. D., 1841,
Pennsylvania College, Philadelphia. Died May 17, 1864. Grandson of
Peter Lauck, an officer in Morgan's Virginia Riflemen, War of American
Revolution; son of First Lieutenant Lauck, Tucker's Winchester Com-
pany, War of 1812. Practiced medicine in Georgetown, D. C. Married
Miss Anna Jones, niece of Dr. Hezekiah Magruder, *infra*. See Minutes
Med. Society, May 18, 1864.

JANUARY 1, 1849

93. WM. H. SAUNDERS—Born in District of Columbia. M. D.,
1848, University of Penna. Left the District about January, 1854. Died
in Nicaraugua in 1860, during the last and disastrous invasion of that
country by Walker, the "freebooter."

94. SAMUEL CLAGETT BUSEY—Born July 23, 1828, Montgomery
Co., Md. M. D., 1848, Univ. Penna. LL. D., 1888, St. Mary's Univ.,
Emmetsburg, Md.; 1899, Georgetown Univ. President Med. Assn., D. C.,
1875-6. Co-Editor National Medical Journal, Washington. Died Feb.
12, 1901. Author of "Congenital occlusion and dilation of lymph
channels," New York, 1878; "Personal reminiscences," etc., Washing-

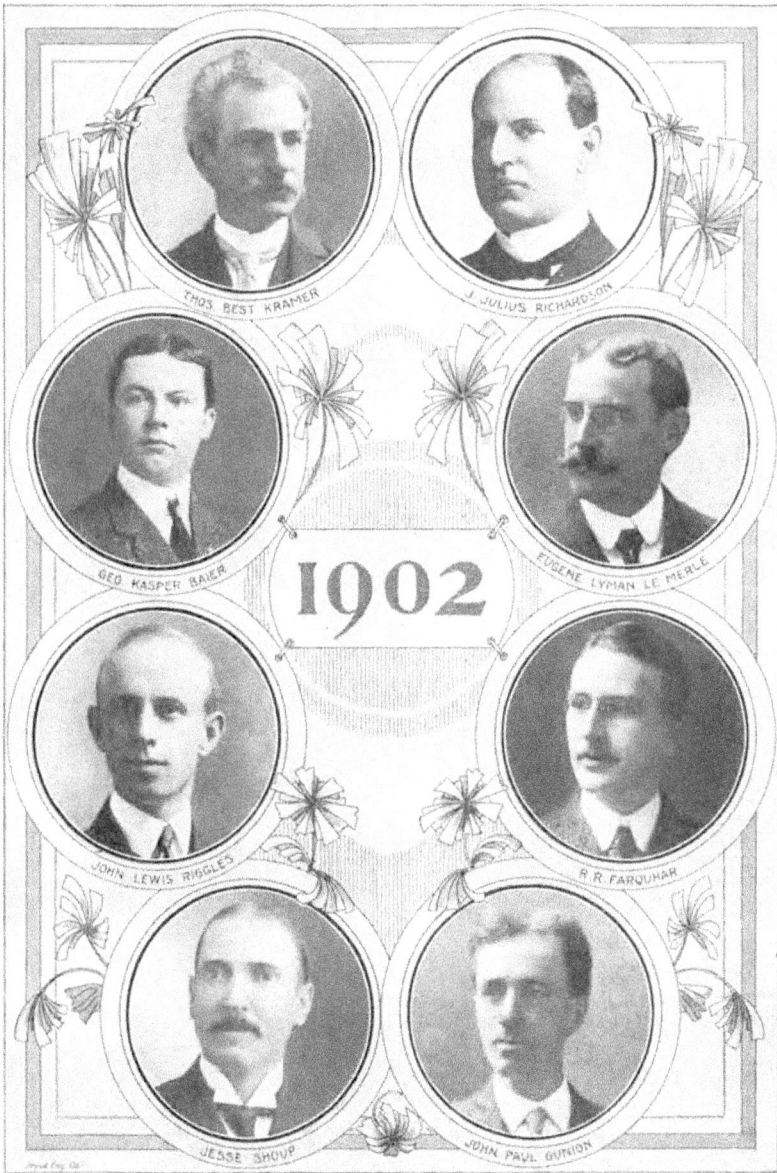

THOS. BEST KRAMER

J. JULIUS RICHARDSON

GEO. KASPER BAIER

1902

EUGENE LYMAN LE MERLE

JOHN LEWIS RIGGLES

R. R. FARQUHAR

JESSE SHOUP

JOHN PAUL GUNION

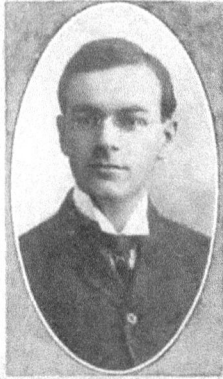

EDGAR P. COPELAND

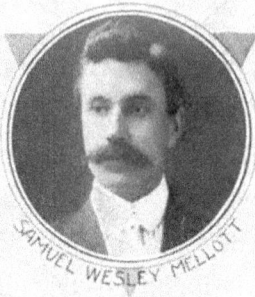

SAMUEL WESLEY MELLOTT

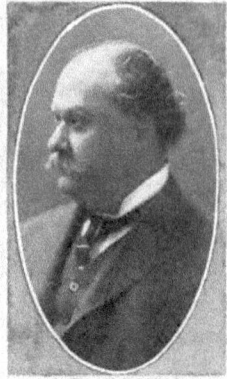

CHARLES ALBERT BALL

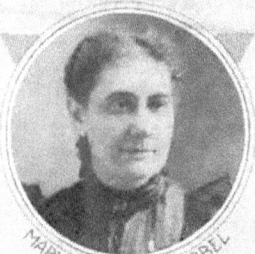

MARY LOUISE STROBEL

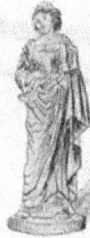

ΨΗΕΙΑ

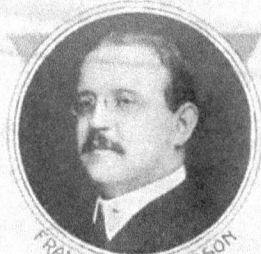

FRANK EUGENE GIBSON

1902

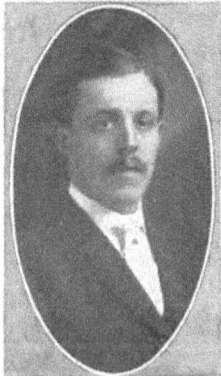

THOS. SANFORD
DUNAWAY GRASTY

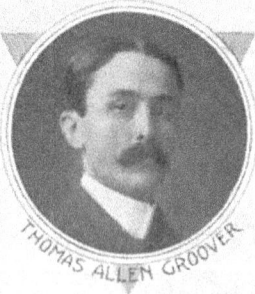

THOMAS ALLEN GROOVER

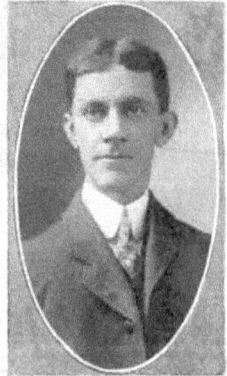

ELIJAH LUMBIA MASON

ton, 1895; "The year 1896," etc., Washington, 1896; "A souvenir,"
etc., Washington, 1896; "Pictures of the City of Washington," Wash-
ington, 1898; "Annual addresses," Washington, 1899; "Physiological
and clinical phenomena of natural labor," Hirst's System of Obstetrics,
Philadelphia, 1888, I; "Chronic inversion of uterus," Mann's System of
Gynecology, Philadelphia, 1888. [Son of John and Rachel Clagett
Busey; born on a farm in Montgomery Co., Md., 1½ miles east of Cabin
John Bridge. Of·Scotch-English descent; his mother the daughter of
Thomas Clagett, seventh in line of descent from Capt. Thomas Clagett,
to whom a tract of land known as Weston was patented by Lord Baltimore.] Attended a country school, afterward the Rockville Academy,
1841-5. Began the study of medicine with Dr. Hezekiah Magruder,
infra; his facilities for study were a Cullen's Treatise on Materia Medica, 37 years old, and a Dissector, 25 years old, several rusty scalpels and
a tooth forceps. Afterwards was a private student of Dr. Geo. B. Wood,
Philadelphia, Pa. After graduation began to practice medicine in Washington. In 1847 married Miss Posey. Was elected a member of the
Common Council. Assisted in the reorganization of the Medical Society
in 1852; an original member of the Pathological Society. In 1853 became Prof. Materia Medica, Georgetown Medical School. In 1858, because of feeble health, gave up his practice in Washington and removed
to a farm named Mount Pisgah, afterward "Belvoir," on the Woodley
Lane Road, where he remained till 1868. He recovered his health, returned to the city and resumed his practice. Was soon engaged in founding a hospital for sick children, assisted by Drs. W. B. Drinkard, F. A.
Ashford and W. W. Johnston. In 1875 was appointed Prof. Diseases of
Children, Georgetown Med. School; in 1876, Prof. of Theory and Practice of Medicine. Aided in establishing a section of Diseases of Children
in Amer. Med. Assn. One of the founders of the American Pediatric Society. Materially assisted in founding Garfield Memorial Hospital. One
of the founders and the first President of Washington Obstet. and
Gynecol. Society; founder of Amer. Gynecol. Society, one of its Vice
Presidents; also founder of Association of Amer. Physicians, its President
in 1890. One of the founders of the Washington Academy of Sciences,
and was on the Board of Managers and Vice President till his death.
Member of Philosophical, Anthropological and Historical Societies of
Washington. Retired from practice in 1895 and devoted himself to literary work. In the matter of the water supply of the city he went before
Committees of Congress and Board of Trade; public meetings were held,
in all of which he took part. So also with the Medical Practice Act;
he was always on the watch, and toward the last he went to the White
House and found in the bill as taken to the President for signature an
interpolation that required that the bill go back to the Senate for correc-
tion. So also with the question of pure milk supply. In 1895 he suf-

16

fered a fracture of the thigh that compelled him to give up out-door work. In 1896 he published an autobiography in which he gave sketches of the lives of many of the founders of the Medical Society and his contemporaries. In 1899 he published a series of annual addresses that he had delivered before the Society. One of these was on "The history of the progress of sanitation in the City of Washington and the efforts of the medical profession in relation thereto." See Minutes Med. Society, Feb. 13, 20, and March 6, 1901; Trans. Med. Society, 1901, VI, pp. 72–92; National Med. Review, 1893-4, II, p. 177; Georgetown University, II, p. 77.

JANUARY 7, 1850

95. HENRY JOHN CROSSON—Born Jan. 19, 1805, Baltimore Co., Md. M. D., 1836, Univ. Maryland. Sometime clerk in Treasury Dept., D. C. Dropped from membership, 1877. Died Nov. 21, 1880, of consumption.

96. RUFUS HOLMEAD SPEAKE—Born April 17, 1807, Alexandria, D. C. M. D., 1829, Washington Med. College, Baltimore. Licentiate M. C. F., Maryland, 1831-2. Died Sept. 20, 1867. Son of Capt. Josias M. Speake, U. S. N. Educated in Alexandria, and in Georgetown College. Studied medicine with Dr. Peregrine Warfield, *supra*. Practiced in Montgomery Co., Md., until 1849; afterwards in Washington till 1863, when poor health compelled him to give up practice, after which he was a clerk in the Second Auditor's Office, Washington. See Minutes Med. Society, Sept. 20, 1867; Trans. A. M. A., 1868, XIX, p. 435; Cordell's Med. Annals, Maryland, 1903, p. 577.

97. HEZEKIAH MAGRUDER—Born May 24, 1804, Montgomery Co., Md. M. D., 1826, Univ. Maryland. Died July 20, 1874. Son of George B. and Charity Margaret Wilson Magruder. Educated at Carnachan's Seminary. Studied medicine with Dr. B. S. Bohrer, *supra*. After graduation practiced in Georgetown, D. C. Member Med. Assn., D. C.; Amer. Med. Assn. Married Miss Alice Crittenden, of Georgetown; afterwards, Miss Mary Chipman, of Georgetown; afterwards, Miss Mary E. Fitzhugh, of Virginia. One son, Dr. Alex. F. Magruder, is Passed Asst. Surg., U. S. N. See Minutes Med. Society, July 21, 1874; Trans. A. M. A., 1880, XXXI, p. 1065; Busey's Reminiscences, p. 157.

JULY 1, 1850

98. AARON WOOLLEY MILLER—Born Aug. 26, 1818, Pittsburg, Pa. M. D., 1846, Columbian. Surgeon, C. S. A. Dropped from membership, 1877. Died Jan. 6, 1881. Received liberal education; served in hospital of U. S. Marine Barracks, Washington. After graduation in medicine practiced in Washington. At the outbreak of the Civil War "went south" and served in hospitals till 1865 ; then returned to Washington and resumed practice. Member Med. Assn., D. C., and Amer. Med. Assn. Son of Isaac Smith Miller who was connected with U. S. Arsenal, Washington, and Abbie Woolley Miller. Married Julia Woodward, daughter of Amon Woodward. See Minutes Med. Society, Jan. 12, 1881 ; Trans. A. M. A., 1881, XXXII, p. 526.

1850

99. JAMES MORRIS WILSON—[Wilson's name appears on the 1885 list as having been a member in 1850. His name is not on the minutes of the Society nor on the Treasurer's book.] Born Nov. 21, 1821, Princess Anne Co., Md. [So stated in the 1885 catalogue, but there is no county of that name in Maryland.] M. D., 1846, Berkshire. Removed from the District about 1858.

100. WILLIAM H. WATERS—[Waters' name does not appear on the minutes of the Society nor on the Treasurer's book. The Society took no action in regard to his death. The list of the Medical Association of 1854 states that he had left the District. The date, 1850, therefore, is tentative.] Born in District of Columbia. M. D., 1841, Columbian. Said to have removed from the city between 1848 and 1854. Died Nov. 7, 1865.

JANUARY 6, 1851

101. ALEXANDER SOMERVILLE WOTHERSPOON—Born 1817, New York City. A. B., 1837, Columbia, N. Y. City; M. D., 1841, Coll. Phys. and Surg., N. Y. City. Asst. Surg., U. S. A., 1843-54. Died May 4, 1854. See Brown's History, p. 293 ; Powell's History, p. 690.

JULY 7, 1851

102. SAMUEL W. EVERETT—Born Aug. 25, 1820, London, England. M. D., 1850, Univ. City of New York. Removed in 1852 to Quincy, Ill. Surgeon, 10th Ill. Vols. and U. S. Vols. Killed at Battle of Pittsburg Landing, April 6, 1862. Son of Chas. Everett, of Boston, Mass. Educated in London and Paris. In 1840 the family came to the United States, and resided at Quincy, Ill. Studied medicine with Dr. Adams Nichols. In 1847-8 was in charge of medical stores at San Antonio, Texas. After graduation in medicine, practiced in Washington. When the Georgetown Med. School was organized he was appointed Prof. Anatomy. In 1852 returned to Quincy; at the outbreak of the Civil War he joined the Union Army; was stationed awhile at Cairo, Ill. In the winter of 1861-2 was Med. Director, Dept. Missouri, and later was ordered to Tennessee. "On the battlefield of Shiloh, April 6, 1862, at about 8 A. M., he fell, pierced by two bullets, one through the forehead and the other through the body; the wounds were instantly fatal. He had been actively engaged in his surgical duties from the commencement of the action, when General Prentiss saw him stop men who were retreating, and induce them to return to the front. A short time afterward he was seen to rally fifty men and lead them personally into the fight, during one of the most critical periods of the engagement. It was at this time, when in near proximity to the enemy, and between the opposing lines, that he was shot dead from his horse." In 1848 he married Miss Mary Smith, of Alexandria, Va. See Trans. A. M. A., 1863, XIV, p. 212.

103. ALEXANDER YELVERTON PEYTON GARNETT—Born Sept. 19, 1820, Essex Co., Va. M. D., 1841, Univ. Penna. Asst. Surg. and Passed Asst. Surg., U. S. N.; Surgeon, C. S. A. President Med. Assn., D. C., 1882–3. President A. M. A., 1887. Died July 11, 1888, Rehoboth Beach, Del. Son of Muscoe and Maria Wills Battle Garnett, who resided on a plantation near the Rappahannock River. Educated by private tutors. After graduation in medicine served in U. S. Navy, finally stationed at the Navy Yard, Washington. Resigned in 1848, and afterwards practiced in Washington. Member of Med. Assn., D. C. ; President Patholog. Society ; member Amer. Med. Assn ; one of the original members Amer. Climatolog. Society. In 1858 Physician to U. S. Penitentiary, Washington ; Prof. Clinical Medicine, Columbian Med. College. During the Civil War was Surgeon, C. S. A., in charge of military hospitals, Richmond, Va. ; member of Board of Med. Examiners, C. S. A. Physician to Jefferson Davis, President of Southern Confederacy ; to Gen. R. E. Lee and family, and to most of the families of the Cabinet Officers of the Confederate Government. At the close of the war he returned to Washington and resumed practice here. Elected Prof. of Practice of Medicine, Columbian Med. College ; resigned in 1870. Member of Board of Directors and Consulting Staff, Columbia Hospital for Women, and Children's Hospital ; of Consulting Staff, Garfield Memorial Hospital ; Consulting Physician to St. Ann's Infant Asylum and Central Dispensary and Emergency Hospital. President Southern Memorial Association. Chairman of Local Committee of Arrangements, Ninth International Med. Congress. Married the daughter of Hon. Henry A. Wise, Governor of Virginia. One son was a physician, Dr. A. Y. P. Garnett, Jr. See Minutes Med. Society, July 13, 1888 ; Jour. Amer. Med. Assn, 1888, XI, p. 105 ; Trans. Amer. Climat. Assn. (1890), 1891, VII, p. 323 ; Atkinson's Phys. and Surg., 1878, p. 113 ; 20th Century Biog. Dict., 1904 ; Busey's Reminiscences, p. 192 ; J. B. Hamilton's Remarks, etc., Washington, 1888.

104. FREDERICK ADOLPHUS WISLIZENUS—Born May, 1810, Koenigsee, Germany. M. D., 1834, Univ. Zürich. Removed to St. Louis, Mo., where he died, Sept. 22, 1889. Said to have served in the

Mexican War. Educated at the Gymnasium at Dörnfeld, Thuringia, at Goettingen, Jena and Wuerzburg. Was compromised in the famous "Frankfuerter Attendat," and had to flee the country. "In the spring of 1833 a conspiracy had been formed in Frankfurt-on-the-Main, to avenge itself on the Federal Diet, which by its severely restrictive press laws had roused the citizens, particularly the younger portion, including many students in the several faculties, to something little short of madness. In this conspiracy Wislizenus, with Matthia and others of the medical *Burschenschaft*, took a leading part, the design being to blow up the Diet. April 3, 1833, the attempt was made. The guard house was carried by storm, and the conspirators were within an ace of effecting their purpose when the military appeared in the nick of time, arrested nine of the youths and put the others to flight. Among those who, after hairbreadth escapes, eluded arrest, was young Wislizenus, who found his way to Switzerland, where, at the University of Zürich he resumed his studies and graduated with distinction, and in 1835 proceeded to the United States. Ultimately settling in practice at St. Louis, he rapidly formed an extensive *clientèle*, of which his compatriots were the nucleus, and realized a handsome income, which enabled him to give time to pure science and also to travel in and beyond the States. He made memorable visits to Mexico and the Rocky Mountains, and published most interesting records of his observations and experiences. By all classes he was looked upon as an enthusiastic and large-minded reformer, and honest and benevolent survivor of the 'Vor Achtundvierziger' men, as the precursors of the revolution of 1848 are familiarly called." See Annual Report of Smithsonian Institution, 1904, pp. 398, 715 ; Lancet, London, 1889, II, p. 936.

JANUARY 2, 1852

105. JAMES M. AUSTIN—Born in Virginia. M. D., 1832, Univ. Penna. First Prof. Materia Medica, Georgetown Med. School ; member Clinico-Patholog. Society. Removed and died.

106. MARTIN VAN BUREN BOGAN—Born Sept. 16, 1829, Woodstock, Va. Son of Maj. Benjamin Lewis and Sarah Ott Bogan. Brother of Dr. S. W. Bogan, *infra*. Father of Dr. J. B. Bogan. M. D., 1851, Columbian. Dropped from membership 1878. Married Naomi Thompson ; in 1859 Charlotte Augusta Gray. Died April 20, 1898.

107. SAMUEL B. BLANCHARD—Born in 1817, in Massachusetts. M. D., 1850, Columbian. Dropped from membership 1872. Died suddenly Aug. 21, 1877. Practiced in Washington. Member Med. Assn., D. C. Unmarried. See Trans. A. M. A., 1878, XXIX, p. 618.

[P. J. Reuss paid the membership fee $5.oo Oct. 26, 1852, but there is no record of nomination, election, or even the granting of a license; nor does the name appear on the list of the Med. Association.]

JANUARY 13, 1853

108. FRANCIS HAMILTON HILL—Born 1826 or 1827, D. C. M. D., 1849, Columbian. Reëlected again about July 7, 1856; the reason does not appear. Dropped from membership. Died Jan. 30, 1906.

109. BENJAMIN FANEUIL CRAIG—Born Jan. 28, 1829, at U. S. Arsenal, Watertown, Mass. A. B., 1849; M. D., 1851, Univ. Penna. Acting Assist. Surg., U. S. A. Author of "Weights and Measures according to the decimal system," &c. New York, 1867; second edition, 1868. "Report relative to steerage passengers on emigrant vessels," Washington, 1874. Died April 10, 1877. Son of Gen. H. K. Craig, Chief of Ordnance, U. S. A. Educated at schools in Boston. After graduation in medicine he studied in London and Paris. Returned to United States in 1853 and was appointed Prof. Chemistry, Georgetown Med. School. In 1858 was placed in charge of Chemical Laboratory, Smithsonian Institution. At the outbreak of the Civil War was made Consulting Chemist to the Medical Purveyor's Dept., U. S. Army. "Dr. Craig also prepared, from material found in the U. S. Patent Office, a monograph on rifled field ordnance, showing the actual condition of the rifled artillery used in the army in the early years of the war. General H. J. Hunt, remarked of this paper that it contained later information by eighteen months than could be found in the War Department files, and was of great use to him in discharging his duties as Chief of Artillery of the Army of the Potomac, and he was much aided by the analyses, made by Dr. Craig, of fuses and other ordnance material." After the close of the war Dr. Craig continued in charge of the chemical laboratory of the Army Medical Department, and in addition supervised and collected the meteorological observations reported by the medical officers at various points. In 1873, at the request of the Secretary of the Treasury, he made two voyages to Europe to make a series of elaborate experiments on the air of the steerages of emigrant steamers, with a view of establishing regulations for the amelioration of the condition of the passengers by these vessels. For a year before his death he was engaged in drawing up a report on the influence of climate on the health of troops, designed as an addition to the Medical History of the War. Member of Amer. Assn. Adv. Science; Secretary of Philosophical Society of Washington, etc. [The Treasurer's book shows that Benjamin Franklin paid $5.oo on March 15, 1853: this is probably intended for Craig, as no one by the name of Franklin appears on the list of licentiates or the Med. Assn.] See Boston Med. and Surg. Jour., 1877, XCVI, p. 590.

110. EDWARD HACKLEY CARMICHAEL—Born in Glasgow, Scotland. M. D., 1817, Univ. Maryland. Died in 1855, in Washington.

[Carmichael, Du Hamel and Palmer attended a meeting, Nov. 19, 1852, and Carmichael and Du Hamel voted, though they were not elected till Jan. 13, 1853, so that the mere fact of attending or even voting, does not prove that the person was a member.]

111. WM. JAMES CHAMBERLIN DU HAMEL—Born June 18, 1827, Maryland. A. M., St. Mary's College, Baltimore; M. D., 1849, Univ. Maryland. Licentiate M. C. F., Maryland. Acting Asst. Surg., U. S. A. Dropped from membership, 1872. Removed to Baltimore. Died in Washington, Aug. 15, 1883. After graduation in medicine, he practiced, in partnership with a Dr. Bayne, for several years. Said to have attended the occupants of the White House for three Presidential terms. Physician to U. S. prisoners, D. C., several years. See Atkinson's Biog., 1880, Supplement, p. 5; Appleton's Biog., 1887, II, p. 251; Cordell's Med. Annals, Maryland, 1903, p. 383.

112. JOHN CAMPBELL RILEY, son of Dr. Joshua Riley, *supra*—Born Dec. 15, 1828, D. C. A. B., 1848; A. M., 1851, Georgetown. M. D., 1851, Columbian. Acting Asst. Surg., U. S. A. President Board of Health two years. Commissioner of Pharmacy. Died Feb. 22, 1879, of Bright's Disease. Author of "Compend of materia medica and therapeutics," Philadelphia, 1869, which was translated into Japanese; Tokio, 1872. After graduation in medicine he practiced in Washington. In 1859 succeeded his father in the chair of Materia Medica, Therapeutics and Pharmacy, Columbian Med. College. Member Med. Assn., D. C.; Amer. Med. Assn.; Philosophical Society of Washington; Secretary of Pharmacopoeia Revision Committee. Consulting Physician Providence Hospital, Central Dispensary and Eye and Ear Infirmary. Married a Miss Howle, afterwards a Miss Wilson. See Minutes Med. Society, Feb. 24, 1879; Atkinson's Phys. and Surg., 1878, p. 234; National Med. Review, 1878-9, I, p. 136; Appleton's Biog., 1889, V, p. 256; Trans. A. M. A., 1879, p. 833; Georgetown University, II, p. 155.

113. WILLIAM GRAY PALMER—Born Feb. 22, 1824, Montgomery Co., Md. M. D., 1844, Univ. Penna. Died Nov. 23, 1893. Came of a family of medical men. Son of a popular physician in Montgomery Co. Studied medicine with his father. After graduation practiced at Bladensburg, Md., until 1853, when he removed to Washington. Member Amer. Med. Assn. See Minutes Med. Society, Nov. 24, 1893; Atkinson's Phys. and Surg., 1878, p. 511; Stone's Biog., 1894, p. 664; Busey's Reminiscences, p. 201.

114. JOHN RICHARDS—Born Oct. 15, 1815, County Antrim, Ireland. M. D., 1834, Univ. Maryland. Father of Dr. F. P. Richards, *infra*. Died in Washington, of pneumonia, Jan. 19, 1862. [Son of Samuel Richards and Rosanna Brown, who came from near Belfast, Ireland; their ancestors came from Scotland in the time of Henry VIII.] Had a classical education and attended medical schools at Univ. Edinburgh and in Paris. Had an uncle, John Richards, who practiced in Alexandria, Va., and who persuaded the Doctor to come to America. He came in 1837 (?) In 1841 married Laura, daughter of Col. Francis Peyton. In 1852 he removed to Washington to practice. Member Med. Association, D. C. See Minutes Med. Society, Jan. 21, 1862.

115. LEOPOLD VICTOR DOVILLIERS—Born Feb. 15, 1818, Paris, France. M. D., 1850, Columbian. Acting Asst. Surgeon, U. S. A. Sometime Prof. French, U. S. Naval Academy, Annapolis. Dropped from membership, 1889. Died Aug. 25, 1892.

116. McCARTHY B. MELVIN—Born 1814, Virginia. M. D., 1849, Univ. Maryland. Dropped from membership, 1875. Died May 21, 1904, District of Columbia.

JANUARY 2, 1854

117. SAMUEL AUCHMETY HARRISON McKIM—Born April 17, 1826, Charlestown, Mass. M. D., 1852, Columbian. Acting Asst. Surg., U. S. A. Dropped from membership. Reëlected Oct. 1, 1861; dropped a second time; reëlected April 3, 1889; resigned Jan. 24, 1900. Died July 26, 1900, of paralysis. [His parents came from England to Washington in 1804; removed later to Massachusetts, and returned to Washington, when his father was appointed Paymaster at U. S. Marine Barracks.] After graduation in medicine he practiced in Washington. In 1861 he organized a company of volunteers for the Union Army and was made Captain; was stationed at Bennings Bridge, D. C. In 1890 was made Surgeon of 3d Battalion, D. C. N. G.; in June, 1893, Surgeon 1st Regt., N. G. For some years was Surgeon B. & O. R. R.; for 30 years Surgeon to Metropolitan Police, D. C.

118. ALEXANDER S. YOUNG—Born in the D. C. M. D. 1850, Columbian. Was elected again Jan. 7, 1856; the reason does not appear. Nothing more known of him.

119. HENRY CONSTANTINE SIMMS—Born, 1828, D. C. M. D., 1855, Jefferson. Elected again Jan. 7, 1856; the reason does not appear. Removed to Brooklyn, N. Y., 1857. Was Coroner of Kings Co., N. Y., 1874-82. Physician to several hospitals. Died Feb. 13, 1883.

S. CLIFFORD COX

NORMAN RICHARDS JENNER

LUTHER HALSEY REICHELDERFER

WM. SAWYER NEWELL

1902

MONTGOMERY HUNTER

HOWARD WILSON BARKER

DEWITT CLINTON CHADWICK

WM. JOHN ARMSTRONG

63

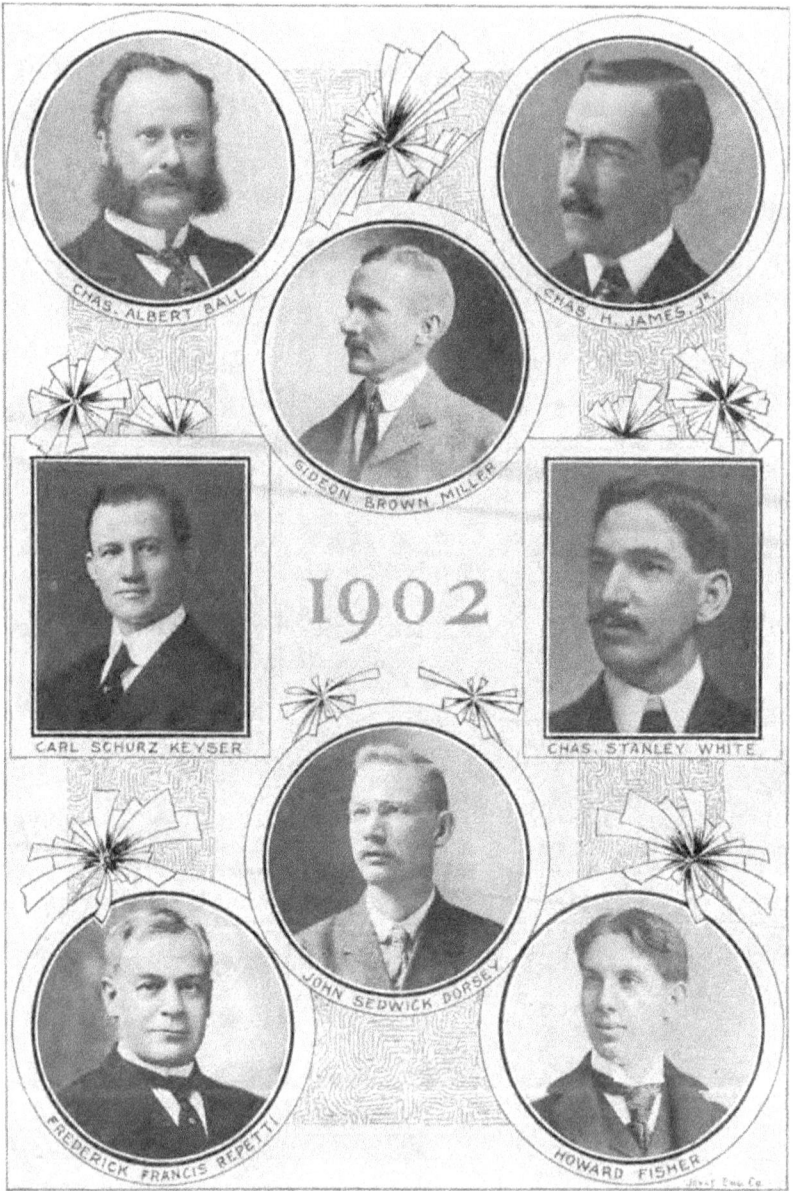

CHAS. ALBERT BALL
CHAS. H. JAMES, JR.
GIDEON BROWN MILLER
CARL SCHURZ KEYSER
1902
CHAS. STANLEY WHITE
JOHN SEDWICK DORSEY
FREDERICK FRANCIS REPETTI
HOWARD FISHER

120. JAMES WM. HAMILTON LOVEJOY—Born Dec. 15, 1824, D. C.
A. B., 1844; A. M., 1847, Columbian. M. D., 1851, Jefferson. President
Med. Assn., D. C., 1870–3. Died March 18, 1901. His ancestors settled
in Maryland about 1600. Son of John Naylor Lovejoy, Jr., of Washington, and Ann Beddo Lovejoy, of Montgomery Co., Md. Educated in
private schools, Washington; taught school a few years. After graduation in medicine, practiced in Washington. 1851-4, was Prof. Chemistry,
Georgetown Med. School; became Prof. Materia Medica in 1880, and of
Practice of Medicine in 1883; resigned in 1898. Was Dean five years
and President of the Med. Faculty ten years. One of the founders and
Consulting Physician, Garfield Memorial Hospital; Director and Consulting Physician and Chairman of Executive Committee, Children's
Hospital; Chairman of Lecture Faculty of Nurses' Training School;
member Amer. Med. Assn., Asst. Secretary in 1868; member Med. and
Surg. Society, D. C.; sometime President Alumni Assn., Columbian
University. Nov. 24, 1858, married Maria Lansing Green, daughter of
Wm. A. Green, of Brooklyn, N. Y. See Minutes, Med. Society, March
20, and April 3, 1901; Tans. Med. Society, 1901, VI, p. 120; Atkinson's
Phys. and Surg., 1878, p. 64; Who's Who in America, 1901-2; Georgetown University, II, p. 74.

121. RALEIGH T. BROWNE—Born in Virginia. M. D., 1836, Univ.
Penna. Died before 1861.

122. ALEXANDER JENKINS SEMMES—Born Dec. 17, 1828, District of Columbia. A. B., 1850; A. M., 1852, Georgetown; M. D., 1851,
Columbian. Removed from D. C. in 1860. Surgeon, 8th Louisiana
(Conf.) Vols.; Surgeon and Med. Insp., C. S. A. Died September, 1898,
at New Orleans, La. [Son of Raphael Semmes, of Nanjemoy, and Matilda Neale Jenkins, of Cobneck, on the Potomac, Charles Co., Md.; his
paternal and maternal grandfathers were officers of the Maryland line of
the Revolutionary Army, direct descendants of Roman Catholic gentry,
who, flying from persecution in England, came to Maryland between
1636 and 1650; some of them settled in the adjoining counties of Virginia.] Cousin of Raphael Semmes, Commander of the Alabama, Confederate Navy. Educated in Georgetown College. Studied medicine with
Dr. Grafton Tyler, *supra*. After graduation, attended medical schools
and hospitals in London and Paris. Practiced medicine in Washington;
was Physician to U. S. Jail. After removal to New Orleans was Resident
Physician Charity Hospital. During the Civil War, served in Hay's
Louisiana Brigade, Army of Northern Virginia; was Surgeon in charge
third division Jackson Military Hospital, Richmond, Va.; Medical Inspector, Department of Northern Virginia; Inspector of Hospitals, De-

partment of Virginia; member of Army Board to examine medical officers; President of Examining Boards of the Louisiana, Jackson, Stuart and Winder Hospitals, Richmond. After the close of the war he returned to New Orleans, and was Visiting Physician to Charity Hospital. In 1867 removed to Savannah, Ga.; 1870 to 1876, Prof. Physiology, Savannah Med. College. Subsequently took orders in Roman Catholic Church and in 1886 became President of Pio Nono College, Macon, Ga. Member of the Georgia Med. Society and Amer. Med. Association, of which he was one of the Secretaries in 1858-9 and 1869, and in 1852 was Corresponding Secretary of the Amer. Med. Society in Paris. Married, Oct. 4, 1864, at Savannah, Ga., Sarah Lowndes Berrien, daughter of John MacPherson Berrien, Attorney General, United States, in Cabinet of President Jackson, and for many years U. S. Senator from Georgia. Author of "Report on the medico-legal duties of coroners," Philadelphia, 1857. See Atkinson's Biog., 1878, p. 271; Appleton's Biog., 1889, V, p. 460; Stone's Biog., 1894, p. 674; Georgetown University, II, p. 158.

[Semmes and Hagner attended the meeting, Jan. 3, 1855, and Semmes was elected Treasurer at that meeting. There is no record of any meeting in July, 1854. Coolidge attended a meeting, July 2, 1855, and was placed on an important committee. Hansmann attended Jan. 7, 1856.]

123. DANIEL RANDALL HAGNER—Born July 19, 1830, D. C. A. B. and A. M., St. John's College, Hagerstown, Md. M. D., 1851, Univ. Penna. President, 1883-4, Med. Assn., D. C. Died March 14, 1893. Son of Peter Hagner, for nearly fifty years Third Auditor, U. S. Treasury Dept. After graduating in medicine he spent a year or more in Europe; then practiced in Washington. Consulting Physician, Providence Hospital and St. Ann's Infant Asylum, 1867-8. Member Board of Health, D. C. Author of "Vaccination and revaccination," Washington, 1864. See Minutes Med. Society, March 15, 1893; National Med. Review, 1893-4, II, p. 21; Atkinson's Biog., 1878, p. 233; Busey's Reminiscences, p. 202.

124. RICHARD HOFFMAN COOLIDGE—Born March 10, 1820, Poughkeepsie, N. Y. M. D., 1841, College Phys. and Surg., N. Y. City. Asst. Surg., Surgeon, Med. Inspector and Med. Director, U. S. A. Died Jan. 23, 1866, Raleigh, N. C. Author of "Statistical report of the sickness and mortality in the army of the U. S." etc., Washington, 1856 and 1860. Studied medicine with his uncle, Dr. Richard Kissam Hoffman. After graduation attended the hospitals of N. Y. City for about two years. Was then commissioned in the Army Med. Corps. Served in Maine and in Indian Territory; in 1848 at Vera Cruz, and afterwards in New Orleans as Medical Purveyor. Jan., 1849, was ordered to duty in the office of the Surgeon General, U. S. Army, at Washington. While there he revised

and republished Dr. Thomas Henderson's (*supra*) "Hints on the examination of recruits;" and was co-editor of Beck's Med. Jurisprudence,
republished in 1860. In 1856-8 was at Ft. Riley, Kansas; 1858-60
again in Washington; 1860-2 on the Pacific coast; 1862-5 was Med. Inspector, serving in the East and South; November, 1865, became Med.
Director, stationed at Raleigh, N. C., where he died. See Brown's History, pp. 286, 288, 293; Powell's History, p. 256; Minutes Med. Society,
Feb. 7, 1866; New York Med. Jour., 1866, II, p. 399. Appleton's Biog.,
1887, I, p. 723; Trans. A. M. A., 1867, XVIII, p. 352.

125. CHARLES FAIRCHILD FORCE—Born Feb. 9, 1827, D. C.
M. D., 1852, Columbian. Acting Asst. Surg., C. S. A. Served during
the Mexican War in Company B, 1st Virginia Infantry. Health Officer
in Washington in 1860 and Surgeon to D. C. Troops. Went South and
joined 5th Alabama Regiment just after first battle of Manassas. Mem-
ber of Gen. R. E. Rodes' staff. Left Virginia and went to Alabama with
Gen. John T. Morgan to raise 51st Alabama Cavalry, and was elected
Captain of Company E. Served in Tennessee campaign under Gens.
N. B. Forrest and Joe Wheeler. Was captured near Shelbyville, Tenn.,
June 29, 1863, and was in prison on Johnson's Island, near Sandusky,
Ohio, until April 22, 1864. Surrendered at Meridian, Miss., at close of
war, after which he lived at Cababa, Ala., until Jan., 1866, then went to
Selma, Ala. Died Aug. 4, 1884. Married .Mary E. Matthews, of Tusca-
loosa, Ala., Jan. 15, 1867.

126. BERNHARD LUDWIG WILHELM THEODOR HANS-
MANN—Born Sep. 21, 1821, Dudesdorf, Germany. M. D., 1850, Göt-
tingen. Resigned from the Society, Jan. 11, 1899. Retired from practice.

JULY 2, 1855

127. SAMUEL JACOBS RADCLIFFE—Born Feb. 2, 1829, D. C. M.
D., 1852; A. M., 1866, Georgetown. Acting Asst. Surg., U. S. A. Asst.
Surg. and Surg., U. S.Vols. Died July 9, 1903. Son of Joseph Radcliffe,
[for twenty years a clerk in the old corporation of Washington], and the
daughter of Thomas Jacobs, Alexandria, Va. Educated at McLeod's
Academy, Rockville, Md., and Georgetown College. Studied medicine
with Dr. J. B. Edelin, *supra*, and Dr. F. Howard, *supra*. After graduation, practiced in Washington. Sometime Physician to the Poor. He
removed to Baltimore, Md., in 1858; was elected a member Med. and
Surg. Society, of Baltimore, in 1859; appointed by the mayor Physician
to the Marine Hospital in 1861. In July, 1862, was appointed Acting
Asst. Surg., U. S. A., and was on duty until Feb., 1864, at U. S. General
Hospital, Annapolis, Md. Was then commissioned Asst. Surg., U. S. V.,

and ordered to the Army of the Potomac. Served through the campaign
to Petersburg, Va., as Surgeon to Field Hospital, 5th Army Corps, and in
Sept., 1864, was ordered to Naval School Hospital, Annapolis.   Promoted to Surgeon, U. S. V., and ordered to North Carolina as Inspector of
Hospitals and Medical Director, 23d Army Corps, until it was disbanded ;
afterwards Surgeon in charge of General Hospital, Smithville, N. C.
Brevetted Lieut. Col.; mustered out, Oct., 1865.   In 1866 appointed Act-
ing Asst. Surg., U. S. A., and assistant to Surgeon Basil Norris, U. S. A.,
the Attending Surgeon at Washington ; and occupied the position many
years. Member Med. Assn., D. C.; Amer. Med. Assn.; National Institute;
Wash. Acad. Sciences and Wash. Microscop. Society.   Married Florence
C., daughter of Dr. Joshua Riley, *supra*. See Atkinson's Biog., 1880,
Supp., p. 12 ; Minutes Med. Society, Oct. 7 and 21, 1903 ; Wash. Med.
Annals, 1903, p. 350 ; Georgetown Univ., II, p. 163.

128. JOSEPH DUNTON STEWART—Born in Peñnsylvania. M. D.,
1837, Univ. Penna. Asst. Surg., 31st and 74th New York Vols. Dropped
from membership, 1875. Died.

JANUARY 7, 1856

129. LOUIS MACKALL—Born April 10, 1831, Prince George Co.,
Md. M. D., 1851, Univ. Maryland. Licentiate M. C. F., Maryland.
Father of Drs. J. McV. and Louis Mackall, *infra*. President, 1876-9,
Med. Assn., D. C. Died April 18, 1906. Son of Dr. Louis and Sarah
Somervell Mackall. His ancestors emigrated from Scotland about 1650
and settled in Calvert Co., Md. He was educated in Abbott's Classical
Seminary, Georgetown, and Georgetown College.   Studied medicine
with his father.   Practiced in Georgetown; member Amer. Med. Associ-
ation; Prof. Clinical Medicine, afterwards Prof. Physiology, Georgetown
Med. School; many years Attending Physician and on Consulting Board
Columbia Hosp. for Women; of Consulting Boards of Garfield and Emergency Hospitals ; member of Common Council and Board of Health
of Georgetown.   Married, in April, 1851, Margaret W. McVean. See
Atkinson's Biog., 1878, p. 76 ; Minutes Med. Society, June 13, 1906 ;
Wash. Med. Annals, 1906-7, V, p. 209; Cordell's Med. Annals of Maryland, 1903, p. 483.

[July 7, 1856, the Society amended the Constitution, authorizing the
President to issue certificates of membership to qualified applicants.
This continued until July 1, 1860, when it was again required that appli-
cation should be made to and the applicant be elected by the Society.
During the four-years interval the record fails to show the *dates* of the
certificates given by the successive Presidents, and apparently it is now

impossible to ascertain the dates. The names of the accessions to membership during the interval are arranged in an order that is explained for each group.]

PROBABLY JULY 7, 1856

130. JAMES M. GRYMES—Born in Norfolk, Va. M. D., 1853, Georgetown. Died in 1862.

[Hill, McCalla, Marbury, Waring and Nichols were nominated Jan. 7, 1856. Apparently McCalla first attended Jan. 30, 1858; Marbury, June 4, 1857; Lippitt, Oct. 27, 1855; Waring, July 13, 1857; Grymes and Snyder attended May 14, 1856, and were appointed on a committee.]

131. JOHN MARSHALL SNYDER—Born Dec. 21, 1828, Charlestown, Va. M. D., 1850, Univ. City of New York. Second Lieut., 4th Kentucky Infantry, Mexican War. Acting Asst. Surg., U. S. A. Father of Dr. A. A. Snyder, *infra*. Died by accident, Aug. 2, 1863. Educated at Sanborn's Academy, Charlestown, Va. Moved to Tennessee. Served one year in war with Mexico; returned at the close of the war with sick and wounded sent back to the United States. Studied medicine with Prof. S. D. Gross, then of Louisville, Ky. After graduation he practiced in Georgetown. In 1853 became Prof. Surgery, Georgetown Med. School; a few years later, Prof. Obstetrics. Member Med. Assn., D. C.; Amer. Med. Assn.; Patholog. Society, D. C. Married, in 1853, Sophia C. Tayloe, daughter of Wm. H. Tayloe, of Mount Airy, Richmond Co., Va. See Trans. A. M. A., 1880, XXXI, p. 1086; Busey's Reminiscences, p. 177.

132. JOHN MOORE McCALLA—Born May 24, 1835, Lexington, Ky. M. D., 1853, Columbian. Resigned Feb. 21, 1877, retiring from practice. Died April 30, 1897.

133. WILLIAM MARBURY—Born Feb. 9, 1824, D. C. A. M., 1843, Georgetown; M. D., 1847, Univ. Penna. Died Dec. 18, 1879. Son of John Marbury, an eminent lawyer of the District. Educated at Georgetown College. Studied medicine with Dr. Grafton Tyler, *supra*. Began practice at Falmouth, Va., but after four years returned to Washington. Attending Physician to Washington Orphan Asylum and Providence Hospital. Member Med. Association, D. C., and Amer. Med. Association. Retired from practice to engage in the oil business in W. Va. Unmarried. See Trans. A. M. A., 1880, XXXI, p. 1066; Busey's Reminiscences, p. 186; Minutes Med. Society, Dec. 18, 1879.

134. WM. FONTAINE LIPPITT—Born Sept. 27, 1833, near Leesburg, Va. Educated at Univ. Virginia. M. D., 1853, Jefferson. Married, 1859, M. Louise Perry, daughter of Judge Perry, of Cumberland, Md. Removed about 1860 to Charlestown, Va., where he died, March 11, 1902. One son, Dr. W. F. Lippitt, Jr., is in Porto Rico.

135. JAMES JOHNSTON WARING—Born Aug. 19, 1830, Savannah, Ga. A. B., 1850, Yale. M. D., 1852, Univ. Penna. Removed to Savannah, 1863. Was Surg. General, Eastern District North Carolina, C. S. A., 1862-3. Died in 1888. Author of "The Epidemic at Savannah, 1877," etc.; Savannah, 1879. See also Report of Committee on Sewerage, Savannah, 1866. Prof. Obstetrics, Columbian Med. College. It is said that he had some connection with the Smithsonian Institution and pledged his private fortune to raise money for it, but eventually was unable to meet the interest on the loans and the notes were closed out. His principal life work was in connection with drainage and sanitation of Savannah during and after the yellow fever epidemic 1876. Alderman in 1877-8.

136. CHARLES HENRY NICHOLS—Born Oct. 19, 1820, Vassalboro, Me. M. D., 1843, Univ. Penna. A. M., 1851, Union College, Schenectady, N. Y. LL. D., 1879, Columbian. Acting Asst. Surg., U. S. A. Supt. of St. Elizabeth Asylum, D. C., 1852-77, then became Superintendent of Bloomingdale Asylum, New York. Name dropped ; reelected Jan. 7, 1867. Died Dec. 16, 1889. Educated in schools in Maine and at Providence, R. I. In 1847 became connected with the State Insane Asylum, Utica, N. Y.; in 1849 Physician to Bloomingdale Asylum. In 1852, at the suggestion of Miss Dorothea Dix, was appointed by President Fillmore to superintend the construction and management of St. Elizabeth Asylum, Washington. For many years was President of Association of Amer. Superintendents of Insane Asylums ; Honorary member British Med.-Psychol. Association. See Atkinson's Phys. and Surg., 1878, p. 693 ; Appleton's Biog., 1888, IV, p. 512 ; Med. Record, N. Y., 1889, XXXVI, p. 687; Amer. Jour. Insanity, 1888-9 ; XLV, p. 446.

PROBABLY BETWEEN JULY, 1856 AND JANUARY, 1857

137. JOHN EDWARD WILLETT—Born June 23, 1834, Rockville, Md. M. D., 1855, Georgetown. Demonstrator Anatomy, Georgetown Med. School. Was ill with some mental disease from 1863 till his death, Jan. 21, 1887.

138. WILLIAM HENRY BERRY—Born Dec. 3, 1827, D. C. A. M., 1847, Princeton; M. D., 1850, Univ. Maryland. Died Feb. 19, 1859. Son of Philip T. Berry and Mary Ann Haw, daughter of John S. Haw. His grandparents were Wm. and Martha Berry, of Prince George Co., Md. He was educated in Georgetown. Studied medicine with Dr. Grafton Tyler, *supra*. After graduation, spent some time in European hospitals; afterwards practiced in Washington. Was Physician to Washington Asylum. See Minutes Med. Society, Feb. 21, 1859; Trans. A. M. A., 1860, XIII, p. 814.

[Berry and Lincoln were nominated Jan. 7, 1856.]

139. JOHN F. KING—Probably A. B., 1852, Georgetown ; M. D., 1855, Jefferson. Died March 25, 1873.

140. NATHAN SMITH LINCOLN—Born April 3, 1828, Gardner, Mass. A. B., 1850; A. M., 1853, Dartmouth ; M. D., 1852, Univ. Maryland. Acting Asst. Surg., U. S. A.; Surgeon, D. C. Vols. President, 1892-3, Med. Assn., D. C. Died Oct. 14, 1898. His great-grandfather, Gen. Jonathan Chase, drew up the articles of surrender for Burgoyne's army at Saratoga, and Gen. Benj. Lincoln received the sword of Cornwallis at the Yorktown surrender. His grandfather, Dr. Nathan Smith, founded the medical schools of Yale and Dartmouth. Dr. Lincoln's parents were Rev. Increase Turner and Eliza Smith Lincoln. He studied medicine with his uncle, Dr. Nathan Ryno Smith, of Baltimore. After graduation he practiced in Baltimore till Jan. 1, 1854, when he removed to Washington. In 1857 was elected Prof. of Chemistry, Columbian Med. College, and afterwards filled the chairs of Theory and Practice of Medicine, Anatomy and Physiology, and Surgery, holding the latter place till 1874, when he resigned. In 1861 was appointed Acting Asst. Surgeon, in charge of the Quartermaster's Hospital, Washington. Member Med. Assn., D. C.; Amer. Med. Association ; Amer. Assn. Advance. Sci.; Philosophical Society of Washington ; Vice President Ninth Internat. Med. Cougress, 1887; President Alumni Association, Univ. Maryland; Surgeon to Providence Hospital, Washington, 1866 to 1875; Consulting Surgeon, Garfield and Children's Hospitals. Married first, Mrs. Margaret E. Ridgate, of Washington; next, Mrs. Nannie Smith, of Baltimore; and third, Jeanie Thomas, daughter of Judge George Gould, of Troy, N. Y. See Minutes Med. Society, Oct. 19 and Nov. 2, 1898; Trans. Med. Soc., III, for 1898, p. 142; Atkinson's Phys. and Surg., 1878, p. 220 ; Stone's Biog., 1894, p. 651 ; National Med. Rev., 1898-9, VIII, pp. 372, 414 ; Med. Record, N. Y., 1898, LIV, p. 594.

141. JOSEPH MEREDITH TONER—Born April 30, 1825, Pittsburg, Pa. M. D., 1850, Vermont Acad. Med. Sci. ; 1853, Jefferson ; A. M. 1867, Ph. D., 1889, Georgetown. President Med. Assn., D. C., 1886-7. President, 1874, Amer. Med. Assn. Honorary member M. C. F., Maryland, 1878. Died at Cresson Springs, Pa., July 30, 1896. Educated at Western University and Mt. St. Mary's College, Md. Practiced successively at Summit and Pittsburg, Pa., Harper's Ferry, Va., and in Nov., 1855, removed to Washington. Member Amer. Public Health Association, its President in 1874 ; one of the Vice Presidents Internat. Med. Congress, Philadelphia, 1876; honorary member New York and California State Med. Societies, and Boston Gynecological Society. Vice President and Registrar Internat. Med. Congress at Washington in 1887. Founder of Providence Hospital and St. Ann's Infant Asylum, Washing-

ton, to which he was Visiting Physician ; and from 1856 was Attending
Physician to St. Joseph's Orphan Asylum. In consideration of the per-
ishable character of much of the early medical literature of this country
Dr. Toner devised a scheme for a repository of medical works that should
be under the control of the medical profession of the United States and
located at the National Capital. His resolution on this subject was
adopted by the Amer. Med. Association in 1868, and resulted in the establishment of the library of that organization. The collection was placed
in the Smithsonian Institution and reached the number of several thousand volumes, including pamphlets. In 1871 he founded the Toner lectures by placing $3,000, afterwards increased to nearly double that amount,
in the hands of trustees charged with the duty of annually procuring two
lectures containing new facts valuable to medical science ; the interest
on the fund, save ten per cent., which was added to the permanent fund,
was paid to the authors of the essays. These lectures were included in
the regular list of publications of the Smithsonian Institution. It was
the first attempt in this country to endow a course of lectures on such
conditions. Dr. Toner devoted much time and research to early medical
literature, collected over a thousand treatises published before 1800, and,
besides publishing numerous monographs, had in preparation a Biographical Dictionary of Deceased American Physicians, of which more than
four thousand sketches were completed. He was an authority on the
medical, biographical and local history of the District of Columbia. He
devised a system of symbols of geographical localities which was adopted
by the United States Post Office Department. Member of numerous
medical, historical and philosophical associations, and published more
than fifty papers and monographs upon subjects of interest to the medical profession. In 1874 he placed a gold medal, struck at the United
States Mint and bearing his likeness, at the disposal of the Faculty of
Jefferson Med. College to be awarded annually to the student producing
the best thesis based upon original research. In the same year he established a medal to be granted annually by the Faculty of the University
of Georgetown, D. C., to the student who should collect and name the
greatest number of specimens in any department of the natural sciences.
In 1882 he gave his entire library, including manuscripts, to the United
States Government ; it consisted of 28,000 books and 18,000 pamphlets.
Author of Address before the Rocky Mountain Med. Association,
Washington, 1877 ; Med. Register, Washington, 1867 ; Anniversary
Oration, Washington, 1869 ; Contributions to Annals of Med. Progress,
Washington, 1874 ; Dictionary of Elevations, etc., New York, 1874 ;
Medical Men of the Revolution, Philadelphia, 1876 ; Notes on the Burn-
ing of Theaters, Washington, 1876. See Minutes Med. Society, Oct. 14
and 21, 1896 ; Atkinson's Biog., 1878, p. 166 ; Northwestern Med. and
Surg. Jour., St. Paul, Minn., 1872-3, III, p. 247 ; Appleton's Biog., 1889,

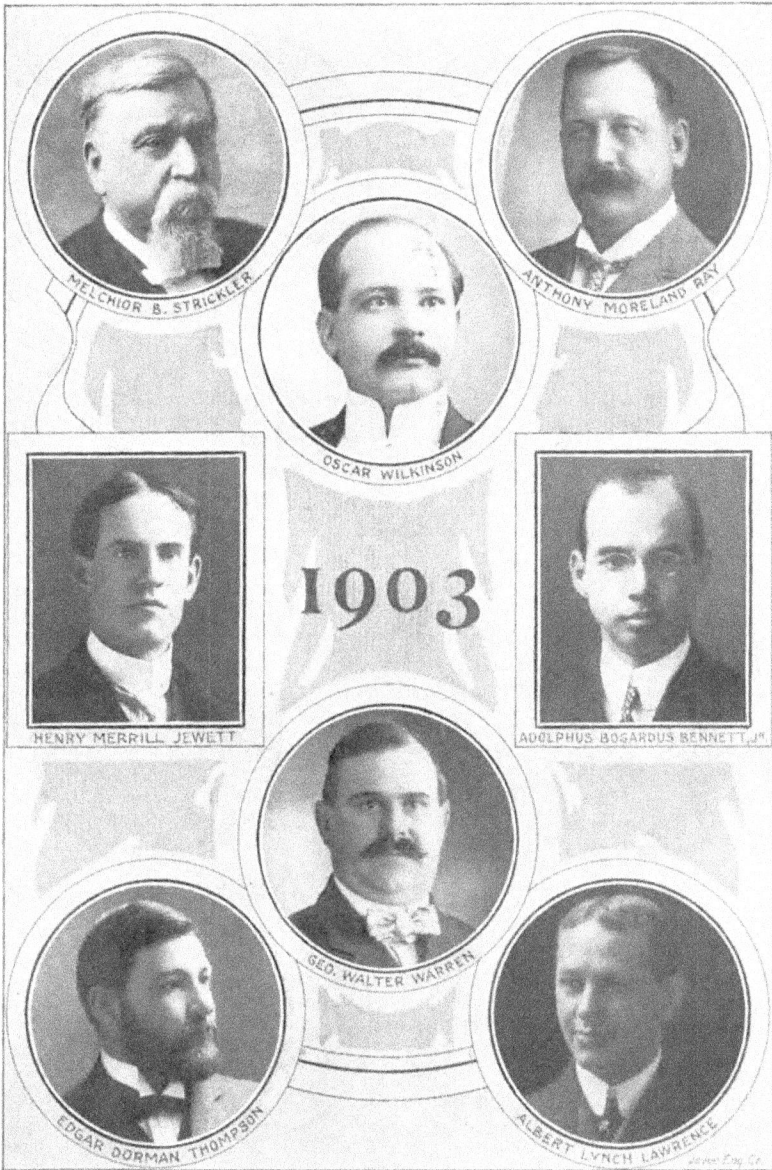

MELCHIOR B. STRICKLER

ANTHONY MORELAND RAY

OSCAR WILKINSON

1903

HENRY MERRILL JEWETT

ADOLPHUS BOGARDUS BENNETT, Jr.

GEO. WALTER WARREN

EDGAR DORMAN THOMPSON

ALBERT LYNCH LAWRENCE

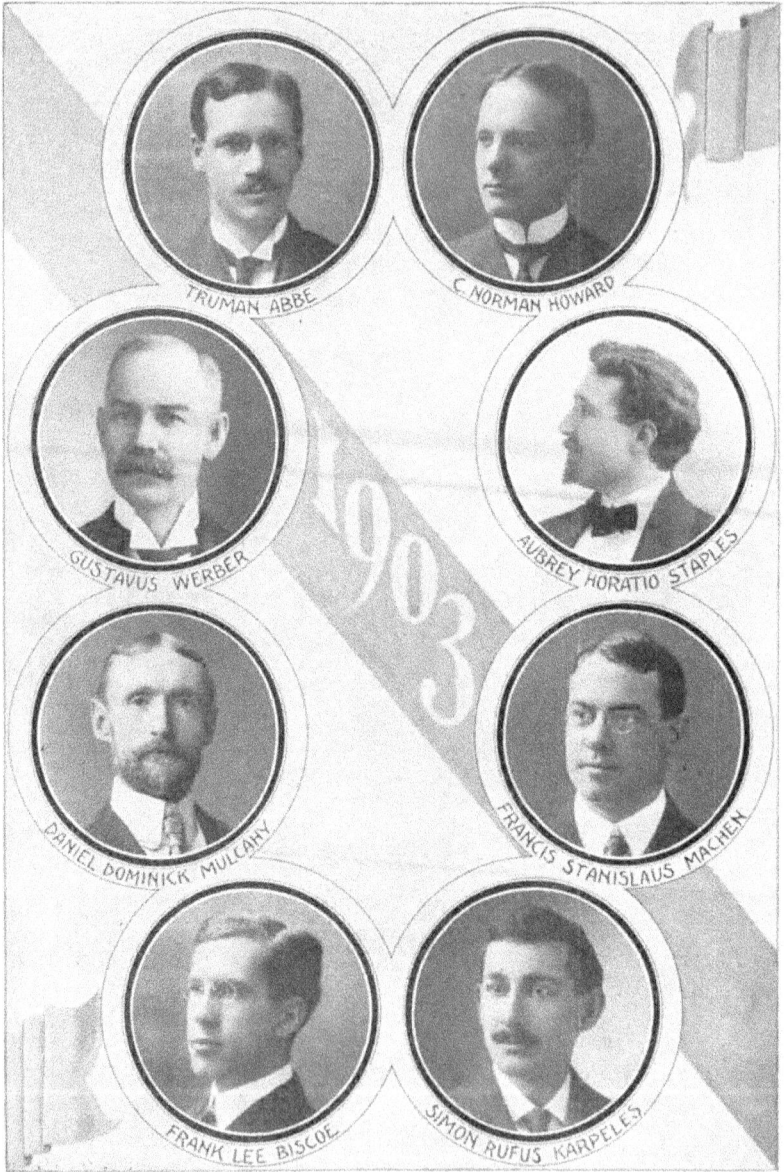

TRUMAN ABBE

C. NORMAN HOWARD

GUSTAVUS WERBER

AUBREY HORATIO STAPLES

1903

DANIEL DOMINICK MULCAHY

FRANCIS STANISLAUS MACHEN

FRANK LEE BISCOE

SIMON RUFUS KARPELES

VI, p. 132 ; National Med. Review, 1896-7, VI, p. 159 ; Stone's Biog., 1894, p. 513; Trans. 75th Anniv. Med. Society, D. C., 1894, p. 22; Georgetown University, II, p. 58; Cordell's Med. Annals Maryland, 1903, p. 598.

142. TOBIAS PURRINGTON—Born March 19, 1801, Windham, Me. M. D., 1826, Bowdoin. Died May 3, 1880. See Minutes Med. Society, May 4, 1880.

143. JOHNSON VAN DYKE MIDDLETON—Born Dec. 15, 1834, D. C. M. D., 1855, Georgetown. Asst. Surg., Surgeon and Deputy Surgeon General, U. S. A. Retired Dec. 15, 1898. Died in D. C., Jan. 29, 1907. Served at Washington Arsenal till May, 1862, then with Army of Potomac in the field till Nov., 1862, and was then detailed for duty in the office of the Medical Director, Department of Washington, where he remained till the close of the Civil War. In November, 1867, was ordered to Texas, and served there at various places till June, 1870, when he was transferred to Baton Rouge, La.; remained there till May, 1873 ; then to Forts Buford and Lincoln, Dakota, till June, 1877, serving with Gen. Terry in October and November, 1876, in an Indian campaign ; then to Forts Schuyler and Wadsworth, N. Y. Harbor, till June, 1881 ; then at Forts Hays and Leavenworth, Kansas, till November, 1886; then to David's Island and Fort Columbus, N. Y. Harbor, as Acting Med. Director, Dept. of the East. To the Pacific coast in 1892, Med. Director and Chief Surgeon of the Department. After his retirement he resumed his residence in Washington. See Brown's History, p. 295 ; Powell's History, p. 481.

PROBABLY BETWEEN JANUARY AND JULY, 1857

144. LEWIS ALLISON EDWARDS—[He attended a meeting June 4, 1857.] Born Sept. 29, 1823, D. C. A. B., 1842, Princeton ; M. D., 1845, Univ. Penna. Asst. Surg., U. S. A., 1846-61 ; Surgeon, 1861-76, and Med. Director, U. S. A., 1876-7. Chief Medical Officer, Bureau of Refugees, Freedmen and Abandoned Lands. Died Nov. 8, 1877, of progressive softening of the brain. Immediately after appointment as Assistant Surgeon he joined the army of invasion and occupation, and served with honor during the Mexican War. Was then stationed at Santa Fé, N. M., till September, 1850; at Fort Washington, Md., till July, 1852 ; and at Fort Towson, Ark., till May, 1854, when he was ordered to duty in the Surgeon General's Office. He remained in Washington, attached to the Bureau, and as Attending Surgeon for officers' families, until August, 1862, when he took charge of the General Hospital at Portsmouth Grove, R. I. In December, 1863, he went to Wilmington, Del., as a member of the Army Retiring Board; returned to the Portsmouth Grove Hospital in May, 1864, and in December, 1864, to January, 1866, was

17

again on the Retiring Board. Was next stationed at Baltimore, Md., as medical officer of the recruiting station, till August, 1866, when he was appointed chief medical officer of the Bureau of Refugees, Freedmen and Abandoned Lands. In March, 1869, became Medical Director, Department of Louisiana, and in April, 1870, Department of Texas. In October, 1872, transferred to Madison Barracks, New York, as Post Surgeon, and in April, 1875, went on sick leave, which continued till his death. Was appointed Lieutenant Colonel and Colonel by brevet, to date from March 13, 1865, for faithful and meritorious services during the Civil War. See Brown's History, pp. 288, 293; Powell's History, p. 298; Trans. A. M. A., 1879, XXX, p. 817.

PROBABLY JULY, 1857, TO JANUARY, 1858

145. JOHN C. GRAYSON—[Grayson attended the meeting, July 13, 1857.] Born in Kentucky. M. D., 1854, Med. Col. Va. Removed from D. C. about 1863. Was at Stevensburgh, Va., 1890-7, and died there about 1897.

146. CHARLES GIRARD—[Girard attended the meeting January 4, 1858.] Born March 9, 1822, Mülhousen, France. M. D., 1856, Georgetown. Removed from D. C., 1860. Died Jan. 29, 1895. Was educated in Neuchatel, Switzerland, where he was the pupil and assistant of Agassiz. Came with Agassiz to the United States, in 1847, remaining with him until 1850. Then removed to Washington, D. C., and became attached to the Smithsonian Institution. In 1852 was naturalized as an American citizen. After graduating in medicine remained in Smithsonian Institution until 1859, and for some time was engaged with Prof. Spencer F. Baird, in the investigation of reptiles. His many publications were on Natural History; and in connection with collaborative work with Prof. Baird, of the Smithsonian, and the outcome of several exploring expeditions. See Drake's Biog., 1872, p. 363; Bull. No. 41, 1891, U. S. National Museum; Appletons's Biog., 1887, II, p. 659.

ABOUT JANUARY 30, 1858

147. WILLIAM ALFRED BRADLEY—Born Aug. 3, 1831, D. C. M. D., 1854, Columbian. Asst. Surg., U. S. A., 1861-9. Died Feb. 27, 1869, at Point San José, Cal. Was with the Army of the Potomac to December, 1862; on hospital duty, Washington, to February, 1864; in office of Medical Director, Department of Washington, to June, 1869; at Point San José, Cal., until his death. See Minutes Med. Society, March 3, 1869; Brown's History, p. 295; Powell's History, p. 207; Trans. A. M. A., 1870, XXI, p. 494.

[Bradley, Culver, Hellen, Keasbey, Newman and Storrow attended the meeting Jan. 30, 1858. Taylor must have been certified after January 18th, and Butt and Maury after Jan. 27, 1858.]

148. FREDERICK BURR CULVER—Born 1809, Frederick, Ohio. M. D., 1857, Louisville Med. College. Dropped from membership, 1878. Died in D. C., June 12, 1879. Sometime Physician to an Indian Agency.

149. BENJAMIN JOHNSON HELLEN—Born March 20, 1830, D. C. A. B., 1850; A. M., 1854; M. D., 1854, Columbian. Died of tuberculosis, July 2, 1864. Soon after graduation in medicine he became Resident Physician at Washington Infirmary. Several years afterwards was Physician to Providence Hospital. Descendant from the Johnson family of Maryland. See Trans. A. M. A., 1872, XXIII, p. 575; Minutes Med. Society, July 4, 1864.

150. JOHN BRICK KEASBEY—Born August 5, 1833, Salem, N. J. M. D., 1854, Univ. Penna. Surgeon, 2d D. C., Vols. Removed from D. C., 1871, to Woodbury, N. J., where he died Aug. 25, 1886.

151. WILLIAM GEORGE HENRY NEWMAN—Born March 17, 1827, Princess Anne, Md. M. D., 1849, Univ. Md. Father of Dr. H. M. Newman, *infra*. Died Nov. 6, 1883. Descended from an old Maryland family that emigrated from England and settled in the State as early as 1650. Educated at Washington College, Baltimore, and Jefferson College, Washington Co., Pa. Read medicine with Prof. N. R. Smith, of Baltimore. Practiced for some years in Georgetown, then returned to Washington. Was at one time a member of the city Council ; at the time of his death the Physician-in-Chief to St. Ann's Infant Asylum. For many years one of the Surgeons to the D. C. police ; for some years one of the staff of Providence Hospital ; member of the old Board of Health of the city ; for some years on the Board of Visitors to the Washington Asylum ; member Med. Assn. D. C., and Amer. Med. Assn. Married Mary Rider, of Somerset Co., Md. See Minutes Med. Society, Nov. 7, 1883 ; Jour. A. M. A., 1883, I, p. 603.

152. SAMUEL APPLETON STORROW—Born in Virginia. M. D., 1852, Jefferson. Asst. Surg. and Surg., U. S. A. Died July 12, 1879. See Brown's History, p. 295; Powell's History, p. 612.

153. WILLIAM HENRY TAYLOR—Born Jan. 26, 1834, Pottsville, Pa. M. D., 1856, Columbian. Sometime Demonstrator of Anatomy, Columbian. President Med. Assn., D. C. Died Sept. 5, 1889. See Minutes Med. Society, Sept. 7, 1889.

154. WILLIAM BEALE BUTT—Born July 19, 1827, Mechanicsburg, Md. M. D., 1850, Columbian. Died of paralysis, June 28, 1877. Son of Richard and grandson of Proverb Butt, of Maryland. His mother was Sarah Ann Richards, daughter of Samuel Richards, Sr., of Port Tobacco,

Md.   He attended the public schools, McLeod's School and Rittenhouse
Academy, Georgetown.   Studied medicine with Dr. Thomas Miller,
supra.   Resident Student, Washington Infirmary.   Practiced medicine in
Washington.   Member Amer. Med. Association.   Married, May 8, 1862,
Margaret Elizabeth Allyn, daughter of Lucius May Allyn.   See Trans.
A. M. A., 1880, XXXI, p. 1023.

155. THOMAS FOYLES MAURY—Born August 16, 1835, D. C.
M. D., 1856, Univ. Penna.   Asst. Surg. and Surgeon, 1st Virginia Regt.,
C. S. A.   Died of pulmonary consumption, Sept. 19, 1871, at Mt. Holly
Springs, Pa.   Studied medicine with Dr. J. F. May, *supra*.   After graduation, spent a year and a half at the hospitals of Paris and Vienna.
April 27, 1861, was appointed Asst. Surg., 1st Virginia Regiment, with
the rank of Captain.   Was engaged in the first battles of the war, near
Manassas, soon after which he was promoted to Surgeon and appointed
on the staff of General Longstreet, in which capacity he continued until
the surrender at Appomattox Court House, participating in nearly all the
battles of the Army of Northern Virginia.   While on duty at Greenville,
Tenn., with General Longstreet's Corps, he sustained a comminuted
fracture of right femur, from which he never entirely recovered.   He returned to Washington after the close of the war, and resumed his practice, but his health failing, he visited Europe in 1869, to recuperate; after
an absence of six months, returned much improved, and continued his
practice until his death.   Married in 1859.   See Minutes Med. Society,
Sept. 20, 1871; Trans. A. M. A., XXIII, 1872, p. 582.

AFTER FEBRUARY 6, 1858

156. WILLIAM PROBY YOUNG, Jr.—[He attended the meeting
July 5, 1858.]   Born Jan. 19, 1834, Portsmouth, Va.   M. D., 1855, Jeffer-
son.   Asst. Surg. and Surgeon, 4th Georgia, C. S. A.   Resigned from the
Society Jan. 20, 1881, retiring from practice.   Educated at Rittenhouse
Academy and Columbiau College.   Was First Asst. Physician Govt. Hosp.
Insane, Oct., 1855, to March, 1858.   Afterward practiced medicine in
Washington.   In June, 1860, as agent for the U. S. Government and
physician for the American Colonization Society, he sailed from Key
West with a cargo of Africans who had been captured from slave ships,
and delivered twenty per cent. of them to the authorities in Cape Mount,
Liberia.   He served in the Confederate army from 1861 until the sur-
render, in 1865, the command being in the field during the entire period
and participating in thirty-five battles.   Was captured at the battle of
Sharpsburg, Md., Sept. 17, 1862, having been on the field all day attending the wounded of both armies.   About a week after the fight Dr. John
H. Rauch, of General Fitz John Porter's staff, placed him in charge of

100 Confederate wounded in an Episcopal church in that town, and gave him eight Union soldiers as nurses. He returned to Washington in 1865 and "dropped into trade." He was a Director of the Children's Hospital, and for fifteen years Secretary of the Board. Has been Secretary of the Game and Fish Protective Association of the District since its formation, and is actively interested in preventing the pollution of the Potomac River and its tributaries. At present is Secretary of Franklin Fire Insurance Co., Washington.

AFTER APRIL 7, 1858

157. BENJAMIN RHETT—Born March 23, 1826, Charleston, S. C. A. B., 1846, and M. D., 1848, College of Charleston. Surgeon, C. S. A. Removed from D. C., about 1861, to Summerville, S. C., where he died June 9, 1884. Entered the Medical Department, C. S. A., in the fall of 1861; served for a few weeks with Boyce's Battery; next as Surgeon to the Marine Hospital, Charleston; then as Surgeon in Battery Wagner, during the siege, terminating in the night assault of the 18th of July. Was Surgeon in Fort Sumter during the siege, under Cols. Rhett and Elliott. Surgeon to the officers of the U. S. Army imprisoned in Charleston, in the Roper and Marine Hospitals, workhouse, jail and O'Connor house. Then served as Surgeon to a camp of 6,000 Andersonville prisoners. Towards the close of the war was Surgeon to the Arsenal, and upon general duty. While stationed at Charleston, was member of Board of Medical Examiners for sick and furloughed soldiers. He was in active practice at the time of his death.

AFTER MAY 20, 1858

158. GEORGE McCOY—[He attended the meeting July 5, 1858.] Born 1828, Dublin, Ireland. M. D., 1857, Georgetown. Acting Asst. Surg., U. S. A. Died Oct. 8, 1880. See Minutes Med. Society, Oct. 8, 1880.

FEBRUARY 5, 1859

159. THOMAS ANTISELL—Born Jan. 16, 1817, Dublin, Ireland. A. B., Trinity College, Dublin; Ph. D., 1881, Georgetown; M. D., 1839, Royal College Surgeons, London, and Dublin Lying-In Hospital. Surgeon, U. S. Vols.; Med. Director, 12th Army Corps. Absent in Japan from 1871 to 1876. Died, D. C., June 14, 1893. [Son of Christopher Antisell, of Kings County, Ireland, a distinguished barrister, and Queen's Counsel—his ancestry going back to Sir Bertine Entwyssel, who accompanied Henry II to Ireland—and Margaret Daly, daughter of Surgeon Daly, of Dublin.] Educated at Trinity College, Dublin; studied medicine at Dublin School of Medicine, Peter Street, and Irish Apothecary's Hall; pupil and afterwards assistant to Sir Robert Kane, from 1839 to 1843. In

1844 pursued his chemical studies in Paris and Berlin, under Pelouze, Biot, Dumas and Berzelius. Practiced medicine in Dublin from 1845 to 1848; Lecturer on Chemistry in "Original School of Medicine." Extra professor to Royal Dublin Society, 1845-48. Member Royal College of Surgeons, England, Royal Dublin Society and Geological Society of Dublin. As one of the "Young Ireland Party," was sentenced to exile and imprisonment, but a friend procuring for him a position as Surgeon on an outgoing vessel, he sailed for America. Landed at New York City, Nov. 22, 1848. Practiced medicine there until 1854, when he became Geologist of the Pacific R. R. Survey on the thirty-second parallel, under Lieut. Parke, Topographical Engineer, U. S. A. Made a geological reconnaissance of Southern California and Arizona Territory, published in the seventh volume of U. S. Reports of Explorations and Surveys, 1856. In 1848 was Professor of Chemistry in Berkshire Med. College and in 1854 Professor of Chemistry at the medical colleges at Woodstock, Vt., and Pittsfield, Mass. From June 1, 1856, to Sept. 30, 1861, was Examiner in Chemistry in U. S. Patent Office. He then resigned, to enter the army. During the war, 1861-5, was Brigade Surgeon; Surgeon, U. S. Volunteers; Med. Director, 12th Army Corps; Surgeon in charge Harewood Hospital, Washington, D. C.; Surgeon in charge of sick and wounded officers in Washington, D. C.; President of Board of Examiners for Surgeons and Assistant Surgeons of Volunteers. Brevetted Lieut. Colonel for faithful and meritorious services during the war; and mustered out of service in October, 1865. From 1866 to 1871, was Chief Chemist in U. S. Bureau of Agriculture. In 1869-70, Professor of Chemistry, Maryland Agricultural College. In 1871, at the invitation of the Japanese Government, he became technologist of a government commission to develop the resources of the northern islands of that empire. Returned to the United States in 1876. While in Japan he was offered the position of President of the College of Cairo, Egypt, which he declined. In appreciation of his valuable services to Japan, he was decorated by the Emperor with the "Order of the Rising Sun of Meijii." While on the ocean *en route* to Japan the opportunity offered to become President of the College, Lancaster, Pa., which he appreciated and would have accepted, but had already contracted with the Japanese Government for five years. May 10, 1877, he was again appointed Examiner in the U. S. Patent Office and held the position until July, 1890, when, his health failing, he was reduced to a first-class clerkship, and finally removed, Sept. 30, 1891. From 1855 to 1893, excepting the interval of army service and while in Japan, he lived in Washington. All his life he was a medical teacher, his specialty being analytical and technical chemistry. Member Med. Association, D. C.; Philosophical Society of Washington; corresponding member Academy of Natural Sciences, Philadelphia, and Geographical Society, New York City; Fellow American Assn. Advance.

Science. Except at intervals, was connected with Georgetown Med. College for many years; Prof. Chemistry and Toxicology, Military Surgery, and Physiology and Hygiene. The sanitary investigation of the National Hotel and the ventilation of the Capitol were public interests that were benefited by his scientific knowledge. He was one of the founders of the Training School for Nurses, and the first President of that school. Author of Suggestions towards improvement of sanitary condition of the metropolis, Dublin, 1847 ; The manufacture of photogenic or hydrocarbon oils, N. Y., 1859. Married twice : Eliza Anne Nowlan, of Dublin, in 1841; Marion Stuart Forsyth, of Detroit, daughter of Paymaster Forsyth, U. S. A., in 1854. See Atkinson's Phys. and Surg., 1878, p. 16 ; Minutes Med. Society, June 15, 1893 ; Bull. Philos. Soc., Washington, XIII, 1896, pp. 367-434; Year Book Department of Agriculture, 1899, p. 238; Annual Report Smithsonian Institution, 1904, pp. 453 and 690; Jour. A. M. A., 1893, XXI, p. 93; Georgetown University, II, p. 80.

JULY 4, 1859

160. JOHN L. GIBBONS—Born, Jefferson Co., Va., between 1790 and 1800. M. D., 1841, Washington University, Baltimore, Md. Licentiate M. C. F., Maryland. Practiced at Pikesville, Md., many years, then in Baltimore a short time, then in Washington, D. C. Left Washington in 1862. Was delegate to Amer. Med. Assn. in 1847. Was also a minister in the M. E. Church. Died about 1870 (?). See Cordell's Med. Annals Maryland, 1903, p. 408.

JULY 12, 1859

161. WEBSTER LINDSLY—Born Oct. 6, 1835, D. C. Son of Dr. Harvey Lindsly, *supra*. M. D., 1857, Harvard. Asst. Surg., U. S. A. Died Aug. 8, 1866. His mother was Emeline Webster Lindsly. He studied medicine with his father. After graduation he spent two years in study in Europe. Practiced some time in Washington. In August, 1859, took back to Africa a shipload of Africans captured from slavers. See Brown's History, p. 295 ; Minutes Med. Society, Aug. 8, 1866.

162. REUBEN CLEARY—Born April 27, 1835, Alexandria, D. C. M. D., 1859; A. M., 1860, Georgetown. Asst. Adjt. General, C. S. A. Soon after the close of the war of 1861-5 he removed to Brazil, where he was employed as civil engineer building a railroad ; afterward practiced medicine at Lages and Rio Janeiro. About 1890 was appointed Sanitary Inspector in U. S. Marine Hospital Service at Rio Janeiro and held this position until his death, Feb. 12, 1898. Married March 12, 1870, Wilhelmina Schmitt.

163. FRANCIS W. MEAD—Born Sept. 23, 1838, N. Y. City. M. D., 1858, Georgetown. Surg., 2d D. C. Vols.; Surg., U. S. M. H. S. Dropped from membership, 1873.

AFTER APRIL 3, 1860

164. JOHN W. DAVIS—Born Aug. 8, 1825, Lenoir Co., N. C. M. D., 1847, Univ. Penna. Asst. Surg., 6th and 24th Indiana, and First Lieut., 20th Ind. Vols. After graduation practiced a short time at Seven Springs, Wayne Co., N. C., then removed to Goldsboro. Was in D. C. in 1860, but remained only a short time. Returned to North Carolina, locating again at Goldsboro, where he died Jan. 23, 1869.

165. RICHARD C. CROGGON—[Croggon attended the meetings, May 9 and July 1, 1860.] Born July 15, 1839, Charles Co., Md. M. D., 1860, Georgetown. Acting Asst. Surg., U. S. A. Died Sept. 23, 1872. Came to Washington at an early age ; was sometime clerk in drug store. Studied medicine with Dr. Joseph Borrows, *supra*. Practiced in Washington. During the Civil War served as Acting Asst. Surgeon in military hospitals, Washington. See Minutes Med. Society, Sept. 24, 1872; Trans. A. M. A., 1873, XXIV, p. 340.

166. PHILIP CHAPMAN DAVIS—Born in Virginia. M. D., 1856, Columbian. Asst. Surg. and Surg., U. S. A. Died Oct. 2, 1871, at Ft. Benton, Montana. See Brown's History, pp. 289, 295; Powell's History, p. 275.

AFTER MAY 16, 1860

167. FRANCIS C. CHRISTIE—Born in New York. M. D., 1859, Georgetown. Died between 1860 and 1870. [Christie attended the meeting Aug. 6, 1860.]

[Since July 1, 1860, the Society has required that an applicant for membership should make formal application and be regularly elected.]

JANUARY 5, 1861

168. JOHN GEORGE FREDERICK HOLSTON—Born, 1809, Hamburg, Germany. A. M., Washington and Jefferson College, Pa.; M. D., 1846, Cleveland. Surgeon, U. S. Vols.; Actg. Asst. Surg., U. S. A. Died of paralysis, May 1, 1874. His father and grandfather were physicians; the son came to America at an early age; landed at New Orleans, La.; was among the planters about a year. Then visited the East Indies, China, and other countries. Returning, he landed at Philadelphia during the cholera epidemic, and served as nurse in hospital. Finally became a student at the Washington and Jefferson College. After graduation in

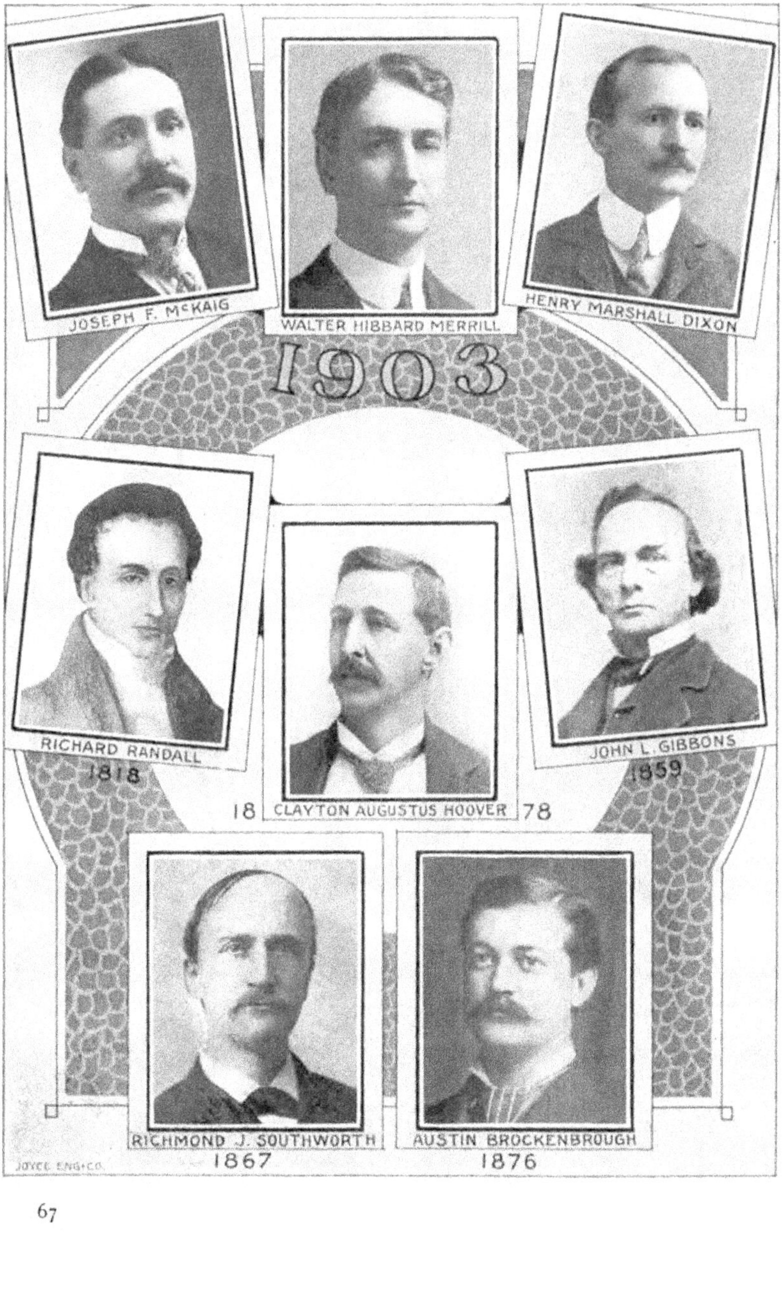

JOSEPH F. McKAIG

WALTER HIBBARD MERRILL

HENRY MARSHALL DIXON

1903

RICHARD RANDALL
1818

CLAYTON AUGUSTUS HOOVER
18 78

JOHN L. GIBBONS
1859

RICHMOND J. SOUTHWORTH
1867

AUSTIN BROCKENBROUGH
1876

JOYCE ENG.CO.

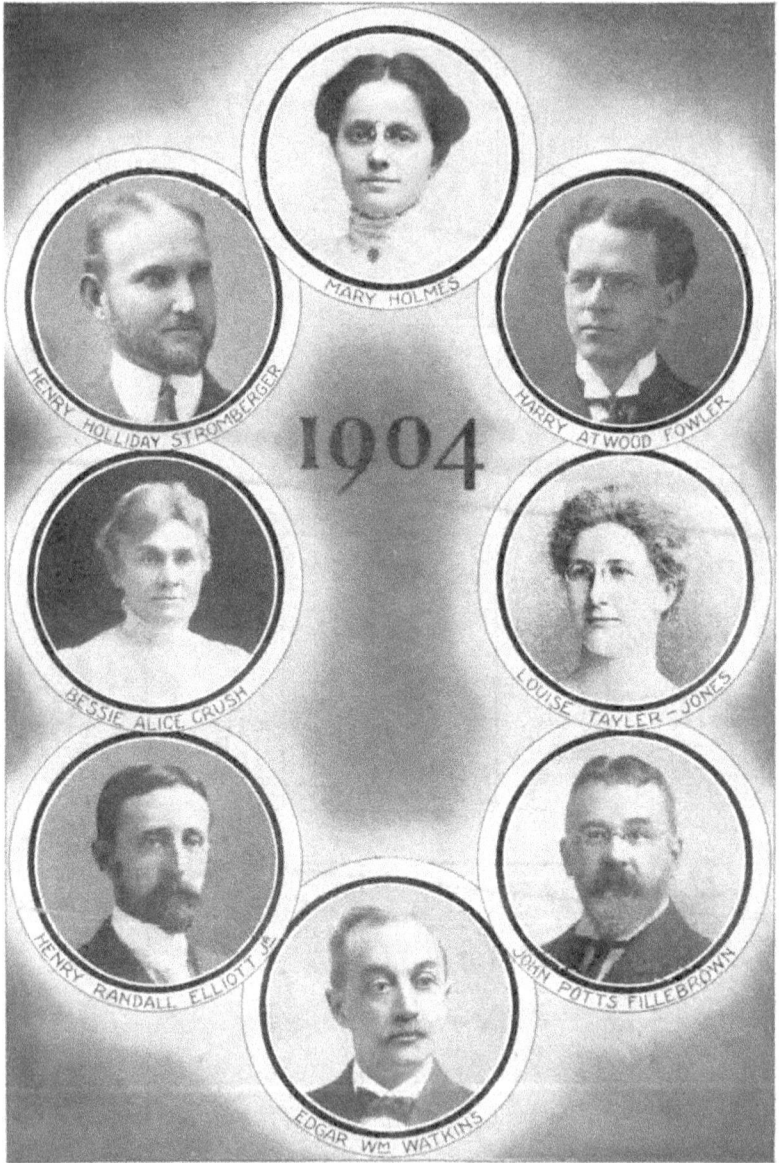

MARY HOLMES

HENRY HOLLIDAY STROMBERGER

HARRY ATWOOD FOWLER

1904

BESSIE ALICE CRUSH

LOUISE TAYLER-JONES

HENRY RANDALL ELLIOTT JR.

JOHN POTTS FILLEBROWN

EDGAR WM WATKINS

medicine he practiced in Ohio until he removed to Washington. In 1857 became Prof. Surgery, Columbian Med. College. In the war, 1861-5, he served in the U. S. Vols.; was sometime Medical Director on the staff of Gen. U. S. Grant. At the close of the war he returned to Zanesville, Ohio; afterwards returned to Washington and became Prof. Anatomy, Georgetown Med. College, 1870-2; in the latter year was paralyzed. He left a son of the same name, practicing at Zanesville. See Minutes Med. Society, May 2, 1874; Trans. A. M. A., 1875, XXVI, p. 454.

JANUARY 7, 1861

169. HOAR BROWSE TRIST—Born Feb. 20, 1832, D. C. M. D., 1857, Jefferson. Asst. Surg., U. S. N.; Brigade Surg., C. S. A. Removed to Baltimore, Md. Died April 5, 1896, in Washington. [Son of Hon. N. P. Trist and Virginia Randolph Trist; she was a granddaughter of Thomas Jefferson.] Educated in Europe. After serving in the Navy he settled in Washington until the outbreak of the Civil War. In 1874-5 was Prof. Anatomy, Washington Med. College, Baltimore. Member Amer. Med. Association, and Pathological Society, of Baltimore. Married, 1861, the daughter of Dr. W. R. Waring, of Savannah, Ga. See Atkinson's Phys. and Surg., 1878, p. 421.

ABOUT JULY, 1862

170. JOHN W. D. STETTINIUS—Born, 1826, D. C. M. D., 1848, Columbian. Died July 20, 1863. [Stettinius appears to have joined about the date named; he attended a meeting Aug. 20, 1862.]

FEBRUARY 1, 1864

171. FRANCIS P. RICHARDS--Born in Virginia. M. D., 1863, Georgetown. Son of Dr. John Richards, *supra*. Said to have died in Washington; apparently before 1867.

172. ANDREW JACKSON BORLAND—Born Nov. 19, 1825, York, Pa. M. D., 1861, Columbian. Dropped from membership, 1877. Died Dec. 5, 1880.

173. HENRY HARRISON LOWRIE—Born July 9, 1841, Newport, Ky. M. D., 1863, Georgetown. Removed, 1874, to Plainfield, N. J.

174. HENRY ELISHA WOODBURY—Born Jan. 1, 1827, Barrington, N. H. M. D., 1863, Georgetown. Acting Asst. Surg., U. S. A., 1864-5. Dropped from membership, 1877. Died in Washington, Jan. 15, 1905, of chronic bronchitis. Came of Revolutionary stock. Educated at Dartmouth College. For some years was employed in the Treasury Dept., Washington. Practiced medicine in Washington, 1865 to 1882, in which year he had a severe accident, from which he never fully recovered.

175. JOSIAH ADAMS CHAMBERLIN—Born March, 1833, Acton, Mass. M. D., 1863, Georgetown. Father of Dr. F. T. Chamberlin, *infra.* Surgeon of the Treasury Guard and Acting Asst. Surg., U. S. A. Died Sept. 27, 1868, Manchester, N. H. His mother was Abigail Adams. He was educated at New Ipswich, N. H., and Appleton Academy. At first practiced dentistry in Manchester; then removed to Washington and graduated in medicine. Soon afterward returned to Manchester. Married, Aug. 13, 1862, Georgette, daughter of Franklin Tenney, of Manchester; she was a descendant of Dr. Isaac Watts.

176. GEORGE PHILIP FENWICK—Born April 26, 1838, D. C. M. D., 1859, Columbian. Acting Asst. Surg., U. S. A. Died June 14, 1905. Grandson of Philip, son of John Fenwick, of southern Maryland. Educated at Gonzaga College, Washington. Was sometime connected with the Washington Infirmary ; served for some months in Armory Square Military Hospital, Washington. Practiced in south Washington; served on Board of Health, 1861–1871; member Med. Association, D. C.; Wash. Obstet. and Gynecol. Society. In 1866, married Miss Mary Agnes Stewart, of Washington. See Minutes Med. Society, July 3, 1905; Wash. Med. Annals, September, 1905, p. 264.

177. WARWICK EVANS—Born Sept. 15, 1828, Portsmouth, N. H. M. D., 1852, Georgetown. Was sometime Demonstrator of Anatomy, afterwards Prof. Anatomy at Georgetown Med. College Practiced in Washington. Hon. President Alumni Society, Georgetown Med. College.

178. ARMISTEAD PETER—Born Feb. 22, 1840, Montgomery Co., Md. M. D., 1861, Columbian. Acting Asst. Surg., U. S. A. Died of angina pectoris, Jan. 28, 1902. His ancestors were owners of much real estate in Georgetown, Md. Son of Major George Peter, U. S. Army, and member of Congress from Maryland. Educated by private tutor and at Carnahan's Academy. Studied medicine with Dr. Joshua Riley, *supra;* after graduation, practiced in Georgetown. Had a defect in his speech and hearing. During the Civil War he served in the Seminary (military) Hospital, Georgetown. For many years was a member of Board of Health, Georgetown; Physician to Smallpox Hospital in 1866. In 1861, married Miss Martha C. Kennon, daughter of Commodore Beverly Kennon. See Minutes Med. Society, January 29 and Feb. 5 and 18, 1902; Atkinson's Phys. and Surg., 1878, p. 430 ; Wash. Med. Annals, March 1902, p. 68.

179. CHARLES MASON FORD—Born May 15, 1840, near Troy, N. Y. M. D., 1861, Univ. Penna. Acting Asst. Surg., U. S. A., and Acting Asst. Surg., U. S. N. Died Feb. 15, 1884, of rheumatic fever. Studied medicine with Dr. Alfred Watkins, of Troy. After graduation he served nine months in the Navy; was on the "Huntsville," one of the blockading fleet. Soon after resigning he came to Washington, and served in Cliffbourne Hospital and at the old Capitol prison. Afterwards practiced medicine in Washington; for several years was Visiting Physician to Washington Asylum Hospital ; was on the staff of Providence Hospital and Surgeon to B. and O. R. R. and Wash. and Fredericksburg R. R. See Minutes Med. Society, Feb. 16, 1884; Maryland Med. Jour., 1883-4, X, pp. 763 and 835; Busey's Reminiscences, p. 191.

MARCH 7, 1864

180. JOSEPH THEOPHILUS HOWARD—Born July 7, 1832, D. C. M. D., 1859, Georgetown. Father of Dr. J. T. D. Howard, *infra*, and Dr. Arcturus L. Howard. Educated in Henshaw's School and at Rezin Beck's Academy. Studied medicine with Dr. Eliot Craig. Since graduation has practiced in Washington. In 1861 was Physician to the Poor. Member Med. Association, D. C., and Amer. Med. Association. Married Miss Elizabeth M. Davidson, of Salem, N. J.

181. CHARLES ALLEN—Born July 6, 1836, Portsmouth, Va. M. D., 1861, Georgetown. Dropped from membership, 1877. Died of paralysis, Dec. 24, 1908, in Washington, D. C. Came to Washington in 1853 ; was sometime clerk at U. S. Arsenal. After graduation in medicine practiced in Washington. Was sometime Ward Physician and also conducted a drug store. Compiled a hymn book for use in Baptist Church. Married.

182. JAMES EWINGS DEXTER—Born, 1822, Groton, N. Y. M. D., 1861, Univ. City of New York. Principal of Collegiate Institute, Rochester, N. Y. Surgeon, 40th N. Y. Vols.; Med. Inspector, 3d Army Corps. Secretary Board of Health, Washington, 1869; Commissioner to Philadelphia Exposition, 1876. Acting Asst. Surg., U. S. A. Dropped from membership, 1877. Died June 17, 1902.

APRIL 5, 1864

183. GEORGE N. HOPKINS—Born in D. C. M. D., 1863, Columbian. Dropped from membership, 1873. Sometime druggist in Washington.

184. ADOLPHUS PATZE—Born April 4, 1804, Stettin, Prussia. M. D., 1838, Univ. Berlin. Surgeon, 4th Pennsylvania Reserves. Removed to Soldiers' Home, Hampton, Va., where he died Oct. 24, 1886. Author of Ueber Bordelle, etc., Leipzig, 1845; translated : The moral depravity of mankind, 1873. See Busey's Reminiscences, p. 159.

185. WILLIAM HERBERT COMBS—Born Aug. 4, 1841, D. C. M. D., 1862, Columbian. Acting Asst. Surg., U. S. A. Died May 16, 1873. See Minutes Med. Society, May 17, 1873.

[Leonard Baum paid $5 April 16, 1864, and there is no record on the Treasurer's books of its having been returned to him. But there is no record of his nomination or election, nor even of his being granted a license.]

JULY 4, 1864

186. THOMAS CROGGON SMITH—Born Aug. 16, 1842, D. C. M. D., 1864, Georgetown. Educated in public schools and Gonzaga College, Washington. Since graduation in medicine has practiced in Washington. Corresponding Secretary of Med. Society over twenty years ; President Obstet. and Gynecolog. Society, 1897-9 ; Consulting Obstetrician, Freedmen's Hospital. A son, Dr. Hugh M. Smith, is Deputy Commissioner Bureau of Fisheries. See Lamb's History, p. 134.

187. JOSEPH FORD THOMPSON—Brother of Dr. Benedict Thompson, *infra*. Born March 20, 1837, St. Mary's Co., Md. M. D., 1857, Univ. Maryland. Acting Asst. Surg., U. S. A. President, 1881-2, Med. Assn., D. C. Son of Charles and Ann Eliza Yates Thompson; of Scotch-Irish descent. Educated in public and private schools in St. Marys Co., and Rittenhouse Academy, Washington. After graduation in medicine he began practice in Washington in partnership with Dr. M. V. B. Bogan, *supra*. During the Civil War, served in the military hospitals of Washington. Was Prof. Anatomy, Columbian Med. College; afterwards Prof. Surgery, serving in the latter chair over twenty years. Surgeon to Providence Hospital, Emergency Hospital, Columbia Hospital for Women, Children's Hospital, George Washington Univ. Hospital and Garfield Memorial Hospital. Member Med. Assn., D. C.; Amer. Med. Assn.; Amer. Surg. Assn. Retired from practice in 1907. In 1860, married Marion Virginia Grieves, of Washington. See Univ. Maryland, 1907, II, p. 327; Atkinson's Phys. and Surg., 1878, p. 671.

188. LOUIS WARFIELD RITCHIE—Son of Dr. Joshua A. Ritchie, *supra*. Born March 4, 1843, D. C. Studied medicine with his father. M. D., 1863, Georgetown. Acting Asst. Surg., U. S. A.; served at Antietam. Attending Physician at Fort Myer, Va. Dropped from membership, 1879. Died of Bright's disease, Sept. 9, 1901.

189. SETH JEWETT TODD—Born Aug. 3, 1842, D. C. M. D., 1862, Columbian. [His name does not appear in the Columbian Catalogue.] Acting Asst. Surg., U. S. A. Died March 13, 1874. His father was a prominent citizen of Washington; his wife was a daughter of Dr. George M. Dove, *supra*. Studied medicine with Dr. J. J. Waring, *supra*, and spent some time in the hospitals of Philadelphia and Paris before graduation. Was sometime a member of the Auxiliary Faculty of Columbian Med. College; member and Secretary Clinico-Pathological Society of Washington. His health failed and he retired from practice; became Secretary of Arlington Fire Insurance Co. See Minutes Med. Society, March 14, 1874; Trans. A. M. A., 1874, XXV, p. 525.

190. ALBERT FREEMAN AFRICANUS KING—Born Jan. 18, 1841, at Hamlet of Blackthorn, Oxfordshire, England. M. D., 1861, Columbian; 1865, Univ. Penna.; A. M., 1883; LL. D., 1904, Univ. Vt. Acting Asst. Surg., U. S. A.; President Med. Assn., D. C., 1903-4. Son of Edward and Louisa Freeman King. Educated at Maley's school and the Bicester Diocesan school in England. Served for three months in 1864 as Acting Asst. Surgeon. Prof. Obstetrics and Diseases of Women and Children, Med. Dept., Columbian Univ., for 37 years; holds the same chair in the Univ. of Vt.; President Washington Obstet. and Gynecol. Soc., 1885-7; Fellow British Gynecol. and Amer. Gynecol. Socs.; Consulting Physician Children's Hospital, Washington; Obstetrician, Columbian Univ. Hospital; member Wash. Acad. Sciences; Fellow A. A. A. S.; Associate Member Philosoph. Soc. of Great Britain; member Med., Philosoph., Anthropol. and Biol. Societies of Washington, etc. Author of a manual of obstetrics, twelve editions; Ligation and management of the umbilical cord, Washington, 1867. Married, Oct. 17, 1894, Ellen Amory Dexter, of Boston, Mass. See Who's Who in America; Amer. Men of Science, 1906; Amer. Biog. Directory, Washington, 1908.

191. JOHN S. CHAPMAN—Born, 1826, in Maryland. M. D., 1847, Univ. Maryland. Licentiate M. C. F., Maryland. Resided in Baltimore, then removed to Washington. Died July 15, 1871, Plainfield, N. J. See Cordell's Med. Annals, Maryland, 1903, p. 347.

192. SAMUEL WILLIAM BOGAN—Born Oct. 15, 1840, D. C. M. D., 1860, Columbian. Brother of Dr. M. V. B. Bogan, *supra*. Father of Dr. Fred M. Bogan, U. S. Navy. Dropped from membership, 1881.

OCTOBER 3, 1864

193. JOSEPH WELLS HERBERT—Born Oct. 3, 1837, St. Marys Co., Md. M. D., 1859, Georgetown. Died Oct. 21, 1903. See Minutes Med. Society, Oct. 21 and Nov. 4, 1903; Wash. Med. Annals, November, 1903, p. 352.

194. GEORGE SYLVESTER—Born in D. C. M. D., 1863, Georgetown. Served as Contract Surgeon, U. S. A., at Gettysburg, Pa. Kept a drug store many years. Dropped from membership, 1872. Died about 1879.

195. RALPH WALSH—Born Nov. 4, 1841, Harford Co., Md. M. D., 1863, Georgetown. Acting Asst. Surg., U. S. A. Father of Dr. F. C. Walsh, *infra*. Co-editor, afterwards editor of Walsh's Retrospect, 1880–2. Son of John C. and Sarah A. Lee Walsh, of Irish-American descent. Educated in private and academic schools in Maryland and Pennsylvania. Was on duty as Medical Officer at Gettysburg after the battle; returned to Washington and served in military hospitals here, especially the Carver and Armory Square. Was. Prof. Physiology, in 1873, Georgetown Med. College. Retired from practice in 1901 and became President of National Vaccine and Antitoxin Company. Married Jeanie Patterson, of Mississippi. Dr. Walsh says : "I may mention that during this period [1865] I was also placed in immediate charge of the Army Medical Museum, then located on H Street, between Thirteenth and Fourteenth. Said Museum, when I assumed charge, consisted of two large rooms filled with empty cases, a back building in which was stored a number of dry and moist specimens in barrels and alcohol, to be mounted by Mr. Schafhirt, who was employed for that purpose. There was also a mass of written histories, numbered to correspond with the specimens. Under my supervision the specimens were mounted, numbered and placed in the cases, and the histories condensed and recorded. In other words, I think I can make a just claim, though I have never heretofore done so, to have started the Army Medical Museum. I mention as a. possibly interesting fact, that most of the alcohol used for the preservation of the moist specimens was procured by distillation of contraband liquors seized on the Long Bridge. These liquors ran from beer and blackberry wine to straight alcohol, and were packed in many peculiar vessels. Frequently women were arrested with belts under their skirts, to which were attached tin sectional cans holding from a quart to a gallon, and, in a number of cases, false breasts, each holding a quart or more." See Georgetown University, II, p. 83.

196. WILLIAM ELDER ROBERTS—Son of Dr. J. M. Roberts, *supra*. Born Aug. 9, 1839, D. C. M. D., 1864, Bellevue. Acting Asst. Surg., U. S. A. Served at Lincoln Hospital, Washington. Did an enterorrhaphy, July, 1865, thirteen days after incised wound of colon; patient died one week afterwards. Married Rebecca Worthington Naylor, daughter of Col. Naylor. Served on staff of Providence Hospital, D. C., many years. Died April 13, 1892. See Minutes Med. Society, April 15, 1892.

NOVEMBER 15, 1864

197. GEORGE L. RICE—Born May 8, 1838, North Adams, Mass. M. D., 1863, Columbian. Acting Asst. Surg., U. S. A. Removed to Framingham, Mass., about 1874; afterwards to North Adams. Member of Cassius M. Clay's Battalion from the inauguration of Lincoln until the arrival of troops, about April 20, 1861; guarded the President, Navy Yard, Long Bridge, etc. Med. Cadet, U. S. A., April to October, 1863; afterward 1st Asst. Surg., 2d Tenn. Heavy Artillery, at Columbus, Ky., till May, 1864. Acting Asst. Surg., 1865, Savannah, Ga.

198. CHARLES A. RAHTER—Born Aug. 8, 1839, near Minden, Westphalia, Prussia. M. D., 1864, Long Island College Hospital. Acting Asst. Surg., U. S. A., and Staff Surg., Franco-Prussian War. Removed to Harrisburg, Pa., about June, 1865, and is still practicing there. President, 1876, Dauphin Co. Med. Soc., Penna. Educated at public schools and Pennsylvania College, Gettysburg. After graduation in medicine served in the Civil War till June, 1865; served also during the Franco-Prussian War, 1870-1, in the military hospital at Coblentz, and the barrack hospital at St. Johann-Saarbruecken. In 1873, received from the German Emperor a medal for service. Member Penna. State Med. Society. For five years was Examining Surgeon of Pensions. Married, Nov. 11, 1875, Mary R., daughter of P. B. Keffer, Esq., of Harrisburg. See Atkinson's Phys. and Surg., 1878, p. 348; Stone's Biog., 1894, p. 668; Watson's P. and S., 1896, p. 658.

DECEMBER 12, 1864

199. JOHN WELLS BULKLEY—Born Dec. 12, 1824, Williamstown, Mass. M. D., 1844, Berkshire. President, 1887-8, Med. Assn., D. C.

200. DANIEL WEBSTER PRENTISS—Born May 21, 1843, D. C. B. Ph., 1861; A. M., 1864, Columbian; M. D., 1864, Univ. Penna.; Acting Asst. Surg., U. S. A. President, 1899-1900, Med. Assn., D. C. Father of Drs. D. W. and E. C. Prentiss, *infra*. Died Nov. 10, 1899. Son of Wm. Henry Prentiss and Sarah Cooper (daughter of Isaac Cooper) Prentiss, of Washington; grandson of Caleb Prentiss, of Cambridge, Mass. Educated at public schools and Columbian College. After graduation in medicine practiced in Washington. Prof. Materia Med. and Therapeutics, 1879-1899, Columbian Med. School; member Med. Assn., D. C.; Wash. Obstet. and Gynecol. Society; Philosophical, Biological and Anthropological Societies of Washington; Amer. Med. Association; Amer. Assn. Adv. Sci.; Assn. Amer. Physicians; delegate to International Med. Congress, 1884, at Copenhagen, and, 1890, at Berlin. Delivered many lectures under various auspices, more especially of the U. S. National

Museum. Member Board of Health of Washington, 1864; Lecturer on Dietetics, etc., Nurse's Training School, Dean of Faculty, 1878-1883; Trustee, 1880-4; President of the Board, 1884. Physician, Eye and Ear Service, Columbia Dispensary, 1874-8; Visiting Physician, Providence Hospital, 1882; Commissioner of Pharmacy, D. C., President from 1888. Married Emilie A. Schmidt, Oct. 12, 1864, daughter of Frederick Schmidt, of Rhenish Bavaria. Author of Clinical history of croupous pneumonia, Washington, 1879; Revision of U. S. Pharmacopoeia, Washington, 1880; Coues and Prentiss, Avifauna, Washington, 1883. See Minutes Med. Society, Nov. 22, 1899; Atkinson's Phys. and Surg.; 1878, p. 305; Trans. Med. Society, 1899, IV, p. 185; Nat. Med. Review, 1899-1900, IX, p. 542; Stone's Biog., 1894, p. 412.

201. JAMES THOMAS YOUNG—Born June 2, 1839, D. C. M. D., 1864, Bellevue. President, 1889-90, Med. Assn., D. C. Died July 3, 1901. After graduation in medicine served as Interne for two years at Bellevue Hospital, N. Y., then returned to Washington and practiced. One of the founders of Clinico-Pathological Society; Lecturer, 1888, on Diseases of Heart and Lungs, Columbian Med. School. Sometime Attending Physician Providence Hospital and Columbia Hosp. for Women. In 1870, married Miss Helen Miller, at Constableville, Lewis Co., N. Y. See Minutes Med. Society, Oct. 2, 1901; Trans. Med. Soc., 1901, VI, p. 228.

202. HORACE PECHIN MIDDLETON—Born Nov. 1, 1839, D. C. M. D., 1863, Univ. Penna. Died of organic heart disease, Oct. 27, 1867. Son of Daniel Wesley Middleton, Clerk of U. S. Supreme Court, and Henrietta, daughter of Col. Wm. Pechin, of Baltimore, Md. Educated at Columbian College. Studied medicine with Dr. J. J. Waring, *supra*. Sometime Resident Physician Episcopal Hospital, Philadelphia; afterward practiced in Washington. One of the founders of Clinico-Pathological Society, Washington. Lecturer on Diseases of Children, Columbian Med. School. Member Med. Association, D. C. See Minutes Med. Society, Oct. 29, 1867; Trans. A. M. A., XIX, 1868, p. 434.

JANUARY 23, 1865

203. PATRICK CROGHAN—Born in Ireland. M. D., 1859, Queen's College, Cork. L. S. A., Ireland, and Lying-in Hospital, Dublin. Acting Asst. Surg., U. S. A. Died suddenly, March 28, 1874. Sometime Surgeon in English merchant service. Came to America in 1859. During the Civil War, 1861-5, served first as enlisted man, afterwards as medical officer. Practiced medicine in Washington. See Minutes Med. Society, March 30, 1874; Trans. A. M. A., 1874, XXV, p. 526.

JAMES FARNANDIS MITCHELL

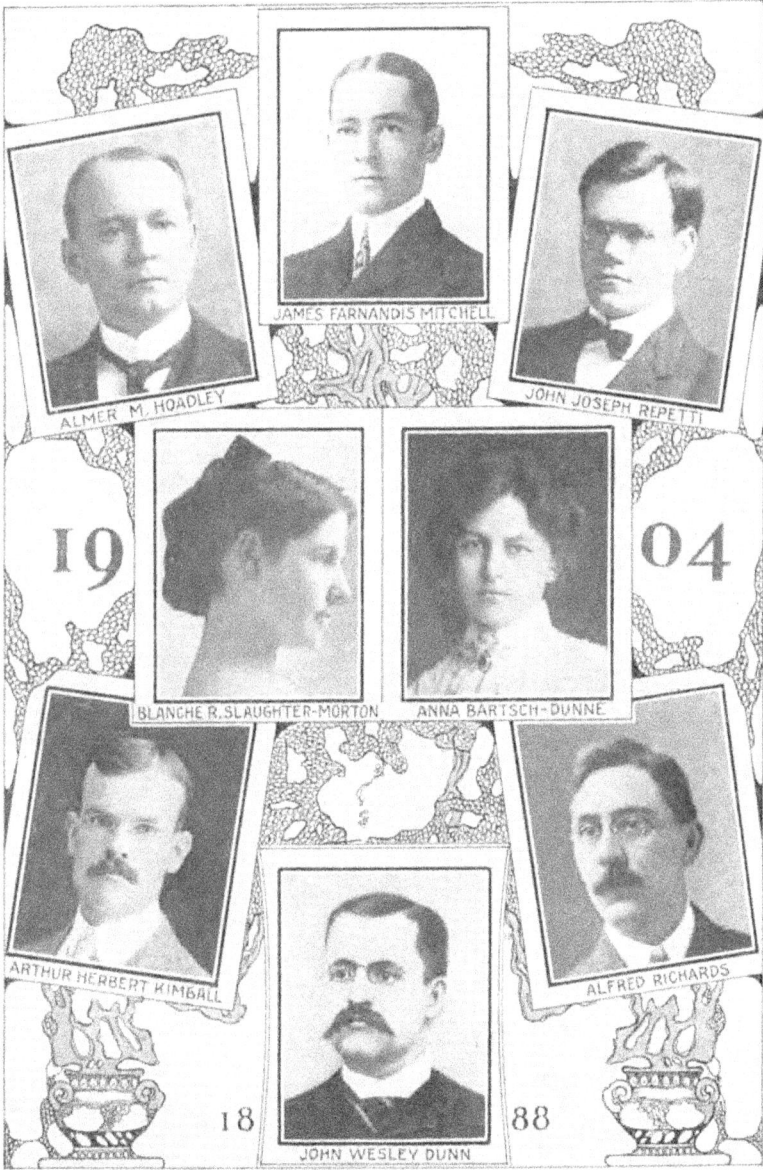

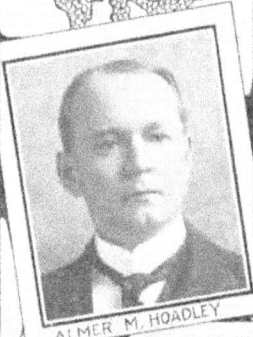

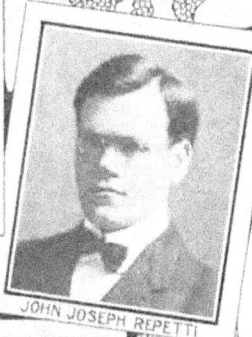

ALMER M. HOADLEY

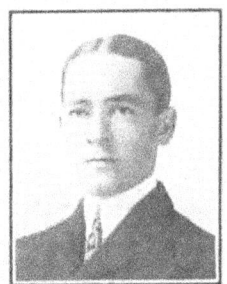

JOHN JOSEPH REPETTI

19

04

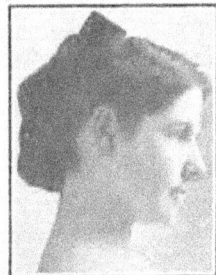

BLANCHE R. SLAUGHTER-MORTON

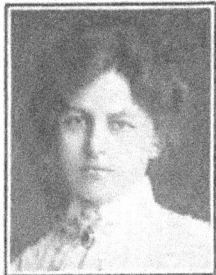

ANNA BARTSCH-DUNNE

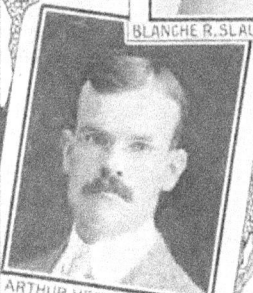

ARTHUR HERBERT KIMBALL

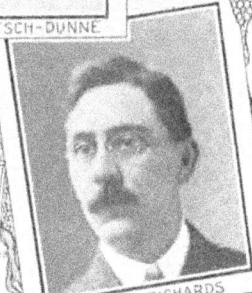

ALFRED RICHARDS

18

88

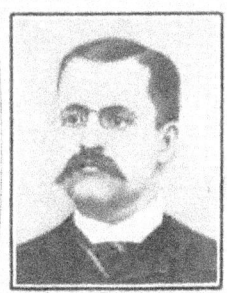

JOHN WESLEY DUNN

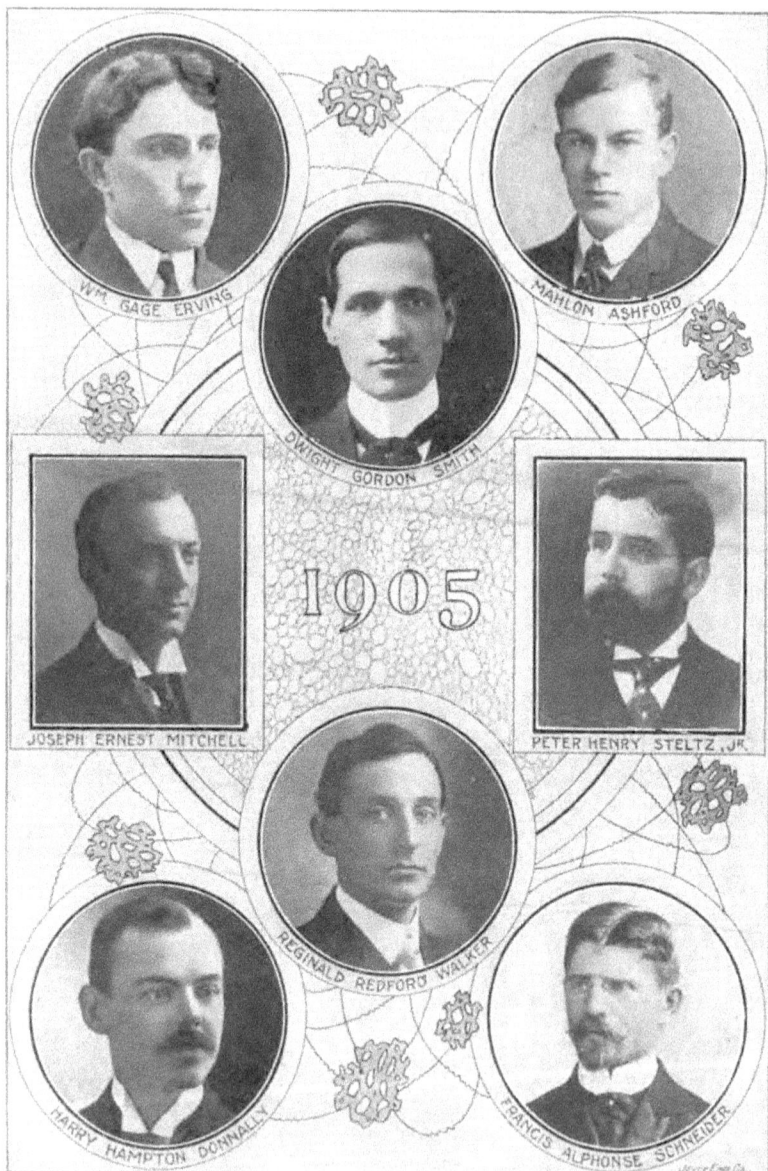

WM. GAGE ERVING

MAHLON ASHFORD

DWIGHT GORDON SMITH

JOSEPH ERNEST MITCHELL

1905

PETER HENRY STELTZ, JR.

REGINALD REDFORD WALKER

HARRY HAMPTON DONNALLY

FRANCIS ALPHONSE SCHNEIDER

70

FEBRUARY 8, 1865

204. WILLIAM HARRISON TRIPLETT—Born Sept. 15, 1836, Mt. Jackson, Va. M. D., 1859, Jefferson. Acting Asst. Surg., U. S. A. Died March 27, 1890, at Woodstock, Va. Author of Life, Washington, 1878; The laws and mechanics of circulation, etc., N. Y., 1885. Came from a family of physicians. Paternally descended from Col. Triplett, of Middleburg, Va., and of Revolutionary fame; maternally from Dr. J. Irwin, a refugee of the Irish Rebellion of 1798. Grandson of Dr. W. H. Triplett, of Front Royal, Va.; son of Dr. L. Triplett, of Mt. Jackson, Va.; brother of Drs. J. J. and A. V. M. Triplett. After graduation in medicine he practiced one year at Harrisonburg, Va.; then at Woodstock, Va., whence, in 1873, he removed to Washington. His specialty was surgery. Member Med. Assn., D. C.; Prof. Anatomy, 1875, Georgetown Med. College. Married, June 1, 1867, Kathleen McKay. See Atkinson's Biog., 1878, p. 113; Minutes Med. Society, April 2, 1890.

APRIL 5, 1865

205. JAMES PHILLIPS—Born in England. M. D., 1854, College of Surgeons, London; 1858, Univ. Mexico. Acting Asst. Surg., U. S. N. Dropped from membership, 1872. Removed to N. Y. City about 1874; was there in 1906.

206. CHARLES McCORMACK—Born Feb. 19, 1841, D. C. M. D., 1861, Georgetown. Acting Asst. Surg., U. S. A. Died in Georgetown, D. C., July 30, 1868, of tuberculosis. [Son of Wm. J. and Eveline B. (Martin) McCormack, of Washington. He was for eighteen years Postmaster of the House of Representatives.] Educated at Washington Seminary. In 1858 was Resident Student, Washington Asylum. After graduation in medicine practiced in Washington. During the Civil War, 1861-5, he served in the field and hospital as medical officer, and in June, 1863, assisted Dr. Thos. Antisell, *supra*, as Attending Surgeon of sick and wounded officers. At the close of the war resumed practice. Sometime Physician to the Poor; member Board of Health, Georgetown; member Med. Assn., D. C. Married, in February, 1866, Miss M. L., daughter of James C. and Anna Balch Wilson, of Georgetown. See Minutes Med. Society, Aug. 1, 1868; Trans. A. M. A., XXI, 1870, p. 481.

APRIL 12, 1865

207. JOHN HARRY THOMPSON—Born about 1828, London, England. M. D., 1858, College Phys. and Surg., N. Y. City. Surg., U. S. Vols.; Surg., 139th N. Y. Vols. Father of Dr. J. H. Thompson, *infra*. Surgeon in charge, Columbia Hospital, 1865 to 1878; Clinical Prof. Surg.,

18

Dis. Women, and Physiology and Hygiene, Georgetown Med. College, 1869–73. Author of Report of Columbia Hospital for Women, etc., Washington, 1873. Removed, 1878, to Rome, Italy, where he died.

MAY 3, 1865

208. WILLIAM LEE—Born March 12, 1841, Boston, Mass. M. D., 1863, Col. Phys. and Surg., N. Y., Acting Med. Cadet, U. S. A. Co-editor National Med. Journal, 1871-2. Died March 1, 1893. Son of Wm. Barlow and Ann (Whitman) Lee ; descendant of John Lee, of Agawam (Ipswich), Mass. (1634). Educated in Boston. In 1861, was Acting Med. Cadet in military hospital, Washington; in 1862, Assistant at Govt. Hosp. Insane, Washington ; 1863–5, Interne at Bellevue Hospital, N. Y. Afterwards practiced in Washington. Member Clinico-Pathological Society; Amer. Med. Association, its Librarian for some years; Lecturer on Microscopic Anatomy, 1865-7, Columbian Med. College, and Adjunct Prof. Anatomy; Prof. Physiology, 1872–1893; member Board of Health, Washington, 1871; Visiting Physician for some years to Columbia Hospital Dispensary ; Attending Physician, Central Dispensary and Emergency Hospital. Married. Author of Report on the disposition of night soil; etc., Washington, 1870 ; contributor to Billings' National Med. Dictionary. See Atkinson's Biog., 1878, p. 111; Minutes Med. Society, March 3, 1893 ; Busey's Reminiscences, p. 200; Nat. Med. Review, 1893–4, II, p. 20; Bull. Philosoph. Society, Washington, 1890, XIII, p. 405.

209. FRANCIS ST. CLAIR BARBARIN—Born Aug. 21, 1832, Newport, R. I. M. D., 1856, Georgetown. Acting Asst. Surg., U. S. A. Dropped from membership, 1874. Died March 29, 1900. He was for many years an officer of the Corcoran Art Gallery, Washington ; at the time of his death was curator.

210. FLORENCE O'DONOGHUE—Born, 1832, D. C. M. D., 1855, Univ. Maryland. Captain and Med. Storekeeper, U. S. A. Died June 29, 1882. See Brown's History, p. 298; Powell's History, p. 511.

MAY 17, 1865

211. BROWER GESNER—Born in New York. Attended, 1853-5, but did not graduate, at Coll. P. and S., New York. Asst. Surg., 38th New York, and Surg., 10th New York Vols.; Acting Asst. Surg., U. S. A. Not known what became of him after 1867.

JULY 5, 1865

212. BODISCO WILLIAMS—Born, 1840, D. C. M. D., 1863, Columbian. Asst. Surg., C. S. A. Died Dec. 23, 1873. Educated in Georgetown, D. C. Studied medicine with Dr. Joshua Riley, *supra*. After the close of the Civil War, practiced in Georgetown. See Minutes Med. Society, Dec. 24, 1873; Trans. A. M. A., 1874, XXV, p. 525.

AUGUST 16, 1865

213. SAMUEL SUPER BOND—Born July 18, 1834, Upper Darby, Pa. Hospital Steward, U. S. A. M. D., 1865, Georgetown. Dropped from membership, 1872; reëlected the same year; dropped again in 1881. Died July 4, 1899.

AUGUST 30, 1865

214. JOHN M. DUNCAN FRANCE—Born, 1842, D. C. M. D., 1865, Georgetown. Removed to St. Joseph, Mo., about 1874, and died there, May 9, 1906.

215. RICHARD M. REYNOLDS—M. D., 1859, Philadelphia Coll. Med. and Surg. Asst. Surg., 50th N. Y. Engineers. Removed to Kansas; was at Motor in 1882, Alton in 1886, Laton in 1890-3. Died about 1902.

216. FREDERICK WOLFE—Born in Austria. M. D., 1853, Univ. Prag. Is said to have removed to St. Louis, Mo. Died before 1870.

SEPTEMBER 13, 1865

217. H. MARIUS DUVALL—Born in Maryland. M. D., 1848, Univ. Penna. Asst. Surg. and Med. Director, U. S. Navy; retired in 1880. Died Feb. 9, 1891. See Hamersly's Officers of the Navy, 1890, p. 252.

SEPTEMBER 27, 1865

218. JOSEPH ALOYSIUS MUDD—Born Sept. 10, 1842, Millwood, Mo. M. D., 1864, Univ. Md. Asst. Surg., Provisional Army, C. S. A. Removed to St. Charles, Mo., about 1866, thence to Hyattsville, Md., where he is now practicing.

219. JAMES OTEY HARRIS—Born 1840, Alexandria, D. C. Brother of Dr. Robert Harris, *infra.* M. D., 1861, Univ. Penna. Said to have served in C. S. A. Dropped from membership, 1881. Died of epilepsy, Dec. 9, 1882, in D. C.

220. E. V. B. BOSWELL—Born May 31, 1839, Montgomery Co., Md. M. D., 1865, Georgetown. Was also a druggist in Washington. Died Dec. 9, 1878.

221. JOHN KEARNEY WALSH—Born 1845, D. C. Son of Dr. Joseph Walsh, *supra*. M. D., 1865, Georgetown. Acting Asst. Surg., U. S. Navy. Removed from D. C. in 1883. Asst. Surg., Soldiers' Home, Ft. Leavenworth, Kansas. Dropped from membership, 1883. Died Jan. 14, 1894, D. C.

OCTOBER 4, 1865

222. CHARLES HENRY BOWEN—Born May 30, 1838, D. C. M. D., 1862, Columbian. Med. Cadet and Acting Asst. Surg., U. S. Army. Dropped from membership, 1895; reëlected, April 1, 1896. Died March 12, 1901, at Fortress Monroe, Va. Son of James G. Bowen. Educated in public school. Served during the Civil War in military hospitals, Washington, and at Fort Stevens, D. C. After the war closed, he served on the frontier. See Minutes Med. Society, March 20 and 27, 1901; Trans. Med. Society, 1901, VI, p. 113.

223. JAMES ROSS REILY—Born March 23, 1835, Philadelphia, Pa. M. D., 1859, Univ. Penna. Asst. Surg., Pa. Reserve Corps; Surg., 127th and 179th Pa. Vols.; Acting Assist. Surg., U. S. A., on duty at the U. S. A. Arsenal, Washington. Dropped from membership, 1879. Died at College Park, Md., Oct. 12, 1904.

224. CARLOS CARVALLO—Born, Santiago, Chili. M. D., 1862, Univ. Berlin. Asst. Surg., U. S. A. Died July 23, 1882, Boston, Mass. Author of Ten days in Army of Potomac, 1864. See Brown's History, p. 297; Powell's History, p. 235.

225. ALEXANDER MATTHEWS—Born May 27, 1825, D. C. M. D., 1847, Univ. Maryland. Removed to Oxford, Md. Died Oct. 5, 1891. [Matthews is recorded as having attended the meetings Oct. 4, 1865, and Jan. 17, 1866. The 1867 list gives his residence as 51 Congress Street, Georgetown. The 1870 list does not give any residence, so that presumably he had already removed to Oxford, Md. He is provisionally placed here as elected October 4th.]

NOVEMBER 22, 1865

226. HENRY ALFRED ROBBINS—Born Feb. 9, 1839, St. Louis, Mo. M. D., 1861, Univ. Penna. Acting Asst. Surg., U. S. A. Surgeon, National Guard of France. [Son of Zenas C. and Mary Byrd Tylden Robbins, of Revolutionary stock.] His parents removed to Washington in 1844. Educated at Betts Academy, Stamford, Conn., Jones' Academy, Bridgeport, Conn., and Norwich University, Vt. Studied medicine with

Dr. W. P. Johnston, *supra*. Served as medical officer through the Civil War; afterwards practiced in Washington. Examining Surgeon for Pensions. Ward Physician two years; for four years had medical charge of Soldiers' and Sailors' Home. Went to Paris in 1870; served as Surgeon (rank of Major) in the National Guard of France. Afterwards attended lectures and clinics at Guy's Hospital, London, assisting Prof. Walter Moxon ; also externe to London Hospital ; attended the cancer wards, Middlesex Hospital. Afterwards attended clinics at Charité Hospital, Berlin, and Allgemeine Krankenhaus, Vienna. Returned to Washington in 1883. In 1884 was President Microscopical Society, Washington. Had charge for several years of Dermatological and Venereal Clinic, Central Dispensary ; Clinical Professor, Georgetown Med. School ; afterwards Prof. Dermatology and Syphilology, Howard Med. School. Member Med. Association, D. C., and Amer. Med. Association; Med. Director, Army Potomac, G. A. R.; President of Union Soldiers' Alliance, 1894. On the staff of Washington Hosp. Foundlings. Sometime President Therapeutic Society, Washington.

DECEMBER 6, 1865

227. JOSEPH SCHOLL—Born March 12, 1823, Carlsruhe, Germany. M. D., 1850, Tübingen. Sometime Coroner at Newark, N. J. Died June 6, 1902, D. C., of hemorrhage from gastric ulcer. Student Surgeon in the war between Prussia and Denmark in 1846; in Revolution of 1848, was Provost Marshal of small town in Germany, which was the reason of his being required to leave his native country. In 1851, came to America, and located for a short time in Salem, Mass., then removed to Newark, N. J., where he practiced medicine nine years ; was Coroner, and with others established the first free hospital in that city. In 1861, came to Washington ; one of the founders and incorporators of Central Dispensary. See Minutes Med. Society, June 11, 1902 ; Wash. Med. Annals, September, 1902, p. 316.

228. DOCTOR WILLARD BLISS—Born Aug. 18, 1825, Brutus, N. Y. M. D., 1845, Western Reserve. Surgeon, 3d Mich. Vols. and Surgeon, U. S. Vols. Dropped from membership, 1873. Died Feb. 21, 1889. Was named after Doctor Willard, of N. Y. City. Practiced medicine in 1846 in Iona, Mich., afterwards at Grand Rapids, Mich. In 1861-2 was in the field with the Army of the Potomac; afterwards in military hospitals, Washington, till the close of the war ; built and conducted Armory Square Hospital. Member Board of Health, Washington. One of the physicians who attended President Garfield. Exploited for a time the drug Condurango as a cure for cancer. See Stone's Biog., 1894, p. 49.

ABOUT DECEMBER 18, 1865

229. WILLIAM JOSEPH CRAIGEN—[There is no record of his election. He paid the required fee Dec. 18, 1865.] Born Sept. 17, 1837, Hampshire Co., Va. M. D., 1859, Univ. Penna. Assistant Surg. 2d D. C., Vols. Removed in 1868 to Emporium, Pa., thence to Cumberland, Md., in 1876, and to Baltimore in 1903. Licentiate M. C. F., Md., 1892. Son of Jacob S. Craigen. Was Coroner of Cameron Co., Pa.; Pension Examiner; Physician to Insane Asylum, Alms House and Jail, Alleghany Co., Md. Vice President Tri-State Med. Assn., 1899. See Cordell's Med. Annals, Maryland, 1903, p. 365.

JANUARY 3, 1866

230. MAURICE TUCKER—Born in Penna. M. D., 1862, Georgetown. Surgeon, 30th U. S. C. T. Died before 1882.

JANUARY 24, 1866

231. GEORGE LOWRIE PANCOAST—Born Dec. 9, 1838, Burlington Co., N. J. M. D., 1859, Jefferson. Assistant Surg., 3d Penna. Reserves. Surg., U. S. Vols. Died of consumption, Dec. 16, 1868. Son of Samuel Abbott and Rachel (Newbold) Pancoast. The family removed to Hampshire Co., Va., while he was a child. Educated at Hallowell's School, Alexandria, Va. Studied medicine with his uncle, Dr. Joseph Pancoast, Prof. Anatomy, Jefferson Med. College, Philadelphia, Pa. After graduation served as Physician to the "Saranack," sailing between Philadelphia and Liverpool. Afterwards practiced in Philadelphia until the outbreak of the Civil War. Was in the seven days' fight of the Peninsular campaign; Second Bull Run campaign; was next Med. Director Stoneman's Cavalry Corps. In February, 1864, was transferred to Washington and given charge of Finley (Military) Hospital. At the close of the war began to practice in Washington, associated with Dr. W. P. Johnston, *supra*. His health failing, he spent a year in southern Europe. Returned in 1868. See Trans. A. M. A., 1872, XXIII, p. 578.

FEBRUARY 4, 1866

232. CHARLES TRAUTMANN—Born in Germany. M. D., 1862, Univ. Maryland. Asst. Surg., U. S. Vols. Said to have removed, about 1867, to Baltimore, and thence to Philadelphia, where he died. Is said to have been the father of Dr. Barthold Trautmann, of Philadelphia, but to a letter of inquiry to the latter no reply was received.

MARCH 14, 1866

233. EPHRAIM CARLOS MERRIAM—Born Dec. 9, 1838, Pittsburg, Pa. M. D., 1863, Dartmouth. Med. Cadet, U. S. A.; Asst. Surg., 40th Mass. Vols. Father of Dr. A. C. Merriam, *infra*. Name dropped; re-elected Oct. 1, 1873. Died Nov. 27, 1895. Son of Dr. Marshall and Sarah (Shook) Merriam. Educated at Merrimack and at Appleton Academy, New Ipswich, N. H., Amherst and Dartmouth. In 1862, was Medical Cadet at Columbian Military Hospital, Washington; afterwards served in the 40th Mass. Vols., and in December, 1864, was transferred to hospital, Washington, where he remained on duty till 1866. Afterwards practiced in Washington. See Minutes Med. Society, Nov. 27, 1895.

234. BEDFORD BROWN—Born Jan. 17, 1825, Caswell Co., N. C. M. D., 1848, Transylvania; 1853, Jefferson. Resided in Alexandria, Va. Surgeon and Medical Director, C. S. A. Was also an honorary member of the Society. Died at Alexandria' Sept. 13, 1897. Son of Bedford Brown, U. S. Senator from North Carolina. After graduating in medicine he practiced in Yanceyville, N. C., thence removed to Alexandria, where he continued to practice. Member and ex-President Med. Society of Virginia; of Med. Examining Board of Virginia; ex-President Southern Surg. and Gynecol. Association; member Pan-American Med. Congress; Amer. Med. Association. See Watson's Biog., 1896, p. 447; Atkinson's Phys. and Surg., 1878, p. 389; Stone's Biog., 1894, p. 592.

MARCH 21, 1866

235. OLIVER A. DAILEY—Born in D. C. M. D., 1855, Georgetown. Resigned, 1877. Died Jan. 5, 1896, at Kansas City, Mo.

236. THOMAS WASHINGTON WISE—Son of John Wise, of Washington. Born Feb. 22, 1846, D. C. Studied medicine with Dr. J. E. Morgan, *supra*. M. D., 1866, Georgetown. Practiced several years in Kentucky, then returned to Washington. Acting Asst. Surg., U. S. A., on duty in the Library of the office of Surgeon General. Died Feb. 17, 1891. See Nat. Med. Rev., 1892-3, I, p. 7; Georgetown University, II, p. 192.

MARCH 28, 1866

237. SAMUEL A. AMERY—Born, 1844, Charles Co., Md. M. D., 1866, Georgetown. Removed to Quincy, Ill., about 1869, thence to Cincinnati, Ohio, about 1875. Died there, August, 1881.

238. ROBERT MILLS WHITEFOOT—Born, 1840, in Pennsylvania. M. D., 1866, Georgetown. Removed to Montana. Surgeon General of Montana. Health Officer of Bozeman, Mont., where he died, July 25, 1906.

239. WILLIAM BEVERLY DRINKARD—Born Dec. 7, 1842, Williamsburg, Va. M. R. C. S., 1865, Royal College Surgeons, England; M. D., 1866, Columbian. Died Feb. 13, 1877. Son of Wm. R. Drinkard, Secretary of War under President Buchanan, and Mary Frances Martin, daughter of Wm. Beverly Martin; granddaughter of Dr. Scott Martin, a Surgeon in the Revolutionary War. The family moved to Washington in 1857. He was educated at Young's school. In May, 1860, went to Europe; attended the Lycée Impériale, Orleans, France. Thence went to Paris to study medicine; assisted the famous Desmarres in ophthalmology; was Hospital Interne. In July, 1865, went to London, and then returned to Washington and began to practice, giving especial attention to the diseases of the eye and ear. Demonstrator of Anatomy and, in 1872, elected Prof. Anatomy, Columbian Med. College. One of the founders of Children's Hospital, and Secretary of the Medical Board; Consulting Physician, Louise Home; Attending Physician, Washington Orphan Asylum; one of the Consulting Board, Columbia Hospital; member Med. Assn., D. C.; Amer. Med. Association; Clinico-Path. Society, Washington; Washington Med. Journal Club. Was the first physician in Washington who practiced ophthalmology as a specialty. His pathetic death is graphically described by Dr. Busey. See Atkinson's Biog., 1878, p. 568; Nat. Med. Review, 1878-9, I, p. 63; Busey's Reminiscences, p. 183; Minutes Med. Society, Feb. 14, 1877; Trans. A. M. A., 1878, XXIX, p. 638.

240. ADAJAH BEHREND—Born July 1, 1841, Hanover, Germany. Hospital Steward, U. S. Army. M. D., 1866, Georgetown. Dropped from membership 1873. Reëlected April 4, 1894. Father of Dr. E. B. Behrend, *infra*.

241. LLEWELLYN ADELBERT BUCK—Born Aug. 17, 1840, Buckfield, Me. Hospital Steward, U. S. Army. Served in the Civil War, 1861-5. M. D., 1866, Georgetown. Removed in 1870 to Augusta, Kansas, in 1876, to Peabody, Kansas. President, 1888, Kansas Med. Society. Local Surgeon, Rock Island R. R. Died Dec. 13, 1906, at El Reno, Okla. See Jour., Kansas Med. Society, Feb., 1907, p. 691.

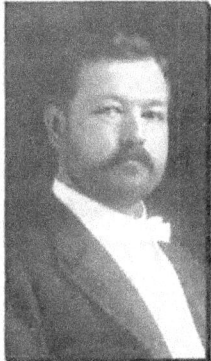

GEO. WASHINGTON BOYD

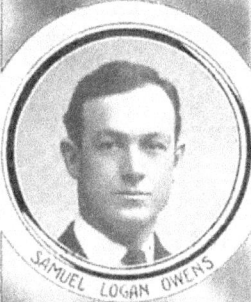

SAMUEL LOGAN OWENS

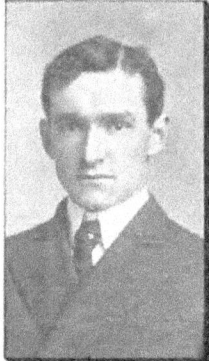

ADAM KEMBLE

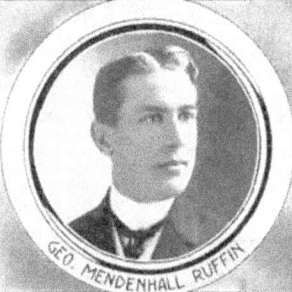

GEO. MENDENHALL RUFFIN

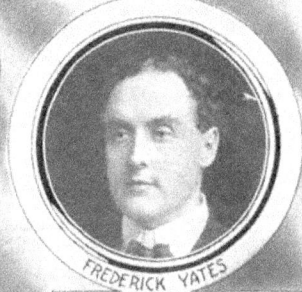

FREDERICK YATES

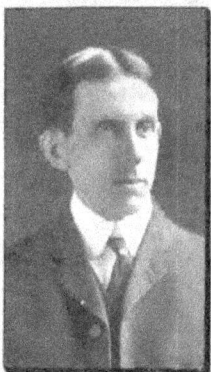

CHAS. WILBUR HYDE

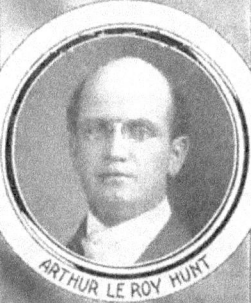

ARTHUR LE ROY HUNT

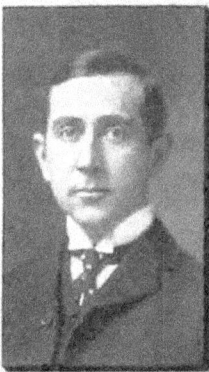

ROBT. CONRAD RUEDY

1906

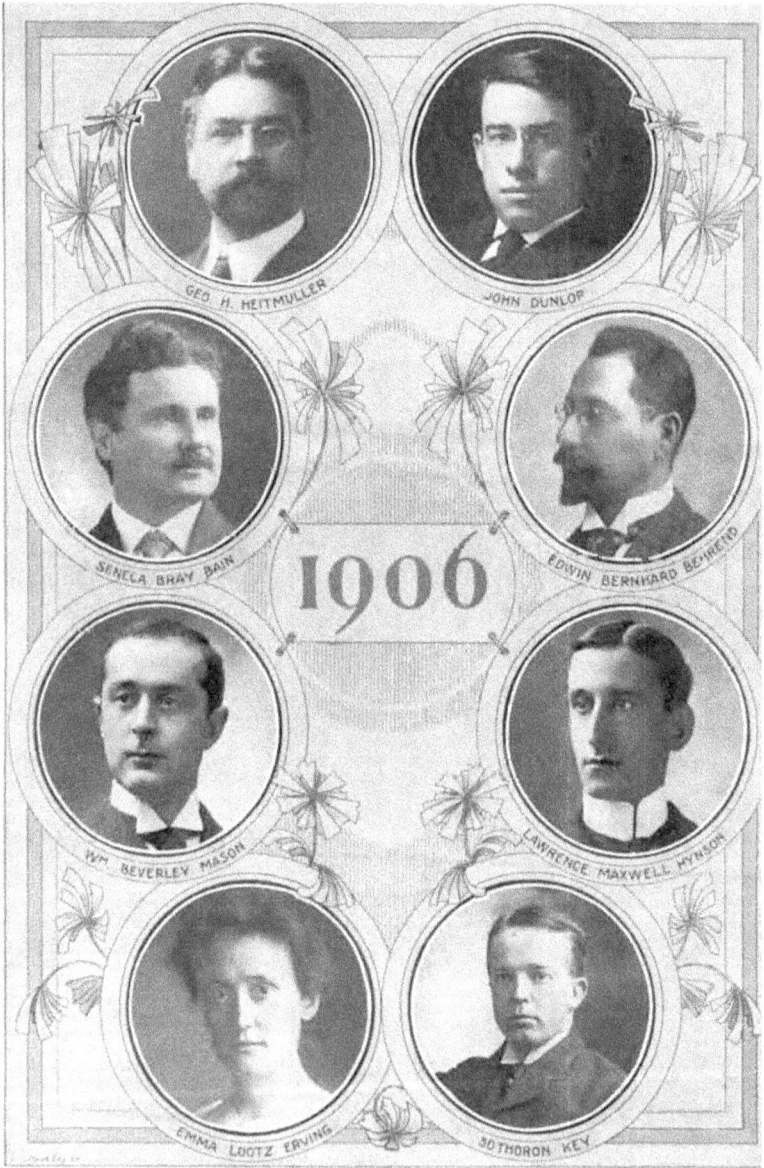

GEO. H. HEITMULLER

JOHN DUNLOP

SENECA BRAY BAIN

EDWIN BERNHARD BEHREND

1906

WM. BEVERLEY MASON

LAWRENCE MAXWELL MYNSON

EMMA LOOTZ ERVING

SOTHORON KEY

OCTOBER 17, 1866

242. FREDERICK WILLIAMS RITTER—Born Aug. 6, 1843, Pough-keepsie, N. Y. M. D., 1866, Univ. Penna. Dropped from membership, 1873. LL.B. and LL.M., National Univ., D. C. Was Med. Cadet, U. S. A., in 1865. After graduation in medicine practiced in Washington until 1874, since which he has practiced law.

243. THOMAS EMORY—Born Dec. 11, 1841, Philadelphia, Pa. Son of General Wm. A. and Matilda Emory. M. D., 1862, Richmond Med. Coll. Asst. Surg., C. S. Navy. Removed in 1870, to Syracuse, N. Y., retired from practice and went into business. Died Aug. 31, 1908, near Annapolis, Md.

244. LEMUEL JAMES DRAPER—Born May 14, 1834, Milford, Del. M. D., 1854, Univ. Penna. Acting Asst. Surg., U. S. A. Asst. Surg., U. S. Navy. Dropped from membership, 1877. Died in St. Louis, Mo., Aug. 31, 1879. Son of Samuel and Anna T. Draper. Educated at the Milford Academy. Served in the Navy in the early part of the Civil War. After the war closed he practiced in Washington and was Examin-ing Surgeon for Pensions, member Med. Assn.,D.C., and Amer. Med. Assn. In July, 1879, was ordered by the Secretary of the Navy, to St. Louis, to serve on an examining board, and died while there. Was married twice; first, to Mary Ellen Mudd, daughter of Thomas and Ellen Taylor Mudd, Oct. 18, 1860 ; second, in Feb., 1870, to Miss Mary E. Owen, daughter of Andrew Balmain and Amy E. Denham. See Trans. A. M. A., 1880, XXXI, p. 1037.

DECEMBER 12, 1866

245. JOHN LEWIS CROUSE—Born, 1833, Maryland. M. D., 1859, Univ. Maryland. Asst. Surg., 118th Pa. Vols. Dropped from member-ship, 1872. Died June 30, 1889, at St. Elizabeth Asylum, D. C.

JANUARY 16, 1867

246. WASHINGTON KILMER—M. D., 1860, Albany Med. Coll. Surgeon, 16th W. Va. Vols. Removed to Orlando, Florida ; was there 1890–6.

247. ROBERT REYBURN—Born Aug. 1, 1833, Glasgow, Scotland. M. D., 1856, Philadelphia Coll. Med. and Surg. ; A. M., 1871, Howard. Acting Asst. Surg., 1862-3, and Asst. Surg., U. S. A., 1867; Asst. Surg., 1863, and Surg., U. S. Vols., 1863-7. Chief Med. Officer, Freedmen's Bureau, 1871-2. President Board of Health, Washington, 1870-1. Re-signed from Med. Society June 8, 1870 ; reëlected Oct. 1, 1873. Died

March 25, 1909. Son of James and Jane (Brown) Reyburn. Was brought by his widowed mother to Philadelphia in 1843. Educated in public schools of that city. Studied medicine with Dr. Lewis D. Harlan. Practiced in Philadelphia until May 7, 1862, when he was appointed Acting Asst. Surgeon; in June, 1863, was commissioned. Mustered out in 1867, as Bvt. Lieut. Col., U. S. Vols., and began to practice in Washington. Surgeon in charge Freedmen's Hospital, 1867–75; Prof. Clinical Surgery, 1866–7, Georgetown Med. College ; Prof. Surgery, Howard Med. School, 1868–73; Prof. Anatomy, Georgetown Med. School, 1878 ; Prof. Physiology and Clinical Surgery, Howard Med. School, 1880–1902, and Preventive Medicine and Hygiene, 1902–9; Dean of Howard Med. Faculty, 1902–9. Member Med. Assn., D. C.; Amer. Med. Association, its Librarian in 1870; President Medico-Legal Society, Washington ; President Amer. Therap. Society; Vice President, 1891–2, National Microscop. Society ; member Microscop., Anthropolog. and Biolog. Societies, Washington; Association Amer. Anatomists ; Consulting Surgeon, Providence and Freedmen's Hospitals; Visiting Physician, St. John's Church Orphanage; member Board of School Trustees, Washington, 1877–9 ; of Board of Council, Georgetown, 1865. One of the Attending Surgeons to President Garfield, 1881. Married, 1854, Catherine White. Three children are physicians, though not practicing—Drs. Robert Reyburn, Jr., Ella Frances Reyburn and Eugenia Reyburn. Author of Types of disease among the freed people of the United States, Washington, 1891; Assassination of President Garfield, Washington, 1905; Fifty years in the practice of medicine, Washington, 1907. See Stone's Biog., 1894, p. 422; Atkinson's Biog., 1878, p. 83; Lamb's History, p. 109; Brown's History, p. 297; Powell's History, p. 550 ; Who's Who in America ; History City Washington, 1903, p. 437; Amer. Biog. Direct., 1908.

248. WILLIAM R. RUSSELL—Born July 21, 1836, Wedmore, Somersetshire, England. M. D., 1860, Rush. Practiced medicine in Beloit, Wis. Served in Civil War, 1861–2. Dropped from membership, 1879. Died April 21, 1883.

FEBRUARY 27, 1867

249. OTHO MAGRUDER MUNCASTER—Born Oct. 12, 1843, Baltimore, Md. M. D., 1866, Univ. Md. Dropped from membership, 1877. Reëlected Oct. 8, 1884.

MARCH 20, 1867

250. JOHN C. NORRIS—Born in Kentucky. M. D., 1863, Univ. Penna. Nothing known of him after 1868.

251. CHARLES MORGAN TREE—Born July 17, 1845, D. C. M. D., 1867, Georgetown. Died Dec. 4, 1881. See Minutes Med. Society, Dec. 5, 1881.

MARCH 27, 1867

252. ALEXANDER BARTON McWILLIAMS—Born, 1827, D. C. Son of Dr. A. McWilliams, *supra*. M. D., 1846, Columbian. Dropped from membership, 1872. Was many years Physician to the U. S. Jail, D. C. Died May 17, 1898. See Busey's Reminiscences, p. 132.

APRIL 3, 1867

253. JOHN E. SMITH—Born March 25, 1840, D. C. M. D., 1867, Georgetown. Son of Col. John L. Smith, a Washington attorney. Died in N. Y. City, Jan. 22, 1907.

254. AMOS N. WILLIAMSON—Born near Fayetteville, N. C., 1828. M. D., 1859, Columbian. Dropped from membership, 1879. Died Dec. 22, 1884.

APRIL 10, 1867

255. RUFUS CHOATE—Born Jan. 31, 1847, D. C. M. D., 1867, Georgetown. Acting Asst. Surg., U. S. Army. Dropped from membership. Was Resident Physician, 1865-6, at Washington Asylum, during an epidemic of typhus fever; 317 cases of the disease in the Asylum. Served many years as Medical Officer to U. S. troops.

APRIL 24, 1867

256. BENJAMIN RALEIGH RAINES—M. D., 1867, Georgetown: Removed about 1869, to St. Derwin, Neb.; thence to Rockport, Mo., about 1870; to Corning, Mo., in 1872; thence to Stony Creek, Va. Member, Missouri Med. Association.

257. EDWARD DEWELDEN BRENEMAN—Born Aug. 14, 1839, Lancaster, Pa. M. D., 1861, Univ. Penna. Asst. Surg., 30th Pa. Vols. Asst. Surg., U. S. Army. Died Oct. 11, 1870. Son of Abraham N. and Mary DeWelden Breneman. After the Civil War ended he resigned from the U. S. Army and practiced in Washington. Is said to have been an accomplished linguist. Married, Sept. 27, 1866, Marion D., daughter of Wm. and Huldah Wilson, of Washington. See Minutes Med. Society, Oct. 12, 1870; Brown's Hist., p. 296; Trans. A. M. A., 1872, XXIII, p. 581.

258. FRANCIS ASBURY ASHFORD—Born Sept. 19, 1841, Fairfax Co., Va. First Lieut., C. S. A. M. D., 1867, Columbian. Father of Dr. Mahlon Ashford, *infra*. Another son, Dr. Bailey K. Ashford, is an

Asst. Surgeon, U. S. Army. Died May 19, 1883. Was wounded and captured at Petersburg, Va., just before the close of the Civil War. Studied medicine with Dr. Thomas Miller, *supra.* After graduation was appointed Resident Physician, Columbia Hospital ; afterwards was Asst. Surgeon and one of the Directors ; assisted in organizing the Dispensary service of the hospital ; assisted also in establishing the Children's Hospital, was Attending Surgeon thereto, and gave especial attention to diseases of joints. At the reorganization of the Faculty of Georgetown Med. School in 1876, he was made Prof. Surgery. Was the principal person establishing Garfield Memorial Hospital, and, according to Dr. Busey, was practically the founder. Member Med. Assn., D. C. ; Amer. Med. Assn. ; Clinico-Patholog. Society, Washington. Married a daughter of Hon. Moses Kelly, of Washington. See Busey's Reminiscences, p. 188 ; Minutes Med. Society, May 20, 1883; Maryland Med. Jour., 1883-4, X, p. 417 ; Atkinson's Phys. and Surg., 1878, p. 78 ; In Memoriam, Washington, 1883 ; Georgetown University, II, p. 91.

MAY 1, 1867

259. JOSEPH TABER JOHNSON—Born June 30, 1845, Lowell, Mass. A. M., 1869, Columbian ; Ph. D., 1890, Georgetown ; M. D., 1865, Georgetown ; 1868, Bellevue ; 1871, Diploma in Obstetrics, Vienna. Acting Asst. Surg., U. S. Army. Father of Dr. L. B. T. Johnson, *infra.* Resigned June 8, 1870 ; reëlected Oct. 1, 1873. Honorary member M. C. F., Maryland, 1890. Son of Lorenzo Dow and Mary (Burgess) Johnson ; grandson of Jeremiah Johnson, soldier of the Revolutionary War ; descendant of John Alden and Priscilla Mullens, of the " Mayflower." Attended Rochester Academy, Plymouth Co., Mass., and Columbian College, Washington. Studied medicine with Dr. Wm. G. Palmer, *supra,* and Dr. Austin Flint, N. Y. City. Served at Freedmen's Hospital, Washington, 1868-73. Prof. Obstetrics and Gynecology, Howard Med. School, 1868-73 ; Lecturer 1874, Prof. Obstetrics 1876, afterwards Prof. Gynecology and Abdominal Surgery, Georgetown Med. School, till the present time ; President of the Med. Faculty ; President of Board, and Gynecologist, Georgetown Univ. Hospital. Surgeon in Charge of Sanitorium for cases of gynecology and abdominal surgery, built by himself, 1887. Was Gynecological Surgeon, Columbian and Providence Hospitals. Consulting Gynecologist Central Dispensary. Member Med. Assn., D. C. One of the founders Wash. Obstet. and Gynecolog. Society, President in 1888-9, and of Amer. Gynecolog. Society, Secretary and Editor " Transactions, " 1888-91 ; President, 1898-9 ; President Southern Surg. and Gynecol. Assn., 1898-9 ; Fellow British Gynecolog. Society ; member Mass. Med. Society ; Med. Society Virginia ; Amer. Med. Assn. ; Wash. Philosoph. and Anthropolog. Societies.

Author of Surgical diseases of ovaries and tubes, in Dennis' System of Surgery. Director Great Falls and Old Dominion R. R. Married in 1873, Edith Maud, daughter of Prof. W. F. Bascom, of Washington. See Atkinson's Biog., 1878, p. 231 ; Stone's Biog., 1894, p. 252 ; Watson's Biog., 1896, p. 405 ; Appleton's Biog., 1887, III, p. 446 ; Who's Who in America ; Amer. Biog. Directory, Washington, 1908 ; Lamb's History, p. 108 ; Georgetown University, II, p. 89 ; Cordell's Med. Annals, Maryland, 1903, p. 456.

MAY 29, 1867

260. GRANVILLE MALCOM—Born April 2, 1839, Boston, Mass. M. D., 1867, Georgetown. A. M., 1896, Bucknell Univ., Lewisburg, Pa. Resigned from Society, Jan. 1, 1872. Removed to Denver, Colorado, and went into real estate business.

261. HENRY GRAY—M. D., 1867, Coll. P. and S., N. Y. Died between 1867 and 1870.

262. ALONZO MORRIS BUCK—Born Jan. 24, 1826, Glens Falls, N. Y. Hospital Steward, U. S. Army. M. D., 1866, Georgetown. Practiced sometime in Michigan, then returned to Washington, and was employed in Surgeon General's Office. Dropped from membership. Died Sept. 29, 1905, Hyattsville, Md.

263. WILLIAM E. POULTON—Born May 16, 1840, D. C. M. D., 1864, Georgetown. Dropped from membership 1873.

264. DAVID PHILIP WOLHAUPTER—Born April 6, 1840, Woodstock, N. B. M. D., 1862, Bowdoin ; A. B., Sackville College, Nova Scotia. Acting Asst. Surg., U. S. A. Father of Dr. W. E. Wolhaupter, *infra*. Served in military hospitals during Civil War, afterwards practiced medicine in Washington. Died July 12, 1900. See Minutes Med. Society, Oct. 3, 1900.

JUNE 12, 1867

265. RICHMOND JOSEPH SOUTHWORTH—Born in 1841, in Wisconsin. M. D., 1866, College Phys. and Surg., N. Y. ; LL. B., 1873, Columbian. Resigned Oct. 7, 1868, from Medical Society. Acting Asst. Surg., U. S. Army. Died in Washington, July 27, 1900. Son of Mrs. E. D. E. N. Southworth, the authoress. Educated at schools in Wisconsin. After graduation in medicine practiced in N. Y. City, till 1867, when he removed to Washington. After graduating in law he removed to Yonkers, N. Y. Returned to Washington in 1890. Married Miss Blanche Porter, daughter of Dr. James J. Porter. See Lamb's History, p. 117.

JULY 3, 1867

266. SAMUEL S. TURNER—Born in 1834, in Tennessee. M. D., 1863, Georgetown. Acting Asst. Surg., U. S. A. Removed to Fort Buford, afterwards to Yankton, Dakota. Died Dec. 11, 1904, while *en route* from Fort Columbia, Washington, to Washington, D. C.

JULY 31, 1867

267. SAMUEL W. CALDWELL—Born in Penna. Hospital Steward, U. S. A. M. D., 1867, Georgetown. Dropped from membership, 1872. Removed to Philadelphia, Pa. [Was there in 1886.]

AUGUST 14, 1867

268. WILLIAM HENRY WHITLEY—Born in New Jersey. M. D., 1866, Georgetown. Removed to Paterson, N. J., about 1874, and died there after 1890.

AUGUST 21, 1867

269. CARL HERMANN ANTON KLEINSCHMIDT—Born Oct. 12, 1839, Petershagen, Prussia. M. D., 1862; Ph. D., 1889, Georgetown. Asst. Surg., C. S. A. President, 1895-6, Med. Assn., D. C. Died May 20, 1905. Educated at Royal College, Minden, Westphalia, Prussia. Came to America in 1857. After graduation in medicine served in the Confederate Army, 1863-5, with the "Texas Rangers," in most of the engagements in Northern Virginia, at Gettysburg, in the "Wilderness," and finally at Appomattox, whence he walked to Georgetown, D. C. He then took a medical course at the Univ. Berlin. Returned to Georgetown and began practice. In 1876 was appointed Prof. Physiology, Georgetown Med. School; was the first President of Board of Med. Examiners, D. C., under the law of 1896, and also President of Board of Med. Supervisors; member Wash. Acad. Sciences; on the staff of Georgetown Univ. Hospital; member Med. Assn., D. C.; Amer. Med. Association. Author of The necessity for a higher standard of medical education, Washington, 1878. See Minutes Med. Society, May 24, 1905; Atkinson's Biog., 1878, p. 531; Wash. Med. Annals, September, 1905, p. 260; Georgetown University, II, p. 84.

270. ABRAHAM BOHRER SHEKELL—Born Oct. 4, 1838, D. C. M. D., 1863, Georgetown. Acting Asst. Surg., U. S. A. Dropped from membership, 1883.

SEPTEMBER 11, 1867

271. SILAS LAWRENCE LOOMIS—Born May 22, 1822, North Coventry, Conn. A. M., Howard; M. D., 1857, Georgetown. Acting Asst. Surg., U. S. A. Father of Dr. C. L. Loomis, *infra*. Died June 22, 1896. Brother of Dr. L. C. Loomis, of Washington. Son of Silas and Esther (Case) Loomis. When five years old his father died and he early assumed the care of his mother, brother and sister. Taught school in Massachusetts and Rhode Island, 1837-43, in this way being able to work his way through college, graduating in 1844 at Wesleyan University, Middletown, Conn. The same year, with his brother Charles, he established the Adelphian Academy, North Bridgewater, now Brockton, Mass. Was married in 1848 to Betsy Ann Tidd, who died in 1850. Married in 1851 to Abigail Paine. Member Amer. Assn. Advance. Sci., in 1852. In 1854 removed to Washington, D. C., and opened the Western Academy, southwest corner Seventeenth and I Streets, N. W. Appointed, in 1857, Astronomer to the Lake Coast Survey. In 1860 was Special Instructor in Mathematics at U. S. Naval Academy, Annapolis, and was ordered on a cruise at sea. In 1861, elected Prof. Chemistry and Toxicology, Georgetown Med. College; resigned in 1867. During the war of 1861-5 was an Acting Asst. Surg., U. S. A.; served in Army of Potomac on staff of General McClellan, and also in several military hospitals in Washington. In 1862, became member Amer. Med. Association. At the close of the Civil War he was Chief Clerk, Bureau of Statistics, Treasury Department. Was associated with others in founding Howard University, and is said to have suggested the University instead of a College; organized the medical department; Dean of Med. Faculty, sessions 1868-70. In 1870 was chairman of a special committee on examination of mathematical and chemical instruments for use of Internal Revenue Bureau; in 1871, member of Board of Health of Washington. In 1878 was employed by the U. S. Bureau of Agriculture collecting special statistics of food products of the United States. Estimated the population of the United States for 1880, and was in error by only 18,000. In 1878 discovered a process and invented machinery for making textile fiber from varieties of the palm. Removed to Fernandina, Fla., in 1882. Author of Normal arithmetic, 1859; Analytical arithmetic, 1860. See Appleton's Biog., 1888, IV, p. 19; 20th Cent. Biog. Dict.; Lamb's History, p. 108.

SEPTEMBER 25, 1867

272. DANIEL SMITH LAMB—Born May 20, 1843, Philadelphia, Pa. A. B., 1859, A. M., 1864, Central High School, Philadelphia. Hospital Steward, U. S. A.; Acting Asst. Surgeon, U. S. Army. M. D., 1867, Georgetown. Co-Editor Washn. Med. Annals. Husband of Dr. I. H.

Lamb, and father of Dr. R. S. Lamb, *infra*. Author of " History of Med. Dept., Howard Univ.," 1900; "Rules of Health," 1900 (with Dr. I. H. Lamb); and contributed to "Witthaus' Med. Jurisprudence." Son of Jacob Matlack and Delilah (Rose) Lamb; descended from a number of families that peopled New Jersey, and from Revolutionary soldiers. Educated in public schools, Philadelphia, Pa. Enlisted in 81st Penna. Vols., in 1861; in hospital in Alexandria, 1862 to 1865; Hospital Steward, U. S. A., 1864–1868; Acting Asst. Surg., U. S. A., 1868–1892. On duty at Army Med. Museum, Washington, 1865, to the present time; Pathologist since 1892. Sometime Professor of General Pathology, U. S. College Veterinary Surgeons, Washington; member Med. Assn. D. C. and Amer. Med. Assn.; President Assn. Actg. Asst. Surgeons, U. S. A., for many years; many years Secretary Assn. Amer. Anatomists; Treasurer Woman's Clinic, Washington; Councilor Ninth International Medical Congress, 1887; Secretary Anatomical Section Pan-American Med. Congress, 1893; President Anthrop. Society, Washington; Vice President Washington Academy of Sciences; Prof. Materia Medica and Med. Jurispr. Howard Med. School, 1873–7, of Anatomy since 1877; Chairman Editorial Committee Washington Med. Annals, since 1902. Made post mortem examination of President Garfield, the assassin Guiteau, and Vice President Henry Wilson. Married May 20, 1868, Lizzie Scott, daughter of Robert Scott, Philadelphia; and July 3, 1899, Isabel Haslup, *infra*. See Stone's Biog., 1894, p. 649; Watson's Biog., 1896, p. 503; 20th Cent. Biog. Dict., 1904; Amer. Men. Science, 1906; Who's Who in America; Amer. Biog. Directory, Washington, 1908; Lamb's History, p. 121; Genealogy of Lamb and Others, 1904.

NOVEMBER 13, 1867

273. VALENTINE McNALLY—Born Oct. 18, 1839, Scotland. M. D., 1867; A. M., 1869; LL.D., 1889, Georgetown; LL. D., 1886, College St. Francis Xavier, N. Y. Captain and Major of Ordnance, U. S. Army. See Powell's History, p. 474. Now Colonel, U. S. A., Retired.

274. GEORGE P. HANAWALT—Born Sept. 11, 1836, Ross Co., Ohio. M. D., 1864, Georgetown. Hospital Steward, 1862–4, and Acting Asst. Surgeon, U. S. Army, 1864–8. Removed, 1868, to Des Moines, Iowa. Of German ancestry. Member and Vice Pres. Alumni Society Georgetown Med. College, 1869–70; Secretary Iowa Med. Society, 1870–3; President Polk Co., Med. Society; Surg. 3d Iowa Nat. Guard; member Board of Pension Examiners; Division Surgeon, Chicago, Rock Island and Pacific R. R.; Surgeon, Des Moines and Fort Dodge R. R. In Oct., 1871, married Emma Agnes, daughter of James C. Jordan, of Des Moines. See Atkinson's Biog., 1878, p. 432.

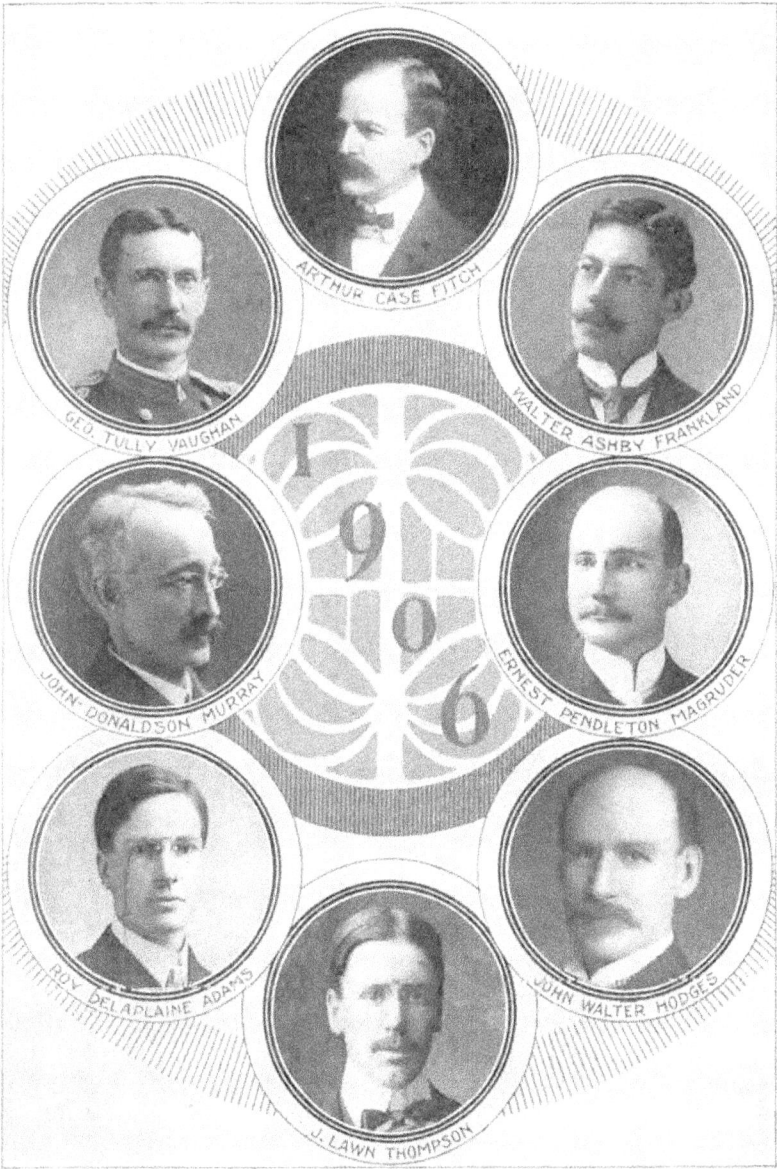

ARTHUR CASE FITCH

GEO. TULLY VAUGHAN

WALTER ASHBY FRANKLAND

JOHN DONALDSON MURRAY

ERNEST PENDLETON MAGRUDER

ROY DELAPLAINE ADAMS

JOHN WALTER HODGES

J. LAWN THOMPSON

1906

73

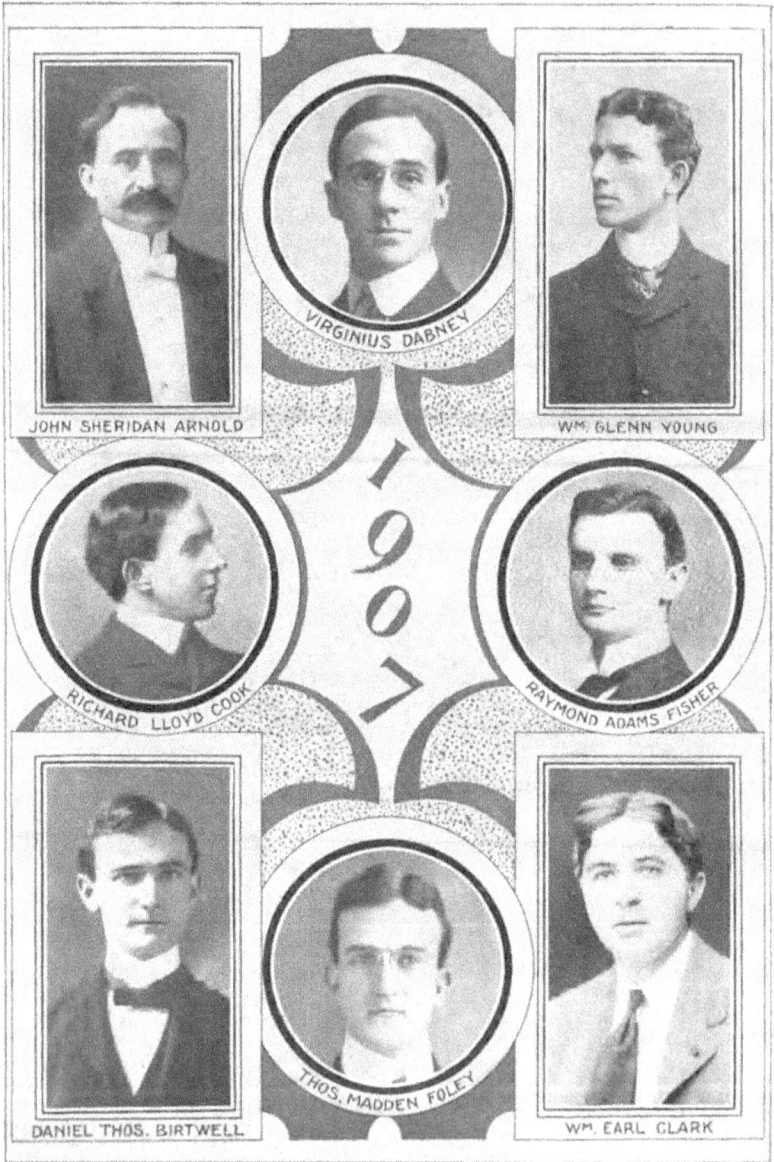

JOHN SHERIDAN ARNOLD

VIRGINIUS DABNEY

WM. GLENN YOUNG

RICHARD LLOYD COOK

RAYMOND ADAMS FISHER

DANIEL THOS. BIRTWELL

THOS. MADDEN FOLEY

WM. EARL CLARK

1907

74

275. JOSEPH DEANE BARNES—Born in 1844, in North Carolina. M. D., 1867, Univ. Penna. Acting Asst. Surg., U. S. A. Dropped from membership 1872. Was the son of Surgeon General J. K. Barnes, U. S. A. Died May 13, 1882.

DECEMBER 4, 1867

276. DeWITT CLINTON PATTERSON—Born Aug. 3, 1826, Berkshire Co., Mass. M. D., 1851, Western Reserve. Surgeon, 124th Ohio Vols. Acting Asst. Surg., U. S. A. President, 1885-6, Med. Assn., D. C. Many years Coroner of D. C. Father of Dr. A. C. Patterson, *infra*. Died Dec. 20, 1893. See Minutes Med. Society, Dec. 21, 1893 ; Lamb's History, p. 120.

1867

277. BENJAMIN B. BABCOCK—Born in Pennsylvania. M. D., 1867, Georgetown. Died Jan. 21, 1868. See Minutes Med. Society, Jan. 22, 1868.

278. JOSEPH NELSON CLARK—Born Nov. 12, 1839, near Dillsbury, Pa. Served in the army in the war, 1861-5. M. D., 1867, Georgetown. Removed to Harrisburg, Pa., where he kept a drug store and was President of the People's Savings Bank.

[Babcock was nominated April 10, 1867, and Clark May 29, 1867. There is no record of the election of either, but they were recognized as members, and, Jan. 29, 1868, the Secretary was instructed to record the election of Babcock and sign his name to the constitution.]

JANUARY 15, 1868

279. EDWIN WALTER LATIMER—Born June 6, 1826, Prince William Co., Va. M. D., 1860, Columbian. Was in C. S. A. Removed from D. C. to Prince William Co., Va. Died of meningitis April 20, 1880, in D. C. See Minutes Med. Society, April 21, 1880.

MARCH 25, 1868

280. CORNELIUS VAN NESS CALLAN—Born July 19, 1844, D. C. M. D., 1868, Georgetown. Was attending Physician, Providence Hospital and St. Ann's Infant Asylum, Washington.

281. ANDREW ROTHWELL BROWN—Born May 31, 1847, in D. C. M. D., 1868, Georgetown. Dropped from membership, 1877. Died Dec. 16, 1900. Was associated for a while with his uncle, Dr. Borrows, *supra;* then ceased to practice medicine and became a patent attorney.

19

282. GEORGE ARTHUR FITCH—Born July 30, 1846, Morgantown, Va.   M. D., 1868 ; A. M., 1869, Georgetown.   Died of tuberculosis, Nov. 30, 1875. Educated at Monongahela Academy. Studied medicine with Dr. Johnson Eliot, *supra*, Member Med. Assn., D. C., and Amer. Med. Association. See Minutes Med. Society, Dec. 1, 1875 ; Trans. A. M. A., 1878, XXIX, p. 654.

APRIL 1, 1868

283. BENEDICT THOMPSON—Born April, 1843, St. Mary's Co., Md. M. D., 1868, Columbian. Brother of Dr. J. Ford Thompson, *supra*, and father of Dr. J. Lawn Thompson, *infra*. Died of typhoid fever, July 22, 1875. Son of Charles and Eliza Thompson. Attended Georgetown College, 1857-61. Studied medicine with his brother. After graduation became Assistant Physician at Columbia Hospital, and subsequently House Physician to Providence Hospital, Washington. In 1870 married the daughter of James P. Lawn, of Baltimore. Was an active member of the Medical Society, and during a trying time in its history was instrumental in reviving the interest of its members in its meetings and did much toward improving the efficiency of its organization. Served for some time on a committee appointed to edit the transactions of the Society, and filled other offices. Member of Med. Assn., D. C. Sometime President of Carroll Institute, Washington. See Minutes Med. Society, July 23, 1875 ; Lamb's History, p. 120 ; Busey's Reminiscences, p. 200; Trans. A. M. A., 1878, XXIX, p. 722.

APRIL 29, 1868

284. JESSE LEE ADAMS—Born Aug. 6, 1841, D. C. Served in D. C. Volunteers during Civil War. M. D., 1868, Georgetown. Dropped from membership, 1879. Had a son, Dr. J. L. Adams, Jr. Was Ward Physician several years; member Med. Assn., D. C. Died April 16, 1905. See Georgetown University, II, p. 194.

285. CHARLES FRANCIS NALLEY—Born, 1849, D. C. M. D., 1868, Georgetown. Dropped from membership, 1873. Died March 4, 1876. See Minutes Med. Society, March 6, 1876.

JUNE 10, 1868

286. GEORGE RICHARD MILLER—Born Jan. 10, 1846, D. C. Son of Dr. Thomas Miller, *supra*. M. D., 1868, Univ. Penna. Died in Washington, June 5, 1872, of tuberculosis. [His mother was Virginia C. Jones, daughter of General Walter Jones.] He had a college education ; studied medicine with his father. After graduation, practiced in Washington. Apparently as the result of too close attention to practice, his

health failed and he retired to his father's farm near Leesburg, Va.
Member Med. Assn. and Clinico-Patholog. Society, D. C.   See Minutes
Med. Society, June 7, 1872.   Trans. A. M. A., 1873, XXIV, p. 340 ; and
1880, XXXI, p. 1076.

NOVEMBER 4, 1868

287. EDGAR ARMISTEAD DULIN—Born Dec. 19, 1843, D. C.   M.
D., 1865, Georgetown.   Medical Cadet, U. S. Army ; Acting Asst. Surg.,
U. S. Navy.   Removed in 1869 to Lexington, Mo. ; afterwards to Nevada,
Mo.   President Med. Soc., Vernon Co., Mo. ; and John T. Hodgen Med.
Society.   Member U. S. Board of Pensions.

NOVEMBER 25, 1868

288. ROBERTSON HOWARD—Son of Dr. Flodoardo Howard, *supra*.
Born Dec. 12, 1847, D. C.   M. D., 1867 ; A. M., 1870 ; LL. B., 1874,
Georgetown.   Removed to St. Paul, Minn., and practiced law.   Died
there, Dec. 1, 1899.

DECEMBER 2, 1868

289. WILLIAM WARING JOHNSTON—Born Dec. 28, 1843, D. C.
Eldest son of Dr. W. P. Johnston, *supra*.   Med. Cadet, U. S. A.   M. D.,
1865, Univ. Penna.   President Med. Assn., D. C., 1888-9.   Brother of Dr.
G. W. Johnston, *infra*, and father of Dr. W. B. Johnston.   Died March 22,
1902, at Atlantic City, N. J.   [His mother was Mary Elizabeth, daughter
of Bernard Hooe, of Prince William Co., Va.]   He was educated by Mr.
Hector Munro, at a Washington school, and at St. James College, near
Baltimore, till 1862 ; then by Mr. Chas. B. Young, Washington.   After
graduating in medicine served as Interne at Bellevue Hospital, N. Y.,
one year, during the cholera epidemic ; a fellow student, his room mate,
died of the disease.   He next attended the Univ. Edinburgh and was a
private pupil of Dr. John Hughes Bennett; and next the Paris hospitals.
Returned to Washington in 1868 and began practice with his father.   In
1871, became Prof. Theory and Practice of Medicine, Columbian Med.
School, and held the position till his death.   His practice included many
patients connected with the U. S. Government, Cabinet Officers, Justices
of Supreme Court, Senators and others.   He was on the staff of the Children's Hospital, Providence Hospital, Columbia Hospital, Garfield Memorial Hospital, Emergency Hospital and, finally, the Columbian Univ.
Hospital.   One of the founders of Children's Hospital and Garfield
Memorial Hospital and a member of the Board of Directors of each;
Consulting Physician to Washington Asylum Hospital, to Episcopal Eye
and Ear Hospital and Government Hospital for Insane.   Chairman of
Committee on Public Health of Board of Trade.   Was married three
times.   Author of Diarrheal diseases and dysentery, in Hare's system of

practical therapeutics, Philadelphia, 1897, IV; The Eureka Springs, Arkansas, St. Louis, 1885; see Medical Society, D. C., Report on typhoid fever, Washington, 1894. See Minutes Med. Society, March 24 and April 9, 1902; Atkinson's Biog., 1878, p. 319; Stone's Biog., 1894, p. 253; In Memoriam, Washington, 1902; American Medicine, 1902, III, p. 500; Boston Med. and Surg. Jour., 1902, CXLVI, p. 349; Jour. A. M. A., 1902, XXXVIII, p. 835; Medical News, 1902, LXXX, p. 616; N. Y. Med. Jour., 1902, LXXV, p. 558; Physician, Detroit, 1902, XXIV, p. 188; Wash. Med. Annals, May, 1902, pp. 151-175.

JANUARY 20, 1869

290. JAMES B. LITTLEWOOD—Born June 25, 1843, Ashton, England. M. D., 1868, Georgetown. Was Examiner of Patents, U. S. Patent Office, Washington. Married, Sept., 1900, Florence Buckingham, of Baltimore, Md. Died Feb. 7, 1906.

APRIL 7, 1869

291. CHARLES EVELYN HAGNER—Born Aug. 14, 1847, Norfolk, Va. M. D., 1869, Univ. Penna. Father of Dr. F. R. Hagner, *infra*. Dropped from membership 1902. Was Attending Physician Providence Hospital; member Med. Assn., D. C., and Wash. Obstet. and Gynecolog. Society.

MAY 5, 1869

292. JOHN WESLEY VAN ARNUM—Born 1840, Manitou, Mich. Hospital Steward, U. S. A. M. D., 1867, Georgetown. Sometime druggist. Dropped from membership 1878. Died Nov. 9, 1884, as the result of an accident.

JUNE 30, 1869

293. CHARLES ADAMS GRAY—Born in N. Y. City. M. D., 1869, Bellevue. Removed to Sioux Falls, Dakota; was there 1886; thence to Brattleboro, Vt., and Hinsdale, N. H., 1890-6.

294. WILLIAM WARREN POTTER—Born Dec. 31, 1838, Strykersville, N. Y. M. D., 1859, Univ. Buffalo. Asst. Surgeon 49th and Surgeon, 57th N. Y. Vols. Sometime Coroner, D. C. Removed to Buffalo, N. Y. Editor Buffalo Med. Jour., since July, 1888. [His father was Dr. Lindorf Potter, of Sheldon, Wyoming Co., N. Y. Son of Dr. Benjamin Potter, formerly of Rhode Island, but who located in Western N. Y. in the early years of the nineteenth century, and was one of the first physicians in the Holland Purchase.] Educated at seminaries at Arcade and Lima, N. Y. After graduation in medicine practiced with his uncle, Dr. M. E. Potter, at Cowlesville, N. Y. Served as Asst. Surgeon, 49th N. Y. Vols., in 1861-2. Accompanied the regiment throughout its early career with the Army of the Potomac, during the peninsular campaign, under McClellan in Maryland, and under Burnside in the Fredericksburg disaster. Was left in charge of wounded soldiers while the army was retreating to Harrison's Landing ; captured in June, 1862, confined in Libby prison, but released among the first exchanges and rejoined his regiment after an absence of three weeks. In December, 1862, just after the battle of Fredericksburg, was promoted to Surgeon, and served with the 57th New York Vols. during the Chancellorsville and Gettysburg campaigns. Soon after the battle of Gettysburg was assigned to the charge of 1st Division Hospital, 2d Army Corps, and continued on that duty until mustered out of service with his regiment at the close of the war. Brevetted for faithful and meritorious service, Lieutenant Colonel, U. S. Vols. He remained a few years in Washington, then practiced awhile at Batavia, N. Y. Soon afterwards he removed to Buffalo, where he is still practicing medicine, mainly surgery and diseases of women. Member of Amer. Med. Assn. ; Med. Society of New York, its President in 1891 ; Medical Society of Erie Co., President in 1893 ; of Buffalo Med. and Surg. Assn., President in 1886 ; President of Buffalo Obstetrical Society, 1884-6 ; Secretary Amer. Assn. Obstet. and Gynecol. from 1888 ; Pan-Amer. Med. Congress, 1893; Examiner in Obstetrics N. Y. State Med. Examining Board ; President of National Confederation of State Med. Examining Boards ; Surgeon to Hospitals, etc. Married, March 23, 1859, Emily A. Bostwick, daughter of Wm. H. Bostwick, Lancaster, N. Y. See Stone's Biog., 1894, p. 411 ; Watson's Biog., 1896, p. 150 ; Who's Who in America ; Men of New York, 1898.

295. ARTHUR CHRISTIE—Born Jan. 13, 1830, London, England. M. D., 1866, Univ. Maryland. Dropped from membership, 1880. Died June 24, 1891, D. C.

NOVEMBER 17, 1869

296. RALPH V. AULICK—Born, 1839, D. C. M. D., 1867, Univ. Penna. Died Oct. 3, 1872, with symptoms of apoplexy. Son of Commodore Aulick, U. S. N. Studied medicine with Dr. D. R. Hagner, *supra*. After graduation practiced in Washington. In 1870 had inflammation of the brain and never recovered his health again. He collected many medical engravings and portraits of medical men, and also devoted much time to entomology. See Minutes Med. Society, Oct. 9, 1872; Trans. A. M. A., 1873, XXIV, p. 341.

297. ALBERT B. NORTON—Born 1823, Massachusetts. M. D., 1849, Berkshire. Died July 5, 1873, of hemoptysis.

298. JOHN HOLLINS McBLAIR—Born Nov. 12, 1843, D. C. M. D., 1869, Georgetown. 1st Lieut., U. S. A. Dropped from membership, 1891; reëlected April 4, 1894. Died Dec. 3, 1899. See Powell's History, p. 459; Minutes Med. Society, Dec. 6 and 13, 1899; Trans. Med. Society, 1899, IV, p. 212.

299. GEORGE W. WOOLEY—Born in Pennsylvania. M. D., 1836, Med. Coll., Ohio. Removed in 1893 to Williamsport, Md., where he died Nov. 6, 1893.

DECEMBER 8, 1869

300. ALBERT SPERRY PIERCE—Born, Madison, Indiana, Feb. 6, 1839. M. D., 1867, Georgetown. Removed to Kirksville, Mo., in 1873; to Hastings, Neb., in 1885; to Omaha, Neb., in 1903. Had a common school education. Was Hospital Steward, 27th Mo. Vols., 1861-5. In 1896-7 was Med. Director, Grand Army Republic of Nebraska; 1897-8, Surgeon General, National G. A. R.

301. WILLIAM F. CADY—Born June 30, 1826, Keesville, N. Y. M. D., 1853, Albany Med. College, N. Y. Surgeon, 12th Illinois Vols. Removed in 1873 to Lafayette, Ind., where he died, Dec. 24, 1883. Was principal of a school at Oswego, N. Y., 1847-51; a pioneer agitator for free schools. After graduating in medicine he practiced at Rock Island, Ill., 1853-61. Served during the Civil War from the beginning to the close. In the three months' service, was Asst. Surg., 12th Ill. Vols. He was mentioned in dispatches on account of bravery in attending the wounded on the firing line at battle of Fort Donelson. Suffered from chronic diarrhea a long time, and a post mortem examination revealed a cicatricial condition of almost the entire intestinal tract. From 1869 to 1873 was Chief Clerk, U. S. Indian Bureau, Washington, D. C., and also served a short time as Indian Agent.

DECEMBER 29, 1869

302. FRANCIS SALTER—Born in England, 1831. L. R. C. P. and S., Edinburgh (1850) and Glasgow. Surgeon, 7th Ohio Vols., and Surgeon, U. S. Vols. Dropped from membership, 1873. Sometime Med. Referee, U. S. Pension Bureau, Washington. Died May 3, 1879. Buried at Flood Hill, Va. See Powell's History, p. 816.

[There is no record of any one having been elected a member in 1870. Dr. Christian Miller paid the fee of $1.00, March 7, 1870, and June 30th, Drs. W. T. S. Duvall and Basil Norris also paid the fee. But there is no record of their election, nor is there any record of the fee having been returned. The name of W. Noxton appears in the printed list of 1870,

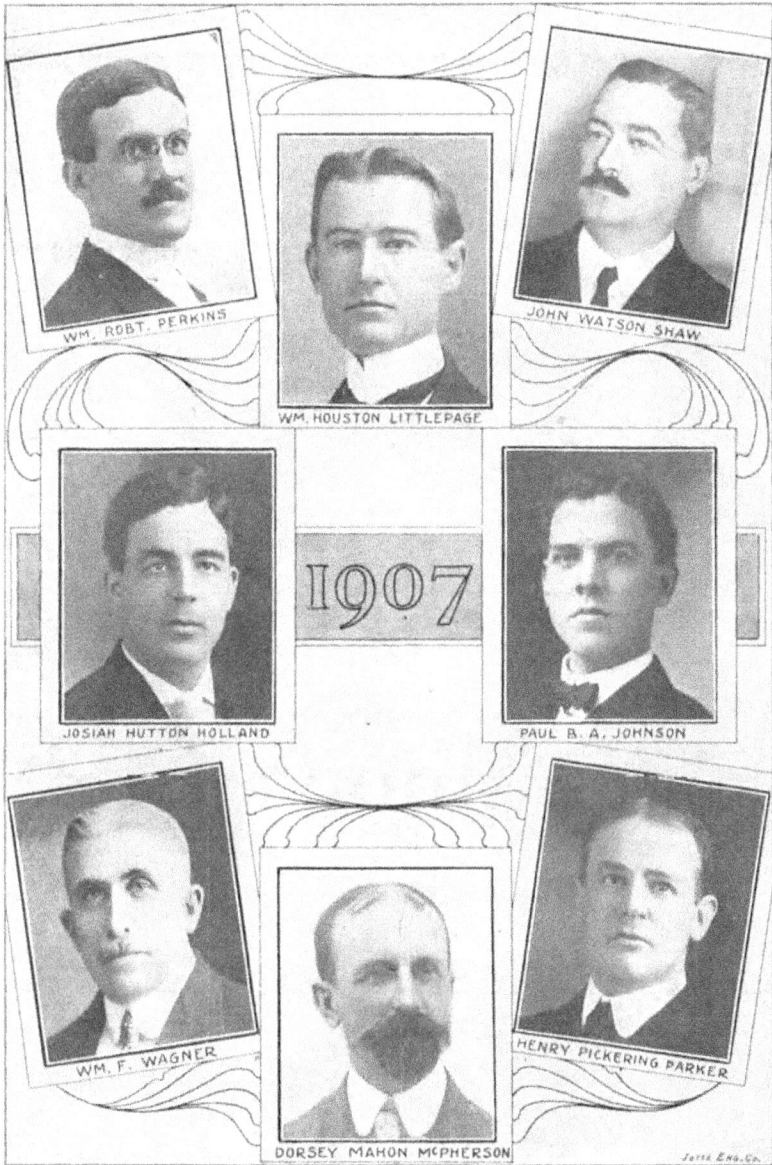

WM. ROBT. PERKINS

WM. HOUSTON LITTLEPAGE

JOHN WATSON SHAW

1907

JOSIAH HUTTON HOLLAND

PAUL B. A. JOHNSON

WM. F. WAGNER

DORSEY MAHON McPHERSON

HENRY PICKERING PARKER

JOHN ENG. CO.

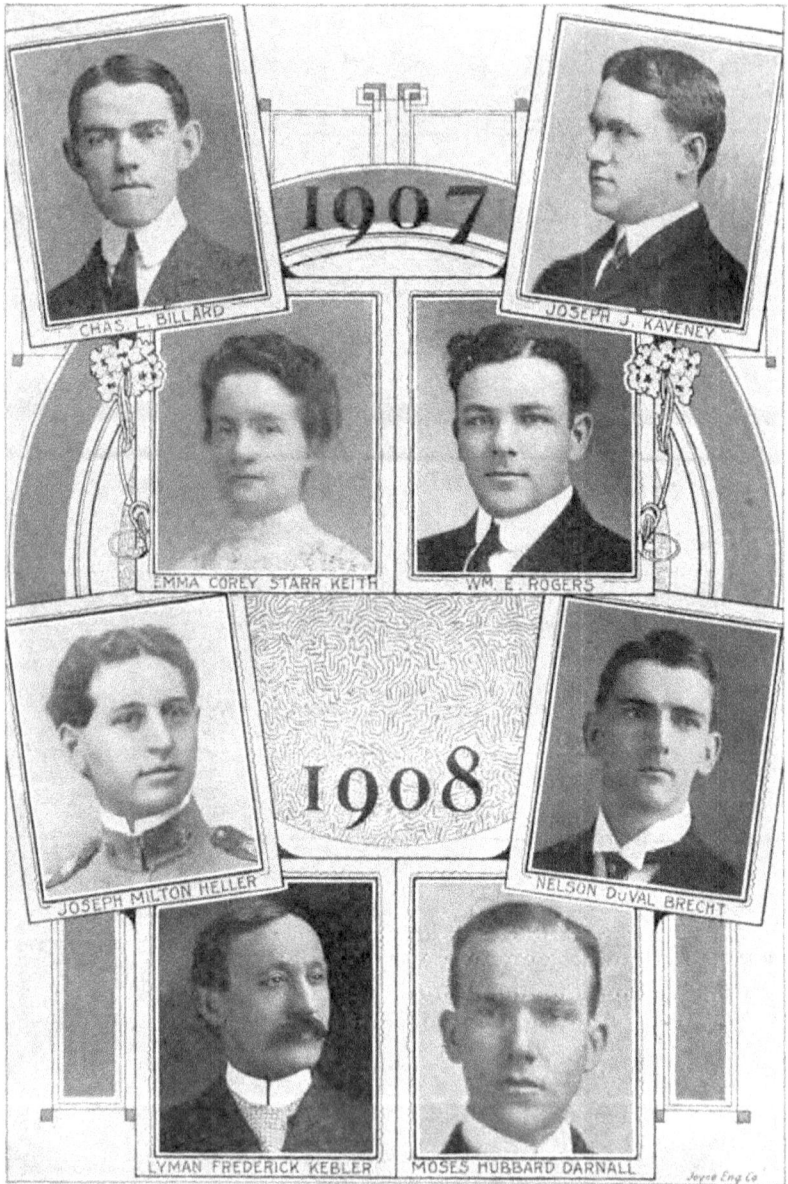

1907

CHAS. L. BILLARD

JOSEPH J. KAVENEY

EMMA COREY STARR KEITH

WM. E. ROGERS

1908

JOSEPH MILTON HELLER

NELSON DUVAL BRECHT

LYMAN FREDERICK KEBLER

MOSES HUBBARD DARNALL

Joyce Eng Co

and W. Norton in the lists of 1882 and 1885, but the name does not appear anywhere on the minutes of the Society, nor on the Treasurer's book. It is possible that the name is a mistake for W. W. Hoxton, but he had died in 1855.]

[January 5, 1870, the constitution was amended to require that candidates for active membership should make their applications in January or July, their papers to be referred to the Board of Censors, and the election to be held in October or April.]

JULY 5, 1871

WOOD—[The minutes state that —— Wood was elected a member. This must be a mistake.]

OCTOBER 11, 1871

303. JOSHUA OTIS STANTON—Born Oct. 22, 1837, Strafford, N. H. M. D., 1862, Bowdoin. Acting Asst. Surg., U. S. A.; Surg. U. S. Vols. President Med. Assn., D. C., 1890-1. Surg. Gen. N. G., D. C. Died April 9, 1891. Educated at Strafford and Wolfboro Academies, N. H. As Acting Asst. Surg. he served in Washington, June, 1862, to Feb., 1865, when he was appointed Surg., U. S. Vols., and attached to the Bureau of Provost Marshal General, U. S. A.; served there until Oct., 1865. Afterward practiced in Washington, making a specialty of diseases of women. Was a member Med. Assn., D. C.; Gynecolog. Society of Boston (corresponding member); Advisory and Consulting Board of Physicians and Surgeons, Columbia Hospital for Women, Washington; Consulting Physician, Providence Hospital; Examining Surgeon for Pensions. In May, 1870, married Ida M., daughter of Dr. Wm. Brooke Jones, of Washington. See Atkinson's Biog., 1878, p. 355; Minutes Med. Society, April 10, 1891.

304. JAMES FRENCH HARTIGAN—Born Dec. 20, 1843, Limerick, Ireland. Hospital Steward, U. S. A. M. D., 1868, Georgetown. Died Jan. 31, 1894, at Trieste, Austria, where he was serving as U. S. Consul. Had yellow fever while a prisoner of war at Newbern, N. C., in 1864; and in 1888 was sent by Surgeon General Hamilton to Florida towns, as an Inspector of the Marine Hospital Service, to investigate their condition. In the performance of this duty his health gave way, and he was appointed consul at Trieste, partly in the hope that the warm climate of that place would be beneficial to him. Was for many years Coroner's Physician, D. C.; assisted in the *post mortem* examination of the assassin Guiteau. Co-author of Report of post mortem examination of Guiteau, Washington, 1882; Lockjaw of infants, N. Y., 1884. See Jour. A. M. A., 1894, XXII, p. 235; Georgetown University, II, p. 195.

305. WALTER CLARKE BRISCOE—Born Dec. 16, 1837, D. C. M. D., 1869, Georgetown. Surgeon, Central Dispensary. Died May 16, 1896. See Minutes Med. Society, May 18, 1896.

306. WALTER BOWIE TYLER—Son of Dr. Grafton Tyler, *supra*. Born Sept. 19, 1846, D. C. M. D., 1870, Columbian. Served in C. S. Army. Died March 6, 1889, Summerville, S. C., where he had gone for his health. His mother was Mary M. Tyler. He was educated at Georgetown College. At the close of the Civil War he studied medicine with his father. Married Kate Moffat Stansbury, daughter of Dr. C. F. and Ellen R. Stansbury, of Washington. See Minutes Med. Society, March 9, 1889.

307. HOWARD HINES BARKER—Born Sept. 13, 1848, D. C. M. D., 1870, Georgetown; LL. D., 1890, National University, Washington. President, 1904-5, Med. Assn., D. C. Father of Dr. H. W. Barker, *infra*. Was the son of James William and Sarah Ann Rozelle (Hines) Barker. Educated at Union Academy, Everett Institute and Columbian College. Married, Sept. 12, 1872, Fannie Rozelle Wilson, of Washington. Practiced in Washington. Was Prof. Obstetrics and Gynecology, and Dean Med. Department, National University, Washington, from 1884; Demonstrator of Anatomy, 1871-3; Lecturer on Anatomy, 1874-5, Georgetown Med. College; charter member Washington Obstet. and Gynecolog. Society; member of Clinico-Patholog. Society; President Therapeutic Society, D. C., and Amer. Therapeutic Soc.; member Amer. Med. Assn.; Resident Physician, Columbia Hospital for Women in 1871; in charge Diseases of Women and Children, Central Dispensary and Emergency Hospital, 1872-7; Consulting Physician, Eastern Dispensary and Casualty Hospital; also Surgeon to Sibley Memorial Hospital. Author of Open letter to S. C. Busey, etc., Washington, 1895. See Who's Who in America; Amer. Biog. Direct., 1908.

308. MOSES BRÜCKHEIMER—Born April 2, 1836, Kilsheim, Baden, Germany. M. D., 1868, Columbian. Dropped from membership, 1879; reëlected Oct. 1, 1902. Died Aug. 7, 1903. Emigrated from Germany about 1860. Served in 66th New York Vols. from April 19, 1861; afterward in 155th N. York V.; was discharged for disability. Then studied medicine. Married Henrietta Fuchs, of Badigheim, Germany, whom he knew in the old country. After graduation took a post-graduate course at Jefferson Med. College, Philadelphia, and then returned to Washington and practiced there until his death. See Minutes Med. Society, Oct. 7 and Dec. 16, 1903; Wash. Med. Annals, January, 1904, p. 488.

309. JAMES LITTLETON SUDDARTH—Born Dec. 13, 1841, Albemarle County, Va. M. D., 1868, Columbian. Dropped from membership, 1877. Reëlected April 7, 1886.

310. JOHN STEARNS—Born in Massachusetts. M. D., 1860, Harvard. Surgeon, 4th Mass. Heavy Arty. Acting Asst. Surg., U. S. A. Dropped from membership, 1879. Died Aug. 28, 1898.
[Stearns was nominated March 27th and elected April 3d. The name became mixed up with that of Dr. S. S. Stearns.]

OCTOBER 2, 1872

311. CHARLES VERNON BOARMAN—Born March 2, 1851, D. C. A. M., 1874, Gonzaga College, Washington; M. D., 1871, Georgetown. Died Nov. 2, 1901. Was a descendant of the Boarmans and Morgans, of England; the latter from Monmouthshire; the former received grants of land from Lord Baltimore, and the latter also settled under proprietor's grant in Maryland previous to 1647. Member Med. Assn., D. C.; Medical Society of Alumni of Georgetown College ; Lecturer in Summer School of Medicine in said College; afterward Demonstrator of Anatomy. One of the Physicians of Central Dispensary, and also City Physician. Surgeon, Penna. R. R., and member of Board of Med. Examiners, U. S. Pension Bureau. See Atkinson's Biog., 1878, p. 383; Minutes Med. Society, Nov. 6 and 15, 1901; Trans. Med. Society, VI, 1901, p. 271.

312. JAMES KNOX POLK GLEESON—Born June 6, 1844, London, N. H. M. D., 1869, Columbian.

APRIL 2, 1873

313. JOHN THOMAS WINTER—Born April 26, 1842, Petersville, Md. M. D., 1870, Georgetown. Brother of Dr. E. C. C. Winter, *infra*. Died June 22, 1902. Son of Thomas and Elizabeth Fortney Winter ; grandson of Benjamin Winter. Educated at Petersville Academy. Clerk in Quartermaster's Department, U. S. A., during most of the Civil War. Oct. 20, 1869, married Miss Alphonsa R. Hirst, daughter of Rev. Wm. Hirst, of the M. E. Church. In 1871 began to practice in Washington. Member of Med. Assn., D. C. ; Amer. Med. Assn. ; Washington Obstet. and Gynecolog. Soc.; charter member and President Washington Therapeutic Society; one of the Commissioners of Pharmacy, D. C., and President of the Board, 1894 to 1902; was on the staff of Eastern Dispensary, and Sibley Hospital; Physician to Meth. Episc. Home for Aged Women. In 1884 he organized the Med. Dept., National University, Washington; was President of the school till his death ; Prof. Materia Medica and Therapeutics, 1884-92, and of Practice of Medicine, 1892-1902. See

Minutes Med. Society, Oct. 1 and 22, 1902; Wash. Med. Annals, November, 1902, p. 387; Watson's Biog., 1896, p. 575; Georgetown University, II, p. 196.

OCTOBER 1, 1873

314. WILLIAM HENRY ROSS—Born July 17, 1844, New York City. M. D., 1869, Georgetown. Removed, 1880, to N. Y. City. President, 1886, Harlem (N. Y.) Med. Society. Died Nov. 20, 1900. See Minutes Med. Society, D. C., Dec. 5, 1900; Trans. Med. Society, V, 1900, p. 228.

315. CHARLES WILLIAM FRANZONI—Born Aug. 15, 1837, D. C. Ph. B., 1858; M. D., 1869, Columbian. President, 1891-2, Med. Assn., D. C. Son of John Clement and Ann Dunbar Franzoni; grandson of Carlo Franzoni, the distinguished Italian sculptor, whose work appears in the Statuary Hall, U. S. Capitol, Washington. Dr. Franzoni was educated at private schools, the Union Academy and Columbian College, Washington. Married, Oct. 25, 1876, Sarah Cecilia Saunders, of Cleveland, Ohio. Has practiced in Washington since 1869; Treasurer of Med. Society since 1874. See Amer. Biog. Direct., 1908.

316. GEORGE LLOYD MAGRUDER—Born Nov. 1, 1848, D. C. A. B., 1868, Gonzaga College, D. C.; A. M., 1871; M. D., 1870, Georgetown. [Son of Thomas Contee and Elizabeth Olivia Morgan Magruder. His earliest American ancestor on the paternal side was the immigrant, Alexander McGregor, who came from Scotland about 1650 and settled in Maryland, and changed his name to Magruder soon after his arrival. Dr. Magruder's father was Paymaster on the Washington Aqueduct and Capitol Extension, and Disbursing Officer under Quartermaster General M. C. Meigs.] Educated at private and public schools and by private tutors. Since graduation in medicine has practiced in Washington. Sometime Prosector in Minor Surgery, afterwards Prof. Materia Medica, 1883 to 1906, and Dean and Treasurer of Medical Faculty, now Emer. Prof. Mat. Med. and Therap., Georgetown Med. School; Physician to the Poor, 1871-2; Physician to Police and Fire Depts., 1883-7; Chairman of Committee of Med. Society on typhoid fever in D. C., 1894, the outcome of which was the present filtration plant. Delegate to Internat. Med. Congress, Berlin, 1890, and Pan-American Med. Congress, 1893. Secured an investigation by the Department of Agriculture, Washington, into water supplies of dairy farms, 1906-7; also in 1907 secured the appointment of the Milk Commission of the District; also the investigation of the milk industry of the District, and the publication of Bulletin 41, Hygienic Laboratory, "Milk and its relation to public health," under auspices Bureau Public Health and Marine Hosp. Service together with the Department of Agriculture. One of the founders of Central Dispensary, and of Georgetown Univ. Hospital; Consulting Physician, Central Dispensary and Providence Hospital; member Med. Assn., D. C.; Wash. Obstet. and Gynecol. Society; Amer. Pub. Health Assn ; Washington Acad. Sciences; Board of Visitors, Govt. Hosp. Insane, D. C. Married, Nov. 22, 1882, Belle, daughter of Gen. W. W. Burns, U. S. A., and Priscilla R. Atkinson Burns. Has a son, a 1st Lieut., Coast Artillery Corps, U. S. A. See Atkinson's Biog., 1878, p. 369; Stone's Biog., 1894, p. 656; Amer. Biog. Direct., 1908; Georgetown University, II, p. 88 ; Who's Who in America.

OCTOBER 8, 1873

317. WILLIAM OLIVER BALDWIN—Born April 9, 1827, Prince George County, Md. M. D., 1852, Columbian. Acting Asst. Surg., U. S. A. Surgeon, 2d D. C. Vols. Dropped from membership in 1879. Died Dec. 21, 1894.

APRIL 8, 1874

318. CHARLES BITTINGER—Born May 19, 1852, D. C. M. D., 1873, Georgetown. Resigned November 8, 1876. Died Aug. 31, 1879.

319. GIDEON STINSON PALMER—Born June 14, 1815, Gardiner, Me. A. B., Bowdoin, 1838 ; A. M., Howard ; M. D., 1841, Maine Medical. Surgeon, 3d Maine Vols., and Surg., U. S. Vols. Died in Washington, Dec. 8, 1891. Educated at the Gardiner Lyceum. Sometime Principal of the Lyceum. Practiced medicine for twenty years in Gardiner and other towns of southern Kennebec County, Me.; and during this time served successively as Councilman, Alderman, and Representative in the State Legislature. During the Civil War, after Oct. 5, 1861, served as Brigade Surgeon and Medical Director until Oct. 12, 1865, when he was mustered out. Was brevetted Lieut. Col., U. S. Vols., for meritorious service. Resumed practice at Gardiner. In 1869, by request of General O. O. Howard, U. S. A., he took the chair of Physiology and Hygiene in the Med. Department, Howard University, and, 1871-81, was Dean of the Faculty. From 1875 to 1881 was also Surgeon in Charge of Freedmen's Hospital, Washington. Nov. 17, 1869, married Susan, widow of Charles Henry Coolidge, of Boston, Mass. See Stone's Biog., 1894, p. 364 ; Lamb's History, p. 112 ; Minutes Med. Society, Dec. 9, 1891.

320. THOMAS MICHAEL HEALEY—Born June 16, 1840, Cumberland, Md. M. D., 1866, Long Island Medical College. Asst. Surg., 2d Maryland Vols., 1861-5. Dropped from membership, 1878. Removed to Cumberland. Died Aug. 13, 1892.

321. PATRICK JOSEPH MURPHY—Born Oct. 10, 1844, Dublin, Ireland. Studied at Maynooth College. A. M. and M. D., 1873, Georgetown. For many years was Surgeon in Charge of Columbia Hospital for Women, Washington. Died Oct. 3, 1891. He is said to have done the first successful ovariotomy (June 16, 1878) in Washington. Author of Chylous ascites, Washington, 1887. See Georgetown University, II, p. 90; Minutes Med. Society, Oct. 7, 1891.

322. JOSEPH ASBURY TARKINGTON—Born Nov. 25, 1837, in Indiana. M. D., 1870, Georgetown. Was Ward Physician ; Asst. Physician, Central Dispensary. Died May 1, 1902, at Greensburg, Ind.

323. ZACHARIAH TURNER SOWERS—Born Dec. 15, 1846, Clark Co., Va. Ph. B., 1869 ; A. M., 1874, Columbian ; M. D., 1869, Columbian; 1870, Bellevue. Educated at Berryville Academy, Clark Co., Va., and Columbian College, Washington. Settled at Round Hill, Loudoun Co., Va., but removed to N. Y. City in 1870. Was Asst. Interne in Bellevue Hospital; Asst. Examining Physician to Bellevue and Charity Hospitals; Asst. Resident Physician to Contagious Hospital, Blackwell's Island, N. Y. City. Returned to Washington, and in 1872 was appointed Demonstrator of Anatomy, Columbian Med. College; Curator of the museum and Lecturer on Minor Surgery. Member of Med. Assn., D. C., Secretary in 1874. In 1876 and 1877 was member of Advisory Board of Physicians and Surgeons to the Columbia Hospital, D. C. Assisted in the post mortem examination of the assassin, Guiteau. Has long been President of the Washington Hospital for Foundlings. Author of Report of *post mortem* examination of Guiteau, Washington, 1882. Father of Dr. W. F. M. Sowers, *infra*. See Atkinson's Biog., 1878, p. 323; Amer. Biog. Direct., 1908.

OCTOBER 6, 1874

324. EDWARD MARTIN SCHAEFFER—Born September 30, 1843, Jamaica, L. I., N. Y. M. D., 1868, Columbian. Hospital Steward and Acting Asst. Surgeon, U: S. Army. Dropped from membership in 1886 ; reëlected Oct. 6, 1886. Dropped again in 1899. Son of Dr. George C. Schaeffer, of Washington.

325. ROBERT HARRIS—M. D., 1860, Univ. Penna. Brother of Dr. J. O. Harris, *supra*. Died Dec. 26, 1880. See Minutes Med. Society, Dec. 27, 1880, and Jan. 3, 1881.

326. JAMES SHIELDS BEALE—Born Nov. 14, 1844, D. C. M. D., 1869, Georgetown. Father of Dr. R. S. Beale, *infra*. Died Feb. 12, 1884, of apoplexy at Providence Hospital, Washington, where he had gone to perform an operation. Son of Robert Beale. Served in Maryland Battery, C. S. Army. After graduating in medicine attended special courses in Paris, London and Vienna. Afterwards practiced in Washington, preferably doing surgical work. Was on the staff of Providence Hospital; Prof. Anatomy, 1876–1883, Georgetown Med. School ; Professor in Washington Training School for Nurses ; member Med. Assn., D. C., and Washington Obstet. and Gynecol. Society. See Minutes Med. Society, Feb. 13, 1884; Maryland Med. Jour., 1883-4, X, pp. 763 and 835; Jour. A. M. A., 1884, II, p. 614.

327. WILLIAM TYLER RAMSEY—Born April 18, 1847, Frederick, Md. M. D., 1871, Columbian. Dropped from membership 1878. Practiced in Washington, until July, 1880; was then appointed Surgeon on Pacific Mail Steamer. Removed to Washington Guernsey County, Ohio, May 1, 1881, and to Cambridge, the county seat, April 1, 1883, where he has since practiced. Member U. S. Pension Examining Board.

328. GEORGE MARTIN KOBER—Born March 28, 1850, Alsfeld, Hesse Darmstadt, Germany. M. D., 1873; LL. D., 1906, Georgetown. Educated at the grand ducal Realschule of his native town. In April, 1867, emigrated to United States ; secured an assignment to Hospital Corps at Carlisle Barracks, Penna.; commenced his medical studies under Dr. J. J. B. Wright, U. S. A., and in January, 1870, was appointed Hospital Steward, and ordered to Frankford Arsenal, near Philadelphia ; there he continued his studies until October, 1871, when he was ordered to duty in the office of the Surgeon General, at Washington. He studied medicine under Drs. Johnson Eliot and Robert Reyburn, *supra*, and was the first graduate of a post-graduate course, instituted by Drs. Thompson, Busey, Ashford and others, at the Columbia Hospital for Women, in 1873. In 1874 he assisted in the reorganization of the Central Dispensary and in providing a German-speaking staff for the benefit of his suffering countrymen. In July, 1874, he was appointed Acting Asst. Surg., U. S. A.; was Post Surgeon at Alcatraz Island, Cal., to November, 1874 ; Post Surgeon, Fort McDermit, to July, 1877; was in the field, in southeastern Nevada, expedition against the Indians in the fall of 1875 ; and in the Nez Percés expedition and in charge of the field hospital at Kamiah, on the Clearwater, Idaho, from July to October, 1877 ; Post Surgeon at Camp near Spokane Falls and Fort Coeur d'Alène, to November, 1879; Fort Klamath, Oregon, to June, 1880 ; and at Fort Bidwell, Cal., to November, 1886. While at Fort Bidwell was engaged extensively in practice among civilians until June, 1887, when he traveled extensively in this country and Europe, returning to Fort Bidwell in 1888. The same year he returned to Washington, and in 1889 was appointed Professor of State Medicine, Georgetown Med. School. In August, 1890, was a member of the 10th Internat. Med. Congress, Honorary Secretary of one of its sections. In December, 1890, returned to Fort Bidwell, Cal. In 1894 established his permanent residence in Washington. Fellow Amer. Assn. Advance. Sci.; Amer. Assn. Physicians; Amer. Med. Assn.; Honorary Member Assn. Military Surgeons; member Medical and Surgical Society, D. C. (President, 1889); Med. Assn., D. C. (President, 1898); Washington Academy of Sciences; Washington Anthropological Society (President, 1907); President of Association Amer. Med. Colleges, 1906; author of the standard medical curriculum. In 1890 he directed attention to the pollution of the Potomac water as a factor in the undue prevalence of typhoid fever in Washington, and in 1895, at the request of the Health Officer and the District Commissioners, he investigated the causes of typhoid fever in Washington, and was the first to point out the agency of flies in carrying the germs. His report was published in 1895; his public addresses on the relations of water supply and sewers to the health of the city, as well as his researches into the relative merits of slow-sand and mechanical filtration, helped to secure the necessary sanitary legislation and requisite appropriation by Congress. One of the principal promoters of the Washington Sanitary Improvement Company, offering to capital a safe 5 per cent. investment and at the same time securing to wage earners, and others of moderate resources, sanitary homes at reasonable rentals. Has been a member of the consulting staffs of nearly all the hospitals in this city. In May, 1907, was appointed a member of the President's Homes Commission; as Chairman of the Committee on Social Betterment, prepared a monograph on Industrial hygiene and social betterment, published in 1908 as Senate Document No. 644. This, with his monograph on Milk in relation to public health, published in 1902 as Senate Document No. 441, and his work on Urinology and its practical applications, are his most important writings. See also Conservation of life and health, Washington, 1908; History and development of the housing movement in Washington, Washington, 1907. In 1908 he was invited to represent the medical profession at the Conference on the Conservation of Natural Resources, held at the White House, Washington, May 13th, and presented an address on The conservation of life and health by improved water supply. See Who's Who in America; Watson's Biog., 1896, p. 46; Amer. Men of Science, 1906; Georgetown University, II, p. 61.

329. JAMES McVEAN MACKALL—Son of Dr. Louis Mackall, *supra*. Brother of Dr. Louis Mackall, Jr., *infra*. Born Jan. 25, 1852, D. C. A. B., 1870, A. M. and M. D., 1873, Georgetown. Dropped, 1886, from membership. Was Acting Asst. Surg., U. S. A., in Spanish-American War. Died June 25, 1909.

330. LEWIS E. NEWTON—Born Sept. 3, 1840, D. C. M. D., 1868, Georgetown. Died Feb. 3, 1889.

331. BENJAMIN M. BEALL—Born April 17, 1854, D. C. M. D., 1873, Georgetown. Dropped from membership in 1878.

332. HORACE TURNBULL PORTER—Born March 11, 1849, Chester, Pa. M. D., 1870, Georgetown. Removed, 1878, to Philadelphia, where he died Aug. 14, 1879. [Son of Dr. James Jefferson Porter, who practiced for years in Philadelphia, but removed to Washington in 1860, and of Elizabeth, daughter of Dr. Michael Leib, of Philadelphia.] Studied medicine with his father. After graduation he practiced in Georgetown, D. C. Sometime physician at Columbia Hospital for Women, Washington ; member Med. Assn., D. C.; sometime Physician to the Poor. See Trans. A. M. A., 1881, XXXII, p. 538.

333. DAVID BLAIR—Born March 17, 1831, Kippenross, Scotland. Hospital Steward, U. S. Army. M. D., 1872, Howard. Dropped from membership 1881. Died Nov. 25, 1885. Served in U. S. Army from Oct. 22, 1852, to Dec. 17, 1874, for twelve years as Hospital Steward. Married Dec. 6, 1866. Was sometime on duty at Freedmen's Hospital, Washington. See Lamb's History, p. 118.

334. JAMES MORSELL GASSAWAY—Born Jan. 7, 1848, D. C. M. D., 1872, Columbian; 1882, Jefferson. Asst. Surg., Passed Asst. Surg., and Surg., U. S. M. H. S.

335. ARTHUR C. ADAMS—Born April 14, 1847, D. C. A. B., 1870; A. M., 1873, Univ. Mich. ; M. D., 1873, Columbian. Shot himself at his home, Dec. 31, 1904, while laboring under mental aberration, and died at Providence Hospital, Jan. 1, 1905. Served in 24th N. Y. Cavalry during the Civil War. Taught some time at Howard University before studying medicine. Was Prosector to Chair of Anatomy, Columbian Med. College, 1878-9, and Demonstrator of Anatomy, 1879-89 ; member Med. Assn., D. C., and Amer. Med. Assn. In 1878 married a Miss Schneider, who died in 1888. After some years interval married a Miss Heitmuller. See Minutes Med. Society, Jan. 25 and Feb. 1 and 15, 1905; Wash. Med. Annals, May, 1905, p. 136; Lamb's History, p. 232.

336. R. ARNOLD PAGE—Born in D. C. M. D., 1871, Georgetown. Removed to New York City, where he died in 1878.

337. SMITH TOWNSHEND—Born Dec. 13, 1836, Prince George Co., Md. Capt., 32d Ill. Vols., during the Civil War. M. D., 1870, Columbian. Sometime Health Officer, D. C. Died Feb. 25, 1896. See Minutes Med. Society, Feb. 26, 1896; Nat. Med. Rev., 1896, V, p. 21.

338. JAMES THOMAS SOTHORON—Born July 9, 1842, near Charlotte Hall, Md. M. D., 1865, Georgetown. Med. Cadet, U. S. A. Father of Dr. E. H. Sothoron, *infra*. Died Sept. 27, 1897. His ancestors were among the first settlers of southern Maryland. He was educated at the grammar school, Washington Select School and Georgetown College. In 1862 was a tutor at Charlotte Hall. Studied medicine with Dr. Thos. Antisell, *supra*. After graduation practiced in Washington. Member Med. Assn., D. C.; Amer. Med. Assn., and 9th Internat. Medical Congress ; also of Board of Managers of Associated Charities ; member and many years Vestryman and Treasurer of St. Paul's Episcopal Church. See Stone's Biog., 1894, p. 477; Minutes Med. Society, Feb. 28, 1897 ; Georgetown University, II, p. 192.

339. PARKE GEORGE YOUNG—Born Feb. 21, 1852, D. C. M. D., 1872, Georgetown. Sometime Ward Physician. Died July 30, 1906. See Minutes Med. Society, Oct. 3 and 24, 1906; Wash. Med. Annals, V, 1906, p. 301.

340. JOHN D. PARSONS—Born in D. C. M. D., 1870, Georgetown. Was sometime House Physician Central Dispensary. Dropped from membership 1879. Removed to Chicago, Ill.

341. HENRY A. DUNCANSON—Born March 4, 1847, D. C. Ph. B., 1866, (?) M. D., 1870, Columbian. Acting Asst. Surg., U. S. Army. Died Jan. 28, 1878, at Las Cruces, N. M. Son of John A. M. Duncanson, one of the early settlers of the District of Columbia. Educated at Columbian College. After graduation in medicine practiced in Washington. After being appointed Acting Asst. Surgeon he set out for his post of duty, but died on the way. Member of Med. Assn., D. C. Buried in Washington. See Trans. A. M. A., 1878, XXIX, p. 640 ; Minutes Med. Society, Feb. 6, 1878.

342. DAVID HENRY HAZEN—Born Aug. 10, 1846, Upper Mt. Bethel, Northampton Co., Pa. M. D., 1873, Georgetown. Acting Asst. Surg., U. S. A. Dropped from membership 1880. Reëlected April 15, 1903. Died of diabetes Nov. 6, 1906. Buried at his birthplace. Son of David B. and Susan Depue Hazen. Educated in the public schools of his native place, and Belvidere Academy, Belvidere, N. J. Taught school at Upper Nazareth, Pa., and in Oxford Township, N. J. Came to Washington in 1870. Resident Student at Washington Asylum two years, and also at Naval Hospital. Physician to the Poor, 1873-1876. Sometime Acting Asst. Surgeon, U. S. A., on duty at U. S. Arsenal, Washington, after which he practiced as civil physician. Member Med. Assn., D. C.; Amer. Med. Assn., and Board of Education, and Board of Trade, D. C.

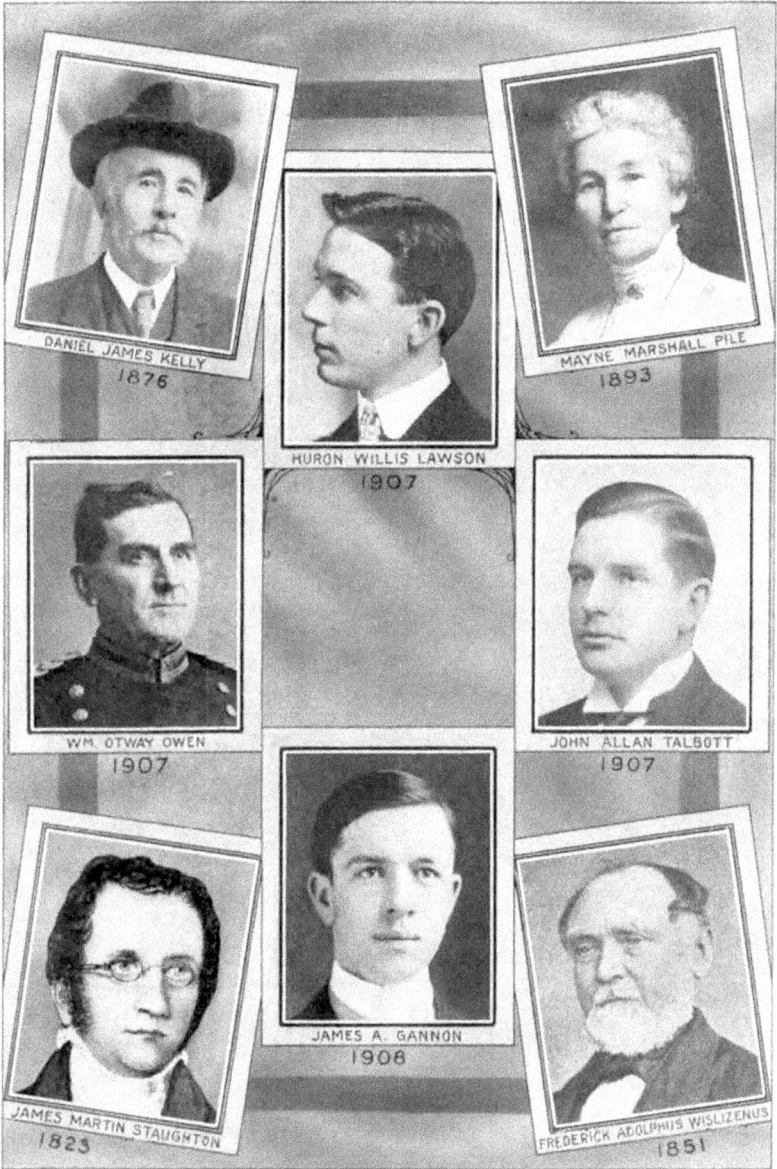

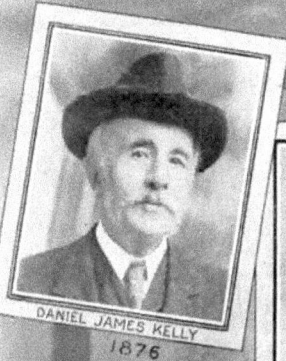

DANIEL JAMES KELLY
1876

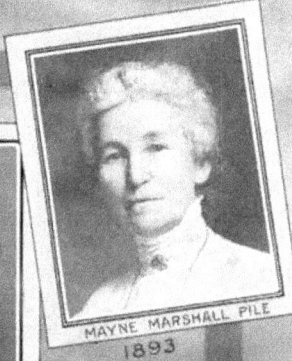

HURON WILLIS LAWSON
1907

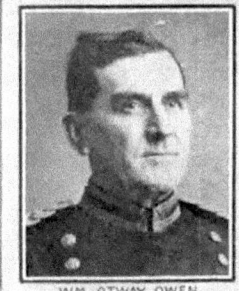

MAYNE MARSHALL PILE
1893

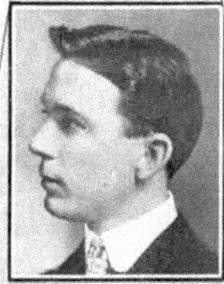

WM. OTWAY OWEN
1907

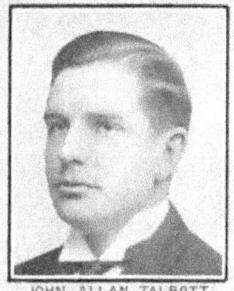

JOHN ALLAN TALBOTT
1907

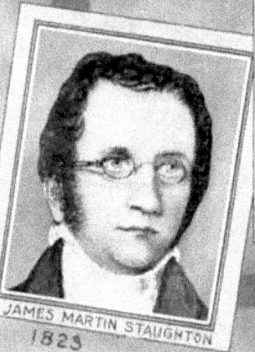

JAMES MARTIN STAUGHTON
1823

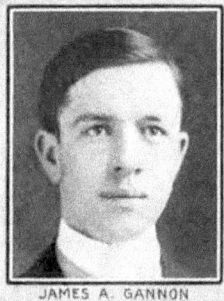

JAMES A. GANNON
1908

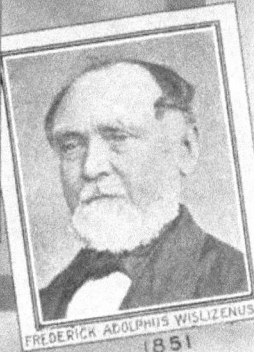

FREDERICK ADOLPHUS WISLIZENUS
1851

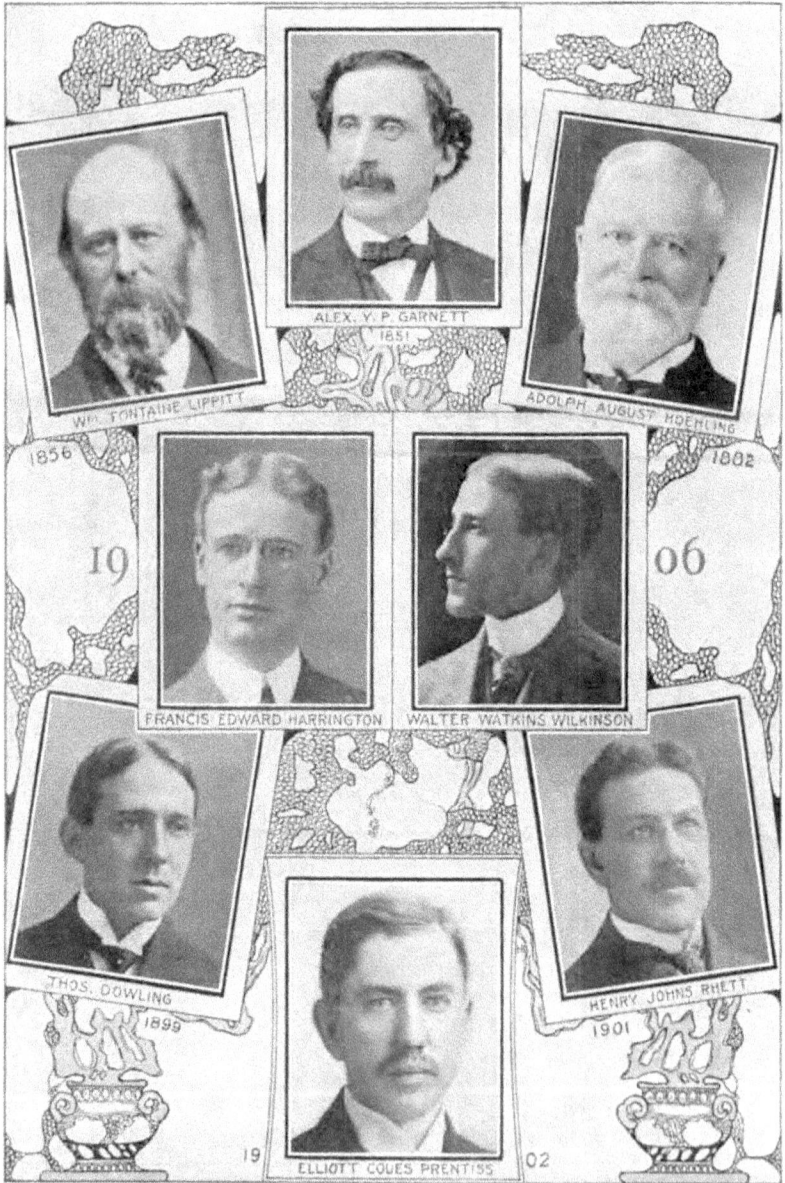

ALEX. Y. P. GARNETT
1851

WM. FONTAINE LIPPITT
1856

ADOLPH AUGUST HOEHLING
1802

19 06

FRANCIS EDWARD HARRINGTON

WALTER WATKINS WILKINSON

THOS. DOWLING
1899

ELLIOTT COUES PRENTISS
19 02

HENRY JOHNS RHETT
1901

Oct. 23, 1878, married Emma Louise Honeyman, daughter of Robert and Margaret Honeyman, of New Jersey. A son, Dr. H. H. Hazen, is now practicing in Washington. See History, City of Washington, 1903, p. 448; Minutes Med. Society, Nov. 14, 1906; Wash. Med. Annals, 1906-7, V, p. 410; Georgetown University, II, p. 203.

OCTOBER 6, 1875

343. JOHN WALTER—Born Sept. 2, 1844, D. C. M. D., 1868, Georgetown. Died at his wife's funeral, Nov. 17, 1906. Son of John Walter, of Washington, one of the founders of the German Orphan Asylum. After graduation in medicine took post-graduate course in Germany. Was several years Ward Physician, D. C.; Prosector of Anatomy, Georgetown Med. School; Physician, Central Dispensary, Washington; member Med. Assn., D. C., and Amer. Med. Assn. See Minutes Med. Society, Nov. 21, 1906; Wash. Med. Annals, 1906-7, V, p. 411.

344. WILLIAM LOVEJOY NAYLOR—Born May 20, 1844, D. C. Educated at Columbian College. M. D., 1869, Univ. Maryland. Was Ward Physician several years. Died June 3, 1890. See Minutes Med. Society, June 4, 1890.

345. RICHARD G. MAUSS—Born Aug. 24, 1842, in Germany. M. D., 1872, Georgetown. Was Ward Physician several years. While in delirium from the grippe he shot himself, and died May 2, 1891. See Minutes Med. Society, May 2, 1891.

346. EDMUND A. ZEVELY—Born Feb. 24, 1845, D. C. M. D., 1865, Univ. Penna. Acting Asst. Surg., U. S. A. Died March 1, 1876. See Minutes Med. Society, March 2, 1876.

APRIL 5, 1876

347. GEORGE W. OFFUTT—Born in 1851, D. C. M. D., 1874, Georgetown. Died Sept. 13, 1878. See Minutes Med. Society, Sept. 14, 1878.

348. THEODORE MEAD—Born Nov. 19, 1838, Ontario, N. Y. M. D., 1869, Georgetown. Dropped from membership, 1881. Sometime Inspector, Health Department, Washington.

349. CHARLES FRANKLIN RAND—Born Jan. 19, 1839, Batavia, N. Y. M. D., 1873, Georgetown. Died Oct. 14, 1908. Educated in Batavia. Sometime reporter on New Orleans Picayune. Said to have been the first volunteer in the Union army of the Civil War, No. 1 in an army

20

of 2,777,450 soldiers. In the seven days battle before Richmond, Va.,
he was shot in the arm and captured; six inches of the humerus were re-
sected while he was a prisoner. After recovering he reëntered the Army,
V. R. Corps, and served till the end of the war. After graduating in
medicine he practiced ten years in Batavia, afterwards in Washington.
On account of the suffering from his old wound he finally gave up practice and was employed in the Post Office Department at Washington.
See Army and Navy Magazine, July, 1906, p. 5 ; Minutes Med. Society,
Oct. 14 and 28, 1908; Wash. Med. Annals, 1908-9, VII, p. 386.

350. JOHN ELY BRACKETT—Born Dec. 31, 1846, Rochester, Ind.
M. D., 1870, Columbian; 1873, Ludwig Maximilian Univ., Bavaria. Acting Asst. Surg., U. S. A. Dropped from membership, 1881 ; reëlected
Oct. 3, 1894. Son of Lyman S. and Eliza Ann Rannells Brackett. Descended paternally from early colonists of New England, and maternally
from Virginians. Educated at the public schools and Emerson Institute, Washington, and the Norwalk (Conn.) Academy. After graduation in medicine he practiced for two years at Rochester. 1872 and 1873
were spent in Europe, at Munich, Vienna, London, etc. Since 1874 has
practiced in Washington. Was Resident Student, Washington Asylum
Hospital, 1868; House Physician, Providence Hospital, Washington, 1874
to 1878; Physician to the Poor, 1874-8; member of Board of Pension Examiners, 1886 to 1890; member Med. Assn., D. C. Served July–August,
1864, in the Home Guard, Washington; in 1880–2 was Surgeon, National
Guard, Washington ; Acting Asst. Surg., in 1898–9, on U. S. Hospital
Ship Missouri, visiting the islands of Porto Rico and Cuba. Married,
Nov. 21, 1878, Jeanie Deans Foster, of Fairfax Co., Va. Professor, 1877
to 1891, of Materia Medica and Therapeutics, and 1891 to 1908, of Practice of Medicine, Med. Dept. Howard University, Washington. See Atkinson's Biog., 1878, p. 366; Lamb's History, p. 123.

351. AUSTIN BROCKENBROUGH—Born Aug. 4, 1846, Chatham,
Westmoreland Co., Va. M. D., 1871, Columbian. Grandson of Dr.
Austin Brockenbrough, of Rappahannock, Va., and son of John Fauntle-
roy Brockenbrough, of Chatham. Was a cadet at Virginia Mil. Inst.
Was in the Signal Corps and later in the Secret Service, C. S. A. After
the Civil War he studied medicine with Dr. Joshua Riley, *supra*. Began
to practice with Dr. Louis Ritchie, *supra*, in Georgetown ; afterwards
was associated with Dr. S. C. Busey, *supra;* was connected with the Columbia Hospital for Women, Outdoor Physician of the Dispensary; Ward
Physician; member of staff of Central Dispensary. Spent two years in
Europe, mainly in Paris, attending clinical lectures. Returned to Washington and resumed practice. Removed, in 1878, to Northampton Co.,
Va., where he has since been practicing.

352. WINFIELD PETER LAWVER—Born Nov. 28, 1848, Stevenson Co., Ill. M. D., 1874, Columbian. Dropped from membership, 1886. Died Aug. 29, 1891, at St. Elizabeth Asylum, D. C. Author of Tables for practical examination of urine, etc., Washington, 1885.

OCTOBER 4, 1876

353. DANIEL JAMES KELLY—Born Sept. 20, 1843, Kilkenny, Ireland. Graduated, 1863, Stonyhurst College, England. A. M., 1873; M. D., 1875, Georgetown. For many years an Examiner in the U. S. Patent Office, Washington. Resigned from Med. Society, Jan. 20, 1909. Educated at Kilkenny College and at Stonyhurst. Studied chemistry at University College, London, and medicine with Mr. Bradley, F. R. C. S., Manchester, England. Was first assistant in Stonyhurst Observatory. Sometime Prof. Chemistry and Physiology in Georgetown University, and Prof. Chemistry and Toxicology in Georgetown Med. School; member Med. Assn., D. C. See Atkinson's Biog., 1878, p. 204.

354. BENJAMIN BELA ADAMS—Born August 15, 1851, Havre, France. M. D., 1875, Howard; 1876, Georgetown. Dropped from membership in 1890. Died Jan. 25, 1897. Son of Rev. Ezra Eastman Adams, the English and American Agent at Havre, during the Crimean War. Attended Freehold (N. J.) Academy, and Crosby's Academy, Nassau, N. H. Taught school at Coleraine, Pa. After graduation practiced medicine in Washington until his death. Married Ella D. Taylor. Had a brother, a physician, Dr. J. O. Adams, of Washington. See Lamb's History, p. 144.

APRIL 4, 1877

355. GEORGE S. KING—M. D., 1857, Coll. P. and S., N. Y.; 1859, N. O. School of Medicine. Removed from D. C. Not known what became of him.

356. WM. MEADE PAGE—Born June 13, 1831, Millwood, Va. Attended University Virginia, going thence in 1853 to Univ. Penna., where he graduated M. D., in 1855. Served as Asst. Surgeon and Passed Asst. Surgeon, U. S. Navy. Surgeon, C. S. Navy, and also served in C. S. Cavalry, 1861-5. Married in 1865; was a farmer in Virginia for some years; was in Washington in 1876-7, and for some time in charge of the Smallpox Hospital. Resigned from Med. Society, Oct. 3, 1877. Went to California and practiced medicine there till 1900. Returned to Virginia and died in Fauquier Co., May 8, 1906.

APRIL 3, 1878

357. CLAYTON AUGUSTUS HOOVER—Born Feb. 25, 1853, D. C. M. D., 1875, Columbian. Removed in 1880 to Montpelier, Idaho. Local Surgeon to Union Pacific and Oregon Short Line R. R., 1882–1905; since July 5, 1905, Medical Supt. of Idaho State Insane Asylum, Blackfoot, Idaho.

358. HAMILTON E. LEACH—Born March 10, 1850, D. C. M. D., 1872, Georgetown. Died of tuberculosis, May 9, 1893. After graduation he practiced in Washington. He is best remembered as an efficient organizer and chief of Hospital Committee during the Grand Army Encampment, Washington, 1892. See Minutes Med. Society, May 10, 1893; Nat. Med. Review, 1893–4, II, p. 49.

APRIL 2, 1879

359. SWAN MOSES BURNETT—Born March 16, 1847, Newmarket, Tenn. M. D., 1870, Bellevue ; Ph. D., 1890, Georgetown. Died Jan. 18, 1906. After graduation in medicine practiced in Knoxville, Tenn., until he removed to Washington, in 1876. Prof. Ophthalmology and Otology, Georgetown Univ., from 1879; President Attending Staff Central Dispensary and Emergency Hospital; member of staff of Children's and Providence Hospitals; member Washington Academy Sciences and Philosophical and Anthropological Societies, Washington. Said to have been the first to introduce Japanese art into this country. Married Miss Frances Eliza Hodgson, the authoress. They were divorced; he afterward married Miss Margaret Brady, of Washington. Author of Translation of Landolt's manuel d'ophthalmoscopie, Philadelphia, 1879 ; Diseases of conjunctiva and sclera, Norris and Oliver's System of Diseases of Eye, Philadelphia, 1898; Principles of refraction, Philadelphia, 1904. See also J. S. Billings, National Medical Dictionary, Philadelphia, 1890; E. Landolt, The introduction of the metrical system into ophthalmology, London, 1876. See Atkinson's Biog., 1878, p. 187 ; Who's Who in America ; Amer. Biog. Direct., Washington, 1908 ; Minutes Med. Society, Jan. 24, 1906 ; Wash. Med. Annals, 1906–7, V, p. 57; Georgetown University, II, p. 95.

360. WALTER SCOTT WELLS—M. D., 1854, Univ. City New York. Editor of Summary of Medical Science, 1861 ; also Editor National Medical Review, Washington, 1878–9. Author of Epitome of Braithwaite's Retrospect, etc., 2 Vols., N. Y., 1860. Removed, 1881, to N. Y. City, where he died March 4, 1897. Was member of N. Y. Co. Med. Assn.

361. WILLIAM LAUCK HUDSON—Born July 20, 1850, Luray, Va. M. D., 1874, Louisville Med. College. Removed, 1881, from D. C., to Luray, where he practices medicine and was sometime Coroner.

362. HARRY CRÈCY YARROW—Born Nov. 19, 1840, Philadelphia, Pa. M. D., 1861, Univ. Penna. Asst. Surg., 5th Pa. Cavalry. Acting Asst. Surgeon, U. S. A. Son of John and Caroline Crècy Yarrow. Educated at private schools in Philadelphia, and Geneva, Switzerland. Studied medicine with Drs. J. L. Ludlow and J. J. Woodward, Philadelphia. Was Med. Examiner of Recruits from April to July, 1861. Served with 5th Penna. Cavalry till Jan., 1862. Afterwards Executive Officer in Military Hospital, Philadelphia. In 1866, served with troops at Atlanta, Ga., and Tybee Island, Ga., during a cholera epidemic, and in 1867, in a similar epidemic in New York Harbor. In 1872-6 was Surgeon and Naturalist in the Wheeler exploring expedition. On duty in 1876 at the Exposition in Philadelphia. 1877-1888 on duty at Army Med. Museum, Surgeon General's Library and Soldiers' Home Hospital, Washington. 1888-1893 at the Army Dispensary, Washington. Has also been connected with U. S. National Museum, Washington, 1872-80. Member of Med. Assn., D. C.; Amer. Med. Assn.; Anthropolog. and Philosoph. Societies, Washington ; N. Y. Society Natural History ; Amer. Assn. Adv. Science; Zoölogical Society, London, etc. Professor Dermatology, George Washington Univ. Med. Dept., and Consulting Surgeon to several hospitals. Married, April 10, 1862, Miss Anna Provand Dryburgh, Philadelphia. Author of Introduction to the study of mortuary customs among the North American Indians, Washington, 1880. See also Report of Geological Surveys, 1879 ; Reference handbook medical sciences ; Proceedings U. S. Nat. Museum ; also publications of Coues, Henshaw and Rothrock ; and Billings Nat. Med. Dict., 1890. See Appleton's Biog., 1889, VI, p. 638 ; Stone's Biog., 1894, p. 705 ; Who's Who in America ; Watson's Biog., 1896, p. 683; Amer. Biog. Direct., Washington, 1908.

363. JOHN HARRY THOMPSON, JR.—Son of Dr. J. H. Thompson, *supra.* Born June 1, 1852, London, England. M. D., 1875, Georgetown; 1877, College Physicians and Surgeons, New York. Removed, 1882, to Kansas City, Mo.

364. HENRY DAVIDSON FRY—Born April 11, 1853, Richmond, Va. M. D., 1876, Univ. Maryland. Of English descent; among his ancestors was Col. Joshua Fry, of the Virginia Colonial period. Dr. Fry was the son of Hugh Walker Fry, Jr., of Richmond, and Mary L. Davidson, daughter of John Davidson, of Georgetown, D. C. Educated in Richmond and Washington. After graduating in medicine was Interne in Jersey City Charity Hospital. Since 1878 has practiced in Washington ; for fourteen years was associated with Dr. W. W. Johnston, *supra*. In 1890 spent some time in European hospitals ; in 1890, also, he did the first successful Cæsarean operation in this District; he also did the first successful symphysiotomy in the District. Prof. Obstetrics, Georgetown Med. School ; Attending Gynecologist and Obstetrician at Garfield Hospital ; sometime Obstetrician to Columbia Hospital for Women ; sometime President Washington Obstet. and Gynecolog. Society ; member of local and national medical societies ; Vice-President Amer. Gynecolog. Society, 1904. Author of Maternity, Washington, 1907. See History City of Washington, 1903, p. 431 ; Who's Who in America; Amer. Biog. Direct., Washington,' 1908.

OCTOBER 8, 1879

365. FRANCK HYATT—Born March 28, 1851, Bladensburg, Md. M. D., 1872, Univ. Maryland. Member Amer. Laryngological Society, and Med. Assn., D. C.

366. WILLIAM OCTAVIUS EVERSFIELD—Born Nov. 4, 1840, College Park, Md. M. D., 1860, Univ. Va.; 1861, Univ. Penna. Acting Asst. Surg., U. S. A. Removed, 1880, to Branchville, Md. Died Jan. 20, 1908, at College Park, from influenza. Educated at Edge Hill School, Princeton, N. J., and St. John's College, Annapolis, Md. Attended Agnew's School of Surgery, Philadelphia; was Surgeon at Blockley and U. S. Military Hospitals, Philadelphia ; Acting Asst. Surg., U. S. A., during Civil War; Surgeon, Panama Railroad, 1866–7; Surgeon, Pacific Mail S. S. Co. Removed to Washington about 1878. Ex-President Med. Assn., Prince George Co., Md. Was in Panama during an epidemic of yellow fever ; contracted the disease and, after recovery, returned to Maryland. See Maryland Med. Jour., 1908, LI, p. 439.

APRIL 7, 1880

367. STEPHEN OLIN RICHEY—Born April 12, 1849, Woodstock, Va. M. D., 1876, Chicago Med. College. Son of Rev. Francis Hartman and Eliza Jones Richey. Educated at private school and by tutors. Taught sometime a country school and read law. Studied medicine with Dr. Nicholas Brewer, of Dawsonville, Md. Asst. Aural Surgeon to several hospitals in Chicago, 1876–8. Since 1878 has practiced ophthalmology and otology in Washington ; sometime Ophthalmic and Aural Surgeon, Providence Hospital ; member Amer. Med. Assn.; Amer. Ophthalmolog. Society ; American Otolog. Society; Washington Biolog. Society ; Congress Amer. Phys. and Surgeons since 1888 ; International Med. Congress ; Amer. Public Health Association ; Washington Philosophical Society. Married, in 1878, Miss Sarah R. White, who died the following year. In 1884 married Mina, daughter of Hon. Montgomery Blair, and granddaughter of Francis Preston Blair. See Watson's Biog., 1896, p. 387.

368. ETHELBERT CARROLL MORGAN—Born Feb. 10, 1856, D. C. Son of Dr. J. E. Morgan, *supra ;* brother of Dr. J. D. Morgan, *infra.* A. B., 1874, Gonzaga, D. C. ; M. D., 1877, Univ. Penna. ; Ph. D., 1889, Georgetown. President, 1888, Amer. Laryngolog. Association. Died May 5, 1891. In childhood he showed a decidedly mechanical turn. After graduating in medicine spent some months in Vienna, Paris and London, in laryngological study. Began to practice in Washington in 1879. Sometime Prof. Laryngology, Georgetown Med. School ; member of many medical organizations. See Minutes Med. Society, May 7, 1891 ; Trans. Amer. Laryngological Assn., 1891 (1892), XIII, p. 147 ; Busey's Reminiscences, p. 197; Georgetown University, II, p. 121.

369. FREDERICK C. VAN VLIET—M. D., 1876, Univ. Vermont. Resigned Oct. 25, 1882. Removed, 1883, to Red Bank, N. J.

370. HARRISON CROOK—Born April 13, 1850, Prince George Co., Md. M. D., 1878, Georgetown.

371. LACHLAN TYLER—Son of John Tyler, President of the United States. Born Dec. 7, 1851, Charles City County, Va. M. D., 1876, Coll. Phys. and Surg., N. Y. Removed, Nov. 23, 1888, to Elkhorn, W. Va., to become Surgeon of a mining company. Afterward to N. Y. City, where he died Jan. 27, 1902. One of the founders of Eastern Dispensary, Washington ; Attending Physician, Protestant Orphan Asylum. Member Med. Assn., D. C.; Amer. Med. Assn.; Wash. Obstet. and Gynecolog. Society. Examining Surgeon for Pensions ; Deputy Coroner, D. C.

372. HENRY MARTEL NEWMAN—Son of Dr. W. G. H. Newman, *supra.* Born Aug. 19, 1856, D. C. M. D., 1876, Georgetown. Dropped, 1886, from membership ; reëlected April 3, 1895. Educated at Rock Hill College, Md., and Spencerian Business College, Washington. Sometime Physician to the Poor, D. C.; Attending, afterwards Consulting Physician, Providence Hospital ; Attending Physician, St. Ann's Infant Asylum. Member Med. Assn., D. C. and Amer. Med. Assn.

OCTOBER 13, 1880

373. SAMUEL SHUGERT ADAMS—Born July 12, 1853, D. C. A. B., 1875; A. M., 1878, Univ. West Va.; M. D., 1879, Georgetown. President, 1900–1, Med. Assn., D. C.; sometime President Amer. Pediatric So-

ciety. Son of George Roszell and Mary Ann Adams. Since graduation in
medicine has practiced in Washington. Has lectured in the medical
schools of Georgetown University, National University and Columbian
University, and at present holds the Chair of Theory and Practice of
Medicine and Diseases of Children in Georgetown University. Attending
Physician, Children's Hospital and Garfield Memorial Hospital; Consult-
ing Physician, Sibley Hospital, Georgetown University Hospital, Wash-
ington Hospital for Foundlings and Woman's Hospital and Dispen-
sary. Member of Congress of Amer. Physicians; Amer. Pediat. Society;
Amer. Med. Assn. and Med. Assn., D. C.; Wash. Obstet. and Gynecolog.
Society; Washington Acad. Sciences. Married, April 30, 1890, Lida
Winslow Hollister. Author of Evolution of pediatric literature in U. S.,
Washington, 1897. See Med. Mirror, St. Louis, 1893, IV, p. 380; Who's
Who in America; American Men of Science, 1906; Amer. Biog. Direct.,
1908.

374. THOMAS HENRY TROTT—Born Oct. 1, 1843, D. C. M. D.,
1867, Georgetown; 1869, Bellevue. Resident Physician, Providence
Hospital. Member Med. Assn., D. C. Died April 23, 1896. See Minutes Med. Society, April 29 and May 6, 1896.

375. THOMAS EUGENE McARDLE—Born April 12, 1852, D. C.
A. B., 1874; A. M., 1879, St. Mary's University, Baltimore. M. D.,
1879, Georgetown. Co-editor of National Medical Review. Son of
Owen and Ann Toumey McArdle. After graduation in medicine,
practiced in Washington. Married, June 14, 1888, Marion V. Thompson,
daughter of Dr. J. Ford Thompson, *supra*. Was Asst. Editor, Washington
Retrospect, 1880; Co-editor and Publisher, National Medical Review
from 1898. Member Washington Acad. Sciences; Med. Assn. D. C.;
Amer. Med. Assn.; Medalist, Georgetown Med. School. See Who's
Who in America; Amer. Biog. Directory, Washington, 1908.

APRIL 6, 1881

376. GEORGE WYTHE COOK—Born at Front Royal, Va., Oct. 28,
1846. [Son of Giles Cook (a distinguished lawyer of the Valley of Virginia) and Elizabeth (Van Meter Lane) Cook. Descended on paternal
side from Mordecai Cooke, who came from England and settled at
"Mordecai's Mount," Gloucester Co., Va., in 1650. His maternal progen-
itors emigrated from Holland and settled in Ulster Co., New York, in
1662. The Van Meters became large land owners in New Jersey, Pennsylvania, Maryland and the Valley of Virginia.] Educated at the Front
Royal Academy. Served in the 7th Virginia Cavalry, C. S. A.; severely
wounded at the battle of Hawe's Shop, Hanover Co., Va., May 28, 1864.

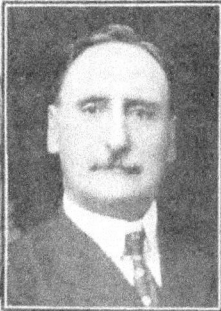

DANIEL OLIN LEECH
1888

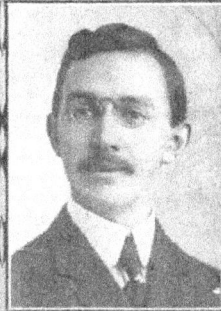

HENRY WOOD TOBIAS
1905

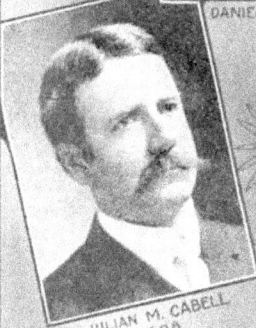

JULIAN M. CABELL
1908

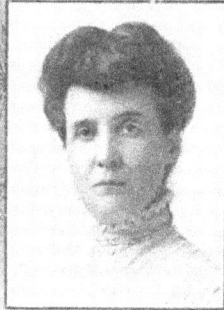

MARY O'MALLEY
1908

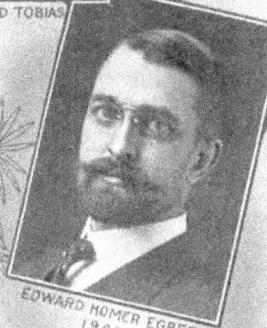

EDWARD HOMER EGBERT
1908

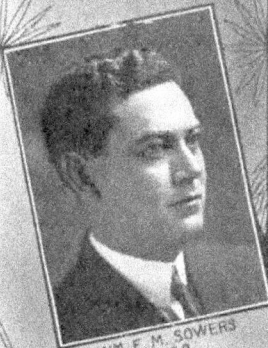

WM. F. M. SOWERS
1909

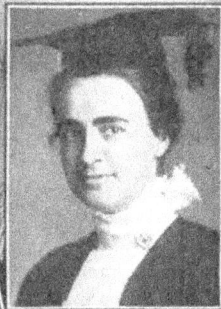

MARTHA M. H. LYON
1909

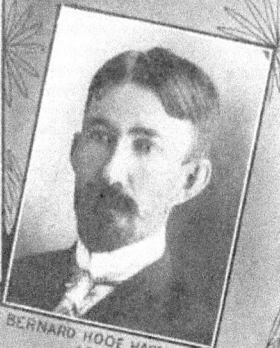

BERNARD HOOE HARRISON
1909

79

Graduated from Med. Dept., Univ. Maryland, 1869, and was an Interne in the Hospital of that University. Began practice at Front Royal, and after two and a half years removed to Upperville, Fauquier Co., Va., where he continued practice for seven years, removing to Washington in 1878. In 1890, received the degree of LL. D. from the National University, in the medical department of which institution he was formerly Professor of Physiology. Was Attending Physician to George Washington Univ. Hospital; Physician to Washington Home for Incurables; President Board of Med. Examiners, D. C.; Acting Asst. Surg., U. S. A., stationed at Washington during the Spanish-American war. Is Professor Clin. Med., George Washington University; Attending Physician Garfield Memorial Hospital; Physician to Louise Home; Consulting Physician, Government Hospital for Insane; Consulting Physician, Episcopal Eye, Ear and Throat Hospital; Treasurer, U. S. Pharmacopoeial Convention; member Amer. Med. Association; of Medical Association, D. C., President, 1897-8, Chairman of its Board of Counsellors and its Delegate to the Amer. Med. Association; member Washington Obstet. and Gynecolog. Society, President, 1902-3 (two terms), Corresponding Secretary, 1887-91, and Recording Secretary, 1891-6; Association Military Surgeons of United States; Washington Academy of Sciences. Honorary member Clinico-Patholog. Society. Author of a number of medical papers and monographs published in various current medical journals. Member Medical History Club. See Report on typhoid fever, Med. Society, 1894. In 1877, married Rebecca Lloyd, daughter of Richard Lloyd, Esq., of Alexandria Co., Va. Has one son, Dr. Richard Lloyd Cook, *infra*. See Who's Who in America; National Medical Review, 1892-3, I, p. 184; Univ. Maryland, Cordell, p. 337; Amer. Biog. Direct., Washington, 1908.

377. ORLANDO CRISMAN KETCHAM—Born Jan. 30, 1839, Northumberland, Co., Pa. M. D., 1871, Georgetown. Dropped, 1886, from membership. Sometime Physician to the Poor, D. C.; afterwards clerk in the departmental service. Member Med. Assn., D. C. Died July 30, 1892, in D. C.

NOVEMBER 2, 1881

378. ALEXANDER MILLER STOUT—Born July 26, 1853, Louisville, Ky. M. D., 1880, Georgetown. Removed, 1882, to Chicago, Ill.

379. BENJAMIN GEORGE POOL—Born Aug. 24, 1854, Fairfax County, Va. M. D., 1879, Columbian. Sometime Inspector, Health Office, D. C. Co-editor, Washington Med. Annals.

380. HORATIO RIPLEY BIGELOW—Born June 18, 1844, Boston, Mass. Lieut., U. S. Marine Corps. M. D., 1879, Columbian. Removed, about 1883, to Philadelphia. Sometime U. S. Consul, Rouen, France.

Died Feb. 20, 1909, in D. C. Buried at Boston, Mass. Author of Hydrophobia, Philadelphia, 1881 ; Gynecological electro-therapeutics, London, 1889 ; also German translation, 1890 ; Plain talks on electricity and batteries, etc., Philadelphia, 1891. See also, International system of electro-therapeutics, Philadelphia, 1894 and 1901.

APRIL 12, 1882

381. FRANCIS BOOTT LORING—Born July 18, 1850, Boston, Mass. M. D., 1874, Harvard. Member Amer. Ophthalmol. Society; Amer. Otolog. Society; Internat. Ophthalmol. Society; Pan-American Ophthalmol. and Otolog. Society ; Amer. Med. Association. Late Professor Diseases Eye and Ear, National Med. College, Washington ; Surgeon in charge Washington Eye and Ear Infirmary ; late on staff New York Eye and Ear Infirmary. Ophthalmic Surgeon, Providence Hospital ; Ophthalmic and Aural Surgeon, Children's Hospital; Ophthalmic Surgeon, St. Ann's Infant Asylum ; U. S. Expert in Guiteau and Star Route cases ; Consulting Surgeon, Diseases of Eye and Ear, to Woman's Dispensary. Member Med. Assn., D. C.; Alternate Delegate to Congress of American Physicians and Surgeons. See E. G. Loring's Text Book of Ophthalmology, N. Y., 1891.

382. WILLIAM NICHOLSON—Born May 16, 1853, Camden, Ark. M. D., 1879, Columbian. Removed, 1886, to Massachusetts, where he died Oct. 3, 1896. Sometime Ophthalmic Surgeon, St. Ann's Infant Asylum, Washington; member Med. Assn., D. C.

383. GEORGE NICHOLAS ACKER—Born Oct. 5, 1852, D. C. A. B., 1872 ; A. M., 1875, Pennsylvania College, Gettysburg ; M. D., 1874, Columbian ; 1877, Univ. Berlin. President, 1902-3, Med. Assn., D. C. Son of Nicholas Acker, of Washington. Since graduation in medicine has practiced in Washington. Clinical Professor of Medicine and Diseases of Children, Columbian Med. College; member Med. Association, D. C.; President Gynecolog. and Obstet. Society, D. C. ; member Amer. Med. Assn.; Amer. Pediatric Society; Amer. Microscop. Society; Washington Acad. Sciences; Anthropolog. Society, Washington. See Who's Who in America.

384. WM. VINCENT MARMION—Born May 27, 1843, Harper's Ferry, Va. A. B., 1859, Emmettsburg, Md. A. M., 1883, Georgetown ; M. D., 1866, Univ. Penna. Asst. Surg. and Passed Asst. Surg., U. S. Navy, 1866-71. Dropped, 1902, from membership in Med. Society. Pursued the study of medicine sometime at the Univ. Vienna. Began practice in Washington in 1872; specialty, ophthalmology. For many years Ophthalmic Surgeon, Children's Hospital, Washington. See Atkinson's Biog., 1878, p. 312; Stone's Biog., 1894, p. 315.

OCTOBER 4, 1882

385. ADOLPH AUGUST HOEHLING—Born March 5, 1839, Philadelphia, Pa. M. D., 1860, Univ. Penna. Asst. Surgeon, Surgeon and Med. Inspector, U. S. Navy. Resigned from Med. Society, Nov. 17, 1896. See Hamersly's Officers of Navy, p. 257.

386. WILLIAM FRANCIS BYRNS—Born Aug. 6, 1847, Bolton, Mass. A. B., 1868, A. M., 1890, Holy Cross College, Worcester, Mass. M. D., 1873, Georgetown. Son of Jeremiah and Catherine Murray Byrns. Educated in public schools. Came to Washington about 1872. Practiced in Manchester, N. H., 1874 to 1878; member of School Board, and N. H. Med. Society. Returned to Washington in 1878, since which has practiced here. Member Med. Assn., D. C.; Amer. Med. Assn. Married Miss Anna R. French; afterwards Mrs. Mary A. Berry. See Georgetown University, II, p. 200.

387. JAMES CLARK BIRD—Born July 1, 1828, Delaware. A. B., 1849; A. M., 1852, Delaware College, Newark, Del. M. D., 1853, Univ. Penna. Dropped from membership 1885; reëlected April 7, 1886. Member Med. Assn., D. C. Died Dec. 5, 1904. See Minutes Med. Society, Dec. 7 and 14, 1904; Wash. Med. Annals, 1904-5, III, p. 454.

OCTOBER 3, 1883

388. HENRY LOWRY EMILIUS JOHNSON—Born Nov. 11, 1858, D. C. M. D., 1882, Columbian. President, 1901-2, Med. Assn., D. C. Trustee, Amer. Med. Assn. Son of Henry L. and Emily E. Johnson; nephew of Charles Goodyear, patentee of India rubber. Since graduation in medicine, Dr. Johnson has practiced in Washington. Sometime Prof. Gynecology, Med. Dept., Columbian University, D. C.; connected with various hospitals. Vice President, International Executive Commission, Third Pan-American Med. Congress; Chairman, Committee on National Legislation, Amer. Med. Association; member Amer. Therapeutic Society; Vice President Pan-American Medical Congress; Vice President First, Second and Third International Sanitary Conventions of American Republics. Member Chicago, Ill., Med. Society; Deputy Governor Society Colonial Wars; member Society Descendants Colonial Wars. Married Miss Eugenie Reel Taylor, of St.

Louis, Mo. See Who's Who in America ; Amer. Biog. Direct., Washington, 1908 ; Genealogy of the Goodyear family ; Americans of gentle birth and their ancestors.

389. JOSIAH ROBSON BROMWELL—Born Sept. 10, 1843, Frederick Co., Md. M. D., 1871, Univ. Maryland.

390. GEORGE BYRD HARRISON—Born Aug. 30, 1844, Ampthill, Cumberland Co., Va. M. D., 1879, Univ. Va. President, 1894-5, Med. Assn., D. C. Died July 19, 1898, Cape May, N. J. Son of Wm. Byrd Harrison, of "Brandon," on the James River, Va., and Mary Randolph Harrison, of "Clifton," Cumberland Co., Va. Educated under private tutors, at William and Mary College, Williamsburg, and Washington College, Va. Served in the C. S. A., 1863-5, after which he farmed for awhile. After graduation in medicine he attended the College of Physicians and Surgeons and Univ. City of New York, and private courses. Began practice in Washington in 1880. Member Washington Obstet. and Gynecolog. Society, for two years its president ; one of the founders of the Med. and Surg. Society, Washington, and of the Eastern Dispensary ; Physician to Garfield Memorial Hospital ; member of staff and Board of Directors, Central Dispensary and Emergency Hospital ; Physician to Washington City Orphan Asylum from 1882 till his death; Physician to Epiphany Church Home ; Professor of Diseases of Children, Columbian Med. College ; member of Faculty of Washington Training School for Nurses. Nov. 22, 1876, married Jeannie L. Stone (daughter of Dr. R. K. Stone, *supra*, and Margaret Ritchie Stone). See Trans. Med. Society, III, 1898, p. 129 ; Minutes Med. Society, Oct. 5 and 12, 1898; Nat. Med. Review, 1898-9, VIII, p. 335.

391. JOHN LLEWELLIN ELIOT—Son of Dr. Johnson Eliot, *supra*. Born Aug. 2, 1853, D. C. A. M., 1869, Rock Hill College, Md. Hospital Steward, U. S. A., 1871-4. M. D., 1874, Georgetown. President, 1893-4, Med. Assn., D. C. His mother was Mary John Llewellin. He was educated at Gonzaga College, Washington. While studying medicine he also attended the Georgetown School of Pharmacy ; was drug clerk, 1870-1. Resident Physician, Washington Asylum; Assistant Physician, Central Dispensary ; Surgeon at Casualty Hospital ; Physician to St. Ann's Infant Asylum ; Consultant at Providence Hospital ; Medical Inspector, Health Department, D. C.; Resident Physician, in 1882, at Smallpox Hospital, and Physician in charge of same, 1894-'06 ; Clinical Professor of Medicine, sometime Prosector Anat. and Surg., Georgetown Med. College. Member Council of Pathology, 9th Internat. Med. Congress ; Pan-Amer. Congress: Wash. Pharm. Assn.; member Med. Assn., D. C. ; Amer. Med. Assn. ; Amer. Public Health Assn. ; Med. and Surg.

Soc., D. C. ; Med. Society of Georgetown University, and Med. Society of Charles Co., M d. April 15, 1885, married Mary Spruance Lancaster, of Maryland. Author of Historical roster of Med. Association, D. C., Washington, 1899. See Nat. Med. Review, 1893-4, II, p. 39; Amer. Biog. Direct., Washington, 1908.

392. IRVING COLLINS ROSSE—Born Oct. 20, 1843, East Newmarket, Dorchester Co., Md. A. M., 1889, Georgetown ; M. D., 1866, Univ., Maryland. F. R. G. S., England. Cadet at West Point. Acting Asst. Surgeon, U. S. Army. Died May 3, 1901. Descendant of Rev. John Rosse, Rector of All Hallows, Md., and son of Dr. Zadock H. Rosse. Educated at St. John's College, Annapolis, Md. Studied medicine with Dr. Alexander H. Bayly, Cambridge, Md. After graduation he attended Univ. City of New York and N. Y. Post-Graduate School; also lectures in Edinburgh, London, Paris and Berlin. Was Clinical Assistant, Baltimore Infirmary ; Medical Officer, U. S. Army, 1866 to 1874, during which time he served at various posts with cavalry, infantry and artillery; in cholera epidemic at Tybee Island, Ga.; Quarantine Officer at Savannah, Ga., and Brazos and Santiago, Texas ; Post Surgeon at Point Isabel ; served at Artillery School, Fort Monroe, Va., and during the Ku-Klux troubles in North Carolina. In the Surgeon General's Office, Washington, 1870-74, in connection with the preparation of the Med. and Surg. History of the War of the Rebellion ; prepared Circular No. 3, a report of the surgical cases treated in the army of the U. S. from 1865 to 1871. Afterwards was Med. Examiner, U. S. Pension Bureau, Washington. Surgeon to Revenue Marine Bureau, 1877 to 1883. In Africa during the Zulu War. Circumnavigated the coast of the U. S. and the Great Lakes. Made voyages on training ship "Chase," also two polar expeditions on the " Corwin," in search of the exploring yacht " Jeannette ;" was the first to climb Herald Island, and Wrangel Land ; this achievement won recognition from the Royal Geographical Society, England. Was Executive Officer of Red Cross Hospital, Washington, 1887 ; juror to Paris Exposition, 1889 ; sometime President of U. S. Examining Board, Washington. Member of Med. Association, D. C.; Med. Society, D. C.; Amer. Med. Association ; the Amer. Congress Physicians and Surgeons ; the Amer. Anthropometric Society ; Amer. Neurolog. Association; Congress International d'Anthropologie Criminelle. Special correspondent of the New York Herald, Chicago Times and San Francisco Examiner. Contributed to Appleton's Cyclopedia, Reference Handbook Medical Sciences, and Witthaus' Med. Jurisprudence. A number of his contributions have been translated and published abroad. He had a record as an all round athlete. Was Prof. of Nervous Diseases, Med. Dept. Georgetown University, which was the specialty that he practiced. Married Miss Florence James, daughter of

Horace James, of New York. See Minutes Med. Society, May 8 and 22, 1901 ; Trans. Med. Society, 1901, VI, p. 165 ; Atkinson's Biog., 1880, p. 11, Supplement ; Georgetown University, II, p. 100 ; Stone's Biog., 1894, p. 433.

[The catalogue of 1885 contains the name of J. H. Baxter, as elected in 1883. There is no record of his nomination or election, nor of any fee paid to the Treasurer. Nor did he sign the constitution. The name is therefore omitted from this list.]

APRIL 2, 1884

393. LEON LEIGH FRIEDERICH—Born Sept. 3, 1857, D. C. M. D., 1881, Columbian. Resident Physician, Providence Hospital ; Hosp. Assistant, Central Dispensary.

APRIL 9, 1884

394. THOMAS TAYLOR—Born April 22, 1820, Perth, Scotland. M. D., 1882, Georgetown. Son of Thomas and Anne Kennedy Taylor. Educated in Scotland, including a scientific course at Anderson University, Glasgow, 1835-8, special studies in chemistry, frictional electricity, galvanism, etc. Invented the first interleaved electric condenser, as improvement on Leyden jar, 1841 ; pneumatic battery for igniting explosives for mining and blasting, 1850 ; safety lamp for coal mines ; rotary galvanic battery. Came to U. S. in 1851. Demonstrated that electricity could be transmitted across sea to given point without wires ; became connected with Ordnance Dept., U. S. A. ; had charge of rifle-shell branch, Washington Arsenal, during Civil War ; invented improved rifle projectiles. Invented and patented rubber to supersede wax molds for plate work. Studied and became specialist on fungoid diseases of plants. Was Chief of Division of Microscopy, U. S. Dept. Agriculture, 1871-95 ; Fellow A. A. A. S. ; Hon. member Micros. Sect. Royal Institute, Liverpool, England, and International Med. Society of Hygiene, Brussels ; member Amer. Chemical Society and French Chemical Society. One of the founders of Washington Chemical and Biolog. Societies. Author of Food products, Washington, 1893-4; Student's handbook, mushrooms of America, edible and poisonous, Washington, 1897-8 ; The diseases of plants ; Edible and poisonous mushrooms, U. S. Jan. 4, 1909, Dr. Taylor's dues were remitted for the rest of his life. See Who's Who in America; Amer. Biog. Directory, Washington, 1908.

395. WILLIAM WARD—Born Sept. 15, 1842, Prince George Co., Md. M. D., 1871, Georgetown. Dropped from membership, 1905. Died April 19, 1909. Educated in the county schools. During the Civil War served in Breathet's Battery, C. S. A.; afterwards in Stuart's Artillery. Married Miss Anna J. Webb, daughter of Joseph Warren Webb, of Washington.

396. JOHN BROWN HAMILTON—Born Dec. 1, 1847, Jersey Co., Ill. M. D., 1869, Rush. Asst. Surg., U. S. A.; Asst. Surgeon, Surgeon and Supervising Surgeon General, U. S. M. H. S. Died Dec. 24, 1898, of perforation of intestines. Editor Jour. Amer. Med. Association. He spent his early life on the farm, in a village printing office and in a drug store. Served in the Union Army, 1864-5. After graduation in medicine he served again till 1876, when he entered the U. S. Marine Hospital Service, becoming finally Supervising Surgeon General. Was also Prof. of Surgery, Med. Dept. Georgetown University. In 1892 he resigned as Surgeon General of the Marine Hospital Service and removed to Chicago, becoming Prof. of Surgery in Rush Medical College; was also connected with the hospitals. He became also editor of the Journal A. M. A. In 1896, resigned from the Marine Hospital Service. In 1896-7, was Supt. Northern Illinois Hosp. for Insane. He is said to have been the first to make visual examinations of pilots and the first physical examination of seamen preliminary to shipment; was largely instrumental in the passage of the national quarantine acts, and it is said that he had the largest private surgical library west of the Alleghenies. Sometime Lecturer on Surgery, Columbian Med. College; Surgeon to Providence Hosp. and St. Ann's Infant Asylum. Author of Lessons in longevity, Washington, 1884; Lectures on tumors, delivered 1891, Philadelphia, 1898; Surgery of the lymphatic system, in Warren and Gould's international text book of surgery, Philadelphia, 1899. See also Mansell-Moulin's Surgery, Philadelphia, 1893, 1895. See Powell's History, p. 351; Stone's Biog., 1894, p. 196; 20th Century Biog. Dict.; Med. Record, N. Y., 1898, LIV, p. 956; N. Y. Med. Jour., 1898, LXVIII, p. 968; Virginia Med. Semi-Monthly, 1899-1900, IV, p. 293; Jour. A. M. A., 1898, XXX, p. 1575.

OCTOBER 8, 1884

397. JOHN HODGES MUNDELL—Born Aug. 29, 1827, Upper Marlboro, Md. M. D., 1849, Univ. Maryland. Died May 12, 1900. Educated at Rockville, Md. Academy. Studied medicine with Dr. Henry Brooke, Marlboro. Practiced in Upper Marlboro five years; in Washington from 1871 till his death. Married Miss Louise Mulliken. See Minutes Med. Society, May 16 and June 6, 1900; National Med. Review, 1900-1, X, p. 383; Trans. Med. Society, 1900, V, p. 127.

398. LEROY M. TAYLOR—Born 1838, N. Y. M. D., 1860, Georgetown. Druggist. Asst. Surgeon 4th Texas Mounted Troops, C. S. A. Resigned from Med. Society, Nov. 25, 1896. Died Sept. 27, 1904.

APRIL 1, 1885

399. RAYMOND THOMAS HOLDEN—Born April 23, 1860, D. C. M. D., 1881, Georgetown. Son of Thomas and Catherine Gleeson Holden. Member Med. Association, D. C., and Clinico-Patholog. Society. Married, Oct. 7, 1896, Celeste Selma Moritz. See Georgetown University, II, p. 222.

400. CHARLES MASSEY HAMMETT—Born Aug. 4, 1835, St. Mary's Co., Md. M. D., 1856, Georgetown. Father of Dr. C. M. Hammett, *infra;* brother of Dr. Whit. Hammett, D. D. S., of Washington. Health Officer, 1891–4, and Coroner, 1894–7, D. C. Died Nov. 22, 1898. Son of Robert Hammett, of England, and of the daughter of Governor Blackistone, of Maryland. Educated at Charlotte Hall, Md. Married Miss Julia Maddox, of St. Mary's Co., Md. See Minutes Med. Society, Nov. 23 and 30, 1898 ; Trans. Med. Society, 1898, III, p. 173; Nat. Med. Review, 1898–9, VIII, p. 435; Georgetown University, II, p. 166.

401. GEORGE WILLIAM WEST—Born Jan. 18, 1845, Buckingham County, Va. M. D., 1868, Richmond Med. Coll. Died of sunstroke, July 23, 1901. Son of John S. West, whose ancestors settled in Virginia in 1609. Was educated at Buckingham College. Served in the C. S. Army, 1862–5, and for some months was prisoner of war at Point Lookout, Md. After graduating in medicine he attended lectures for several years in London and Paris, giving especial attention to diseases of the eye. On his return home was appointed Demonstrator of Anatomy, Richmond Med. College. Was charter member of Richmond Med. Society; member Virginia State Med. Society and Association. In 1877, married Blanche Claughton, daughter of H. O. Claughton, Esq., of Washington. In 1882 removed to Washington, where he afterward practiced until his death. One of the founders of the Med. Dept. National University, and many years Prof. Anatomy there. Member A. M. A. and Assn. Amer. Anatomists. See minutes Med. Society, Oct. 2, 1901 ; Trans. Med. Society, 1901, VI, p. 229 ; Atkinson's Biog., 1878, p. 494.

402. THOMAS VICTOR HAMMOND—Born Feb. 28, 1861, Berlin, Md. M. D., 1882, Jefferson. Resident Physician, afterwards Consulting Physician, Providence Hospital, Washington.

OCTOBER 7, 1885

403. LOUIS KOLIPINSKI—Born Nov. 3, 1859, D. C. Phar. D, 1880, National College Pharmacy, D. C. M. D., 1883, Georgetown. Resident Physician, Children's Hospital, D. C. ; Prof. Surgery, National Univ. Med. College, D. C.

404. SAMUEL BACKUS LYON—Born, 1841, Palmer, Mass. M. D., 1879, Columbian. Resigned from Med. Society, Jan. 11, 1888. Sometime Assistant at Govt. Hosp. for Insane, Washington. In 1890 appointed Supt. Bloomingdale Insane Asylum, N. Y. City.

405. THOMAS ATTAWAY REEDER KEECH—Born March 28, 1833, Harford County, Md. M. D., 1856, Univ. Maryland. After graduation practiced in Harford Co.; 1863 to 1873 in Prince George Co., Md.; since Nov. 1, 1873, in Washington.

406. GEORGE CLARKE OBER—Born April 11, 1860, D. C. M. D., 1882, Georgetown. Resident Physician, Children's Hospital; Physician, Eastern Dispensary; Prof. Materia Medica, afterwards Practice of Medicine, National Univ. Med. College.

OCTOBER 14, 1885

407. CHARLES LINCOLN LOOMIS—Born Sept. 9, 1859, D. C. M. D., 1882, Univ. Vermont. Resigned Jan. 11, 1888. Died April 6, 1888, at Denver, Col. Son of Dr. Lafayette C. Loomis, of Washington, and nephew of Dr. Silas L. Loomis, *supra*. Educated at Alleghany College, Meadville, Pa. Attended the Faculté de Med., Paris. After graduation he spent some time in Europe at the hospitals and in traveling. See Lamb's History, p. 252.

[1885. The names William D. Stewart and S. J. Waggaman appear in only one list of the Society, namely, 1885. There is no record of their election, they did not sign the constitution and their names do not appear on the Treasurer's book up to 1886. It is very doubtful if they were ever members.]

APRIL 7, 1886

408. FRANK BAKER—Born Aug. 22, 1841, Pulaski, N. Y. A. M., 1888; Ph. D., 1890, Georgetown; M. D., 1880, Columbian. Resigned from Med. Society, Dec. 18, 1889. Son of Thomas C. and Sybil S. Weed Baker. Was Sergeant, 37th New York Vols., 1861-3. Prof. Anatomy, Georgetown Med. School, since 1883; Supt., National Zoölogical Park, Washington, since 1890; Asst. Supt., U. S. Life-saving Service, 1889-90; Editor American Anthropologist, 1891-8; F. A. A. S. (Secretary Section H, 1888, Vice President, 1890); member Amer. Naturalists; Assn. Amer. Anat. (President, 1897); Philadelphia Zoölog. Society; Washington Academy of Sciences (Secretary since 1890); Washington Biolog. Society; Washington Anthrop. Society. Married, Sept. 13, 1878, at Sedgwick, Me., May E. Cole. Has a son in Medical Corps, U. S. Army. Has

21

contributed articles to Wood's Reference Handbook Med. Sciences ; Billings' National Med. Dictionary ; Standard Dictionary ; International Encyclopedia. See Amer. Men of Science, 1906 ; Who's Who in America; Amer. Biog. Directory, Washington, 1908 ; Georgetown University, II, p. 96.

409. FRANK CLINTON FERNALD—Born Portsmouth, N. H. M. D., 1884, Harvard. Member Wash. Obstet. and Gynecolog. Society. Died June 17, 1889.   See Minutes Med. Society, Sept. 11, 1889.

410. HARRY MADISON CUTTS—Born Sept. 4, 1858, D. C.   A. B., 1880 ; A. M., 1883, Princeton ; M. D., 1883, Harvard. Resigned, Sept. 28, 1887, and removed to Brookline, Mass.

411. WILLIAM MAY—Born Sept. 6, 1850, D. C.   Son of Dr. J. F. May, *supra;* M. D., 1874, College Phys. and Surg., N. Y. Dropped from membership, 1897; reëlected, Oct. 6, 1897. Removed to New York City.

OCTOBER 6, 1886

412. DANIEL PERCY HICKLING—Born Sept. 19, 1863, D. C.   M. D., 1884, Georgetown. Son of Daniel P. and Sarah A. Hickling. Attended Emerson Institute and the Columbian Preparatory School, Washington.   After graduation in medicine took special courses in Boston, Chicago and the medical centers of Europe.   Since then has practiced in Washington. Was Prof. Clin. Surg., Electro-therapeutics, Clinical Prof. of Neurolog., Georgetown School of Medicine ; Visiting Physician, Washington Asylum Hospital ; member Consulting Staff, Providence Hospital and Government Hospital for the Insane ; member A. M. A.; Fellow, Amer. Electro-therapeutic Association ; member Med. Association, D. C.   In charge of Neurolog. and Electro-therapeutic Clinic, Eastern Dispensary and Casualty Hospital ; Consulting Neurologist, Washington Home for Incurables ; in charge Department Neurology, Georgetown University Hospital. Member Washington Chamber of Commerce ; Washington Acad. Sciences ; Med. and Surg. Society, D. C.   Chairman, Committee on Public Health, Washington Board of Trade.   Vice President, Society Nervous and Mental Diseases, D. C., and Med. Society, Casualty Hospital ; President, Med. Society, Georgetown Med. College.   Also member of the Vestry, Pro-Cathedral Church of the Ascension.   Sept. 5, 1894, married Harriet Frances Stone. See Amer. Biog. Direct., Washington, 1908; Georgetown University, II, p. 322.

413. BENJAMIN FRANKLIN MADISON—Born Sept. 1, 1852, Edgefield, S. C.   M. D., 1884, Georgetown. Dropped, 1900, from membership.

414. JEROME HENRY KIDDER—Born Oct. 26, 1842, Baltimore Co., Md. A. B., 1862; A. M., 1865, Harvard; M. D., 1866, Univ. Maryland. Med. Cadet, U. S. A. Asst. Surg., U. S. Navy, 1866-71; Passed Asst. Surg., 1871-76, and Surgeon, 1876 to 1884. Resigned June 18, 1884. Curator of Laboratory and Exchanges, Smithsonian Institution. Died April 8, 1889. About 1862, was placed in charge of the Sea Island plantations, near Beaufort, S. C.; contracted yellow fever, and was obliged to return north early in 1863. On recovery enlisted in Tenth Maryland Infantry, and served as private and non-commissioned officer for about a year. Was then appointed Med. Cadet and served in hospitals near Washington until the Civil War ended. His first detail in the Navy was to the Naval Asylum, Philadelphia; remained a little over a year. From 1867 to 1870 was Asst. Med. Officer, U. S. Ship "Idaho," then stationed off Nagasaki, Japan, as the general hospital for the Asiatic Squadron. While there he received from the King of Portugal the decoration of the Military Order of Christ, in recognition of professional services to a distressed vessel of the Portuguese Navy; and during the memorable typhoon of Sept. 21, 1868, he made a careful chart of the track of the storm. In 1874-5 served on U. S. Steamer "Swatara," as Surgeon and Naturalist of the Transit of Venus Expedition to Kerguelen Island, and in 1877-8 as Surgeon, U. S. Steamer "Alliance," in the Mediterranean. On the latter cruise he was married at Constantinople, Sept. 18, 1878, to Anne Mary, daughter of Hon. Horace Maynard, U. S. Minister to Turkey. During the summer of 1878-9 was on special duty with the small Naval Steamers "Bluelight" and "Speedwell," engaged in fishery investigations on the New England coast, and in December, 1882, became the first Surgeon of the Fish Commission Steamer "Albatross," on which he remained until the following April. His shore service was performed mainly at the Naval Hospital and Laboratory, Brooklyn, from 1871 to 1874, and at the Bureau of Medicine and Surgery, Washington, from 1879 to 1882. See Smithsonian Collections; Billings' National Med. Dictionary, Philadelphia, 1890; also Minutes Med. Society, April 17, 1889; Bull. Philosoph. Soc., Washington, 1892, XI, p. 480.

415. MILLARD FILLMORE THOMPSON—Born Nov. 17, 1857, D. C. D. D. S., 1879, Baltimore Coll. Dental Surgery; M. D., 1884, Columbian. Sometime Prof. Anatomy, Med. Dept., National University, D. C.

416. GEORGE WOODRUFF JOHNSTON—Born Sept. 17, 1858, D. C. Son of Dr. W. P. Johnston, *supra*. A. M., 1879, Princeton; M. D., 1882, Univ. Pa. Co-editor National Medical Review. Resigned from Med. Society, April 17, 1901. Gynecologist, Central Dispensary; member Wash. Obstet. and Gynecol. Society.

324   MEDICAL SOCIETY

417. MIDDLETON FULLER CUTHBERT—Born July 5, 1860, in
Pennsylvania. M. D., 1883, Columbian. Was Resident Physician and
Gynecologist, Providence Hospital ; member Wash. Obstet. and Gyne-
col. Society.

418. WILLIAM WHITNEY GODDING—Born May 5, 1831, Winchendon, Mass. A. B., 1854, Dartmouth ; M. D., 1857, Castleton.
Superintendent, Government Hospital for the Insane, D. C. Died May
6, 1899. Son of Dr. Alvah and Mary Whitney Godding, of English
descent. Educated at the academy at Winchendon, Brown University,
Providence, R. I., Phillips' Academy, Andover, Mass., and Dartmouth
College. Studied medicine first at College of Physicians and Surgeons, N. Y. City, but graduated at Castleton, Vt. Practiced with his
father at Winchendon for eighteen months ; in 1859 became Asst.
Physician at State Hospital for Insane, Concord, N. H. In 1862 resumed
practice, this time at Fitchburg, Mass., but the same year was appointed
Second Assistant Physician at St. Elizabeth Insane Asylum, Wash-
ington. In 1870 was appointed Superintendent of the State Hospital for
Insane at Taunton, Mass. In 1877 returned to St. Elizabeth Hospital
as Superintendent, and continued in charge till his death. During his
incumbency the capacity of the hospital was greatly increased. Married,
Dec. 14, 1860, to Miss Ellen Rowena Murdock, daughter of Elisha
Murdock, of Winchendon. Author of Two hard cases, Boston, 1882.
The rights of the insane in hospital, Philadelphia, 1884. See Minutes
Med. Society, May 10 and June 7, 1899 ; Trans. Med. Society, 1899,
IV, p. 118 ; Proceedings Amer. Med. Psych. Assn., 1899, VI, p. 398 ;
Bull. Philos. Soc., Washington, 1895-1900, XIII, p. 390; Jour. A. M.
A., 1899, XXXII, p. 1073; Jour. Mental Sci., London, 1900, XLVI, p.
404; National Med. Review, Washington, 1899-1900, IX, p. 366.

419. ERNEST FROTHINGHAM KING—Born Nov. 29, 1858, Turner, Maine. A. B., 1880 ; A. M., 1883, Colby College, Watervliet, Me.;
M. D., 1883, Howard.

420. MAGRUDER MUNCASTER—Born Feb. 13, 1859, D. C. Brother of Dr. S. B. Muncaster, *infra.* Phar. D., 1880, National College
Pharmacy, D. C. ; M. D., 1883, Univ. Md. Died Nov. 28, 1901, Rockville, Md. Son of Harriet Magruder and Otho Z. Muncaster and great-
grandson of Col. Zadock Magruder, who was a member of the Committee
of Safety of Maryland, under General George Washington, during the
Revolutionary War. Was educated at Rockville Academy. After graduation in medicine he engaged in the drug business for a few years,

after which he practiced medicine in Washington City. He soon built up quite a lucrative practice. About 1895 his health began to fail. Was one of the U. S. Examining Surgeons for Pensions; member Med. Association, D. C.; Clinico-Patholog. Society, and Amer. Med. Assn. See Minutes Med. Society, Dec. 4 and 11, 1901; Trans. Med. Society, 1901, VI, p. 324.

421. JOHN WESLEY BOVÉE—Born Dec. 31, 1861, Clayton, N. Y. M. D., 1885, Columbian. Editor of The Practice of Gynecology, Philadelphia, 1906. Son of Wm. Henry and Sarah Elizabeth Roat Bovée. Educated at public and high schools and by private tutors. Since graduation in medicine has practiced in Washington. Member of House Staff, Children's Hospital and Columbia Hospital, Washington, 1884-88; Visiting Surgeon, Washington Asylum, 1889–97; Surgeon, Columbia Hospital, since 1891; Gynecologist, Providence Hospital, 1891 to 1908, and George Washington Univ. Hospital since its opening; formerly Attending and now Consulting Physician to St. Ann's Infant Asylum; Professor Gynecology, George Washington Univ. Med. School; sometime Chairman, Section of Gynecology and Obstetrics, A. M. A.; member Amer. Urolog. Assn.; Washington Acad. Sciences; Mississippi Valley Med. Assn.; President, Med. and Surg. Society, D. C.; President, Washington Obstet. and Gynecolog. Society and Southern Surg. and Gynecolog. Assn.; Fellow Amer. Gynecolog. Society; honorary member Med. Society, Virginia; member Board of Trustees, Reform School for Girls, D. C.; Consulting Gynecologist, St. Elizabeth Hospital for Insane, D. C. See Who's Who in America; Amer. Biog. Direct., Washington, 1908.

422. JOSEPH HAMMOND BRYAN—Born July 4, 1856, D. C. M. D., 1877, Univ. Va.; 1878, Univ. City of New York. Asst. Surg., U. S. N., 1880-5. Son of Joseph Brooke and Louisa Stearns Hammond Bryan. Has practiced medicine in Washington since 1887. Unmarried. Member Wash. Acad. Sciences; Philosoph. Society, Washington; Amer. Laryngolog. Assn., President, 1902. Author of Diseases of accessory sinuses of the nose, in System of diseases of ear, nose and throat, Philadelphia, 1893. See Who's Who in America; Amer. Biog. Direct., Washington, 1908.

423. CHARLES JOHNSON OSMUN—Born Oct. 10, 1845, Washington, N. J. M. D., 1872, Washington Univ., Baltimore; 1875, College Phys. and Surg., Baltimore. Died Aug. 14, 1894. Came to Washington in 1884, and was the first medical man to take charge of the details in enforcing the law for the prevention of scarlet fever and diphtheria, during which service he contracted and died of diphtheria. See Minutes Med. Society, Aug. 16, 1894; Nat. Med. Review, 1894-5, III, p. 101.

424. ISIDOR SAMUEL LEOPOLD BERMANN—Born Jan. 7, 1845, Hesse Darmstadt, Germany. Educated at Darmstadt and Frankfurt-on-the-Main. Studied medicine at Marburg, Würzburg and Vienna. M. D., 1878, Julia Maximiliana, Würzburg. Was assistant to Prof. Kuelz, Marburg. Physician, 1879–80, to Maryland Eye and Ear Infirmary and Baltimore Eye, Ear and Throat Hospital, 1879–82; Licentiate, M. C. F., Maryland. Afterwards practiced in Washington. Member Wash. Acad. Sciences. See Who's Who in America; Amer. Biog. Direct., Washington, 1908; Cordell's Med. Annals, Maryland, 1903, p. 319.

425. JOHN WOART BAYNE—Born Feb. 9, 1846, "Salubria," Prince George Co., Md. M. D., 1868, Univ. Maryland. Acting Asst. Surg., U. S. A., and Surgeon, U. S. Vols. Died May 17, 1905. Educated at country schools. After graduation in medicine served as Medical Attendant at Fort Foote, Md., 1870 to 1878, when the fort was abandoned. Was then transferred to duty at Washington Barracks, D. C., serving 1878–81. For some years was Surgeon to Metropolitan Police and Fire Department, Washington. In 1881 became Surgeon to Providence Hospital, President of Hospital Board, 1889–1905; in 1883 became Prof. Clinical Surgery, Georgetown Med. School; member of Consulting Board, Episcopal Eye, Ear and Throat Hospital and Casualty Hospital. During the Spanish-American War was Brigade Surgeon, serving at Leiter Hospital, Chickamauga, after which he resumed practice in Washington. Sometime President, D. C. Society, S. A. R. Was grandson of Major Andrew Leitch, of the staff of General Washington, in the war of the American Revolution; and son of Dr. John H. Bayne, of Maryland, a Surgeon in the U. S. Vols. in the war of 1861-5. Married, in 1872, Miss May Ashby, of Fauquier Co., Va. Father of Dr. John Breckenridge Bayne, of Washington. The Bayne family was especially interested in St. Barnabas' Church in Prince George Co., Md. See Minutes Med. Society, May 17 and 24, 1905; Wash. Med. Annals, 1905, IV, p. 257; Georgetown University, II, p. 122.

OCTOBER 6, 1887

426. ARTHUR AUGUSTINE SNYDER—Born June 6, 1859, D. C. Son of Dr. J. M. Snyder, *supra.* M. D., 1882, Univ. City of New York. Acting Asst. Surg., U. S. A. During the Spanish-American War he served in the 1st Divisional Hospital before Santiago, Cuba, and in the Base Hospital at Siboney, near Santiago. Returned with the last regiment of Shafter's Corps, 24th Inf., to Montauk, N. Y. Is Visiting Surgeon to Garfield Memorial Hospital and Clinical Surgeon to George Washington Univ. Hospital.

427. WILLIAM PRICE MANNING—Born Dec. 8, 1844, Virginia. M. D., 1869, Univ. Maryland. Died Feb. 9, 1901. See Minutes Med. Society, Feb. 13, 1901; Trans. Med. Society, 1901, VI, p. 53.

428. HENDERSON SUTER—Born July 1, 1855, D. C. Brother of Dr. W. N. Suter, *infra*. M. D., 1877, Univ. Penna.

429. THOMAS MARSHALL NORTON—Born Nov. 21, 1863, Fauquier Co., Va. M. D., 1885, Univ. Va. Died Jan. 9, 1892, Alexandria, Va. See Minutes Med. Society, Jan. 13, 1892.

430. CHARLES TUFTS CALDWELL—Born Aug. 22, 1855, West Bridgewater, Mass. M. D., 1879, Columbian. Resigned, Feb. 10, 1904.

APRIL 4, 1888

431. WILLIAM FLEET LUCKETT—Born March 6, 1838, Middleburg, Va. M. D., 1860, Univ. Louisville. Surgeon, C. S. A. Father of Dr. L. F. Luckett, *infra*. Died March 30, 1901. Educated at the Frank Minor school. After the close of the Civil War practiced medicine in Frederick, Md., until 1885, when he removed to Washington. Member Med. Assn., D. C.; A. M. A., and Washington Acad. Sciences. Buried at Frederick. See Minutes Med Society, April 3 and 10, 1901, and Trans. Med. Society, 1901, VI, p. 125.

432. WILLIAM EDWARD HANDY—Born Oct. 10, 1858, D. C. M. D., 1885, Columbian. Dropped from membership, 1897. Removed to Manila, P. I.

433. JOHN WESLEY DUNN—Born Dec. 30, 1858, Philadelphia, Pa. Educated in public schools, Washington, and Columbian University. M. D., 1880, Columbian. Afterwards attended Med. Dept., Univ. Penna. Served as Interne at Children's Hospital, Washington. Practiced in Washington from 1883 till his death. Married, Sept. 29, 1886, Miss Helen Margaret McFarland, daughter of John M. and Sarah J. McFarland, Washington. Contracted diphtheria from a patient and died six days afterward, Dec. 30, 1890. See Minutes Med. Society, Dec. 31, 1890.

434. THOMAS COLLINS STEVENSON MARSHALL—Born April 28, 1856, Carlisle, Pa. M. D., 1883, Howard. Attended also the Howard Dental School. Has been in the Government departmental service, Washington. Member Med. Assn., D. C. Prof. Histology and afterwards Pathology, Howard Medical School. See Lamb's History, p. 133.

435. CHARLES WILLIAMSON RICHARDSON—Born Aug. 22, 1861, D. C. M. D., 1884, Columbian, and Univ. Penna. Educated at Columbian College, D. C. Is Prof. Laryngology and Otology, Med. Dept. Columbian Univ.; Trustee of the University ; ex-President Amer. Laryngol., Rhinol. and Otolog. Society; Vice President, Amer. Laryngol. Assn.; member Washington Acad. Sciences ; Anthropol. and Biolog. Societies, Washington; Fellow Academy Oto-Laryngology; member Amer. Climatolog. Society ; Amer. Otolog. Society; A. M. A.; Throat and Ear Surgeon to Providence and Foundling Hospitals, Washington; ex-President, Alumni Assn., Columbian Univ. Contributor to Posey and Wright's Diseases of Eye, Ear, Nose and Throat, to Buck's Reference Handbook and Musser-Kelly Handbook. Son of Charles F. E. and Charlotte A. Richardson. Married, May 27, 1889, Amy Elizabeth Small. See Stone's Biog., 1894, p. 671; Who's Who in America; Amer. Biog. Direct., Washington, 1908.

436. DANIEL OLIN LEECH—Born July 13, 1862, Port Republic, Va. M. D., 1887, Columbian. Brother of Dr. Frank Leech, *infra*. President, 1906-7, Medical Assn., D. C.; President, 1905, Therapeutic Society, D. C.

437. GEORGE WASHINGTON GRINDER, JR.—Born Dec. 1, 1862, D. C. M. D., 1885, National Univ., D. C. Dropped from membership, 1897. Died Dec. 13, 1901. Graduated, 1882, from the Spencerian Business College, Washington. Sometime Demonstrator Anatomy, National Univ. Med. School. See Lamb's History, p. 245.

438. JAMES THOMAS SWEETMAN, JR.—Born June 22, 1862, Philadelphia, N. Y. A. B., 1883; A. M., 1886, Princeton; M. D., 1886, Howard. Dropped from membership, 1891. Removed to Ballston, N. Y. Married. See Lamb's History, p. 220.

439. WILLIAM LEON MILLER—Born Jan. 22, 1859, D. C. M. D., 1883, Columbian.

440. THOMAS FRANCIS MALLAN—Born July 19, 1857, Lynchburg, Va. M. D., 1880, Georgetown. Surgeon to Providence Hospital ; Consulting Surgeon, St. Ann's Infant Asylum ; Attending Physician, Catholic Univ. and Marist College and Seminary, Washington.

441. ROBERT THAXTER EDES—Born Sept. 23, 1838, Eastport, Me. A. B., 1858 ; M. D., 1861, Harvard. Asst. Surg. and Passed Asst. Surg., U. S. N. Removed from D. C., 1891, to Boston, Mass.; thence to Jamaica Plains, Mass. His family is of English descent. His literary education was received at Harvard College. Studied medicine under Dr. Benjamin Cushing. Entered U. S. Navy at beginning of Civil War and served, chiefly in the West Gulf or Mississippi Squadron, until June, 1865. Then visited Europe and supplemented his medical education at Vienna, after which he located at Hingham, Mass., and practiced his profession until 1869; then settled in Boston. In 1886 removed to Washington. Was Attending Physician, Boston City Hospital, 1872 to 1886; at Garfield Memorial Hospital, Washington, 1889–91; Professor Materia Medica, Harvard Med. School, 1871 to 1883, and Jackson Prof. Clin. Medicine, same school, 1883–6. In 1891 became Resident Physician, Adams' Nervine Asylum, Jamaica Plains, Mass. Sometime Lecturer in Med. School, Dartmouth, N. H., and Georgetown and Columbian Med. Schools, Washington. Author of The part taken by nature and time in the cure of disease, prize essay, Boston, 1868; The physiology and pathology of the sympathetic or ganglionic nervous system, New York, 1860; Translation of Alex. Ecker's Die Hirnwindungen des Menschen, etc., New York, 1873; Handbook of U. S. Pharmacopoeia, N. Y., 1883; Intracranial hemorrhage, etc., in Pepper's System of Med., Philadelphia, 1886, V.; Text book of therapeutics, etc., Philadelphia, 1887, 1895; Shattuck lectures, Boston, 1895. See Atkinson's Biog., 1878, p. 496; Stone's Biog., 1894, p. 156; Who's Who in America; 20th Century Biog. Dict.; Amer. Men of Science, 1906.

OCTOBER 3, 1888

442. JAMES DUDLEY MORGAN—Born July 5, 1861, D. C. Son of Dr. J. E. Morgan, *supra*. A. B., 1881; M. D., 1885, Georgetown. Son of James E. and Norah Digges Morgan. Studied medicine some time at Bellevue. After graduation took post-graduate course at Beaujon Hospital and Amphitheatre d'Anatomie, Paris, and in 1902 and 1903, clinical course under Prof. William Osler. Member of Staff of Garfield and Georgetown Univ. Hospitals; Chief of Medical Service, Emergency Hospital. In 1893 was Chairman of Registration Committee, Pan-American Med. Congress; President, Columbia Historical Society, D. C.; Vice President, Washington Acad. Sciences; member Anthropolog. Society, Washington; was Demonstrator of Anatomy, 1888-9, Georgetown Med. School; Prof. Clinical Medicine, 1899; now Associate Prof. Theory and Practice of Medicine. Interne, Children's Hospital, 1885; Lecturer on Differential Diagnosis, 1897-8; Co-editor, Trans. Med. Society, 1898-1900; member A. M. A.; Assn. Amer. Anatomists; Amer. Climat. Assn.; Med. and Surg. Society and Wash. Obstet. and Gynecol. Society, D. C. Author of many medical and historical essays. Married, Dec. 2, 1891, Mary Abell, daughter of E. F. Abell, Baltimore, Md. See Amer. Men of Science, 1906; Amer. Biog. Direct., Washington, 1908.

443. MARY ALMERA PARSONS—Born May 2, 1850, Colebrook, N. H. M. D., 1874, Howard. From Revolutionary stock. Educated at Robinson Female Seminary, Exeter, N. H., graduating in 1870. Since graduation in medicine has practiced in Washington. See Lamb's History, p. 205.

444. PHILIP SEDDON ROY—Born April 15, 1861, Tappahannock, Va. M. D., 1880, Univ. Va.

445. THOMAS MORRIS MURRAY—Born July 5, 1851, Maryland. M. D., 1873, Univ. Maryland; Licentiate, 1876, M. C. F., Maryland. Practiced some time in Baltimore, then removed to Washington. See Cordell's Med. Annals, Maryland, 1903, p. 515.

446. ERNEST AUGUST SELLHAUSEN—Born May 12, 1853, D. C. M. D., 1874, Columbian; 1877, University of Leipzig.

447. ABRAHAM HARMON WITMER—Born April 10, 1845, Lancaster County, Pa. M. D., 1866, Jefferson. Died Jan. 18, 1900. Of American parentage, Swiss descent. Educated at Wilmington, Del. After graduation in medicine practiced at Mt. Joy, Pa. About 1868 to 1872 was Asst. Physician, Insane Dept., Philadelphia Almshouse; was next Steamship Surgeon for a year, after which he returned to duty at the Almshouse. In 1876 became Asst. Physician to St. Elizabeth Insane Asylum, Washington, where he remained till his death; was promoted until finally was First Assistant and at times acted as Superintendent. Member A. M. A.; of Board of School Trustees, D. C. Attended several Medical Congresses abroad. For some time was connected with the Faculty of Georgetown Med. School. Married Miss Roberta Stone, of Washington. See Minutes Med. Society, Feb. 7, and 14, 1900; Atkinson's Biog., 1878, p. 332.

448. THOMAS NOTLEY McLAUGHLIN—Born Aug. 15, 1860, D. C. M. D., 1882, Columbian. President, Med. Assn., D. C., 1909-10.

449. ALBERT CLARK PATTERSON—Son of Dr. D. C. Patterson, *supra.* Born May 8, 1854, Cleveland, Ohio. M. D., 1879, Columbian. Removed from Washington, 1896. Returned and became connected with the Health Dept., D. C.

APRIL 3, 1889

450. EDWIN LEE MORGAN—Born Sept. 29, 1855, D. C. M. D., 1879, Med. College, Va. Son of Edwin Cecil and Evelina Prosser Lee Morgan. Educated at Blackburn and Taylor High School and St. John's

Academy, Alexandria, Va.; was two years at Virginia Military Institute, Lexington ; afterward attended Glenwood Institute, Md. From 1879 to 1886 was Physician to Colville Indian Agency, State of Washington ; during that time was Coroner for two terms. Returned to Washington. Sometime Physician to the Poor; Physician to St. Ann's Infant Asylum. Member Med. Assn., D. C.; A. M. A.; Med. and Surg. Society, Washington ; President, Therapeutic Society, Washington ; member Anthrop. Society, Washington ; President, 1899-1900, Library Association, D. C. Grandson of Col. Richard Bland Lee, U. S. A. Married, Oct. 10, 1893, Mary Garland VanZandt. See Who's Who in America ; Amer. Biog. Direct., Washington, 1908.

451. FRANCIS BESANT BISHOP—Born Aug. 13, 1853, Wilmington, N. C. M. D., 1883, Univ. Maryland.

452. WILLIAM HINES HAWKES—Born Oct. 25, 1845, Meriden, Conn. A. B., 1867, Brown; A. M., 1890, Georgetown; M. D., 1874, Univ. Penna. Acting Asst. Surg., U. S. A. Died suddenly, March 13, 1904. Served some time as Assistant to the Attending Surgeon, U. S. Army officers, Washington. Was Prof. Materia Medica and Therapeutics, and Clinical Prof., Diseases of Children, Georgetown Med. School; Secretary of Attending Staff and Director of Clinic for Diseases of Children, Emergency Hospital; Attending Physician, Garfield Hospital. See Stone's Biog., 1894, p. 636 ; Minutes Med. Society, March 23 and April 13, 1904; Wash. Med. Annals, 1904-5, III, p. 239.

OCTOBER 2, 1889

453. EUGENE CHARLES CURTIS WINTER—Born Aug. 13, 1848, Petersville, Md. Brother of Dr. J. T. Winter, *supra*. M. D. and Phar. D., 1883, Howard. Since graduation has practiced in Washington. Is married. See Lamb's History, p. 230.

454. WILLIAM MERCER SPRIGG—Born April 3, 1864, Petersburg, Va. M. D., 1885, Columbian.

APRIL 2, 1890

455. THOMAS RITCHIE STONE—Born July 18, 1856, D. C. Son of Dr. R. K. Stone, *supra*. M. D., 1884, Univ. Vermont. Died suddenly, May 31, 1902, of acute indigestion. [Born in the "Stone" house, corner Fourteenth and F Streets, N. W., that was built by his grandfather, Wm. J. Stone. His mother was daughter of Thomas Ritchie.] Educated at Emerson Institute, Washington, and William and Mary College, Williamsburg, Va. After graduation in medicine he traveled extensively abroad; then practiced three years in California. Returned to Washington in 1890 and practiced here till his death. Sometime President Clinico-Patholog. Society; on the Staff of Emergency Hospital; member of Faculty of Med. Dept., Columbian College. Married, Jan. 22, 1885, Miss Lelia Whitney, of New Orleans, La. See Minutes Med. Society, June 3, 1902; Wash. Med. Annals, 1902, p. 312.

456. JAMES KERR—Born Dec. 14, 1848, Port Steuart, Co. Derry, Ireland. M. D., M. Ch., 1870, Royal Univ., Belfast, Ireland. Father of Dr. H. H. Kerr, *infra*. Son of Abraham John and Isabella Kerr. Educated at Coleraine Institute. After graduation in medicine was Surgeon, Royal Canadian Mail Service, 1871-3; Surgeon, H. M. Transport "No. XII," Gold Coast Expedition, 1873-4; Chief Surgeon, Canadian Pacific Ry., 1882-8; Surgeon, Canadian Militia, Riel Rebellion, 1885; Prof. Surgery, Manitoba Med. College, and afterward of Georgetown Med. School. Member Wash. Acad. Sciences. Married, at Brantford, Ontario, Canada, July, 1876, Laurie I. Bell, daughter of Alexander Graham Bell. See Who's Who in America; Amer. Biog. Direct., Washington, 1908.

457. GAIUS MARCUS BRUMBAUGH—Born May 7, 1862, Huntingdon Co., Pa. M. E., 1881, M. S., 1897, Juniata College, Huntingdon. M. D., 1885, Howard; 1888, Georgetown. Son of Dr. Andrew B. Brumbaugh (practicing at Huntingdon, 1866-1909), and Maria Frank Brumbaugh. Educated in private schools and Huntingdon Academy. Taught sometime in public schools. Removed to Washington in 1882. Sometime in departmental service; for three years Asst. Chief of Bureau of Animal Industry, Dept. Agriculture. Since 1887 has practiced medicine in Washington. Member of Board of U. S. Pension Examining Surgeons; Med. Association, D. C.; A. M. A.; A. A. A. S.; Lecturer on Materia Medica and Therapeutics, Nurses' Training School, Washington; Trustee, Juniata College. Married, Oct. 1, 1889, Catherine Elliott Brown, daughter of Dr. C. W. Brown, *infra*. See Lamb's History, p. 152; Amer. Biog. Direct., Washington, 1908.

458. GEORGE GIDEON MORRIS—Born Oct. 23, 1860, Mt. Morris, Pa. M. D., 1884, Univ. Maryland. Asst. Surg., U. S. Vols., Spanish-American War.

459. JAMES CLARK McGUIRE—Born Feb. 1, 1853, D. C. A. M., 1887, St. John's College, Annapolis, Md.; M. D., 1879, Columbian. Acting Asst. Surg., U. S. A., 1881-3. Author of Dermatological Notes, Washington, 1888. Prof. Dermatology, Hospital School of Medicine, Louisville, Ky., 1886 to 1888, and Georgetown Med. School, Washington, since 1892.

460. CHARLES ROSCOE LUCE—Born Oct. 17, 1862, in New York. M. D., 1885, Georgetown.

461. HENRY BUCKMASTER DEALE—Born April 16, 1862, in Maryland. A. B., 1882; A. M., 1885, Dickinson; M. D., 1887, Columbian.

462. ARTHUR JOSEPH HALL—Born March 7, 1858, St. Louis, Mo. M. D., 1886, Columbian. Son of Samuel K. and Massie D. Hall. Educated in public schools of St. Louis and Warrensburg, Mo. 1882-1891, was in Government Printing Office, Washington; since then has practiced medicine in Washington. Member Med. Assn., D. C.; A. M. A.; Amer. Therap. Society; Secretary, Therap. Society, Washington. Married.

463. NEIL FERGUSON GRAHAM—Born Feb. 9, 1840, near London, Canada. M. D., 1861, Cleveland. Asst. Surg. and Surgeon, 12th Ohio Vols., and Surgeon, U. S. Vols. Father of N. D. Graham, *infra*. Of Scotch descent. Son of Duncan C. and Mary Graham. Educated at county school, afterwards at Bailey's Academy, London. Taught school until 1859. Was Resident Physician one year, U. S. Marine Hospital, Cleveland; July 13, 1862, was appointed Asst. Surgeon, 12th Ohio Vols.; promoted to Surgeon, Dec. 28, 1862. Served in Peninsular Campaign and battles of Manassas, Bull Run and Falls Church, Va., and in campaign in Maryland and West Virginia; established Seminary Hospital, Clarksburg, W. Va. On detached service a long time as Brigade Surgeon. Was twice captured by the enemy—at Bull Run in August, 1862, and Cloyd's Mountain, W. Va., May, 1864. Mustered out with regiment, July 11, 1864. About Aug. 1, 1864, was appointed Acting Staff Surgeon; in charge of large general field hospital, Sandy Hook, Md. (afterward removed to Harper's Ferry, W. Va., as the Island Hospital), until August, 1865. Served also as Surgeon-in-Chief of Military District of Harper's Ferry. Practiced medicine two years at Xenia, Ohio. In summer of 1867 removed to Minnesota and practiced at Faribault until 1872. Was then appointed Asst. Med. Referee, U. S. Bureau of Pensions, Washington, and Examining Surgeon for Pensions. Resigned as Referee in 1885, since which has practiced medicine in Washington. Is married. Prof. Surgery, 1872 to 1902, Howard Med. College; member Med. Assn., D. C., and Military Order, Loyal Legion. See Who's Who in America; Lamb's History, p. 119; Powell's History; Powell's Officers of Army and Navy, 1893, p. 342; Amer. Biog. Direct., Washington, 1908.

464. FREDERICK SOHON—Born Dec. 29, 1866, D. C. Educated in public schools; in High School was commanding officer of cadet corps. M. D., Georgetown, 1888. Was Resident Physician, Emergency Hospital. In 1890, took special course, Univ. Vienna, and attended clinics in other European cities. Returning home, was appointed for two years First Asst. at Throat and Chest clinic, Central Dispensary, and Instructor in Physical Diagnosis at Georgetown Med. School. Was medically in the auxiliary expeditions of Commander Peary to Arctic regions, 1897, 1903, 1905. Member A. M. A.; Med. Assn., D. C.; Med. Society, Georgetown Med. School; Med. and Surg. Society, D. C.

OCTOBER 8, 1890

465. EDWARD ARTHUR BALLOCH—Born Jan. 2, 1857, Great Falls, N. H. A. B., 1877; A. M., 1891, Princeton; M. D., 1879, Howard. Son of George W. Balloch, late Brigadier General, U. S. Vols. Has resided in Washington since 1866; attended public and private schools. Since graduation in medicine has practiced in Washington. Married in June, 1886. Member Med. Assn., D. C.; Wash. Acad. Sciences; ex-President Alumni, Howard Med. School. Sometime Examining Surgeon for Pensions; Attending Surgeon, Freedmen's and Sibley Hospitals. Served in the chairs of Practical Anatomy, 1880-4; Microscopy, 1884-6; Minor Surgery, 1890-2; Med. Jurisprudence, 1891-5, and Surgery, since 1895, Howard Med. School. See Lamb's History, p. 123.

466. WILLIAM HENRY FOX—Born Nov. 18, 1857, D. C. A. B., 1877; A. M., 1891, Princeton. M. D., 1884, Columbian.

467. FRANCIS XAVIER DOOLEY—Born May 11, 1841, D. C. M. D., 1865, Georgetown. Also Druggist in D. C. Dropped, 1894, from membership.

468. EDWARD OLIVER BELT—Born May 19, 1861, Rock Hall, Frederick Co., Md. M. D., 1886, Univ., Maryland. Licentiate M. C. F., Maryland. Killed in railroad accident, Dec. 30, 1906. [Son of John Lloyd and Sarah Eleanor McGill Belt; descendant of Hon. Wm. Burgess who founded South River, Md., and was member of State Council, Deputy Governor, Justice of High Provincial Court and General of the Military forces of the province.] Attended public schools of Frederick and Montgomery counties, and Frederick College, Maryland. Studied medicine with his brother, Dr. Alfred M. Belt, of Baltimore. Practiced medicine a few months in Frederick Co., then for two years was Resident Physician, Presbyterian Eye, Ear and Throat Hospital, Baltimore. Afterward studied ophthalmology and otology, Univ. Vienna and hospitals of Paris, Berlin and London; next took post-graduate course in Histology and Pathology at Johns Hopkins Univ., Baltimore, and was Visiting Surgeon to the above mentioned hospital. In October, 1889, removed to Washington, where he afterwards practiced his specialty. Member Med. Assn., D. C.; Society of Ophthalmology and Otology, Washington, of which he was President; A. M. A.; the originator and one of the organizers of the Episcopal Eye, Ear and Throat Hospital, Washington, and Surgeon and Executive Officer to the same. Ophthalmologist and Otologist, Freedmen's Hospital, D. C., and Baltimore and Ohio R. R.; Consulting Ophthalmologist to City and Emergency Hospitals, Frederick, Md.; Prof. Ophthalmology and Otology, Howard Med. School. May 18, 1899, married Emily Walker Norvell. See Minutes Med. Society, Jan. 16, 1907; Wash. Med. Annals, 1907-8, VI, p. 53; Watson's Biog., 1896, p. 103; Lamb's History, p. 129; Amer. Biog. Direct., Washington, 1908; Cordell's Med. Annals, Maryland, 1903, p. 317; Univ. Maryland, p. 392.

469. RICHARD SMITH HILL—Born July 9, 1864, Prince George Co., Md. M. D., 1886, Georgetown. Dropped, 1897, from membership. Removed, 1898, to Upper Marlboro, Md., and retired from practice.

470. THOMAS BEAL HOOD—Born March 19, 1829, Fairview, Ohio. A. M., 1874, Ohio Wesleyan Univ.; M. D., 1862, Western Reserve, Cleveland; 1865, Univ. Maryland. Asst. Surg., 76th Ohio; Asst. Surg., and Surg., U. S. Vols; Acting Asst. Surg., U. S. A.; Medical Referee, U. S. Pension Bureau. Died March 15, 1900. Son of Dr. James Hood. Educated at Seminary at Blendon, Robinson's High School, West Rushville, and Ohio Wesleyan Univ., Delaware, Ohio. Next attended Med. Dept., Univ. Maryland, one course; then practiced medicine with his father, at Gratiot, Ohio, afterwards at Columbus, North Lewisburg and Newark, Ohio. Served, 1861-3, at Ft. Donelson, Shiloh, Corinth; resigned in 1863 because of illness, was recommissioned in 1864 and served as Attending Physician to sick and wounded officers, New York City, 1864-5, and in charge of Hospital Transport on the Potomac river, and at the close of the war, dismantled the hospitals of the Army of the Potomac. Surgeon in Chief, Division of Mississippi, 1865-6. Afterwards resumed practice at Newark, Ohio; 1867 to 1874, was Assistant in Provost Marshal General's Office, Washington, and 1874-1885, Med. Referee, U. S. Pension Bureau; Examining Surgeon of Pensions, 1872-1893; member Med. Assn., D. C.; Military Order Loyal Legion; Director, Ohio National Bank, Washington; Prof. Anatomy, Howard Med. School, 1870-1; of Practice of Medicine, 1877-91; Dean of Faculty, 1881-1900. Married, 1850, Margaret, daughter of Samuel Winegarner; June, 1854, Mary, widow of Dr. Eliphalet Hyde, of Columbus, Ohio, and daughter of Wm. C. Boggs. See Minutes Med. Society, March 21 and 28, 1900; Trans Med. Society, 1900, V, p. 60; Lamb's History, p. 115; Nat. Med. Review, 1900-1, p. 156.

APRIL 1, 1891

471. JOSEPH THEOPHILUS DAVIDSON HOWARD—Son of Dr.
J. T. Howard, *supra*. Born Nov. 20, 1866, D. C. M. D., 1889, George-
town. Resigned, Nov. 20, 1901. Removed to Shiloh, N. J., then to
Falls Church, Va. Sometime in the Indian service.

472. CHARLES KNELLER KOONES—Born Oct. 24, 1866, Richmond, Va. M. D., 1887, Columbian.

473. JOHN DUNCAN McKIM—Born Jan. 4, 1864, Staunton, Va.
M. D., 1886, Univ. Va. Died April 23, 1892, of consumption. See Minutes Med. Society, April 27 and May 4, 1892.

474. WILLIAM HOLLAND WILMER—Born Aug. 26, 1863, Pow-
hatan Co., Va. M. D., 1885, Univ. Va. Interne, Mt. Sinai Hospital,
New York, 1885-7; Lecturer on Ophthalmology, New York Polyclinic,
1887-9; one of the attending Ophthalmologists to Bellevue Hospital, out-
door department, 1887-9; Prof. Ophthalmology, Georgetown Med.
School; Attending Ophthalmologist, Episcopal Eye, Ear and Throat
Hospital, and Emergency and Garfield Hospitals, Washington. Member
Amer. Ophthalmol. Society; A. M. A.; Society Ophthalmologists and
Otologists, Washington; Clinico-Patholog. Society, D. C.; Hereditary
Member, Society Cincinnati.

475. LOUIS KELLY BEATTY—Born Jan. 31, 1857, in Iowa. M. D.,
1881, Columbian.

476. JOSEPH LACY BRAYSHAW—Born Jan. 21, 1855, Wethered-
ville, Md. M. D., 1888, College Phys. and Surg., Baltimore. Dropped,
1897, from membership; reëlected, Oct. 6, 1897; dropped again, 1900.
Removed to Parole, Anne Arundel Co., Md.

477. GEORGE JOHN LOCHBOEHLER—Born April 18, 1865, St.
Louis, Mo. Phar. D., 1884, National College Pharmacy, D. C.; M. D.,
1889, Georgetown.

478. WILLIAM KENNEDY BUTLER—Born March 7, 1857, D. C.
A. M., 1879; M. D., 1882, Columbian. Son of Rev. Dr. J. G. Butler. In
charge of Lutheran Eye and Ear Infirmary.

479. ROBERT MAITLAND ELLYSON—Born Jan. 1, 1862, Petersburg, Va. M. D., 1888, Columbian. Resigned Jan. 24, 1900.

480. ARTHUR SNOWDEN—Born Aug. 8, 1862, in Virginia. M. D.,
1883, Jefferson. Resigned Oct. 9, 1895, and removed to Alexandria, Va.

481. WILLIAM T. GILL—Born Feb. 17, 1865, in Kentucky. M. D., 1887, Columbian.

OCTOBER 7, 1891

482. CLIFTON MAYFIELD—Born Feb. 6, 1858, D. C. M. D., 1880, Columbian. Sometime Surgeon, Metropolitan Police; President, 1905-6, Med. Assn., D. C. Resigned from Society, Oct. 7, 1908, and removed to Canarsie, L. I., N. Y.

483. EDMUND LEE TOMPKINS—Born Nov. 18, 1862, Richmond, Va. M. D., 1885, Univ. Va. Resigned Nov. 11, 1903. Removed to Fine Creek Mills, Va.

484. WILLIAM SINCLAIR BOWEN—Born June 14, 1866, Woodville, Prince George Co., Md. Graduated, 1883, Charlotte Hall, Md. M. D., 1888, Univ. Maryland.

485. LOUIS MACKALL, JR.—Born Nov. 25, 1867, D. C. Son of Dr. Louis Mackall, *supra.* M. D., 1890, Columbian. President, Med. Assn., D. C., 1908-9.

486. JOHN FRANCIS PRICE—Born Nov. 23, 1850, Charles Co., Md. M. D., 1875, Washington Univ., Baltimore. Died Nov. 17, 1903, Denver, Colo. Practiced at his Maryland home, 1875 to 1890, when he removed to Washington, where he continued to practice. In 1901 he contracted influenza, on which tuberculosis supervened. See Minutes Med. Society, Nov. 18 and Dec. 2, 1903; Wash. Med. Annals, 1903-4, II, p. 486.

487. JAMES FOSTER SCOTT—Born Jan. 22, 1863, India. A. B., 1884, Yale; M. D., 1888, Edinburgh. Author of Sexual instinct, N. Y., 1899.

488. B. ASHBOURNE CAPEHART—Born April 2, 1865, near Edenton, N. C. M. D., 1886, Univ. Maryland. Dropped from membership, 1904. Died Dec. 20, 1904, New York City. He studied about two years in hospitals in Vienna and Berlin. Married, November, 1898, Mrs. Palmer, great granddaughter of Chancellor Kent, of New York. Practiced about one year in the Bermudas.

489. AMELIA ERBACH—Born Aug. 22, 1860, D. C. M. D., 1889, Columbian.

490. JOHN THOMAS KELLEY, JR.—Born Dec. 7, 1863, D. C. M. D., 1890, Columbian. Gynecologist, Providence Hospital; Associate at Georgetown Univ. Hospital.

22

491. CHARLES W BROWN—Born Oct. 11, 1846, Wyalusing, Pa. M. D., 1871, Long Island Med. College. Son of Daniel Warren and Catharine King Brown. Educated in public schools. Studied medicine with Dr. C. V. Elliott, Mansfield, Pa. After graduation practiced in Mansfield five years; while there, served as Trustee of State Normal School. Removed to Elmira, N. Y., in 1877 and practiced there until he came to Washington, in 1890. Was Physician to Elmira, N. Y., State Reformatory; Surgeon for D., L. & W. R. R.; Health Officer of Elmira two terms; member Tioga Co., Pa., Medical Society (Sec'y and Pres't); Penna. State Medical Society; Chemung Co., N. Y., Med. Society; Secretary, Elmira Acad. Medicine; one of the founders N. Y. State Med. Assn.; Secretary and President, Third District Branch of same; member A. M. A. since 1872; Med. Assn., D. C.; Lecturer on Surgery, Nurses' Training School, Sibley Hospital, Washington. Married Mary E. Elliott, of Mansfield, Pa., Jan. 1, 1866. See Amer. Biog. Direct., Washington, 1908.

492. ELMER HEZEKIAH SOTHORON—Born Oct. 13, 1868, D. C. Son of Dr. J. T. Sothoron, *supra*. B. A., 1887, Ashland College, Ohio. M. D., 1890, Bellevue. Member Med. Assn., D. C.; A. M. A.; ex-President, Med. and Surg. Society, D. C.; member Wash. Obstet. and Gynecol. Society; Examining Surgeon, Bureau of Pensions. See Lamb's History, p. 262.

493. CHARLES HENRY STOWELL—Born Oct. 27, 1850, Perry, N. Y. M. D., 1872, Univ. Mich. Removed, Oct. 1897, to Lowell, Mass. Co-editor, The Microscope, Ann Arbor, Mich., 1881-8. Editor of Trained Motherhood, Food and Practical Medicine. Editor and publisher, National Medical Review, Washington. Author of The student's manual of histology, etc., Detroit, 1881. A healthy body, N. Y., 1892; Primer of health, N. Y., 1894; Essentials of health, N. Y., 1898; The microscopic structure of a human tooth, etc., Ann Arbor, 1888; Stowell and Stowell, Microscopical diagnosis, Detroit, 1882. Son of David P. Stowell. Educated at Genesee Wesleyan Seminary, 1868. After graduation in medicine was Prof. Histology and Microscopy, Univ. Michigan. Practiced medicine in Washington, 1885-97. See Who's Who in America; Appleton's Biog., 1889, V, p. 715.

494. FAYETTE CLAY EWING—Born May 28, 1862, La Fourche Parish, La. M. D., 1884, Jefferson. Removed, about 1890, to Kansas City, Mo. Educated at Univ. of the South, Sewanee, Tenn., and at Univ. Mississippi, at Oxford. After graduation in medicine spent one year at clinics at Charity Hospital, New Orleans. Practiced medicine in Washington till 1892. Then for six months attended New York Polyclinic and Metropolitan Throat Hosp. Removed with his family to London, England, 1893. Attended London Post-Graduate School, Laryngeal and Chest Diseases. Served one year as Clinical Asst. at Central London Throat and Ear Hosp. and London Throat Hosp.; Asst. Surg. on Staff of the latter. Later attended clinics in Vienna. Began the practice of Oto-laryngology, exclusively, in St. Louis in 1893. Was delegate, 1894, from Amer. Med. Assn. to Internat. Med. Congress, Madrid, Spain. In 1899 Delegate from West. Acad. Oto-laryngology, to Internat. Otolog. Congress, London, England ; was Vice Pres. said Society, 1900 ; late Fellow Brit. Rhinol., Laryngol. and Otol. Assn. ; original Fellow Royal Society Med., Great Britain ; was Abstract Editor, The Laryngoscope, St. Louis, for eight years. On staff of various hospitals, St. Louis. Trustee, Univ. of the South. See Who's Who in America; Tri-State Med. Jour., St. Louis, 1897, IV, p. 379.

495. GEORGE ALBERT COGGESHALL—Born March 17, 1843, Portsmouth, R. I. A. M., 1866, Trinity College, Hartford, Conn. M. D., 1879, Bellevue. Removed, 1893, to Oxford, N. C., thence, 1900, to Henderson, N. C.

APRIL 6, 1892

496. WILLIAM CHARLES FOWLER—Born Nov. 24, 1864, D. C. M. D., 1888, Georgetown. Chief Inspector, Health Office, Washington. See Lamb's History, p. 243.

497. JOHN SPEED McLAIN—Born Aug. 9, 1848, D. C. M. D., 1871, Columbian. Acting Asst. Surgeon, U. S. A. Died June 2, 1907. Son of Rev. Wm. and Maria Louisa Mosby McLain. Educated at Rittenhouse Academy, Washington, and by private tutors. After graduation in medicine practiced in Washington for three years; House Surgeon at Providence Hospital in 1873. In 1874, appointed Acting Asst. Surg., U. S. A., and served with 8th U. S. Cavalry in New Mexico ; participated in many expeditions into the Pan Handle of Texas, the "Staked Plains," Indian Territory, and Colorado. Crossed the Rio Grande into Mexico to check cattle stealing. Afterwards served at military posts in Texas till 1879. Was Medical Officer and Botanist in the expedition to survey and explore the country west of the Pecos river, Texas. Continued to serve in Texas and Kansas till 1882, when yellow fever broke out along the Rio Grande; had charge of yellow fever camp. Retired from service Nov. 18, 1883, returned to Washington and resumed practice. Prof. Toxicology, Med. Dept., National University, Washington. Sometime President, Board of Med. Supervisors, Washington ; member Med. Association, D. C.; Therapeutic Society, Washington ; Amer. Med. Association. Unmarried. See Stone's Biog., 1894, p. 308 ;

Who's Who in America; Amer. Biog. Direct., Washington, 1908; Minutes Med. Society, Oct. 2, 1907; Wash. Med. Annals, 1907, VI, p. 393.

498. JEANNETTE JUDSON SUMNER—Born Nov. 15, 1846, Constantine, Mich. Daughter of Dr. Watson and Hester Ann Welling Sumner. M. D., 1883, Woman's Med. College, Philadelphia. Dues remitted, Jan. 16, 1895, because of continued illness. Died Nov. 12, 1906.

499. CHARLES GRANVILLE STONE—Born Nov. 30, 1846, Frederick Co., Md. M. D., 1872, Univ. Maryland. Son of Wm. H. and Cornelia D. Norris Stone—the Stones from Virginia, the Norrises from Maryland. Educated in private schools in Maryland. Studied dentistry with his brother, Dr. Llewellyn Stone, of Baltimore; afterwards medicine with Profs. Miles and Chisholm, of Baltimore. Since graduation has practiced in Washington. Sometime Physician to the Poor; Physician to B. and O. R. R. Co. Relief Association; Surgeon to Brightwood Electric R. R. Co., and Washington R. R. and Electric Co. One of the Directors Casualty Hospital. Member Med. Assn. D. C.; A. M. A.; and Washington Board of Trade. Married, in 1870, Dora L. Higgins; in 1883, Mary Florence Rapley. See Univ. Maryland, 1907, II, p. 348.

500. JAMES JOSEPH CARROLL—Born April 14, 1858, D. C. B. S., 1875, St. John's College, Annapolis, Md.; M. D., 1877, Columbian. Acting Asst. Surg., U. S. A. Died Nov. 5, 1899. See Minutes Med. Society, Nov. 8 and 15, 1899; Trans. Med. Society, IV, 1899, pp. 173 and 181; Nat. Med. Review, 1899-1900, IX, p. 538.

501. ARTHUR CARLOS MERRIAM—Born July 27, 1866, D. C. Son of Dr. E. C. Merriam, *supra*. M. D., 1889, Columbian.

502. CHARLES READ COLLINS—Born Feb. 6, 1862, King George, Va. M. D., 1884, Jefferson.

503. WILLIAM J. DILLENBACK—Born Jan. 30, 1865, N. Y. M. D., 1888, Columbian.

504. IDA JOHANNA HEIBERGER—Born in Washington. M. D., 1885, Woman's Med. College, Philadelphia. One of the founders Woman's Clinic, Washington.

505. JOHN FRANCIS MORAN—Born June 8, 1864, D. C. A. B., 1894; M. D., 1887, Georgetown. Demonstrator of Anatomy, 1891-6; Clinical Prof. Obstetrics, 1896-1900; Prof. Obstetrics, 1900-6, Georgetown Med. School. Obstetrician Columbia Hospital, 1896-1900, and

Georgetown Univ. Hospital, 1900–6. Member Washington Acad. Sciences ; Obstet. and Gynecol. Society, Washington ; Southern Surg. and Gynecol. Assn.; Med. and Surg. Society, Washington. Contributor to Peterson's "Practice of Obstetrics."

506. ISAAC SCOTT STONE—Born March 1, 1851, Sandy Spring, Md. M. D., 1872; Sc. D., 1907, Univ. Maryland. Son of James H. and Martha A. Scott Stone. Educated at Academy, Wilmington, Del., and public schools of Maryland. After graduation in medicine pursued his medical studies in New York City and London, England. Practiced in Virginia and Washington. Prof. Gynecology, Georgetown Med. School, 1892 ; Surgeon to Columbia Hospital for Women and Georgetown Univ. Hospital. Member Wash. Acad. Sciences ; Amer. Gynecolog. Society ; Washington Gynecolog. Society ; A. M. A. ; A. A. A. S. One of the founders Southern Surg. and Gynecolog. Assn. Life member British Gynecol. Society. Married, Nov. 16, 1875, Thomasin J. Taylor, of Virginia. See Who's Who in America ; Amer. Biog. Direct., Washington, 1908 ; Univ. Maryland, 1907, II, p. 349.

507. JOHNSON ELIOT, JR.—Born May 6, 1868, D. C. Son of Dr. Johnson Eliot, *supra*. Graduated, 1886, St. John's College, Washington. A. M., Gonzaga, 1908; M. D., 1890, Georgetown.

OCTOBER 5, 1892

508. FRANCIS ALPHONZO ST. CLAIR—Born July 21, 1861, Albion, N. Y. Phar. D., 1886, Nat. Coll. Pharmacy, D. C. ; M. D., 1890, Georgetown.

509. RICHARD ALOYSIUS NEALE—Born Oct. 15, 1850, D. C. Sometime in the drug business. M. D., 1870, Georgetown. Ward Physician several years. Removed, 1896, to Chicago, Ill.

510. STEUART BROWN MUNCASTER—Born Sept. 16, 1857, D. C. Brother of Dr. Magruder Muncaster, *supra*. M. D., 1885, Georgetown. Licentiate, M. C. F., Maryland, 1892. Practices in Washington. See Cordell's Med. Annals, Maryland, 1903, p. 513.

511. JOSHUA LAMBERT DULANEY—Born Sept. 12, 1838, Baltimore, Md. Asst. Surgeon, C. S. A. M. D., 1868, Univ. Maryland. Resigned Jan. 27, 1908.

512. HENRY LOUIS HAYES—Born Feb. 17, 1867, Brooklyn, N. Y. M. D., 1890, Georgetown. Resigned Jan. 23, 1901, and removed to Hilo, Hawaii.

513. WILLIAM PHILLIPS CARR—Born May 10, 1858, Boydton, Va. M. D., 1888, Columbian. President, 1896-7, Medical Assn., D. C. Father of Dr. W. B. Carr, *infra*. Son of Prof. Wm. B. and Laura Phillips Carr. Educated at Leesburg, Va., Academy, 1870-4; Randolph-Macon College, 1874-6. Was Prof. Physiology, Columbian Univ., D. C.; Prosector and Lecturer on Anatomy in same, 1896-9; sometime Coroner, D. C.; Surgeon, Metropolitan Police and Fire Dept.; Surgeon to Emergency Hospital and University Hospital, Washington; Consulting Surgeon, Wash. Asylum Hosp. and Govt. Hosp. Insane, D. C.; member Med. Assn., D. C.; Wash. Obstet. and Gynecol. Society; Wash. Acad. Sciences; Med. and Surg. Society, D. C.; A. M. A.; Virginia Med. Society; A. A. A. S.; Assn. Amer. Anatomists; Fellow Southern Surg. and Gynecol. Assn. Married at Hamilton, Va., Feb. 15, 1883, Georgia O. Carter. See Who's Who in America; Amer. Men of Science, 1906; Amer. Biog. Direct., Washington, 1908.

514. ROBERT EDMOND HENNING—Born Jan. 22, 1864, D. C. M. D., 1885, Georgetown. Resigned Aug. 31, 1893, and removed to Cheriton, Va.

515. JOSEPH N. GARDNER—Born Feb. 24, 1860, D. C. M. D., 1889, Univ. Maryland. Removed to Baltimore, Md. Dropped, 1895, from membership.

516. WILLIAM CREIGHTON WOODWARD—Born Dec. 11, 1867, D. C. M. D., 1889; LL. B., 1899; LL. M., 1900, Georgetown. Son of Mark Rittenhouse and Martha Jane Pursell Woodward, of Washington. Educated in public schools of Washington; graduated from High School in 1885. Employed in Washington Post Office, 1886-91. Resident Physician, Central Dispensary and Emergency Hospital, 1892; Physician to the Poor, 1893. July 20, 1893, appointed Coroner, D. C. Since Aug. 1, 1894, Health Officer, D. C.; Secretary to Board of Medical Supervisors, D. C., for some years. Prof. State Medicine, Georgetown, Columbian and Howard Medical Schools; Prof. Med. Jurisprudence, Georgetown Law School. Member Med. Assn., D. C.; A. M. A.; Amer. Public Health Assn; Washington Board of Trade. Married, Feb. 14, 1895, Ray Elliott, daughter of Alexander and Mary Lavinia Scaggs Elliott. See Who's Who in America; Amer. Biog. Direct., Washington, 1908; History City of Washington, 1903, p. 76.

517. DANIEL KERFOOT SHUTE—Born Oct. 22, 1858, Alexandria, Va. A. B., 1879; M. D., 1883, Columbian. Son of Samuel Moore and Jane Cecilia Kerfoot Shute. After graduation in medicine took post-graduate course in Ophthalmology at Royal London Ophthalmic Hospital and Univ. Berlin, Germany. Acting Clinical Asst. at London Hospital, 1891. Prosector to Chair of Anatomy, Columbian College Med. School, Washington, 1886-7; Lecturer on Anatomy, 1887-8; Prof. Anatomy since 1888; Consulting Ophthalmologist, Univ. Hospital, Central Dispensary and Emergency Hospital, Providence Hospital, Columbia Hospital and Govt. Hosp. Insane, D. C. Ex-President, Wash. Society Ophthalmologists and Otologists. Member Med. Assn., D. C.; Wash. Acad. Sciences; Wash. Anthropolog. Society; Clinico-Path. Society, Washington; Microscop. Society, Washington; A. M. A.; A. A. A. S.; Assn. Amer. Anatomists; Society of Cincinnati (hereditary member). Author of A first book in organic evolution, Chicago, 1899. Contributor to Reference Handbook Med. Sciences. Married, at Waltham, Mass., Aug. 19, 1896, Augusta Pettigrew. See Who's Who in America; Amer. Men of Science, 1906; Amer. Biog. Direct., Washington, 1908.

518. JAMES HENRY MORGAN BARBER—Born Aug. 4, 1866, Yates Hope, Md. M. D., 1888, Georgetown.

519. JOHN EDGAR WALSH—Born March 16, 1865, D. C. M. D., 1890, Columbian. Son of John J. and Elizabeth Walsh. Educated in public schools, Washington, and St. John's College, Annapolis, Md. Was Physician-Surgeon to Peary Relief Expedition, 1895. Resident Physician, Wash. Asylum Hospital; Attending Physician, St. Ann's Infant Asylum; Bacteriologist and Med. Sanitary Inspector, D. C., since 1895. Invented a lock system for mail boxes and a safety watch-guard device. Married, Nov. 4, 1897, Florence Butler. See Amer. Biog. Direct., Washington, 1908.

APRIL 5, 1893

520. JEFFERSON DAVIS BRADFIELD—Born Feb. 8, 1868, Fauquier Co., Va. Phar. D., 1886, Virginia Board of Pharmacy; M. D., 1891, Georgetown. Son of Cornelius Henry and Annie Elizabeth Holmes Bradfield. Educated in private and public schools, Alexandria, Va. Practiced pharmacy until 1891. Married, Dec. 27, 1893, Flora Johnson. See Georgetown University, II, p. 257.

521. FRANCIS SMITH NASH—Born Nov. 23, 1854, Virginia. A. B., 1876, Hampden-Sidney; M. D., 1877, Univ. Va. Asst. Surgeon, Passed Asst. Surgeon, U. S. Navy. Resigned from Society, May 3, 1905. See Hamersly's Officers of Navy, 1890, p. 279.

522. JOHN VAN RENSSELAER—Born April 4, 1862, Belleville, N. J. A. B., 1882; A. M., 1886, Hobart College, N. Y.; M. D., 1889, Columbian.

523. ALBERT EUGENE JOHNSON—Born Dec. 9, 1840, Cooperstown, N. Y. M. D., 1869, Columbian.

524. SAMUEL LUNT HANNON—Born Sept. 22, 1858, Pomonkey, Charles Co., Md. M. D., 1888, Columbian. Acting Asst. Surgeon, U. S. A., in war with Spain. Dropped from membership, 1901. Removed to La Plata, Md. Son of Charles E. and Elizabeth H. Lunt Hannon [daughter of Samuel H. Lunt, Alexandria, Va.]. Educated at Henry School and Potomac Academy, Alexandria. Engaged sometime in pharmacy. During yellow fever epidemic of 1876-7 was in drug stores in Memphis, Tenn., and Paris, Texas; and in drug store, Washington, from 1879 to about 1883. Was awarded a scholarship, 1885, in Columbian Med. College, Washington. On House Staff, Children's Hospital, Washington, 1885-9, and Garfield Hospital, 1888. Physician to Emergency Hospital, 1891-3. Surgeon at Fort Stevens, North Dakota, in the Indian Bureau, 1889-90. Member of Society of Physicians and Surgeons to the Poor, Washington. Married, Sept. 5, 1881, Hollie E. Hutton, Alexandria, daughter of George Hutton, Liverpool, England. See Watson's Biog., 1896, p. 612.

525. MAYNE MARSHALL PILE—Born Sept. 10, 1850, Somerset, Pa. M. D., 1884, Woman's Med. College, Baltimore.

526. RUFUS DELBERT BOSS—Born April 19, 1861, Riley, Mich. M. D., 1891, Columbian. Acting Asst. Surgeon, U. S. A., in war with Spain. Removed, 1901, to Wacousta, Mich.

527. FREDERICH EDWARD MAXCY—Born May 15, 1853, Gardiner, Me. M. D., 1879, Bowdoin. Died Dec. 25, 1908. Son of Ira and Sarah A. Fuller Maxcy. Educated in the public schools of Gardiner; graduated from the High School, Westbrook (Maine) Seminary, and Cooper Institute, N. Y. City. In 1880 was Interne at Maine General Hospital, Portland. Practiced in Saco, Me., 1881-91, then removed to Washington, D. C. Member, Med. Assn., D. C. Lecturer, Nurses' Training School, Freedmen's Hospital, Washington; Clinical Lecturer, Practice of Medicine, Howard Med. School. Married, Jan. 18, 1883, Estelle A. Gilpatric, of Saco, Me. See Lamb's History, p. 139; Minutes Med. Society, Jan. 20 and 27, 1908 ; Wash. Med. Annals, 1909, p. 71.

528. JOHN HENRY McCORMICK—Born March 25, 1870, D. C. M. D., 1891, National Univ., D. C. Son of John H. and Julia A. McCormick. Educated in public schools and Georgetown College, Washington. Married, in Washington, Sept. 16, 1890, Aimee Sioussat. Was Asst. Surgeon, Johns Hopkins Univ. Med. School, 1891-2 ; Prof. Natural

Sciences, Mt. Vernon Seminary, Washington, 1890–1; and Washington Seminary, 1892–6; Secy., Anthropolog. Society, Washington, 1893–1900; Asst. Secy., Amer. Folk-Lore Society; Asso. Editor, Amer. Antiquarian, 1894–1896. Practiced medicine, Washington, 1890–1904; Secy., 8th Internat. Geograph. Congress, 1904. See Who's Who in America.

529. CHARLES MILTON BUCHANAN—Born Oct. 11, 1868, Alexandria, Va. M. D., 1890, National Univ., D. C. Removed, October, 1894, to Tulalip, Washington. Superintendent of Indian Agency.

530. JOHN WILLIAM CHAPPELL—Born Nov. 22, 1855, D. C. B. S., 1877; M. D., 1881, Columbian. Member Med. Assn., D. C.; Amer. Therapeutic Society; Montgomery Co., Md., Med. Society, and M. C. F., Maryland. Ex-President Therapeutic Society, D. C., and President, 1906–7, of George Washington Univ. Med. Society.

531. WILLIAM PENN COMPTON—Born Aug. 23, 1865, Maryland. M. D., 1889, Georgetown.

532. FRANK TENNEY CHAMBERLIN—Born Dec. 19, 1863, D. C. Son of Dr. J. A. Chamberlin, *supra*. Educated at Georgetown College and St. John's Academy, Alexandria, Va. M. D., 1885, Georgetown. Sometime Prof. Laryngology, Georgetown Med. School. Resident Student, Washington Asylum Hospital, 1881. After graduation in medicine studied in Paris and Vienna. About 1887 became Assistant at Central Dispensary, and sometime afterward aided in founding the Eastern Dispensary. Member Med. Assn., D. C.; A. M. A.; Med. and Surg. Society; Wash. Board of Trade; President San Juan Battista Mining Co., Sonora, Mexico. Sometime First Lieut., 3d Va. Nat. Guard. Married, July 25, 1888, Nannie Lee Naylor. See Georgetown University, II, p. 235.

533. JOHN BENJAMIN BAGGETT—Born Sept. 3, 1844, Mississippi. M. D., 1869, Wash. Univ., Baltimore. Dropped from membership, 1897.

OCTOBER 4, 1893

534. JAMES ALOYSIUS MALONEY—Born Feb. 24, 1846, Baltimore, Md. M. D., 1891, Columbian. Died Oct. 29, 1897. See Minutes Med. Society, Nov. 3, 1897; Watson's Biog., 1896, p. 620.

535. FLOYD VERNON BROOKS—Born Jan. 25, 1856, Newark, N. J. M. D., 1877, Jefferson. Son of James J. (sometime Chief of Secret Service, U. S. Treasury Dept.) and Maria Brooks. Educated in public schools, Philadelphia, Pa. Is Chief Surgeon, Chesapeake Beach R. R. Member Med. Assn., D. C. Married Ada Florence Ash, of Evans City, Pa. See Amer. Biog. Direct., Washington, 1908.

536. GEORGE HENDERSON—Born Aug. 6, 1843, Galena, Ill. M. D., 1885, Howard. Major and Surgeon General, National Guard, D. C., since Dec. 22, 1890. [Grandson of William Henderson, of Aberdeen, Scotland; son of George Henderson, who served in the Indian Wars of the West, having removed from Philadelphia to Wisconsin while it was yet a Territory, and Jemima Haslet, granddaughter of Colonel John Haslet, of Delaware (a personal friend of General Washington), and who was killed at the battle of Princeton, N. J., Jan. 3, 1777, while leading the 1st Delaware regiment. His only son, Joseph Haslet, commanded a regiment of Delaware troops in the War of 1812, and was severely wounded; afterward was twice Governor of Delaware.] Attended public schools and Page's Academy, Lancaster, Wis. Aug. 15, 1861, enlisted in 7th Wis. Vols., one of the regiments of the "Iron Brigade," Army of Potomac. Was twice wounded in second battle of Bull Run and severely wounded at South Mountain, one month later, for which he was discharged from service, Oct. 25, 1862. Since graduation has practiced in Washington. Member Med. Assn., D. C.; A. M. A.; Assn. U. S. Military Surgeons. Author of Preservation of health, etc., Washington. Married, September, 1871, to Miss Mary C. Eels. See Lamb's History, p. 178.

537. CHARLES RICHARD CLARK—Born Nov. 17, 1862, Cuyler, N. Y. M. D., 1889, Columbian. Removed, 1896, to Warsaw, N. Y. In 1898 gave up the practice of medicine because of ill health, and was appointed Post Office Inspector. Removed to San Antonio, Texas.

538. HENRY SKINNER GOODALL—Born May 28, 1866, Greensboro, Vt. A. B., 1887, Williams; M. D., 1890, Columbian. Removed, December, 1895, to Charlemont, Mass., thence to Lake Kushagee, N. Y.

539. FRANK LEECH—Born Jan. 14, 1870, Prince George Co., Md. M. D., 1891, Columbian. Brother of Dr. D. O. Leech, *supra*.

540. CLARENCE RUTER DUFOUR—Born Jan. 1, 1853, Vevay, Indiana. Phar. D., 1873, National College Pharmacy, D. C.; M. D., 1890, Georgetown. He was brother of Dr. J. F. R. Dufour, of Maryland. Practiced pharmacy in Washington some years; afterwards practiced medicine. Has resided in Washington many years. Is married. Was Prof. Pharmacy and Botany, 1883 to 1896, Howard Medical School; Physician in Charge of Eye Dept., Eastern Dispensary; Ophthalmologist and

Otologist, Sibley Hospital; Instructor in Ophthalmol. and Otol., Georgetown Med. School; Chief of Eye and Ear Clinic, Georgetown Univ.
Hospital; Assistant in Eye and Ear Department, Emergency Hospital.

541. OSCAR ADDISON MACK McKIMMIE—Born March 13, 1868,
D. C. M. D., 1891, Columbian. Member Med. Assn., D. C.; Med. and
Surg. Society, D. C.; on Staff of Episcopal Eye, Ear and Throat Hospital.

542. HENRY PERCIVAL PARR THOMPSON—Born Oct. 21, 1868,
Hancock, Md. M. D., 1890, South Carolina Med. College. Resigned,
Jan. 21, 1903, and removed to Hillsboro, Va.

543. HOWARD CARLYLE RUSSELL—Born Sept. 25, 1868, D. C.
M. D., 1891, Univ. Penna. Asst. Surgeon, U. S. M. H. S. Died March
2, 1904, Stapleton, Staten Island.

544. HENRY LIDDELL—Born Dec. 3, 1843, Northumberland, England. M. D., 1891, National Univ., D. C. Removed, December, 1895, to
Brooklyn, N. Y. Son of Henry George and Barbara W. Greetham Liddell. Educated at Burdis Acad., King Edward VI Grammar School,
Newcastle-on-Tyne. Came to America in 1862; served in Nova Scotia
Militia, with rank of Captain, 1863-4; attached to U. S. Sanitary Commission, 1864-5. Married, Boston, 1887, Eva Louise Barnes. Traveled
extensively in Asia and Australia, 1865-82; in service of Japanese Government, 1873-9; attaché foreign military contingent, Shanghai, China,
1879-80; employed in U. S. War Department, 1889-93; made several
visits to extreme north of American Continent, Labrador and the waters
of Hudson's Bay. Member of various European and American scientific
societies. Author of Traces of prehistoric civilization in Australia, 1871-
01; The Islands of the Antarctic, 1873-01; The romance of morning
glory, 1875-01; A cruise toward the North Pole, 1905. See Who's Who
in America.

545. WADE HAMPTON ATKINSON—Born Nov. 4, 1866, Johnston
Co., N. C. M. D., 1889, Georgetown. Resident Physician, Central Dis-
pensary and Emergency Hospital. Member Med. Assn., D. C., and
Med. and Surg. Society, D. C.

APRIL 4, 1894

546. GEORGE NELSON PERRY—Born Oct. 12, 1850, Layman,
Ohio. M. D., 1884, Howard. Attended public schools and Bartlett
(Ohio) Academy and Mt. Union College, Alliance, Ohio. Since graduation has practiced medicine in Washington. Prof. Pediatrics, afterward Obstetrics, Howard Med. School. Married. See Lamb's History,
p. 126.

547. DANIEL BAEN STREET—Born March 10, 1842, Cambridge, Md. M. D., 1874, Georgetown. Father of Dr. Baen Street, *infra.*

548. CHARLES L. MINOR—Born May 10, 1865, Brooklyn, N. Y. M. D., 1888, Univ. Virginia. Removed, 1896, to Asheville, N. C. Director of National Assn. Study and Prevention Tuberculosis ; Vice Pres., Amer. Climatolog. Assn.

549. JOHN RYDER WELLINGTON—Born Oct. 28, 1865, Albion, Me. A. B., 1886; A. M., 1891, Colby; M. D., 1891, Columbian.

550. THOMAS NORRIS VINCENT—Born Nov. 29, 1866, D. C. A. B., 1885; A. M., 1891, Georgetown; M. D., 1889, Jefferson.

551. JOSEPH M. CARROLL—M. D., 1881, Univ. Maryland. Removed to Baltimore, 1896. Resigned from Med. Society, Jan. 20, 1897.

552. JOHN EDMUND TONER—Born March 14, 1859, Loudoun Co., Va. Phar. D., 1887, National College of Pharmacy, Washington ; M. D., 1891, Georgetown.

553. CORNELIUS BRECKENRIDGE BOYLE—Son of Dr. Cornelius Boyle, *supra.* Born June 24, 1864, Gordonsville, Va. M. D., 1891, Columbian. Removed, in 1896, to Hot Springs, S. D.; afterwards to Bozeman, Montana.

554. LARKIN WHITE GLAZEBROOK—Born July 28, 1867, Richmond, Va. M. D., 1890, College Phys. and Surg., N. Y., and Long Island College Hospital, Brooklyn. Son of Rev. Dr. Otis Allan and Virginia Calvert Key-Smith Glazebrook. Educated at Univ. of the South, Norwood's School, Richmond, Va., Episcopal High School, Va., and Univ. Virginia. Sometime Resident Physician, St. Luke's Hospital, South Bethlehem, Pa.; Attending Physician, Emergency Hospital, Washington ; Washington City Orphan Asylum ; Coroner's Physician, D. C., since 1903. Jan. 9, 1894, married Jane Threlkeld Cox. See Amer. Biog. Direct., Washington, 1908.

555. CHARLES VOLNEY PETTEYS—Born May 12, 1847, Palmyra, N. Y. Second Lieut., 138th N. Y. Vols. (Artillery). M. D., 1873, Georgetown. Acting Asst. Surgeon, U. S. A. Dropped from membership, 1898 ; reëlected, Oct. 1, 1902. Son of Martin D. and Jane A. Ketcham Petteys. Educated in country schools, New York, Union Academy, Wayne Co., N. Y., and Spencerian Business College, Washington, and by private instructor. Enlisted when 15 years old ; took part in the battles of the Wilderness and was at the attack on Washington ; was given a medal of honor for gallantry at battle of Cedar Creek, Va. In 1873–84, served with U. S. troops in Crook's and Wilcox's campaigns against the Indians. Member Med. Assn., D. C.; Therapeutic Society, Washington. President, Associated Survivors 6th Army Corps, Washington and New York. Past Medical Director, Dept. Potomac, G. A. R.; Past Dept. Commander, Union Veterans' Union, Washington. See Georgetown University, II, p. 201.

OCTOBER 3, 1894

556. HUGH WILSON BEATTY—Born March 9, 1850, Mifflin Co., Pa. LL. B., 1872, Univ. Mich.; M. D., 1886, Howard. Died April 27, 1897. Graduated at State Normal School, Kirksville, Mo., in 1870. Married Etta Orr, of Kirksville. Removed to Hutchinson, Kansas, in 1876; to Washington in 1883. Practiced medicine in Washington until his death. See Lamb's History, p. 148; Minutes Med. Society, April 28, 1897.

557. ANITA NEWCOMB McGEE—Born Nov. 4, 1864, D. C. M. D., 1892, Columbian. Acting Asst. Surgeon, U. S. A. Resigned from Society, Oct. 11, 1905. Daughter of Prof. Simon Newcomb, of U. S. Naval Observatory, and Mary Carolina Hassler Newcomb. Educated in private schools, Washington, and took special course at Newnham College, Cambridge, England, and Univ. Iowa. Post graduate (medical), Johns Hopkins Hospital. Practiced medicine in Washington, 1892–6. Fellow and ex-Secretary, A. A. A. S.; Surgeon General, Librarian General, Vice-President General and Historian General, National Society, D. A. R.; Director, D. A. R. Hospital Corps, April to September, 1898, selecting trained women nurses for army and navy service. Appointed, Aug. 29, 1898, Acting Asst. Surg., U. S. A., the only woman to hold such a position; assigned to duty in Surgeon General's Office, in charge of army nurse corps of trained women, which she organized. When U. S. Congress approved this work by making the nurse corps of trained women a permanent part of the army, the pioneer stage was passed and she resigned, Dec. 31, 1900. About 2,000 women served during her incumbency. In 1904, as President Society Spanish-American War Nurses and as Representative of Philadelphia Red Cross Society, and by agreement with the Japanese Government, she, with a party of trained nurses, formerly in U. S. Army, served in Japanese Army for six months gratuitously. Was appointed by Minister of War, Supervisor of Nurses, which placed her in same rank as officers of Japanese Army, and inspected and reported on relative nursing conditions. The Emperor of Japan bestowed upon her the Order of the Sacred Crown, a very rare distinction, and she also holds the "special" decoration of the Red Cross of Japan

and the War Medal. After returning from Japan she lectured on A woman's experience in the Japanese Army. Member of United Spanish War Veterans (the only woman eligible) and Assn. Military Surgeons, United States. Founder and first President, Spanish-American War Nurses. Married, 1888, W J McGee. See Who's Who in America; Woman's Med. Journal, Toledo, 1896, V, p. 27; 20th Cent. Biog. Dict.; Amer. Men of Science; Amer. Biog. Direct., Washington, 1908.

558. EMORY WILLIAM REISINGER—Born Sept. 16, 1871, D. C. M. D., 1893, Georgetown. Son of Wm. Wagner and Julia Reisinger. Educated in schools in Washington and in Paris and Nice, France. Demonstrator of Anatomy, Georgetown Med. School, since 1894; Lecturer on Osteology since 1898. Sometime Resident Physician, Emergency Hospital, and Wash. Asylum Hospital. Member Med. Assn., D. C.; A. M. A.; Wash. Acad. Sciences; Assn. Amer. Anatomists. Married, Sept. 27, 1898, Laura Ethel Barnett, of Wisconsin. See Amer. Men of Science, 1906; Georgetown University, II, p. 102.

559. WILLIAM BATES FRENCH—Born Jan. 9, 1855, D. C. M. D., 1885, Columbian.

560. HORACE MORGAN DEERLE—Born July 18, 1851, D. C. M. D., 1880, Columbian. Acting Asst. Surg., U. S. A., 1880–1891. Dropped from membership, 1899.

561. GEORGE BARRIE—Born June 3, 1865, Australia. M. D., 1892, Georgetown.

562. WILLIAM DAVIS HUGHES—Born June 19, 1835, Honey Creek Valley, Miami Co., Ohio. A. B., 1860; A. M., 1863, Ohio Wesleyan Univ.; M. D., 1884, Howard. Attended the district school, classical course at New Carlisle Academy, and Ohio Wesleyan Univ. In 1861-2 was Superintendent of public schools, Fairfield, Ohio; examiner of teachers of Miami Co. public schools. Studied law, and was admitted to the bar in 1864. In the same year opened an office in Troy, Ohio, in partnership with Hon. H. H. Williams, under the firm name of Hughes and Williams. Was elected Mayor of Troy in 1872, and reëlected in 1874. In 1876, removed to Sidney, Ohio, and after the election of President Garfield, in 1880, came to Washington. Since graduation in medicine has practiced in Washington. See Lamb's History, p. 182.

563. ALLEN WALKER—Born July 14, 1852, Hightown, England. M. D., 1886, Univ. Maryland. Dropped from membership, 1897. Medical Examiner, Prudential Insurance Co.

564. ANNE AUGUSTA WILSON—Born Sept. 20, 1859, Baltimore, Md. M. D., 1892, Royal College Phys. and Surg., Edinburgh and Univ. Brussels. Died March 13, 1908, of diabetes. Served as Head Physician at Clapham Maternity Hospital, London, in 1892. In summer of 1893 came to Washington. Largely through her efforts the Dorothea Dix Dispensary was opened. Medical Assistant at Central Dispensary, and for several years on Staff of National Florence Crittenton Home. Also helped to form the Instructive Visiting Nurses' Society and until her death was an active worker therein. See Minutes Med. Society, March 18 and 25, 1908; Wash. Med. Annals, 1908, VII, p. 282.

565. STERLING RUFFIN—Born July 20, 1866, Graham, N. C. M. D., 1890, Columbian. Brother of Dr. G. M. Ruffin, *infra*. Prof. Mat. Med. and Therap., 1899–1902, and of Theory and Practice of Medicine since 1902, Columbian.

566. PRESLEY CRAIG HUNT—Born March 4, 1871, Newport, R. I. M. D., 1891, Georgetown. Educated at Emerson Institute, D. C. Resident Physician, Emergency Hospital, 1892; Asst. Gynecologist, Georgetown Univ. Hosp., 1894–8; in charge Nervous Diseases, Central Dispensary, 1893–5; Neurologist, Providence Hospital, since 1905; Examining Physician, U. S. Volunteers, 1898–9; Ward Physician, 1901. Member Med. Assn., D. C.; Washington Society Mental and Nervous Diseases; Med. Society, George Wash. Univ. Med. School; Med. Society, Georgetown Univ.; Asst. Demonstrator Anatomy, George Wash. Univ. Med. School.

567. LOUIS ALWARD JOHNSON—Born Oct. 6, 1870, D. C. M. D., 1892, Georgetown.

568. JOHN HEPBURN YARNALL—Born Aug. 2, 1856, D. C. M. D., 1881, Columbian.

569. WM. LITTLETON ROBINS—Born Sept. 14, 1869, near Snow Hill, Md. M. D., 1890, Univ. Maryland. Son of James Bowdoin and Ella Anna Purnell Robins; of English descent. Educated in public schools, Berlin and Snow Hill, Md., and Shenandoah Valley Academy, Winchester, Va. In 1894 attended clinics in hospitals of London and Paris. Practiced at Snow Hill one year, then removed to Washington, in 1893. Served during the Spanish-American War. Was Clinical Assistant one year, University Hospital, Baltimore; Resident Physician, Good Samaritan Hosp., Baltimore; Asst. Resident Physician, Maryland Hospital for Insane, Catonsville, Md.; Asst. and in charge of Nervous Diseases, Emergency Hospital, Washington, six years; in charge of Ner-

vous Diseases, Freedmen's Hospital, Washington. Member A. M. A.;
Med. Assn., D. C.; A. A. A. S. Married, Dec. 19, 1894, Elizabeth G.,
daughter of Dr. W. G. Palmer, *supra*. See Univ. Maryland, 1907, II,
p. 413.

570. ROZIER MIDDLETON—Born Sept. 18, 1861, Herndon, Va.
M. D., 1889, Columbian. Died Jan. 31, 1901. See Minutes Med. Society, Feb. 6 and 13, 1901; Trans. Med. Society, 1901, VI, p. 53.

571. JOHN KURTZ—Born April 20, 1848, Ft. Johnson, S. C. Ph. B.,
1866; M. D., 1870, Columbian. Removed to Moorhead, Minn., about
1876; returned to Washington in 1892.

572. JAMES STUART—Born May 28, 1865, Statesburg, S. C. A. B.,
1886, Charleston College, S. C.; M. D., 1892, Columbian. Associate,
Lutheran Eye, Ear and Throat Infirmary, Washington. Son of Benj.
Rhett Stuart, of Charleston.

573. NANCY D. RICHARDS—Born Aug. 27, 1844, Washington Co.,
Pa. M. D., 1880, Wooster. Removed, 1898, to New Philadelphia, Ohio.
Married.

574. HENRY JOSEPH CROSSON—Born March 8, 1870, Minneapolis, Minn. M. D., 1890, Georgetown.

575. JOHN ALBERTSON STOUTENBURG—Born Dec. 7, 1870,
Hyde Park, N. Y. M. D., 1891, Georgetown.

576. ANTON COE—Born Dec. 21, 1848, New Haven, Conn. M. D.,
1888, Columbian. Dropped from membership, 1904. Died Nov. 5, 1908,
at New Haven.

577. GEORGE ROBERT LEE COLE—Born Jan. 19, 1864, D. C.
Phar. D., 1885, National College Pharmacy, D. C. M. D., 1887, Univ.,
Maryland. Acting Asst. Surgeon, U. S. A. Son of Thos. Walter and
Sarah Ann Wilson Cole. Educated in private schools, and St. John's
Military Academy, Alexandria, Va. Interne, 1887-90, Providence Hos-
pital, Washington; Assistant, 1889-90, Emergency Hospital, Wash-
ington. Attended clinics, 1890, St. Thomas' Hospital, London, England.
Surgeon, D. C. N. G., five years. Lectured on Diseases of Rectum,
National Univ. Med. School. Married, Dec. 7, 1900, Minnie Dale Ber-
nard Dorsey. See Univ. Maryland, 1907, II, p. 246.

APRIL 3, 1895

578. WILLIAM FRANCIS WALTER—Born Oct. 18, 1870, D. C. A. M., 1888, St. John's College, D. C.; M. D., 1892, Georgetown.

579. CHARLES MASSEY HAMMETT, JR.—Born Oct. 26, 1871, D. C. Son of Dr. C. M. Hammett, *supra*. M. D., 1892, Georgetown.

580. JOHN E. CARPENTER—Born Feb. 14, 1842, Aberdeen, Ohio. Hosp. Steward, 12th Ohio Vols.; First Lieut., 175th Ohio. M. D., 1866, Charity Hospital Med. College, Cleveland, Ohio; 1893, Univ. Buffalo. Died May 4, 1899. Enlisted Sept. 1, 1861, 12th Ohio Vols.; appointed Hospital Steward, July 1, 1862; transferred, July 1, 1864, to 23d Ohio Vols., and Oct. 10th, appointed First Lieutenant and Adjutant, 175th Ohio. Mustered out, July, 1865. Practiced pharmacy several years in Memphis, Tenn. Then removed to Charleston, Miss., as Judge of Probate Court, Tallahassee Co. About two years afterwards removed to Washington; employed in U. S. Pension Bureau, where he continued till his death. Member of Board of Trustees, Reform School, D. C.; Prof. Pharmacy and Botany, Howard Med. School. See Lamb's History, p. 125.

581. BERNARD AUGUST STORCH—Born Oct. 9, 1843, Swartzburg-Rudolstadt, Germany. Came to United States while a boy. M. D., 1863, Univ. Iowa. Surgeon at Estes House Hospital, Keokuk, Iowa, during part of the Civil War. Afterwards took a special course at Univ. Berlin. Came to Washington in 1890. Died Nov. 30, 1906. A son, Dr. C. M. Storch, practices at Grand Rapids, Mich. See Minutes Med. Society, Jan. 16, 1907; Wash. Med. Annals, 1907-8, VI, p. 55.

582. HOBART SOUTHWORTH DYE—Born Jan. 17, 1848, Bridgewater, Oneida Co., N. Y. M. D., 1876, Columbian. Studied medicine with Dr. Hiram S. Crandall at Leonardsville, N. Y. Began practice at New Berlin, N. Y., May 3, 1876. Was made a member of the Chenango County Med. Society in 1876, President, 1891-2. Removed to Washington, May, 1893. Member Consulting Board of Washington Asylum Hospital; Associate at Episcopal Eye, Ear, Nose and Throat Hospital; Assistant, Eye and Ear, at Emergency Hospital, Washington. Member Med. Assn., D. C.; George Washington Univ. Med. Society; Washington Society of Ophthalmologists and Otologists; A. M. A.; Amer. Laryngolog., Rhinolog. and Otolog. Society.

583. ANTHONY HEGER—Born Dec. 4, 1828, Austria. M. D., 1848, Univ. Penna. Appointed Asst. Surgeon, U. S. A., Aug. 25, 1856; promoted Captain, Aug. 29, 1861; Surgeon and Major, Sept. 17, 1862; Lt. Col., Jan. 24, 1866; Col. and Asst. Surgeon Gen., Jan. 2, 1891; retired

23

Dec. 4, 1892. Advanced in rank to Brig. Gen., U. S. A., retired, by act of April 23, 1904. Brevetted Lt. Col., March 13, 1865, for faithful and meritorious services during the war. Resigned from Med. Society, April 13, 1904. Died Jan. 25, 1908. See Brown's History, p. 294; Powell's History, p. 367; Who's Who in America; Amer. Biog. Direct., Washington, 1908.

584. SAMUEL EDWIN LEWIS—Born March 1, 1838, D. C. M. D., 1864, Med. Coll. Virginia. Asst. Surg., C. S. A. Attended lectures at Columbian Med. College, D. C., 1861-2, studying with Drs. J. C. Riley, *supra*, and N. S. Lincoln, *supra*. Went South in June, 1863, and attended Med. College of Virginia at Richmond, 1863-4, and graduated. Appointed Acting Asst. Surg., Prov. Army, C. S. A., and, July 19, 1864, Asst. Surgeon. April 3, 1865, surrendered at Richmond, and was continued on duty by U. S. Army officers with sick and wounded till April 17th, when he was paroled. Practiced medicine in Baltimore till 1868, and was member of Baltimore Med. Assn. From 1868 to 1884 conducted a pharmacy in Washington. Resumed practice in 1893. Was the first Vice President, 1901-2, and afterwards President, 1907-8, Assn. Med. Officers, Army and Navy of Confederacy.

585. AURELIUS RIVES SHANDS—Born Nov. 5, 1860, Prince George Co., Va. M. D., 1884, Univ. Maryland. Son of Dr. A. R. Shands. Graduated at Univ. School, Petersburg, Va. Prof. Orthopedic Surgery since 1894, Columbian Med. School; Prof. Orthopedic Surgery, Univ. Vermont. Member Wash. Acad. Sciences; Amer. Orthopedic Assn.; Southern Surg. Assn.; Virginia State Med. Society. See Who's Who in America.

586. SAMUEL EVANS WATKINS—Born Feb. 11, 1871, D. C. Son of Louis and Emily H. Evans Watkins. Educated at Emerson Institute, Washington. M. D., 1892, Georgetown. Sometime Demonstrator in . Dermatology, etc., Georgetown Med. School; Associate, Emergency Hosp. Member Med. Assn., D. C. See Georgetown University, II, p. 266.

587. LOUISA MILLER BLAKE—Born June 2, 1853, New Jersey. M. D., 1893, Columbian. Wife of Dr. L. C. Blake, Washington.

588. OSCAR HENRY COUMBE—Born Dec. 31, 1858, D. C. M. D., 1891, National Univ., D. C.

589. AUSTIN J. O'MALLEY—Born Oct. 1, 1858, Pittston, Pa. A. B., 1878, Fordham; A. M., 1888; Ph. D., 1889; M. D., 1893, Georgetown: LL. D., 1895, Notre Dame, Ind. Removed, 1895, to South Bend, Ind.; to Philadelphia about 1904, where he is Ophthalmologist and Pathologist to St. Agnes' Hospital.   Son of William and Catherine Ward O'Malley. Descendant of Diarmuid O'Malley, chieftain, 1415, of Upper and Lower Umhall, West Ireland.   Studied some time in Italy and Germany.   Sometime Instructor in Bacteriology, Georgetown Med. School.   Sometime Prof. English Literature, Notre Dame University.   See Georgetown University, II, p. 265.

590. JOHN THOMAS COLE—Born Oct. 30, 1856, Virginia.   M. D., 1891, Georgetown.

591. FLORENCE DONOHUE—Born Dec. 15, 1842, Killarney, Ireland.   Graduated, 1857, Trumansburg Academy, Tompkins Co., N. Y. Served in Civil War as enlisted man.   Has been Med. Director and Surg. General, G. A. R., and Army and Navy Union, and Surgeon of the "Old Guard."   M. D., Georgetown, 1872.   Died June 24, 1908.

592. TALIAFERRO CLARK—Born May 14, 1867, Virginia.   A. B., Emory and Henry College, Va.;   M. D., 1890, Univ. Va.   Acting Asst. Surg. and Passed Asst. Surgeon, U. S. M. H. S.

593. JOHN AMBROSE DRAWBAUGH—Born Nov. 10, 1863, Cumberland Co., Pa.   Son of Samuel O. and Elizabeth Hamaker Drawbaugh. D. D. S., 1888; M. D., 1890, National Univ., D. C.   Afterward took special course at hospitals, Vienna, Austria.   Married Gertrude Iseman, of Washington.   Died May 27, 1898, Asheville, N. C.   See Minutes Med. Society, Oct. 5 and 12, 1898; Trans. Med. Society, 1898, III, p. 131; National Med. Rev., 1898-9, VIII, p. 361.

594. HARRY THEODORE HARDING—Born Jan. 21, 1870, Binghamton, N. Y.   M. D., 1893, College Phys. and Surgeons, N. Y. City.

595. DUFF GREEN LEWIS—Born Oct. 26, 1869, West Virginia. A. B., Wash. and Lee Univ.; M. D., 1891, Univ. Virginia.

596. JOHN HENRY JUNGHANS—Born Nov. 5, 1868, D. C.   A. B., 1888; A. M., 1891; M. D., 1891, Georgetown.

597. FRANCIS PATTERSON MORGAN—Born Dec. 25, 1867, Danbury, N. H.   A. B., 1890, Harvard; M. D., 1893, College Physicians and Surg., N. Y.   Son of Francis H. Morgan (sometime member of N. H. Legislature, afterward Chief of Division, Second Auditor's Office, Treasury Dept., Washington) and Martha E. Le Bosquet Morgan.   Educated in public schools, Washington; graduated, 1886, at High School.   Instructor in Materia Medica and Demonstrator of Pharmacy, Columbian

Med. School, D. C.; Lecturer, Wash. Training School for Nurses. Member Med. Assn., D. C.; Clinico-Path. Society, D. C. One of the founders Amer. Therapeutic Society. Oct. 1, 1895, married Ida Adele Pearce, daughter of Henry O. and Mary A. Pearce, of Brooklyn, N. Y. See Who's Who in America ; Amer. Biog. Direct., Washington, 1908.

598. WILLIAM EDMUND WOLHAUPTER—Born April 23, 1869, D. C. Son of Dr. D. P. Wolhaupter, *supra*. Phar. D., 1888, National College Pharmacy, D. C.; M. D., 1890, Georgetown. Surgeon, 1890, on Steamer "Fish Hawk." Died Jan. 21, 1896. See Minutes Med. Society, Jan. 22, 1896; National Med. Review, 1896, V, p. 5.

599. MABEL CORNISH—Born Aug. 24, 1867, D. C. A. B., 1889, Vassar; M. D., 1892, Woman's Med. College, N. Y. City. Married, 1897, to S. R. Bond, Washington. Dropped, 1899, from membership.

600. NATHANIEL BOWDITCH MORTON—Born, Wellesley, Mass. M. D., 1887, Harvard. Removed to Santa Catalina Island, Cal. Member of N. Y. County Med. Society ; Med. Legal Society, N. Y. State. See Shepherd Peter, First aid to the injured, N. Y., 1882.

601. ARGYLE MACKEY—Born, 1868, North Carolina. M. D., 1890, Univ. Maryland. Died Aug. 28, 1896, Baltimore, Md.

OCTOBER 2, 1895

602. GEORGE BURTON HEINECKE—Born Dec. 15, 1871, D. C. M. D., 1892, Columbian. Acting Asst. Surg., U. S. A. Educated in the public schools of Washington. 1892-3, Resident Physician, Emergency Hospital ; 1893-4, Surgeon, U. S. Fish Commission Steamer "Fish Hawk." Engaged in private practice since 1895 in Washington, except 1898, when he was Acting Asst. Surgeon, U. S. A., during War with Spain ; at Santiago, Cuba. Member A. M. A.; Alumni Med. Society, George Washington Univ.

603. ALBERT RHETT STUART—Born Aug. 10, 1868, Spartansburg, S. C. Son of Rev. Albert Stuart, D. C. A. B., 1888; A. M., 1891, Trinity College, Hartford, Conn.; M. D., 1892, Univ. Virginia.

604. PHILIP JAISOHN—Born in 1866. M. D., 1892, Columbian. Removed, 1896, to Korea. Was in Primus, Pa., 1900-6.

605. WALLACE JOHNSON—Born May 2, 1867, Middletown, Ohio. Ph. B., 1889; Ph. M., 1892, Wooster Univ., Ohio; M. D., 1892, Med. College of Ohio. Resigned from Society, Nov. 2, 1904, and removed to

Nampa, Idaho. Son of Charles B. and Sarah M. Hanger Johnson. Educated at Middletown public schools and Wooster Univ. Attended Friederich-Wilhelm Univ., Berlin, and K. K. Univ. Austria, Vienna, 1893-4. Married, Wooster, O., July 5, 1900, Magdalene Masters. Externe, 1891-2 ; Interne, 1892-3, Cincinnati Hospital; post-graduate work abroad, 1893-4 ; Asst. Demon. Histology, 1896-9, Demonstrator Pathology and Bacteriology, 1900-4, Georgetown Med. School ; in charge of Clinical Diagnosis Dept., Lionel Laboratory, Central Dispensary and Emergency Hospital, Washington, 1897-1904; Assistant on various services of Central Dispensary, 1895-1904. Practiced medicine, Washington, 1894-1904; now at Bruneau Valley, Idaho. Member Med. Assn., D. C.; A. M. A.; Southern Idaho Med. Society ; Idaho State Med. Society ; Washington X-ray Laboratory. Author, with Dr. M. D'Arcy Magee, *infra*, of Surgery (Medical Epitome series), 1904, L, 12. See Who's Who in America.

606. ROBERT W. BAKER—Born July 5, 1863, Va. M. D., 1887, Univ. Virginia.

607. THOMAS ASH CLAYTOR—Born July 14, 1869, West River, Md. M. D., 1891, Univ. Penna. Acting Asst. Surgeon, U. S. A., in War with Spain. Prof. Materia Medica and Therapeutics, G. W. Univ. Med. Dept ; and Clinical Professor of Medicine.

608. RUDOLPH H. VON EZDORF—Born Aug. 13, 1872, Philadelphia, Pa. M. D., 1894, Columbian. Resigned from Society, July 4, 1898. Asst. Surgeon, Passed Asst. Surgeon, U. S. M. H. S.

609. FRANK PALMER VALE—Born Dec. 18, 1871, D. C. M. D., 1892, Georgetown ; 1894, Univ. Penna. Resident Physician, Providence Hospital, January, 1893, to January, 1894. Served as Police Surgeon seven years, ending July, 1906. Co-author with Dr. J. B. Nichols, *infra*, of Pocket text book on histology and pathology. Awarded first prize of $250 by Med. Society, D. C., for best essay on any medical or surgical subject. Title, An essay on shock. Demonstrator of Pathology, Georgetown Med. School, 1895 to 1900. Awarded Fiske Fund Prize for 1908, ($200) for the best essay : Has surgical treatment lessened the mortality from appendicitis ; Providence, 1908.

610. LOUIS PERCY SMITH—Born Dec. 10, 1871, D. C. M. D., 1893, Coll. Phys. and Surg., N. Y. Post-Graduate, 1894, Vienna. Asst. Surg., U. S. A. Resigned from Society, Oct. 13, 1897. Died Jan. 8, 1901, Manila, P. I. See Powell's History, p. 597.

611. CHARLES WRIGHT FILLER—Born Oct. 6, 1852, Lovettsville, Va. M. D., 1876, Univ. Md. Dropped from membership, 1903. Died March 22, 1905, of epithelioma of tongue.

612. ALBERT SIDNEY MADDOX—Born June 23, 1866, West Va. M. D., 1890, Bellevue. Resigned, Oct. 29, 1902 ; removed to New York City.

613. WILFRED MASON BARTON—Born July 16, 1871, D. C. M. D., 1892, Georgetown. Author, with W. A. Wells, *infra*, of Thesaurus of medical words and phrases, Philadelphia, 1903. Son of William Henry and Harriet Garrison Barton. Educated in public schools, Washington. Sometime Resident at Washington Asylum Hospital ; Interne, U. S. Marine Hospital, Chicago ; House Physician, Columbia Hospital, Washington. Member Med. Assn., D. C.; A. M. A.; ex-President, Clinical Society, Washington ; corresponding member, London Therapeutic Society. Med. Inspector of Schools, Washington ; Asst. Prof. Materia Medica, etc., Georgetown Med. School. Married, 1905, Miss Minnie A. Quinn, of Worcester, Mass. See Georgetown University, II, p. 262.

614. FRANK ROLLINS RICH—Born April 25, 1864, Reisterstown, Md. M. D., 1889, Univ. Maryland. Removed, 1898, to Towson, Md., afterwards to Pittsburg, Pa.

APRIL 1, 1896

615. SOFIE AMALIE NORDHOFF—Born April 24, 1867, Germany. M. D., 1893, Columbian. Married Dr. F. A. R. Jung, *infra*. Educated in Germany and France ; post-graduate medical work at Univ. Munich and Paris École de Med. Member Med. Assn., D. C.; Wash. Acad. Sciences. Married, July 23, 1896. See Who's Who in America ; Amer. Biog. Direct., Washington, 1908.

616. RUPERT NORTON—Born July 21, 1867, Ashfield, Mass. A. B., 1888 ; M. D., 1893, Harvard. Acting Asst. Surg., U. S. A., 1899–1900. Resigned from Society, Jan. 24, 1900, and removed to Paris, France. Was Med. Referee, N. Y. Mutual Life Insurance Co., in Paris, in 1900–6. Then returned to United States. Is Asst. Supt., Johns Hopkins Hospital, Baltimore, Md.

617. FREDERICK OGLE ROMAN—Born June 7, 1866, Belleville, Ill. A. B., St. John's College, Washington ; M. D., 1894, Columbian. Son of Richard and Isabelle Ogle Roman ; descendant of Samuel Ogle, Colonial Governor of Maryland in 1775, and Col. Joseph Ogle, of War of

Amer. Revolution. Educated in public schools and St. John's College, Washington. Practices medicine in Washington. Married, Jan. 28, 1887, Katherine Stanhope Hogan. See Amer. Biog. Direct., Washington, 1908.

618. CHARLES WESLEY KEYES—Born March 17, 1854, Claremont, N. H. M. D., 1890, Howard. Died of apoplexy, Dec. 19, 1905. His family removed from New Hampshire to Vermont while he was yet an infant. When he grew up he was engaged for some years on newspaper work in Farmington, Me. In 1881 was appointed Special Examiner, U. S. Pension Office, Washington. After graduation in medicine he studied law. He finally resigned his office and practiced medicine in Washington. Married Miss Kate Tomlinson, of Washington. One brother, Dr. F. P. Keyes, lives in Brooklyn, N. Y. See Lamb's History, p. 189; Minutes Med. Society, Jan. 1 and 10, 1906; Wash. Med. Annals, 1906, V, p. 55.

619. CLARENCE ARLINGTON WEAVER—Born Jan. 19, 1871, D. C. M. D., 1892, Jefferson. Surgeon, 1st D. C. N. G., and Asst. Surg., D. C. Vols., 1898. After graduation was Resident Surgeon, Jefferson Hospital, Philadelphia, for twenty months. Since then has practiced medicine in Washington. Was commissioned Surgeon, National Guard, D. C., January, 1894; Surgeon, 1st Regt., D. C. N. G., May, 1897, and served as Surgeon, 1st D. C. Infantry, U. S. V., in the Spanish-American War. Is married. See Lamb's History, p. 267.

620. JAMES RAMSAY NEVITT—Born June 25, 1867, Naylor's Hold, Richmond Co., Va. M. D., 1892, Columbian. Son of Robert K. and Mary Ramsay Nevitt. Educated in public schools of Washington and Columbian Univ., from which he graduated in 1889. Sometime employed in the Engineering Dept., D. C. Student at Washington Asylum Hospital, 1891, Resident Physician, 1892; Police Surgeon, 1893, and served during smallpox epidemic, 1894; President of Board of Police Surgeons, 1895. On the staff of Emergency Hospital. Coroner since 1900 and Medical Examiner to Physicians to the Poor. Member Med. Assn., D. C.; A. M. A. Dec. 19, 1894, married Miss Mary C. Hine, daughter of Mr. and Mrs. L. G. Hine, of Washington. See Amer. Biog. Direct., Washington, 1908; History City of Washington, 1903, p. 75.

621. RANDOLPH BRYAN CARMICHAEL—Born June 20, 1869, Fredericksburg, Va. M. D., 1889, Jefferson.

622. EDWIN EMERY MORSE—Born Jan. 7, 1867, Maine. M. D., 1892, Columbian; L. M., Rotunda Hospital, Dublin, Ireland.

623. CHARLES CLAGETT MARBURY—Born July 11, 1870, near Upper Marlboro, Md.   A. B., 1890, St. John's College, Annapolis, Md.; M. D., 1893, Georgetown.   Acting Asst. Surg., U. S. A., in War with Spain.   Son of Fendall M. and Sallie Clagett Berry Marbury.   After graduation in medicine attended N. Y. Polyclinic.   House Physician, Providence Hospital, Washington, 1895–6, Attending Physician since 1897 ; Prof. Clinical Medicine, Georgetown Med. School; Surgeon to Police and Fire Depts. since 1900.   During War with Spain served at Santiago, Cuba ; afterward in command of Leiter U. S. Gen. Hosp., Chickamauga, Ga.   Member Med. Assn., D. C.; A. M. A.; Clinical Society, Washington ; Society of Mental and Nervous Diseases, Washington.   See Amer. Biog. Direct., Washington, 1908.

624. ADA REBECCA THOMAS—Born Aug. 6, 1868, Trenton, N. J. M. D., 1893, Woman's Med. College, Philadelphia.   Daughter of James Reed and Rebecca Dean Thomas.   Graduated at N. J. State Model School, 1885, where later she did post-graduate work.   1893, Interne at Woman's Hospital, Philadelphia.   Resident, 1893–4, at Philadelphia Hospital.   Since Dec., 1894, has practiced medicine in Washington. Sometime Physician to Woman's Clinic ; Associate in Diseases of Children, Emergency Hospital ; Physician to National Florence Crittenton Home ; Lecturer on Obstetrics, Sibley Hospital Training School, since 1899, and on Children's Diseases, at Emergency Hospital Training School, since 1902.   Member Med. Assn., D. C., and A. M. A.

OCTOBER 7, 1896

625. SUSAN JOHNSON SQUIRE—Born March 17, 1841, Baltimore, Md.   M. D., 1889, Howard.   Wife of Dr. Linus T. Squire, Washington. After graduation practiced medicine at Orlando, Fla., from 1889 to 1894 ; since then in Washington, D. C.   See Lamb's History, p. 217.

626. WALTER D. CANNON—Born May 16, 1865, Indiana.   M. D., 1890, Georgetown.   Dropped, 1899, from membership.

627. WILLIAM ROBEY MADDOX—Born March 8, 1855, Erie, Pa. M. D., 1876, Jefferson.   Died Oct. 25, 1899.   Practiced medicine in Philadelphia until 1884 ; then at Fort Hall Indian Agency, Rose Fork, Idaho, five years.   Removed to Washington in 1889, where he practiced until his death.   See Minutes Med. Society, Nov. 1 and 8, 1899 ; Trans. Med. Society, 1899, IV, p. 173 ; Nat. Med. Review, 1899–1900, IX, p. 530.

628. PHEBE RUSSELL NORRIS—Born Feb. 4, 1860, Monrovia, Md. B. E., 1879, Brethren's Normal College, Penna. M. D., 1891, Columbian.

629. ABBIE CUTLER TYLER—Born Nov. 11, 1835, Warren, Mass. M. D., 1868, New England Female Med. College, Boston, Mass. Died Jan. 6, 1906. Educated in schools at Warren, Mass., and Woodstock, Vt. Assisted in hospital work, N. Y. City. Studied one year in London and Paris hospitals. Practiced medicine at Cooperstown, N. Y., and Waukegan, Ill., for ten years ; afterwards in Washington. Buried at Warren, Mass. See Minutes Med. Society, Jan. 24, 1906 ; Wash. Med. Annals, 1906-7, V, p. 56.

630. ALBERT LIVINGSTON STAVELY—Born Sept. 10, 1863, Pa. A. M., 1885, Princeton ; M. D., 1888, Univ. Penna.

631. THOMAS BEAUREGARD CRITTENDEN—Born March 11, 1862, Shackelfords, Va. M. D., 1895, Georgetown. Removed, 1897, to Horton, W. Va.

632. ADELINE ELWELL METCALF PORTMAN—Born Feb. 27, 1860, Ottawa, Ill. A. M., 1876, Mt. Vernon College, Ill.; M. D., 1887, Univ. Iowa. Post-graduate Student at Univ. Iowa, and in London, 1888-94. Asst. Physician, Emergency Hospital, Washington. See Cordell's Med. Annals, Maryland, p. 537.

633. WILLIAM A. CALDWELL—Born Sept. 29, 1862, W. Va. M. D., 1892, Columbian. Died June 6, 1903, Rockville, Md. Of Scotch-Irish descent ; his great grandfather was one of the first settlers near Ft. Henry, now Wheeling, W. Va. Educated in public schools, and taught school. Studied medicine with Dr. John L. Dickey, of Wheeling. Resident Physician, two years, Garfield and Columbia Hospitals ; Prof. Nervous and Mental Diseases, National Univ. Med. College, Washington. In 1899-1901, because of pulmonary tuberculosis, sought relief in the Adirondacks and other places, and became so much better that he was elected Prof. Anatomy and Physiology, West Virginia Univ. Married Miss Kate L. English, Frederick, Md. See Minutes Med. Society, Oct. 7 and Nov. 4, 1903 ; Wash. Med. Annals, 1903-4, II, p. 353.

634. WALTER AUGUSTINE WELLS—Born March 6, 1870, Bladensburg, Md. M. D., 1891, Georgetown. Co-editor Wash. Med. Annals. Prof. Laryngology and Otology, Georgetown Med. School. Son of Charles A. and Mary Lucretia (Hyatt) Wells. Educated, Bladensburg Academy and public schools of Washington; graduated, Wash. High

School, 1889, and Columbian Univ. Post-graduate medical work, Chicago Polyclinic, 1892-3; Univ. Vienna, 1894-5. Resident Student, Washington Asylum, 1891; Interne, Marine Hospital, Chicago, 1892-3; began practice of medicine in Washington, 1895; Surgeon in Charge of Ear and Throat Dept., Garfield Hospital; Associate Attending Physician, Episcopal Eye, Ear and Throat and Georgetown Univ. Hospitals; sometime Demonstrator Laryngology, Georgetown Medical School. Asso. Editor Jour. of Eye, Ear and Throat Diseases, Baltimore, and collaborator for The Laryngoscope, St. Louis. Member American Rhinol., Laryngol. and Otol. Society; Wash. Acad. Sciences. Author, with Dr. Wilfred M. Barton, *supra*, of Thesaurus of medical words and phrases, 1903. Married, June 19, 1899, at Washington, Frances M. Gibson. See Amer. Biog. Direct., Washington, 1908; Who's Who in America.

635. JOHN HITZ METZEROTT—Born Dec. 2, 1865, D. C. M. D., 1891, Columbian. See E. Landesmann, Therapy of the clinics, Chicago, 1897. Member Wash. Acad. Sciences. See Who's Who in America.

636. EDWIN GLADMON—Born Feb. 27, 1859, Virginia. Phar. D.; 1880, National College Pharmacy, D. C.; M. D., 1890, National Univ., D. C. Removed, 1899, to Southern Pines, N. C.

APRIL 7, 1897

637. GEORGE TITUS HOWLAND—Born May 18, 1862, N. Y. M. D., 1886, Bellevue; 1890, Univ. Berlin. Dropped from membership, 1903. Removed from D. C. to the Bermudas.

638. HUGH CLARENCE DUFFEY—Born Jan. 4, 1870, Hillsboro, Md. M. D., 1891, Georgetown.

639. VIRGIL B. JACKSON—Born Oct. 3, 1868, Front Royal, Va. M. D., 1895, Columbian. Co-editor Wash. Medical Annals. Educated in public schools, Front Royal; finished sophomore year at Columbian Univ., Washington. Resident Physician, Washington Asylum Hospital; since then has practiced medicine in Washington. Associate Surgeon, Emergency Hospital; Visiting Physician, Foundling Hospital; Asst. Gynecologist, George Washington Univ. Hospital, 1894-5; Demonstrator Anatomy and Clinical Surgical Assistant, G. W. Univ.; Police Surgeon, 1897. Member Clinical Society; Med. Assn., D. C. See Amer. Biog. Direct., Washington, 1908.

640. WILLIAM LINCOLN MASTERSON—Born Dec. 25, 1868, Coshocton, Ohio. M. D., 1895, Columbian. Post-graduate course at N. Y. Polyclinic, 1905.

641. THOMAS MILLER—Born Oct. 12, 1857, Glasgow, Scotland. M. D., 1884, Howard. Attended Business College, Adrian, Mich. Since graduation has practiced medicine in Washington. Attended special course in Ophthalmology, Georgetown Med. School. Lecturer on Anatomy and Diseases of Children, 1887-91, Howard Med. School. See Lamb's History, p. 128.

642. CHARLES LEWIS ALLEN—Born Sept. 24, 1860, S. C. M. D., 1887, Univ. Maryland. Resigned from the Society, Nov. 29, 1899, removing to Trenton, N. J.; afterwards to Los Angeles, Cal. Is now practicing at Pasadena, Cal.

643. NOBLE PRICE BARNES—Born Aug. 16, 1871, Killbuck, Holmes Co., Ohio. M. D., 1893, Baltimore Med. College. Surgeon, Battery A, Light Artillery, D. C. Son of Dr. E. P. and Sarah M. Barnes. Educated at public schools; graduated 1889, High School, Millersburg, Ohio. Chief of Service, Diseases of Children, Eastern Dispensary and Casualty Hospital, 1898; Prof. Diseases of Children, 1898, Materia Medica and Therapeutics, 1902, Med. Dept. National Univ. Lecturer, Materia Medica and Toxicology, George Washington Univ. Med. Dept., 1905; one of the organizers of Amer. Therapeutic Society, its Secretary eight years; Secretary, Section Therapeutics, Fourth Pan-American Med. Congress. Member National Assn. for Study, Treatment and Prevention of Tuberculosis; A. M. A.; Pres., Therapeutic Society, Washington, and Wash. Med. and Surg. Soc. Married, Sept. 15, 1897, Isabel Cameron McGregor. See Amer. Biog. Direct., Washington, 1908.

644. JOHN DANIEL THOMAS—Born Aug. 13, 1868, Northampton Co., Va. A. B., 1889, Hampden-Sidney; M. D., 1892, Univ. Virginia. Contract Surgeon, U. S. A., Spanish-American War. Prof. Physical Diagnosis, Georgetown Univ.; Ex-President, Clinical Society, D. C.; member Clinico-Patholog. Society, Med. and Surg. Society, and Obstet. and Gynecolog. Society, D. C.

645. FRANCIS LIEBER—Born in 1869, St. Paul, Minn. M. D., 1891, Univ. Penna. Acting Asst. Surgeon, U. S. A. Died Oct. 10, 1898, Nassau, Florida, of typhoid fever. Grandson of Prof. Francis Lieber, the historian; son of Gen. G. N. Lieber, Judge Advocate General, U. S. A. After graduation in medicine was Resident Physician two years at Univ. and Episcopal Hospitals, Philadelphia; afterwards attended hospitals in Berlin and Vienna. Sometime Assistant at Central Dispensary and Emergency Hospital, Washington; Demonstrator Physical Diagnosis, Georgetown Med. School. See Minutes Med. Society, Oct. 12 and 19, 1898; Trans. Med. Society, 1898, III, p. 132; N. Y. Med. Jour., 1898, LXVIII, p. 711; Nat. Med. Rev., 1898-9, VIII, p. 362.

646. EDWIN MARBLE HASBROUCK—Born July 17, 1866, Syracuse, N. Y. M. D., 1895, Georgetown. Son of Cyrus L. and Adeline W. Marble Hasbrouck. Educated at Syracuse University. Asst. Surg., Georgetown Univ. Hospital ; Prosector Anatomy, Georgetown Med. School. Has worked in biological and ornithological fields. Member Med. Assn., D. C.; A. M. A.; Wash. Med. and Surg. Society. Married, April 20, 1897, Harriet Ann Blackistone, St. Mary's Co., Md. See Amer. Biog. Direct., Washington, 1908.

647. FRANK RANDALL HAGNER—Born March, 1873, D. C. Son of Dr. C. E. Hagner, *supra*. M. D., 1894, Columbian.

648. GEORGE WILLIAM WOOD—Born July 25, 1863, Charles Co., Md. M. D., 1894, Georgetown. Med. Officer, U. S. Fish Commission, 1894-5, Steamer "Fish Hawk." Took post-graduate course, 1895, Philadelphia. Assistant, Diseases of Women, 1896-8, Casualty Hospital, Washington.

649. ROBERT FRENCH MASON—Born April 27, 1869, Charlottesville, Va. M. D., 1895, Univ. Maryland.

OCTOBER 6, 1897

650. LEWIS JUNIUS BATTLE—Born Aug. 6, 1865, Raleigh, N. C. Ph. B., 1886, Univ. North Carolina; M. D., 1893, Univ. Penna. Surgeon, B. and O. R. R. Member of Staff of Casualty Hospital, Washington.

651. FRANCIS ANTHONY MAZZEI—Born Dec. 3, 1863, Basilicata, Italy. M. D., 1895, Columbian.

652. FRANZ AUGUST RICHARD JUNG—Born Oct. 9, 1869, Suhl, Germany. M. D., 1893, Univ. Leipzig. Son of Herman and Marie Jung. Member Med. Assn., D. C.; A. M. A.; Wash. Acad. Sciences. Knight Order St. Stanislaus, conferred by Czar of Russia, April, 1902 ; Order of the Crown, conferred by German Emperor, June, 1904. Married, July 23, 1896, Dr. Sofie A. Nordhoff, *supra*. See Who's Who in America; Amer. Biog. Direct., Washington, 1908.

APRIL 6, 1898

653. MURRAY GALT MOTTER—Born Aug. 29, 1866, Emmetsburg, Md. A. B., 1886 ; A. M., 1889; B. S., 1887, Pennsylvania College, Gettysburg, Pa.; M. D., 1890, Univ. Penna. Resigned Oct. 24, 1900 ; reëlected Oct. 1, 1902. Co-editor Wash. Med. Annals. Author, with Dr. Reid Hunt, of Changes in the Pharmacopoeia, Washington, 1905. Now in Hygienic Laboratory, Navy Dept. Sometime Deputy Health Officer, D. C.

654. JAMES RICHARD TUBMAN—Born March 31, 1867, Alexandria, Va. M. D., 1895, Columbian.

655. LINNAEUS SAMUEL SAVAGE—Born Oct. 24, 1871, Whaleyville, Va. M. D., 1893, Baltimore Med. College.

656. HOMER SANFORD MEDFORD—Born Jan. 24, 1873, D. C. M. D., 1895, Columbian.

657. EDMUND BARRY—Born June 22, 1864, D. C. M. D., 1891, Columbian. Acting Asst. Surgeon, U. S. A., 1898-04. Member Board of Police and Fire Surgeons, D. C.

658. JOHN BENJAMIN NICHOLS—Born Feb. 2, 1867, Cazenovia, N. Y. M. D., 1891, Columbian. Son of George C. and Ellen Farr Ingraham Nichols. Attended public schools; graduated 1884, Cazenovia Seminary. Asst. Surgeon, 1894-9, U. S. Soldiers' Home, Washington; Pathologist and Assistant in Med. Dispensary Service, Garfield Memorial Hospital ; Pathologist, Episcopal Eye, Ear and Throat Hospital; Attending Physician, Freedmen's Hospital ; Prof. Histology and Embryology, Columbian University. Member Med. Assn., D. C. ; A. M. A. ; Amer. Climatolog. Assn.; ex-President, Clinical Society, Washington ; member Washington Anthropolog. Society ; G. W. Univ. Med. Society. Author of Manual of clinical laboratory methods, N. Y., 1902; Diet in typhoid fever—Fiske Fund prize essay, Providence, 1907. See also, Nichols and Vale, Histology and Pathology, Philadelphia, 1899. Married, May 27, 1891, Annie Gledhill. See Who's Who in America ; Amer. Biog. Direct., Washington, 1908 ; G. W. U. Annual, 1905, p. 20 ; Columbian Univ. Annual, p. 63 ; G. W. U. Bibliog., 1904, p. 43 ; G. W. U. Bulletin, Oct., 1905, p. 86.

659. GEORGE WINSLOW FOSTER—Born in 1845, Burnham, Me. M. D., 1871, Bowdoin. Removed, 1901, to Bangor, Me., where he died, Jan. 4, 1904.

660. WILLIAM PEYTON TUCKER—Born in 1870. M. D., 1893, Ensworth.

661. ABRAHAM BARNES HOOE—Born April 12, 1871, Va. M. D., 1896, Columbian.

662. LEIGH H. FRENCH—Born in 1863. M. D., 1894, Univ. Minn. Resigned May 16, 1900. Removed to Nome, Alaska.

663. MONTE GRIFFITH—Born Feb. 10, 1862, Jefferson Co., Va. Phar. D., 1890, National College Pharmacy, D. C.; M. D., 1896, Univ. Maryland. Son of Capt. Joseph Thomas and Jane R. Willson Griffith. Educated at Berryville (Va.), High School; Norwood (Va.), High School and College; Univ. of Virginia. Outdoor Physician, Children's Hospital, Washington, 1896-99; Asst. Surgeon, Episcopal Eye, Ear and Throat Hospital, 1897; since 1905, Associate Physician and Surgeon of same. Prof. Physiology, Wash. Dental College and Hospital of Oral Surgery (now Dental School of Georgetown Univ.), 1898-1901. Ophthalmologist and Aurist, Children's Hospital, 1905. Asst. Prof. Ophthalmology, Georgetown Med. School, 1906. Member Med. Assn., D. C., Secretary, 1901-3; A. M. A.; Ophthalmolog. and Otolog. Society; Clinical Society (President, 1902-3); Therapeutic Society; Trustee Southern Industrial Educational Assn. Married, Oct. 11, 1899, Miss Mary Worthington Milnor, of Baltimore, Md. See Amer. Biog. Direct., Washington, 1908; Univ. Maryland, 1907, II, p. 455.

664. MICHAEL D'ARCY MAGEE—Born July 21, 1871, Norfolk, Va. A. B., 1893; A. M., 1895, Rock Hill College, Ellicott City, Md.; M. D., 1896, Georgetown. Son of Michael and Mary Hoban Magee. Sometime Interne and Acting Superintendent, Garfield Memorial Hospital; Demonstrator in Surgery and Lecturer on Minor Surgery, Georgetown Med. School. Member Med. Assn., D. C., and Clinical Society, Washington. Married, April 25, 1899, Margaret Parker, of Portsmouth, Va. See Georgetown University, II, p. 106. See Magee and Johnson, Peterson's Surgery, Philadelphia, 1904.

665. ARCHIE WARD BOSWELL—Born April 22, 1871, Prince George Co., Md. M. D., 1894, Columbian.

OCTOBER 5, 1898

666. JOHN CRAYKE SIMPSON—Born July 12, 1858, Pelius Grove, Pa. M. D., 1882, Univ. Pennsylvania.

667. VICTOR E. WATKINS—Born Nov. 12, 1871, Hawley, Pa. M. D., 1894, Georgetown. Acting Asst. Surg., U. S. A. Resigned from Society, Jan. 13, 1904.

668. MAURICE ERWIN MILLER—Born Jan. 15, 1868, Reading, Pa. M. D., 1895, Jefferson.

669. ISABEL HASLUP—Born Sept. 16, 1864, Laurel, Md. M. D., 1897, Howard. Married, July 3, 1899, Dr. D. S. Lamb, *supra*. Daughter of J. Waters and Susannah Harrison Haslup. Educated in public schools, Baltimore; graduated at State Normal School, and taught in Maryland and Washington schools till 1892. Sometime Externe, Freedmen's Hospital. Since graduation has practiced in Washington. Assistant in Gynecology, Freedmen's Hospital; Med. Inspector, Public Schools; Attending Physician, Woman's Dispensary, 1897-9; Clinician, Woman's Clinic, 1898-1900. Member Therapeutic Society, Washington; Med. Assn., D. C. Co-author of Lamb and Lamb's Rules of health, 1900. See Lamb's History, p. 138; Amer. Biog. Direct., Washington, 1908.

670. JESSE HOUCK RAMSBURGH—Born Sept. 25, 1869, Frederick Co., Md. A. B., 1890; A. M., 1895, St. John's College, Annapolis, Md.; M. D., 1895, Univ. Va. Acting Asst. Surg., U. S. A. Son of John Stephen and Drusilla Hellen Beeson Ramsburgh; descendant of Ramsburghs, who emigrated to Maryland in 1656, and Beesons, who founded Uniontown, Penna.; Thomas Johnson, first Governor of Maryland, and Hon. John Grubb, an officer in the Colonial Wars. Educated at the Frederick Acad. and St. John's College, Annapolis. In 1895 attended post-graduate course, N. Y. Polyclinic and N. Y. hospitals. Resident Physician, 1895-6, Providence Hospital, Washington; Assistant at Emergency Hospital; on Staff of Georgetown Univ. Hospital. During Spanish War served with army in Cuba, Montauk Point and .Plattsburg, N. Y. Received laudatory letter from officers of 16th U. S. Inf. before Santiago, Cuba. Prof. Oral Surgery, Georgetown Med. School; Consultant in Diseases of Throat and Chest, Frederick City (Md.) Hosp.; Chief of Clinic, Free Dispensary for Consumptives, Washington; Secretary and Treasurer, Wash. Sanatorium for Tuberculosis. Member Society Army Santiago de Cuba. Married, Nov. 21, 1900, Edith, daughter of Dr. Wm. E. Roberts, *supra*. See Amer. Biog. Direct., Washington, 1908; Georgetown University, II, p. 113.

APRIL 5, 1899

671. JACOB PRESTON MILLER—Born Jan. 19, 1853, Fayette Co., Pa. M. D., 1878, Med. College, Ohio. Died Jan. 23, 1909. Educated in public schools and by private tutor; taught school four years. Practiced eighteen years at Buckhannon, W. Va.; Vice President, Society of W. Va. Took post-graduate courses in New York, Paris, Berlin and Vienna. Member A. M. A.; Internat. Med. Congress, 1887; Med. Assn., D. C. In service at Dispensary Clinic, Garfield Hospital and Episcopal

Eye, Ear and Throat Hosp., Washington.   In 1891 married Debra Anna Gore, of Clarksburg, W. Va. See Amer. Biog. Direct., Washington, 1908; Minutes Med. Society, March 17, 1909; Wash. Med. Annals, May, 1909, p. 134.

672. JOHN BAILEY MULLINS—Born Feb. 17, 1867, Princess Anne Co., Va. M. D., 1887, Univ. Maryland. Died Feb. 11, 1909. Son of Col. John Mullins, of Mississippi. Educated at Virginia Polytechnic Institute, Blacksburg, Va. In 1894 married Miss Annette B. Kennedy, of Brunswick, Mo. Practiced at Baltimore until 1899, when he removed to Washington. Member Med. Assn., D. C.; A. M. A.; Amer. Laryngol., Rhinol. and Otol. Society ; Clinical Society, Washington. Assistant Physician Emergency Hospital. Sometime Demonstrator Laryngology and Rhinology, Georgetown Med. School. See Minutes Med. Society, March 10, 1909; Wash. Med. Annals, May, 1909, p. 134; Georgetown University, II, p. 123.

673. WILSON PRESTMAN MALONE—Born July 23, 1863, Old Fort, N. C. M. D., 1888, Univ. Maryland. Took post-graduate course, 1892, Presbyterian Eye and Ear Infirmary, Baltimore, Md., and 1897, in Eye and Ear, at Johns Hopkins.

674. CHARLES EMORY FERGUSON—Born Dec. 27, 1873, Rockville, Ind. M. D., 1896, National Univ., D. C.

675. ERNEST W. FOWLER—M. D., 1895, Coll. P. and S., N. Y. City. Removed, 1902, from D. C. Contract Surgeon, U. S. A.

676. BERNARD LAWRISTON HARDIN—Born June 14, 1870, Lexington, Va. B. S., 1890, Va. Mil. Institute ; M. D., 1895, Columbian.

677. WILLIAM GERRY MORGAN—Born May 2, 1868, Newport, N. H. A. B., 1890, Dartmouth ; M. D., 1893, Univ. Penna.

OCTOBER 4, 1899

678. THOMAS DOWLING, Jr.—Born June 26, 1870, D. C. Graduated at Emerson Institute, Washington; M. D., 1898, Columbian. Asst. Med. Examiner, Volunteer Relief Dept., Penna. R. R., 1905-8. Asst. Med. Examiner, and afterward Surgeon, Washington Terminal Co.

679. ROBERT SCOTT LAMB—Born Oct. 15, 1876, D. C. M. D., 1898, Howard. Son of Dr. D. S. and Elizabeth Scott Lamb, *supra*. Attended public schools ; graduated from High School, Washington, in

1893; attended Cornell University, 1893-4. After graduation in medicine practiced two years, was then appointed Med. Inspector in service of Penna. R. R., in Pennsylvania. Studied at Pennsylvania and Wills Eye Hospitals, Philadelphia. Returned to Washington and resumed practice. For some years was Prof. Physiology, U. S. College Vet. Surgeons, Washington. Is Associate Attend. Physician, Episcopal Eye, Ear and Throat Hospital ; Prof. Ophthalmology, Howard Med. School ; Ophthalmic Surgeon, Freedmen's Hosp. Member Med. Assn., D. C. ; A. M. A.; and Wash. Ophthalmolog. Society. Married, Feb. 5, 1901, Sarah Keen, daughter of Geo. J. and Sarah McClosky Keen, Washington. See Lamb's History, p. 137.

680. WALLACE NEFF—Born Oct. 13, 1852, Cincinnati, Ohio. A. B., 1874 ; A. M., 1877, Princeton ; M. D., 1879, Med. College, Ohio. Surgeon, U. S. Vols.

681. WILLIAM E. WHITSON—Born April 19, 1874, Virginia. M. D., 1898, Columbian.

APRIL 4, 1900

682. JOHN RYAN DEVEREUX—Born Dec. 16, 1868, Lawrence, Kansas. B. S., 1889 ; M. A., 1893, Manhattan College, N. Y. ; M. D., 1892, Univ. Penna. Acting Asst. Surg. and Asst. Surg., U. S. A.

OCTOBER 3, 1900

683. GEORGE BOAZ COREY—Born May 28, 1865, D. C. M. D., 1897, Howard. Son of James Weed and Charlotte E. (Caywood) Corey ; descendant of Giles Corey, of Salem Farms, immortalized in Longfellow's "Christus;" of Isaac Preston Corey, author of Corey's Ancient Fragments, the first translation of the Hieroglyphics of Egypt; of Lord Rowton, Montague Corey, biographer of Disraeli ; of Samuel Andrews, an officer under Gen. George Washington ; of Benoni Andrews, of the French and Indian War; and of Anneka-Jans Bogardas, grand daughter of William of Orange. Was educated in public schools and Columbian Univ. Since graduation has practiced medicine in Washington. Married, in 1889, E. Louise Fowler, of Baltimore, Md., who died in 1893. In 1896, married M. Lucia Naylor, of Pekin, Ill. See Lamb's History, p. 160.

684. DANIEL WEBSTER PRENTISS, JR.—Born Sept. 9, 1874, D. C. Son of Dr. D. W. Prentiss, *supra ;* brother of Dr. E. C. Prentiss, *infra.* B. S., 1895 ; M. D., 1899, Columbian. Asst. Prof. Histology, G. W. Univ. Med. School ; Associate in Gynecology, Emergency Hospital ;

24

Visiting Physician, Freedmen's Hospital; Pathologist, Sibley and Emergency Hospitals. Member Med. Assn., D. C. Unmarried. See Amer. Biog. Direct., Washington, 1908.

685. WILLIAM KRAFFT WARD—Born Feb. 18, 1876, D. C. M. D., 1899, Columbian. Asst. Surgeon, U. S. M. H. S.

686. HARRY HURTT—Born Feb. 22, 1873, Kent Co., Md. M. D., 1895, Univ. Maryland. Of English descent; son of James W. and Mary Elizabeth Woodland Hurtt. Educated at village school, Shrewsbury Academy and Washington College. Post-graduate course at Johns Hopkins Hospital, 1895-6. Member Med. Assn., D. C.; A. M. A.; Clinical Society, Washington ; Wash. Acad. Sciences. See Amer. Biog. Direct., Washington, 1908.

687. HENRY ALEXANDER POLKINHORN—Born Feb. 26, 1874, D. C. M. D., 1896, Med.-Chirurg. College, Philadelphia, Pa.

688. AMELIA FRANCES FOYE—Born Aug. 15, 1871, Honeoye, N. Y. M. D., 1898, Howard. See Lamb's History, p. 166.

689. MICHAEL FRANCIS GALLAGHER—Born May 30, 1859, Pennsylvania. M. D., 1889, Georgetown. Sometime Immigrant Inspector, Immigration Service.

690. KATHRYN LORIGAN—Born Nov. 6, 1877, Vermont. M. D., 1897, Bishop's College, Montreal. Dropped from membership, 1904. Removed to Allegheny, Pa.

691. JAMES ROANE—Born in 1860. M. D., 1882, Georgetown. Dropped from membership, 1896.

APRIL 3, 1901

692. HENRY JOHNS RHETT—Born Oct. 10, 1863, Newport, R. I. A. B., 1885, Brown; M. D., 1890, Univ. Penna.

693. HANSON THOMAS ASBURY LEMON—Born Feb. 3, 1869, Baltimore, Md. M. D., 1896, Columbian.

694. ELIZABETH BAILEY MUNCEY—Born Jan. 6, 1858, Bristol, Pa. M. D., 1898, Howard. Educated at Bristol High School and State Normal School, Millersville, Pa. Taught at Bristol High School. Since graduation has practiced medicine in Washington. See Lamb's History, p. 201.

695. JOSEPH CARLISLE DE VRIES—Born May 26, 1869, N. Y. City. M. D., 1895, Univ. City New York. Acting Asst. Surg., U. S. A., Spanish-American War; Acting Asst. Surg., U. S. N, 1903-5. Removed to Watkins, N. Y. Prof. Pathology, Med. Dept., National Univ., Washington, 1899-1903; Attending Gynecologist, Emergency Hospital, 1899-1903; Recorder, Assn. Military Surgeons, U. S.; member Med. Assn., D. C.; A. M. A.; Attending Surgeon, St. Bartholomew's Clinic, N. Y. City, and Attending Gynecologist, Columbus Hospital, N. Y. City; honorary member Indian Med. Assn., Calcutta, India, and Société de Méd. et d'Hygiène Tropicales, Paris, France; Secretary and Treasurer, New York Assn. Med. Examiners.

696. THEODORE YOUNG HULL—Born Aug. 24, 1860, N. Y. City. B. Sc., 1884, Amity College, Iowa; M. D., 1892, Columbian. Removed, 1906, to San Antonio, Texas. Dropped from membership, Jan. 27, 1909.

697. EDWARD F. PICKFORD—Born July, 1868, Schenectady, N. Y. A. B., 1890, Union College, Schenectady; M. D., 1895, Albany.

698. ANDREW DUNBAR FORSYTHE—Born March 31, 1874, Harrodsburg, Ky. M. D., 1897, Hosp. Coll. Med., Louisville, Ky. Died July 31, 1907, of peritonitis. Son of Dr. Matthew Leander and Bettie Griffith Forsythe. Graduated, 1892, Central Univ., Ky. Resident Physician, 1897-8, Louisville City Hospital; Children's Hospital, 1899-1900, Randall's Island, N. Y. Harbor; member Med. Assn., D. C.; A. M. A. Sept. 17, 1903, married Mary D. Asquith, Washington. See Amer. Biog. Direct., Washington, 1908; Minutes Med. Society, Oct. 9, 1907; Wash. Med. Annals, 1907, VI, p. 394.

OCTOBER 2, 1901

699. WILLIAM JULIUS REICHMANN THÓNSSEN—Born March 28, 1851, Cleve, Holstein, Germany. M. D., 1888, Howard. Educated in public schools in Holstein and Altona. Taught school at Chapel Hill and Houston, Texas, and Fredericksburg, Va., 1871-85. Attended postgraduate course at Columbian Med. School, 1892-3. Married, 1877, Miss Marie Catherine Stephan, of Baton Rouge, La. See Lamb's History, p. 223.

700. FERDINAND CLAIBORNE WALSH—Born Jan. 27, 1877, D. C. Son of Dr. Ralph Walsh, *supra*. M. D., 1899, Univ. Va. Removed to Cananea, Sonora, Mexico.

701. WILLIAM NORWOOD SUTER—Brother of Dr. H. Suter, *supra*. Born Oct. 11, 1861, Berryville, Va. A. B., 1883, Univ. Va.; M. D., 1886, Univ. Md. Asst. Surg., U. S. A., 1887-92. Author of Refraction, etc., Philadelphia, 1903; Handbook of optics, N. Y., 1899. See Powell's History, p. 616.

702. CLARENCE AUSTIN SMITH—Born Jan. 24, 1861, Derby, Conn. A. M., 1882, Yale; M. D., 1887, Coll. Phys. and Surg., N. Y. Interne, 1887-9, Bellevue Hospital. Removed to Seattle, Wash., June, 1889; in 1899 was at Elizabeth, N. J.; in 1900 in N. Y. City and at Johns Hopkins. Practiced, 1901-2, in Washington City. Resigned, 1902, from the Society, and returned to Seattle. Editor of Northwest Medicine.

703. WILLIAM RAYMOND MOULDEN—Born Jan. 16, 1877, D. C. M. D., 1900, Columbian. Removed to Manila, P. I., 1901; afterward to Bethesda, Md., where he is practicing medicine.

704. THOMAS SIM LEE—Born Dec. 24, 1868, N. Y. City. A. B., 1891, Harvard; M. D., 1894, College Phys. and Surg., N. Y. City. Son of Dr. Chas. Carroll and Helen Parrish Lee. Educated in private schools, N. Y. City; Stonyhurst College, England. Sometime Interne in N. Y. hospitals; did post-graduate work in hospitals at Vienna and Johns Hopkins. Is Visiting Physician to Home for Incurables, Washington; Asst. Prof. Physiology, Georgetown Med. School. See Georgetown Univ., II, p. 121.

APRIL 2, 1902

705. DANIEL BAEN STREET, Jr.—Born Sept. 15, 1875, D. C. Son of Dr. D. B. Street, *supra*. M. D., 1897, Columbian. Acting Asst. Surg., U. S. A., 1898-9. Dropped, 1905, from membership. Removed to Jersey City, N. J.

706. EUGENE LYMAN LE MERLE—Born Nov. 12, 1864, D. C. M. D., 1897, Columbian. Is in Health Department, D. C.

707. HENRY COOK MACATEE—Born Front Royal, Va., Aug. 4, 1878. Son of Chas. A. and Mary Cook Macatee. Educated in public schools and at Randolph-Macon Academy, Front Royal. M. D., 1900, Columbian. Was successively Externe and Interne at Garfield Memorial Hospital, 1899-1901. Began practice in Washington in 1901. In February, 1903, became Superintendent of George Washington Univ. Hosp. Resigned in July, 1904, and resumed private practice. Instructor in Medicine in George Washington Univ. Med. School, 1902-9, when he resigned. Is Associate in Internal Medicine at Emergency Hospital;

since 1905 has been a Medical Inspector of Public Schools, D. C. Member Med. Assn., D. C.; A. M. A.; Med. and Surg. Society, D. C. In 1906, married Miss Miniana Paxton, of Washington, D. C.

708. NORMAN RICHARDS JENNER—Born July 4, 1862, Olney, Ill. M. D., 1890, Howard; 1891, Georgetown. Demonstrator Anatomy, Howard Med. School; Associate in Nurses' Training School, Freedmen's Hospital. Married, Dec. 29, 1886, Alvira Gertrude Langwill, Rising Sun, Indiana. See Lamb's History, p. 129.

709. JESSE NEWMAN REEVE—Born Sept. 25, 1866, Greenville, Tenn. M. D., 1893, Georgetown.

710. ROBERT SOMERVELL BEALE—Born Dec. 9, 1876, D. C. Son of Dr. J. S. Beale, *supra*. M. D., 1900, Columbian.

711. MARY LOUISE STROBEL—Born May 2, 1854, D. C. M. D., 1896, National Univ., D. C. Sometime teacher in public schools, Washington. Clinician, Woman's Clinic. See Lamb's History, p. 271.

712. ELLIOTT COUES PRENTISS—Born March 19, 1877, D. C. Son of Dr. D. W. Prentiss, *supra;* brother of Dr. D. W. Prentiss, Jr., *supra*. M. D., 1900, Columbian. Resigned from Society, Oct. 16, 1907. Removed to El Paso, Texas.

713. SAMUEL H. GREENE, JR.—Born July 23, 1874, Vt. M. D., 1900, Columbian.

714. FRANK EUGENE GIBSON—Born Nov. 16, 1873, D. C. M. D., 1899, Columbian.

715. S. CLIFFORD COX—Born June 22, 1867, D. C. M. D., 1892, Columbian. Was Lieut. and Asst. Surgeon, 1st D. C. Vols., Spanish-American War.

OCTOBER 1, 1902

716. CHARLES LOFTUS GRANT ANDERSON—Born March 8, 1863, Washington Co., Md. M. D., 1884, College Phys. and Surg., N. Y. City. Licentiate, 1892, M. C. F., Maryland ; Acting Asst. Surg., U. S. A., and Asst. Surg., U. S. A., 1886-8 ; Surg., 29th Inf., U. S. Vols., Spanish War. Resigned membership, Jan. 17, 1906, and removed to Ancon, Panama. Reëlected April 8, 1908. Son of Rev. Geo. Wash. Anderson and Anna Maria Winter Anderson. Educated at Centenary Collegiate Institute, Hackettstown, N. J.; Claversack College, N. Y.,

and Univ. Penna. Studied medicine with Dr. T. M. A'Heron, Glen
Gardner, N. J. Was House Physician, Jersey City Charity Hosp., 1885.
Practiced medicine in N. Y. City, 1886. In 1888 began practice at
Hagerstown, Md. Removed to Washington. Member Washington Co.
Med. Society ; Med. and Chirurg. Faculty, Maryland ; Brooklyn Ethical Association ; Washington Anthropolog. Society. Physician, Isthmian Canal Commission, 1905-7 ; resigned March 1, 1907, and returned
to Washington. See Watson's Biog., p. 398 ; Powell's History, pp. 161,
712 ; Cordell's Med. Annals, Maryland, 1903, p. 301.

717. LOREN BASCOM TABER JOHNSON—Born June 15, 1875,
D. C   Son of Dr. J. Taber Johnson, *supra.* M. D., 1900, Georgetown.

718. L. FLEET LUCKETT—Born Sept. 19, 1871, Md. Son of Dr.
W. F. Luckett, *supra.* M. D., 1895, Columbian.

719. CAMILLO H. MACHINEK—Born Dec. 3, 1869, Freiburg,
Switzerland. M. D., 1892, Howard. Dropped from membership, 1907.
See Lamb's History, p. 195.

720. ROBERT HENDERSON GRAHAM—Born Jan. 29, 1849, Yellow
Springs, Ohio. M. D., 1879, Columbus Med. College. Died Aug. 24,
1903, of peritonitis, following operation for appendicitis. Spent his early
years at Reynoldsburg, near Columbus, Ohio. Served in Union Army
during Civil War. After graduation in medicine practiced at Marysville,
Ohio. Removed to Washington in 1889. Member of Business Men's
Assn. ; Director, Washington Savings Bank; member Med. Assn., D. C.;
Amer. Therapeutic Society. See Minutes Med. Society, Oct. 7 and 21,
1903 ; Wash. Med. Annals, 1903, II, p. 349.

721. CHARLES ALBERT BALL—Born Jan. 24, 1851, Alexandria
Co., Va. M. D., 1877, Columbian. Lieut., N. G. D. C., 1871-4. Son of
Robert and Elizabeth A. Ball. Educated in public schools and Bryant
and Stratton's Business College, Washington. Since graduation in med-
icine has practiced in Washington. 1893-99, was Pension Examining
Surgeon. See Amer. Biog. Direct., Washington, 1908.

722. EDWARD GRANT SEIBERT—Born Aug. 28, 1865, Chambersburg, Pa. Phar. G., 1887, Philadelphia College Pharmacy; M. D., 1893,
Columbian. Acting Asst. Surg., U. S. A., 1901-5. Son of Joseph Warren and Louise Little Seibert. Descendant of soldiers of Amer. Revolution. Graduated, 1881, Chambersburg High School. Post-graduate
medical course, N. Y. City, since which has practiced in Washington.
Medical Examiner, U. S. Civil Service Commission, 1894-1901 ; Expert

Medical Examiner, U. S. Pension Office; Asst. Prof. Chemistry, G. W. Univ.; Chief of corresponding service in Dispensary of G. W. Univ. Hospital. Member A. M. A.; Assn. Pension Examining Surgeons. March 5, 1904, married Jessie Eastman Hopkins. See Amer. Biog. Direct., Washington, 1908.

723. GEORGE CORREL BURTON—Born Feb. 26, 1857, Georgia, Ind. M. D., 1881, Louisville Med. College. Died July 22, 1909, Mitchell, Ind.

724. THOMAS SANFORD DUNAWAY GRASTY—Born Nov. 16, 1879, Fredericksburg, Va. M. D., 1901, Columbian.

725. HOWARD WILSON BARKER—Born Jan. 4, 1875, D. C. Son of Dr. H. H. Barker, *supra.* M. D., 1901, National Univ., D. C.

726. ALBERT JOSEPH CARRICO—Born Oct. 18, 1874, Bryantown, Md. M. D., 1896, Univ. Maryland. Son of Dr. Thos. A. and Anne Priscilla Dent Carrico; of Spanish descent on his father's side. Educated in public and private schools near Bryantown, and at Rock Hill College. After graduation in medicine practiced in Charles County until 1900, when he removed to Washington. Member Med. Assn., D. C., and A. M. A. Married, Oct. 26, 1903, Harriett Anne Thyson, of Washington. See Univ. Maryland, 1907, II, p. 442.

727. ELIJAH LUMBIA MASON—Born Feb. 23, 1871, Virginia. M. D., 1901, Columbian. Pathologist and Bacteriologist, Children's Hospital; Visiting Physician, Washington City Orphan Asylum.

728. THOMAS BEST KRAMER—Born Feb. 18, 1852, Baltimore, Md. M. D., 1887, Howard. Grandson of Lieut. John Jacob Kramer, of war of Amer. Revolution; son of Rev. Samuel Kramer, Major 3d Maryland Vols., 1861-65. Studied medicine with Surg. C. E. Black, U. S. Navy. Attended Philadelphia Coll. Pharmacy. After graduation in medicine practiced sometime in Brooklyn, N. Y.; afterwards in Washington. Married Luanna Crook, daughter of Francis A. Crook. See Lamb's History, p. 189.

729. WILLIAM ALEXANDER JACK, Jr.—Born Dec. 31, 1873, Newport, R. I. M. D., 1896, Howard. Son of Dr. Wm. A. Jack, of Washington. Was Interne, 1896-7, Freedmen's Hospital, Washington, since which has practiced medicine in Washington. See Lamb's History, p. 183.

730. ENRICO G. V. CASTELLI—Born Jan. 27, 1869, Florence, Italy. M. D., 1897, Bologna, Italy ; L. M., 1900, Dublin. Dropped, 1905, from membership. Removed to N. Y. City.

731. GIDEON BROWN MILLER—Born Dec. 27, 1861, Laurel Mills, Va. C. E., 1886; B. Sc., 1887, Va. Mil. Institute ; M. D., 1890, Univ. Virginia. Student, Johns Hopkins Post-Graduate School of Medicine, 1893-94, and Univ. Leipsig, Med. Dept., 1896-97. Interne, Johns Hopkins Hospital, 1894-6, and 1897 to 1901 ; Resident Gynecologist the last 16 months. In charge of Diseases of Women, Emergency Hospital, Washington ; Associate Surgeon, Columbia Hospital; Instructor, Gynecology, G. W. U. Med. Dept.

732. FREDERICK FRANCIS REPETTI—Born Sept. 5, 1858, D. C. M. D., 1895, Georgetown.

733. RAPHAEL BURKE DURFEE—Born Sept. 14, 1875, D. C. M. D. 1900, Georgetown. Resigned Jan. 25, 1905. Removed to Los Angeles, Cal.

734. EDGAR P. COPELAND—Born Nov. 24, 1878, D. C. M. D., 1900, Columbian. Instructor and Clinical Instructor in Pediatrics, G. W. U. Med. School. In charge Surgical Service, Out-Patients Department, Children's Hospital.

735. WM. CLARENCE GWYNN—Born Nov. 10, 1873, D. C. M. D., 1898, Georgetown.

736. De WITT CLINTON CHADWICK—Born Jan. 5, 1858, Camden, Ohio. M. D., 1895, Columbian.

737. JAMES JULIUS RICHARDSON—Born Jan. 23, 1868, Sardis, Ohio. M. D., 1889, Univ. Maryland. Son of R. P. and Elizabeth Richardson. Post-graduate medical courses at N.Y. Post-Graduate Med. School, Univ. Edinburgh, Univ. Vienna and Post-Graduate School, of London. Married. See Amer. Biog. Direct., Washington, 1908.

738. SAMUEL WESLEY MELLOTT—Born Aug. 3, 1861, Beallsville, Ohio. B. S., 1895, Mt. Union College, Ohio ; M. D., 1897, Howard. Dropped from membership, 1907. Assistant Examiner, U. S. Pension Office. See Lamb's History, p. 198.

739. GEORGE KASPER BAIER—Born Jan. 24, 1876, D. C. M. D., 1898, Columbian. LL. B., 1904, National Univ., D. C.

740. NEIL DUNCAN GRAHAM—Born Sept. 22, 1874, Falls Church, Va. Son of Dr. N. F. Graham, *supra*. M. D., 1901, Johns Hopkins.

741. CHARLES H. JAMES—Born March 4, 1874, D. C. M. D., 1897, Columbian. Dropped from membership, Jan. 27, 1909.

742. R. R. FARQUHAR—Born Oct. 1, 1876, Annapolis, Md. Hospital Steward, U. S. Navy, in Spanish-American War. M. D., 1899, Univ. Penna. Acting Asst. Surg., U. S. M. H. S.

743. JOHN LEWIS RIGGLES—Born Aug. 7, 1877, D. C. M. D., 1900, Columbian.

744. CARL SCHURZ KEYSER—Born Feb. 14, 1872, D. C. M. D., 1898, Columbian.

745. BENJAMIN F. TIEFENTHALER—Born Sept. 7, 1869, Wooster, Ohio. M. D., 1899, Columbian. Died Feb. 6, 1908, of Bright's disease. Graduated in and practiced pharmacy in Ohio. Sometime Secretary to Dean of G. W. Univ. Med. School. Married, April 23, 1895, Miss Daisy Oldroyd, daughter of Capt. and Mrs. O. H. Oldroyd, of Washington; after which practiced in Washington. See Minutes Med. Society, Feb. 26, 1908; Wash. Med. Annals, 1908, VII, p. 122.

746. RICHARD SCOTT BLACKBURN—Born April 29, 1875, Virginia. M. D., 1898, Univ. Va. Resigned Dec. 2, 1908.

747. JOSEPH STILES WALL—Born Oct. 3, 1876, D. C. M. D., 1897, Georgetown. Sometime Surg. Police and Fire Depts., D. C.; Med. Examiner, Board Registration, D. C. Married.

748. THOMAS ALLEN GROOVER—Born May 9, 1877, Pidcock, Ga. M. D., 1898, Columbian. Med. Inspector, Public Schools, D. C.

749. WILLIAM PINKNEY REEVES—Born Feb. 6, 1871, Maryland. M. D., 1899, Georgetown.

750. LUTHER HALSEY REICHELDERFER—Born Feb. 4, 1874, Hallsville, Ohio. M. D., 1899, Columbian. Lieut. Col., 1st Regt. D. C. N. G. Supt. and Chief Resident Physician, Garfield Memorial Hospital, 1900-7; member of Faculty, G. W. Univ. Med. School; of Consulting Staff, Woman's Clinic; of Attending Staff, Garfield and Tuberculosis Hospitals, Washington.

751. JOHN SEDWICK DORSEY—Born Feb. 28, 1868, Port Republic, Md.   M. D., 1890, Coll. Phys. and Surg., Baltimore, Md.

752. THOMAS JOHN CHEW—Born Feb. 25, 1846, Maryland.   A. M., 1865, Princeton; M. D., 1868, Univ. Maryland.   Died May 1, 1904. See Minutes Med. Society, May 4, 1904; Wash. Med. Annals, III, 1904-5, p. 282.

753. MONTGOMERY HUNTER—Born May 11, 1864, Alexandria, Va. M. D., 1896, Columbian.

754. HOWARD FISHER—Born Jan. 25, 1866, Wheeling, W. Va.   A. B., 1886; A. M., 1889, Hanover, Ind. ; graduate, 1889, Theology, McCormick Theological Seminary, Chicago ; M. D., 1895, Jefferson.   Son of Rev. D. W. and Amanda Kounts Fisher.   Educated at Hanover College, Ind., and the Theological Seminary.   Medical Missionary sometime in East Indies.   Attended, 1899-1900, Univ. Berlin.   Associate in Children's Clinic, Emergency Hospital, Washington.   Jan. 10, 1896, married S. Katharine Conner.   See Amer. Biog. Direct., Washington, 1908.

755. CHARLES STANLEY WHITE—Born July 1, 1877, D. C.   M. D., 1898, Columbian.   Interne, Columbian Univ. Hospital, 1898-9 ; Columbia Hospital, 1899-1901.   Practiced in Washington, 1901-3.   House Surgeon, Emergency Hospital, 1903-6; Superintendent of same, 1906-8. Post-graduate courses at Harvard, 1903, and Post-Graduate School, Chicago, 1904.   Vice President, Wash. Obstet. and Gynecol. Society, 1907-8; Vice President, George Washington Univ. Med. Society, 1907-8 ; Asst. Prof. Surgery, George Washington Univ. Med. School; Associate in Surgery, Central Disp. and Emergency Hosp.   Co-editor, Wash. Med. Annals.

756. EDITH LYALL MADDREN—Born Jan. 8, 1877, D. C.   M. D., 1899, National Univ., D. C.   Dropped from membership, 1906.   Physician in Indian Service at Cheyenne Reservation, Cherry Creek, S. Dak.

757. JOHN PAUL GUNION—Born Sept. 15, 1876, ;D. C.   M. D., 1899, Columbian.

758. WILLIAM SAWYER NEWELL—Born Oct. 22, 1874, Evansville, Ind. M. D., 1895, Columbian.

759. JOHN ALPHONSO O'DONOGHUE—Born Dec. 18, 1874, D. C. A. B., 1896, Rock Hill College, Ellicott City, Md.; A. M., 1897 ; M. D., 1900, Georgetown.

760. WILLIAM JOHN ARMSTRONG—Born Sept. 15, 1835, Philadelphia, Pa. M. D., 1870, Georgetown.

761. CHARLES M. EMMONS—Born Nov. 11, 1873, D. C. M. D., 1893, Georgetown; LL. B., 1902, National Univ.; LL. M., 1904, Washington College of Law. See Lamb's History, p. 135.

762. JESSE SHOUP—Born Feb. 24, 1865, Ohio. M. D., 1891, Jefferson.

763. ALFRED VANDIVER PARSONS—Born March 19, 1863, Baltimore, Md. M. D., 1889, Univ. Maryland. Son of Eliphalet and Sue F. Warner Parsons, of American ancestry. Educated in private schools, Baltimore. Practiced in Baltimore about a year, then removed to Washington. Member Med. Assn., D. C. Married, June 23, 1891, Minnie C. Losekam. See Univ. Maryland, 1907, II, p. 247.

764. WALTER PRINCE KEENE—M. D., 1900, Georgetown. Acting Asst. Surg., Revenue Marine Service. Resigned. Removed to California.

[Lewis Albert Walker, Jr.—Never qualified and name dropped, Nov. 1, 1905.]

APRIL 15, 1903

765. FRANCIS STANISLAUS MACHEN—Born Dec. 18, 1873, Toledo, Ohio. Educated in common schools and Detroit College, Michigan. M. D., 1901, Georgetown.

766. HENRY MERRILL JEWETT—Born April 26, 1879, Laconia, N. H. M. D., 1902, Columbian.

767. FRANK LEE BISCOE—Born Sept. 9, 1876, D. C. M. D., 1901, Georgetown.

768. TRUMAN ABBE—Born Nov. 1, 1873, D. C. A. B., 1895, Harvard; M. D., 1899, College Phys. and Surgeons, N. Y. Son of Cleveland and Frances M. Abbe. Educated in public schools of Washington. After graduation spent three years at Univ. Berlin and in hospitals, N. Y. City. Taught Physiology and Surgery, 1902-5, Georgetown Med. School; since 1905 at G. W. Univ. Med. School. Practiced in Washington since 1902. April 22, 1905, married Ethel W. Brown. See Amer. Biog. Direct., Washington, 1908.

769. AUBREY HORATIO STAPLES—Born July 21, 1874, Jersey City, N. J. M. D., 1896, Baltimore Med. College. Educated in public schools at Oil City, Pa., and Presbyterian College, New Windsor. After graduation passed New Jersey State Board. Is practicing in Washington.

770. CHARLES HERMAN CLARK—Born July 30, 1866, Mechanicsburg, Ohio. M. D., 1893, Starling Med. College. Resigned. Removed, March 27, 1907, to Cleveland, Ohio. Supt. Ohio State Insane Asylum.

771. ADOLPHUS BOGARDUS BENNETT, JR.—Born Oct. 18, 1879, Brantford, Canada. M. D., 1901, Columbian. Capt., Med. Corps, D. C. N. G.

772. GEORGE WALTER WARREN—Born Dec. 13, 1863, Wilson, N. C. M. D., 1892, Baltimore University.

773. JOSEPH FRANCIS McKAIG—Born Sept. 15, 1869, N. Y. A. B., 1890; M. D., 1893, Georgetown. Son of Thomas and Mary A. Loughran McKaig. Educated in public and parochial schools, and Gonzaga College, Washington. Member Med. Assn., D. C.; A. M. A. Married, Jan. 9, 1899, Catherine Carley. See Georgetown University, II, p. 267.

OCTOBER 7, 1903

774. SIMON RUFUS KARPELES—Born March 1, 1880, D. C. M. D., 1902, National Univ., D. C. Secretary, Therapeutic Society, D. C.

775. ANTHONY MORELAND RAY—Born April 17, 1867, Forest Glen, Md. M. D., 1895, Univ. Virginia.

776. GUSTAVUS WERBER—Born Dec. 18, 1864, Newberry, S. C. A. B., 1882; A. M., 1884, Newberry; M. D., 1894, Columbian. Son of Frederick and Louisa Werber. Since graduation in medicine has practiced in Washington. April 30, 1902, married Catharine Moses. See Amer. Biog. Direct., Washington, 1908.

777. WALTER HIBBARD MERRILL—Born Feb. 17, 1873, Marlboro, N. H. B. L., 1894, Dartmouth; M. D., 1901, Columbian. See Johnson and Merrill, The X rays, Philadelphia, 1900.

778. C. NORMAN HOWARD—Born Sept. 23, 1875, Bethlehem, Pa. M. D., 1898, Columbian. Removed, January, 1907, to Warsaw, Ind. Resigned from Med. Society, Jan. 1, 1908. Graduated from City Hospital, Blackwell's Island, N. Y. City, Aug. 1, 1902—course of twenty months. Substituted at Nursery and Child's Hospital, in 1900, and Gouverneur Hospital, N. Y. City. Took X-Ray course, Johns Hopkins Hospital, 1903. N. Y. State license, 1902. Asst. Attending Physician of Emergency Hospital, G. W. Univ. Hospital, Episcopal Eye, Ear and Throat Hospital, Washington. Member Board of Directors, Woman's Clinic, Washington. Served during Cuban campaign as Financial Secretary to Brig. Gen. William Ludlow, Chief Engineer on General Miles' Staff. In office Adjutant General, U. S. A., 1899–1900.

779. MELCHIOR B. STRICKLER—Born May 21, 1834, Pennsylvania. M. D., 1861, Univ. Penna.

780. DANIEL DOMINICK MULCAHY—Born Aug. 7, 1871, near Ellicott City, Md. Phar. D., 1893, Nat. Coll. Pharmacy, D. C. ; M. D., 1899, Georgetown.

781. LAURA MARIE REVILLE—Born Nov. 1, 1847, Ohio Co., Ind. M. D., 1890, Woman's Med. College, Philadelphia, Pa.

782. SAMUEL FRY—Born Oct. 26, 1870, New Orleans, La. M. D., 1902, Columbian.

783. ALBERT LYNCH LAWRENCE—Born June 22, 1864, Columbus, Ohio. Phar. D., 1885, Nat. Coll. Pharmacy, D. C. ; M. D., 1896, Columbian. Member Med. Assn., D. C., and A. M. A.

784. HENRY MARSHALL DIXON—Born Dec. 9, 1870, Yazoo, Miss. M. D., 1895, Columbian.

[William Bernard Johnston — Son of Dr. W. W. Johnston, *supra.* Failed to qualify.]

OCTOBER 14, 1903

785. OSCAR WILKINSON—Born Aug. 31, 1870, Mississippi. M. D., 1896, Tulane.

786. EDGAR DORMAN THOMPSON—Born Oct. 10, 1871, Doe Run, Pa. A. B., 1893; A. M., 1896, Franklin and Marshall College, Lancaster, Pa.; M. D., 1896, Long Island Coll. Hospital.

APRIL 6, 1904

787. CHARLES M. BEALL—Born Sept. 22, 1877, D. C. M. D., 1900, Columbian. Inspector, Health Dept., D. C.

788. BLANCHE ROSALIE SLAUGHTER—Born Oct. 28, 1873, Lynchburg, Va. M. D., 1897, Woman's Med. College, Philadelphia. Married, 1906, Baxter Morton. Resigned membership, Oct. 17, 1906, and removed to N. Y. City. Editor, etc., Daughters of Aesculapius, Philadelphia, 1897.

789. JOHN JOSEPH REPETTI—Born Feb. 6, 1875, D. C. M. D., 1897, Georgetown. Asst. Surg., U. S. Vols. Acting Asst. Surg., U.S.A.

790. TAYLOR BOYD DIXON—Born March 30, 1876, Baltimore, Md. M. D., 1900, Columbian.

791. JOSEPH CLARENCE TAPPAN—Born May 31, 1871, D. C. M. D., 1899, Columbian.

792. ALMER M. HOADLEY—Born Nov. 4, 1861, Avoca, N. Y. M. D., 1902, Columbian. Died of uremia, Dec. 8, 1907. Was associated some time with his father in management of Belvidere Hotel, Washington. After graduation in medicine practiced in Washington. Buried at Avoca. See Minutes Med. Society, Jan. 6 and 15, 1908; Wash. Med. Annals, 1908, VII, pp. 124, 125.

[W. W. Richardson was elected but failed to qualify.]

OCTOBER 5, 1904

793. B. ALICE CRUSH—Born Oct. 11, 1848, Newcastle, Va. M. D., 1894, Columbian.

794. HENRY HOLLIDAY STROMBERGER—Born Feb. 20, 1866, D. C. M. D., 1899, Columbian. Acting Asst. Surg., U. S. A.

795. GEORGE ALTICK CURRIDEN—Born July 4, 1866, Shippensburg, Pa. M. D., 1892, Univ. Penna. Acting Asst. Surgeon, U. S. A. Removed, Sept. 15, 1905, to Chambersburg, Pa. Died April 15, 1908, at Grand Rapids, Mich.

796. JOHN POTTS FILLEBROWN—Born Sept. 23, 1858, D. C. M. E., 1880, Lafayette College; M. D., 1897, Bellevue.

797. HENRY RANDALL ELLIOTT, JR.—Born July 18, 1874, D. C. M. D., 1895, Univ. Va.

798. EDWARD ELLIOTT RICHARDSON—Born Feb. 19, 1873, Rockingham, Vt. B. S., 1904; M. S., 1905; M. D., 1895, Columbian. Physician to the Poor, 1895-9. Med. Inspector, Public Schools, D. C., 1899. Asst. Demons. Anatomy, 1898, Columbian; Prosector, 1899-1901.

799. EDGAR WILLIAM WATKINS.—Born Aug. 26, 1857, Fairfax Co., Va. M. D., 1896, National Univ., D. C. Member A. M. A., and Nat. Therap. Assn. On Staff of Casualty Hospital, D. C.

800. JAMES FARNANDIS MITCHELL—Born July 1, 1871, Baltimore, Md. A. B., 1891; M. D., 1897, Johns Hopkins.

801. MARY HOLMES—Born March 15, 1874, New Lexington, Ohio. M. D., 1900, National Univ., D. C.; 1901, Woman's Med. Coll., Philadelphia, Pa. Clinician, Woman's Clinic and Woman's Dispensary, Washington.

802. ALFRED RICHARDS—Born Sept. 29, 1872, D. C. M. D., 1897, Georgetown. Acting Asst. Surg., U. S. A.; Surg. Met. Police and Fire Depts., D. C.

803. HARRY ATWOOD FOWLER—Born Sept. 22, 1872, Boston, Mass. B. S., 1895, Univ. Minn.; M. D., 1901, Johns Hopkins. Prof. Genito-Urinary Diseases, Howard Univ. Med. School, D. C.

804. ARTHUR HERBERT KIMBALL—Born March 13, 1875, D. C. B. S., 1897; A. M., 1903, Amherst; M. D., 1902, Johns Hopkins.

805. LOUISE TAYLER-JONES—Born Nov. 14, 1870, Youngstown, Ohio. B. S., 1896, Wellesley; M. S., 1898, Columbian; M. D., 1903, Johns Hopkins.

806. CHARLES ALEXANDER CRAWFORD—Born Feb. 28, 1875, Natchez, Miss. M. D., 1897, Univ. of Va. Passed Asst. Surg., U. S. N.

807. ANNA BARTSCH—Born Dec. 18, 1876, Silesia, Germany. M. D., 1902, Howard. Graduated at High School, Burlington, Iowa. Was Resident Physician, Lying-in Charity Hospital, Philadelphia, 1902-3; Associate Prof. Histology and in charge Physiological Laboratory, Quiz Master in Obstetrics, and Obstetrical Clinician, Howard Univ. Med. School, Washington; Clinician, Woman's Clinic. Married Dr. H. E. Dunne, of Ridgway, Pa., and removed there in 1908. See Lamb's Hist., p. 234.

808. ROBERT JOHN McADORY.—Born Aug. 15, 1872, Mobile, Ala. Attended St. John's College, Annapolis, Md.; Corcoran Scientific School, D. C.; Stanford Univ., Cal. M. D., 1897, Univ. City N. Y. Acting Asst. Surgeon, U. S. A. ; Surgeon of Revenue Cutter.

809. JAMES GEORGE McKAY—Born July 26, 1871, Stockton-on-Tees, England. M. D., 1895, Univ. Penna. Asst. Surg., U. S. Vols., 1901-2. Acting Asst. Surgeon, U. S. A.

810. EDWARD HIRAM REEDE—Born June 3, 1875, N. Y. M. D., 1902, Johns Hopkins. Was Resident Physician, St. Luke's Hospital, N. Y. City. Dropped from membership, 1907.

APRIL 5, 1905

811. PETER HENRY STELTZ, JR.—Born Dec. 8, 1868, Allentown, Pa. M. D., 1888, Univ. Penna. Was Resident Physician, German Hospital, Philadelphia. Med. Examiner, Penna. R. R. ; Med. Examiner and Surgeon, Washington Terminal.

812. CARL LAWRENCE DAVIS—Born July 9, 1878, Vermontville, Mich. M. D., 1903, Columbian.

813. BUCKNER MAGILL RANDOLPH—Born Aug. 21, 1871, Co lumbia, Pa. M. D., 1898, Med. College Va.

814. JOSEPH ERNEST MITCHELL—Born Dec. 25, 1871, Tyaskin, Md. M. D., 1903, Columbian. Resident Physician, Washington Asylum Hospital, 1903-4.

815. HARRY HAMPTON DONNALLY—Born Sept. 4, 1877, Georgetown, Ky. A. M., 1897, Gallaudet; B. S., 1896; A. M., 1897; M. D., 1903, Columbian.

816. DWIGHT GORDON SMITH—Born Aug. 26, 1873, St. Louis, Mo. A. B., 1896, Williams; M. D., 1903, Columbian. Member Med. Assn., D. C.; Therapeutic Society ; Hippocrates Society. Interne and Resident Physician, Children's Hospital ; on Dispensary Staff, Emergency Hospital.

817. HENRY WOOD TOBIAS—Born May 8, 1876, Donaldson, Pa. B. E., 1895, Millersville College, Pa.; M. D., 1901, Columbian. Externe, Garfield Memorial Hospital ; Resident Physician, Casualty Hospital, University (Columbian) Hospital, and Wills' Mountain Sanatorium, of

Cumberland, Md. Physician to Tubercular Clinic, Associated Charities; Assistant to Nose and Throat Dispensary and Surgical Dispensary, Emergency Hospital. Married, April 30, 1907, Harriet B. Hamill.

818. JOSEPH DECATUR ROGERS—Born Nov. 23, 1880, Hamilton, Va. M. D., 1902, Columbian. Son of Samuel E. and Elizabeth C. Rogers. Educated at Washington High School and Columbian Univ. Postgraduate work in N. Y. hospitals, since which has practiced medicine in Washington. Was Resident Physician, Columbia Hospital and G. W. Univ. Hospital. Unmarried. See Amer. Biog. Direct., Washington, 1908.

819. WILLIAM FOWKE RAVENEL PHILLIPS—Born July 13, 1863, Bedford Co., Va. M. D., 1890, Columbian. Son of Dinwiddie P. and Nannie F. Walden Phillips. Educated in school, Chatham, Va. Med. Climatologist, 1895-1904, U. S. Weather Bureau; 1904-9, Dean, Med. Dept., G. W. Univ.; in 1891-2, and since 1895, Prof. Hygiene in same; President, 1905, Amer. Climatolog. Assn.; Secretary, Anatom. Board, D. C., since 1902. Sometime Editor of Climate and Health, official publication of Weather Bureau. Unmarried. See Who's Who in America; Amer. Men of Science, 1906; Amer. Biog. Direct., Washington, 1908.

820. LEWIS HARVIE TAYLOR—Born July 26, 1875, Chula, Va. M. D., 1903, Columbian.

821. JOHN BRADFORD BRIGGS, Jr.—Born Feb. 17, 1877, Cambridge, Mass. B. S., 1898, New York Univ.; M. D., 1902, Johns Hopkins.

822. LEON ELLERY STORY—Born July 8, 1879, Franklin, N. H. M. D., 1901, Georgetown. Removed to St. Johns, afterwards to Portland, Oregon. Inspector of public schools, Portland. Son of Dr. J. J. Story, of Washington, D. C.

823. REGINALD REDFORD WALKER—Born March 5, 1877, D. C. M. D., 1900, Georgetown.

OCTOBER 4, 1905

824. WILLIAM HITE HOUGH—Born Oct. 31, 1877, Waterford, Va. Phar. D., 1897, National Coll. Phar., D. C.; M. D., 1899, Georgetown. Assistant Physician, Govt. Hospital Insane, D. C.

825. MAHLON ASHFORD—Born March 24, 1881, D. C. Son of Dr. F. A. Ashford, *supra*. M. D., 1904, Georgetown. Resigned Jan. 15, 1909. Now Asst. Surgeon, U. S. A.

25

826. HARRY REID HUMMER—Born Jan. 27, 1879, D. C. M. D., 1899, Georgetown. Sometime Asst. Physician, St. Elizabeth Hospital, Washington. Removed to Caxton, South Dakota. Supt. of Insane Asylum.

827. BENJAMIN RUSH LOGIE—Born Oct. 8, 1867, Kearneysville, W. Va. M. D., 1890, Univ. Md. Assistant Physician, Govt. Hospital Insane, D. C.

828. FRANCIS ALPHONSE SCHNEIDER—Born Feb. 27, 1870, Herbstein, Germany. A. B., 1890, St. Mary's, North East, Pa.; M. D., 1901, Coll. Phys. and Surg., N. Y.; 1902, Univ. Berlin; Asst. Surgeon, Vanderbilt Clinic, N. Y., 1902-4; Asst. Eye and Ear Infirmary, N. Y., 1903-4; Asst., Georgetown Univ. Hosp., and Episcopal Eye, Ear and Throat Hosp., Washington.

829. FRANK FREMONT-SMITH—Born Sept. 13, 1856, Hillsboro, N. H. A. B., 1880, Dartmouth; M. D., 1883, Univ. Pa. Member Amer. Climat. Assn.; Wash. Acad. Sciences.

830. WILLIAM GAGE ERVING—Born Aug. 11, 1877, Hartford, Conn. B. A., 1898, Yale; M. D., 1902, Johns Hopkins. Husband of Dr. E. L. Erving, *infra*. Prof. Orthopedic Surgery, Howard Med. School; Orthopedic Surgeon, Providence and Freedmen's Hospitals; Member Amer. Orthopedic Assn.

APRIL 4, 1906

831. GEORGE TULLY VAUGHAN—Born June 27, 1859, Arrington, Va. M. D., 1879, Univ. Va.; 1880, Bellevue. Asst. Surg., 1888; Passed Asst. Surg., 1892; Surgeon, 1900, and Asst. Surg. General, 1902, U. S. M. H. S.; resigned in 1905; Brigade Surg., U. S. Vols., in Spanish War. Is of Welsh descent. Son of Dr. Washington L. and Francis Ellen Shields Vaughan. Educated at private schools and at Kenmore Univ. High School, Amherst, Va. Post-graduate medical courses at N. Y. Polyclinic Hospital, Jefferson Med. College, Philadelphia, and Univ. Berlin. Practiced at Lowesville and Farmville, Va., 1880-8. Prof. Surg., 1897, Georgetown Med. School; Chief Surg., Georgetown Univ. Hospital; Surgeon, Emergency Hospital; Consulting Surg., St. Elizabeth Asylum. Fellow Amer. Surg. Assn.; President, Assn. Mil. Surgeons; Corresponding member Society French Mil. Medicine; member Med. Society, Va.; Honorary member Vanderburg Co. Med. Society, Indiana; member Wash. Acad. Sciences. Married, 1883, May Townsend, daughter of W. G. Venable, Farmville, Va. Author of Principles and practice of surgery, Philadelphia, 1903-5. See Who's Who in America ; Stone's Biog., 1894, p. 693 ; Amer. Biog. Direct., Washington, 1908 ; Georgetown Univ., II, p. 105.

832. SOTHORON KEY—Born Jan. 29, 1873, Leonardtown, Md. B. S., 1894; M. S., 1897, Maryland Agricult. College ; M. D., 1899, Columbian.

833. GEORGE WASHINGTON BOYD—Born Nov. 18, 1859, D. C. Phar. D., 1880, National College Pharmacy, D. C.; M. D., 1895, College Phys. and Surg., Baltimore, Md.

834. HOMER G. FULLER—Born Jan. 10, 1879, Derby, Conn. Ph. B., 1901, Yale ; M. D., 1904, Columbian.

835. JOHN DUNLOP—Born July 4, 1876, D. C. B. S., 1898, Princeton; M. D., 1902, Johns Hopkins.

836. ERNEST PENDLETON MAGRUDER—Born Oct. 23, 1875, Upper Marlboro, Md. A. B., 1895, Johns Hopkins ; A. M., 1900; M. D., 1902, Columbian. Son of Caleb Clark Magruder and Elizabeth Rice Nalle ; grandson of Dr. Richard Thomas Nalle, of Virginia ; descendant of Alex. Magruder, immigrant, of the Clan Gregor, Scotland. Educated at Upper Marlboro Academy and Georgetown Univ. Was Asst. Demonstrator Anatomy, George Washington Univ., 1907-8 ; Asst. in Surgery, Georgetown Univ. Med. School, 1907-8 ; Med. and Surg. Associate, Emergency Hospital, 1907-8 ; now Superintendent Emergency Hosp. Member A. M. A.; Med. Assn., D. C.; Internat. Congress Tuberculosis.

837. ROBERT CONRAD RUEDY—Born July 12, 1876, Lenawee Co., Mich. M. D., 1904, Columbian.

838. SENECA BRAY BAIN—Born Feb. 10, 1874, Gatesville, Texas. D. D. S., 1898 ; M. D., 1899, National Univ., D. C. Son of Seneca McNeill and Annie M. Bain. Educated at Willis College and High School, Willis, Texas, and Trinity (Texas) Normal School. Taught one year in public school, Texas. For ten years in employ of U. S. Govt. 1899-1905, Special Agent, Dept. Labor. Member Med. Assn., D. C. ; A. M. A. ; Amer. Electro-Therapeut. Assn. ; Honorary member National Capital Dental Assn. Sept. 20, 1900, married Rosalind Moore, of Washington. See Amer. Biog. Direct., Washington, 1908.

839. JOHN WALTER HODGES—Born Dec. 8, 1856, Baltimore, Md. M. D., 1892, Baltimore Med. College. Educated in Baltimore public schools. In drug business, Annapolis, Md., 1885-91, and in Washington,

1891–1905, since which has practiced medicine in Washington. President, 1888, Maryland Pharm. Assn.; 1889–90, President, Business Men's Assn., Annapolis. Member Med. Assn., D. C.; A. M. A. Oct. 28, 1880, married Rosella Burgess. See Amer. Biog. Direct., Washington, 1908.

840. RICHARD MITCHEL LITTLE—Born Sept. 9, 1877, Mercer, Pa. M. D., 1902, Columbian.

841. SAMUEL LOGAN OWENS—Born Jan. 14, 1879, Washington, La. M. D., 1903, Georgetown.

842. THOMAS F. LOWE—M. D., 1902, Georgetown.

843. GEORGE MENDENHALL RUFFIN—Born Sept. 12, 1876, Wilson, N. C. Brother of Dr. Sterling Ruffin, *supra*. M. D., 1902, Columbian.

844. ROY DELAPLAINE ADAMS—Born Oct. 26, 1881, Circleville, Ohio. M. D., 1904, Georgetown. Resident Physician, Georgetown Univ. Hosp., 1904–5 ; Lecturer on Embryology, Georgetown Med. School ; in Surgical Service, Georgetown Univ. Hosp.

845. ARTHUR CASE FITCH—Born April 7, 1867, Delhi, N. Y. Phar. D., 1893, National College Pharmacy, D. C.; M. D., 1903, Columbian. Assistant Physician, Govt. Hospital Insane, D. C.

846. J. LAWN THOMPSON—Born Oct. 16, 1874, D. C. Son of Dr. Benedict Thompson, *supra*. M. D., 1904, Columbian.

847. LOUIS CHARLES LEHR—Born Feb. 17, 1876, Baltimore, Md. A. B., 1898; M. D., 1902, Johns Hopkins.

OCTOBER 3, 1906

848. ADAM KEMBLE—Born Nov. 11, 1878, Tower City, Pa. Phar. D., 1901, National College Pharmacy, D. C.; M. D., 1905, Columbian.

849. FREDERICK YATES—Born Dec. 21, 1878, Manchester, England. LL. M., 1903, National Univ., D. C.; M. D., 1902, Howard; 1904, Columbian.

850. EDWIN BERNHARD BEHREND—Born Sept. 2, 1871, D. C. Son of Dr. A. Behrend, *supra*. A. B., 1892, Johns Hopkins; M. D., 1894, Georgetown.

851. WALTER WATKINS WILKINSON—Born Sept. 10, 1876, Halifax Co., Va. M. D., 1905, Columbian. Resident Physician, 1905-6, Garfield Hospital, D. C.; Asst. Pathologist, Garfield, 1906; Instructor in Physical Diagnosis, George Washington University, 1907. Member G. W. U. Med. Society.

852. GEORGE H. HEITMULLER—Born Nov. 15, 1869, Arkenberg, Hanover, Germany, during a temporary residence abroad of his parents, Anton C. T. and Henrietta Horstkamp Heitmuller. Attended Columbian Preparatory School, 1884-7, Columbian College and Johns Hopkins University. A. B., 1891, Johns Hopkins; M. D., 1894, Univ. Penna. Served some time in Roxborough Hospital, then returned to Washington and began practice. In 1895 attended Univ. Berlin, and clinics, Royal London Ophthalmic Hospital; Clinical Assistant to Messrs. Treacher Collins and Quarry Sillcock over a year. In 1897, married Alice Florence, daughter of John and Mary Medhurst Pelham, of Sussex, England. Is Clinical Assistant, Eye Clinic, Casualty Hospital ; Medical Inspector, Public Schools, and Secretary, Wash. Med. and Surg. Society.

853. LAWRENCE MAXWELL HYNSON—Born Feb. 6, 1879, Still Pond, Kent Co., Md. M. D., 1904, Columbian. Son of Nathaniel Thornton and Lucy Weston Tiffey Hynson. Educated in public schools, Maryland and Washington. Was five years Assistant Secretary, National Geographic Society. Member Med. Assn., D. C.; G. W. Univ. Med. Society ; Hippocrates Society. Unmarried. See Amer. Biog. Direct., Washington, 1908.

854. WILLIAM BEVERLY MASON—Born July 26, 1874, Marshall, Va. M. D., 1899, Med. College Virginia.

855. CHARLES WILBUR HYDE—Born Dec. 30, 1877, Sullivan, Ohio. M. D., 1904, Columbian.

856. WALTER ASHBY FRANKLAND—Born Dec. 10, 1867, Baltimore, Md. M. D., 1896, Columbian.

857. JOHN DONALDSON MURRAY—Born Oct. 3, 1866, San Francisco, Cal. Son of ex-Surgeon General, U. S. A., Robert Murray. M. D., 1899, Coll. Phys. and Surg., N.Y. At present attending Univ. Edinburgh.

858. EMMA LOOTZ ERVING—Born Sept. 26, 1875, Boston, Mass. A. B., 1897, Smith ; M. D., 1902, Johns Hopkins. Wife of Dr. W. G. Erving, *supra*.

859. HENRY CLAY COBURN, Jr.—Born Aug. 5, 1878, D. C. B. S., 1900; M. D., 1903, Columbian. Resigned Oct. 14, 1908. Asst. Surgeon, U. S. A.

860. FRANCIS EDWARD HARRINGTON—Born June 19, 1879, Norfolk, Va. B. S., Gonzaga, 1907; M. D., 1904, Columbian. Med. Inspector, Health Dept., D. C. Married, Jan. 9, 1908, Maye L., daughter of Dr. L. Eliot, *supra*.

861. ARTHUR LE ROY HUNT—Born Jan. 7, 1877, Lewiston, Me. A. B., 1898, Bowdoin; M. D., 1905, Columbian. Med. Inspector, Health Dept., D. C.

862. CARLISLE P. KNIGHT—M. D., 1904, Columbian. Dropped from membership Jan. 27, 1909. Appointed Acting Asst. Surg., P. H. and M. H. S., in Nov., 1908, for duty at Kobé, Japan.

863. CHARLES L. WATERS—M. D., 1905, Columbian.

APRIL 3, 1907

864. DANIEL THOMAS BIRTWELL—Born May 24, 1874, Chester, Pa. M. D., 1900, Columbian.

865. JOHN SHERIDAN ARNOLD—Born Dec. 4, 1865, Port Trevoston, Pa. M. D., 1896, Coll. Phys. and Surg., Baltimore. Medical Inspector, Public Schools, Washington. Member Med. Assn. D. C.; A. M. A.

866. RICHARD LLOYD COOK—Son of Dr. G. Wythe Cook, *supra*. Born in Washington, Nov. 5, 1878. Educated at Friends' Select School, at the University School, by private tutor, and at the University of Virginia. M. D., 1904, Univ. Virginia. On House Staff at Garfield Memorial Hospital; afterward took special study in Obstetrics, at New York Lying-in Hospital. Was Resident Physician at Wills Mountain Sanatorium.

867. VIRGINIUS DABNEY—Born Feb. 2, 1878, Loudoun Co., Va. M. D., 1902, Univ. Virginia. Acting Asst. Surg., U. S. Navy. Now practicing in Washington.

868. WILLIAM ROBERT PERKINS—Born May 17, 1876, Chestertown, Md. M. D., 1901, Columbian; Phar. D., 1897, National Coll. Pharmacy, D. C. Resident Physician, 1903, Emergency Hospital, D. C.; House Surgeon, 1904, Lying-in Hosp., New York City; Interne, Willard Parker and Reception Hospital, 1905.

869. PAUL BOWEN ALDEN JOHNSON—Born March 23, 1878, D. C. B. A., 1901, Yale; M. D., 1905, Georgetown. Resigned July 5, 1909.

870. JOSEPH ALEXANDER MURPHY—Born Nov. 23, 1878, D. C. M. D., 1905, Columbian.

871. HENRY PICKERING PARKER—Born June 24, 1875, Annapolis, Md. A. B., 1896; M. D., 1901, Johns Hopkins. Prof. Practice of Medicine, Howard Med. School.

872. JOSIAH HUTTON HOLLAND—Born May 6, 1880, D. C. Phar. D., 1901, National Coll. Pharmacy, D. C.; M. D., 1905, Columbian.

873. EDGAR SNOWDEN—Born April 2, 1880, Alexandria, Va. M. D., 1903, Columbian.

874. WILLIAM HOUSTON LITTLEPAGE—Born March 21, 1879, Washington, Ark. M. D., 1905, Columbian. Q. M. Sergt., 1st D. C. Vols.

875. RAYMOND ADAMS FISHER—Born Jan. 6, 1883, D. C. M. D., 1905, Columbian.

876. THOMAS MADDEN FOLEY—Born Dec. 14, 1876, Philadelphia, Pa. M. D., 1905, Columbian.

877. JOHN WATSON SHAW—Born Jan. 31, 1866, Lewistown, Pa. M. D., 1890, Univ. Penna. Resident Physician, 1890-1, St. Joseph's Hospital, Philadelphia.

878. PRENTISS WILLSON—Born Aug. 2, 1882, Fredonia, N. Y. M. D., 1905, Georgetown. Resident Physician, Georgetown Univ. Hosp., 1905-6; Anesthetist at same; Asst. to Chair Obstetrics, Georgetown Med. School; Physician to Home for the Blind.

879. WILLIAM F. WAGNER—Born Jan. 25, 1865, Hartleton, Pa. Ph. G., 1886, Philadelphia Coll. Pharmacy; M. D., 1890, Univ. Penna.

880. JOSEPH J. KAVENEY—Born, 1880. M. D., 1904, Georgetown. Educated at High Schools and St. Dunstan's College, Canada. Hospital service at Naval Hospital and N. Y. Lying-in Hospital. Asst. to Surgical Clinic, Emergency Hospital, Washington.

881. CHARLES WALKER ALLEN—M. D., 1902, Jefferson.

882. WILLIAM GLENN YOUNG—Born Dec. 1, 1878, Trion, Ga. M. D., 1904, Columbian.

883. WILLIAM EARL CLARK—Born Sept. 16, 1879, Philadelphia, Pa. M. D., 1904, Columbian.

OCTOBER 2, 1907

884. JOHN ALLAN TALBOTT—Born May 27, 1882, Forest Glen, Md. M. D., 1905, Columbian. Physician, Out-patient Dept., Providence Hospital, and Resident Physician, same hospital, 1905-7.

885. EMMA COREY STARR—Born Aug. 19, 1876, D. C. M. D., 1904, Howard. Resident Physician, 1904-6, Navajo Indian Hospital, New Mexico ; Clinician, Woman's Clinic, Washington. Married A. B. Keith.

886. WILLIAM OTWAY OWEN—Born July 6, 1854, Broylesville, Tenn. M. D., 1878, Univ. Va. Asst. Surg., 1882-98, Surgeon, 1898-1905, U. S. A. Son of Robt. Latham and Narcissa Clarke Chisholm Owen. Educated at Govanstown, Md., 1866-71, and Virginia Mil. Institute, 1873-5. Practiced medicine, 1878-82, Lynchburg, Va. Resigned from the army because of disability incurred in line of duty. Demonstrator of Anatomy, G. W. Univ. Member Board of Incorporators, Garfield Memorial Hospital, Chairman Executive Committee. Member Med. Assn., D. C.; A. M. A.; Cincinnati Acad. Medicine.

887. WILLIAM ELWIN ROGERS—Born Oct. 2, 1878, Alexandria, Va. M. D., 1904, Georgetown. Died Nov. 22, 1908. Resident Physician, Providence Hospital, 1904 to 1906; afterwards connected with X-ray Department, Georgetown Univ. and Casualty Hospitals, and with Dispensary at Providence Hospital. See Minutes Med. Society, Dec. 16, 1908, and Jan. 27, 1909; Wash. Med. Annals, 1909, VIII, p. 72.

888. DORSEY MAHON McPHERSON—Born May 24, 1857, Baltimore, Md. M. D., 1877, Howard ; 1884, Columbian. Acting Asst. Surgeon, U. S. A., October, 1878, to November, 1883. Medical Examiner, U. S. Bureau Pensions and Board Pension Appeals since October, 1890. Member Assn. Acting Asst. Surgeons, U. S. A. Married. See Lamb's History, p. 196.

889. CHARLES L. BILLARD—Born May 13, 1878, D. C. M. D., 1904, Univ. Penna. Resident Physician, 1904-5, Allegheny General Hospital, Pa.; Asst. Physician, Episcopal Eye, Ear and Throat Hospital and Lutheran Eye, Ear and Throat Infirmary, Washington.

890. H. H. KERR—M. D., 1904, McGill. Son of Dr. James Kerr, *supra*. In Dispensary Service, Providence Hospital; Instructor in Clin. Surg., Howard Med. School.

891. GLENN I. JONES—M. D., 1905, Columbian.

892. GRAFTON D. P. BAILEY—M. D., 1896, National Univ., D. C.

893. SETH EASTMAN MOORE—Born Oct. 6, 1875, D. C. M. D., 1898, Univ. Penna. Married, 1902, Elizabeth E. Smith. Served three years at Prot. Epis. Hosp., Philadelphia, Pa.; some time at Agnew Sanitarium, Atlantic City, N. J.

APRIL 1, 1908

894. LYMAN FREDERICK KEBLER—Born June 8, 1863, Lodi, Mich. Ph. C., 1890; B. S., 1891; M. S., 1892, Univ. Mich.; M. D., 1906, Columbian. Educated in parochial and public schools. Took courses, especially in chemistry, at Jefferson College and Temple College, Philadelphia, Pa., 1892-1902. Was Chief Chemist, Pharmaceutical Manufacturing Company, Philadelphia. Taught Chemistry in Iowa Agricult. College, 1888–99; Instructor in Chemistry, 1901-2, Univ. Mich. Member of Jury of Awards, National Export Exposition, 1898, Philadelphia; Amer. Chem. Society; Society Chem. Industry; Amer. Pharm. Assn.; Franklin Institute; National College of Pharmacy. President Chem. Section, Franklin Institute, 1902; Chairman, 1902, Scientific Section, Amer. Pharm. Assn.; now Chief of Division of Drugs, Bureau of Chemistry, U. S. Dept. Agriculture. Married, 1893, Miss Ida E. Shaw, of Ypsilanti, Mich. See Amer. Biog. Direct., Washington, 1908.

895. WILLIAM H. SYME—M. D., 1904, Columbian.

896. JOSEPH MILTON HELLER—Born Jan. 29, 1872, Staunton, Va. M. D., 1896, Georgetown. Acting Asst. Surg., U. S. A.; Major and Surgeon, U. S. Vols. Son of Joseph and Pauline Frank Heller. Educated at public schools and Fisher's Academy, Washington. Post-graduate course, N. Y. Polyclinic. Asst. Demonstrator of Anatomy, Georgetown Med. School; Clinical Asst., Emergency Hospital and Garfield Hospital Dispensary; Resident Physician, 1896-7, Garfield Hospital. Served, 1898-1902, in War with Spain, largely in the Philippines. Was in charge of the Manila water supply during the cholera epidemic, 1902. Officer of Military Order of Carabao; Past Commander, Henry W. Lawton Camp, United Spanish War Veterans; Officer, Military Order of Foreign Wars.

Member Assn. Military Surgeons, United States; Medical Assn., D. C.; Medical Society, Georgetown University. See Amer. Biog. Direct., Washington, 1908; Georgetown University, II, p. 285.

897. EDWARD MASON PARKER—Born June 27, 1860, Middlebury, Vt. A. M., 1881, Middlebury College; M. D., 1884, Univ. City N. Y. Practiced at Brockton, Mass., 1884-5; New Bedford, Mass., 1886-90; Asst. Resident Surgeon, 1891-4, Johns Hopkins Hospital. Has practiced in Washington since 1894. Associate Surgeon, Emergency Hospital, 1894-6; Bacteriologist, Providence Hospital, 1894-1908; Surgeon to same since 1908; Acting Asst. Surg., U. S. A., 1898, at Montauk Point, L. I.

898. JOHN WESLEY SUTHERIN—Born June 27, 1869, East Palestine, Ohio. M. D., 1902, Howard. Graduated from East Palestine High School, 1887. See Lamb's History, p. 264.

899. HURON WILLIS LAWSON—Born March 15, 1873, Disco, Mich. B. S., 1895, Mich. Agricultural College; M. D., 1903; M. S., 1904, Columbian. Son of James S. and Paulina T. Cannon Lawson. Supt. Public Schools, Lawton, Mich., 1896-7; Principal of High School, Illinois, 1898; 1898-1908, Associate Editor, Experimental Station Record, U. S. Dept. Agriculture; 1905 to date, Associate Prof. Bacteriology and Pathology, G. W. U. Med. School; Resident Physician, 1907-8, Columbia Hospital. See Amer. Biog. Direct., Washington, 1908.

900. NELSON DU VAL BRECHT—Born Jan. 10, 1885, D. C. M. D., 1906, Columbian; Graduate Washington High School; sometime Anatomist, Army Med. Museum; member Med. Assn., D. C.; A. M. A.; Therapeutic Society, Washington.

901. STANTON WREN HOWARD—Born May 2, 1880, Wheeling, W. Va. A. B., 1899, Mt. St. Joseph's College, Baltimore, Md.; M. D., 1903, Georgetown. Externe, Children's Hosp., 1902-3; Foundling Hosp., 1903; Providence Hosp., 1903-5; Kingston Hosp., N. Y., 1905-6. Asst. Dem. Pathology and Bacteriology, Georgetown Med. School.

902. ELWIN C. SCHNEIDER—M. D., Georgetown, 1905.

903. HAMILTON K. WRIGHT—M. D., 1875, McGill.

904. EDMUND T. M. FRANKLIN—M. D., Columbian, 1905.

905. GRANT S. BARNHART—M. D., Columbian, 1904.

906. HARRY M. KAUFMANN—M. D., 1901, Johns Hopkins.

907. JAMES A. GANNON—Born March 8, 1884, New York City. Educated, Georgetown College. M. D., 1906, Georgetown. Clinical Assistant, Diseases of Children, Georgetown Univ. Hospital; Clinical Assistant, Surgery, Casualty Hospital; Surgeon to Great Falls and Old Dominion R. R.; Attending Physician, Deer Park Hotel; Interne, Casualty Hospital, 1903–6; Resident Physician, Georgetown Univ. Hospital, 1906–7; Lecturer on Anatomy and Physiology, Georgetown Training School for Nurses. Married, April 14, 1909, Miss Mildred Lambert, of Washington.

OCTOBER 7, 1908

908. JULIAN M. CABELL—Born Dec. 21, 1860, Richmond, Va. M. D., 1885, Univ. Va. Educated in private schools, Richmond College and Univ. Va. Appointed Asst. Surgeon, U. S. A., April 14, 1887; served in the field in South Dakota through the Sioux campaign, 1890–1; appointed Asst. Prof. Army Med. School when it was organized. Retired for disability in 1897, and began private practice in New York City, 1897–8. In 1898, was Asst. to Chief Surgeon, 8th Army Corps, in Philippines; appointed Brigade Surgeon March, 1899; was Medical Superintendent, Columbia Hospital, Washington, 1899 to 1904. In South Africa in Boer War, 1899–1900, Chief Surgeon, Hospital Corps.

909. MEAD MOORE—M. D., Columbian, 1906.

910. MARY O'MALLEY—Born in Medina, N. Y. M. D., 1897, Niagara Univ. Attended Normal School at Brockport and High School at Medina. Served one year as Interne, Buffalo Hospital. In October, 1898, appointed Asst. Phys., Binghamton State Hosp. for Insane, N. Y. In September, 1905, Asst. Phys., Govt. Hosp. Insane, Washington.

911. JOHN R. BUCK—M. D., 1904, Columbian.

912. CARL HENNING—M. D., 1905, Columbian.

913. MOSES HUBBARD DARNALL—Born in Weston, Collin Co., Texas, Sept. 6, 1882. Educated at Collin Co. Public School; Grayson College, Texas, and Kentucky University. M. D., 1907, Columbian. Interne, Government Hospital Insane, Aug. 1, 1907, to February, 1908. Began to practice in Washington, Feb. 1, 1908.

914. HOWARD HUME—M. D., 1905, Univ. Virginia.

915. JOSEPH JAMES KINYOUN—Born Nov. 25, 1860, North Carolina. M. D., 1882, Bellevue; Ph. D., 1894, Georgetown. Son of Dr. J. H. and Bettie A. Conrad Kinyoun of Centre View, Mo. Was Prof. Hygiene and Bacteriology, 1890-2 ; Pathology and Bacteriology, 1892-99, George-town Med. School. Sometime Passed Asst. Surg., U. S. M. H. S. Fellow A. A. A. S.; Member Assn. Pathologists and Bacteriologists; Assn. Amer. Physicians; Prof. Pathology, G. W. U. Med. College. See Amer. Men of Science, 1906 ; Watson's Biog., p. 378.

916. EDWARD HOMER EGBERT—Born South Bend, Ind., May 5, 1881. Attended grammar schools, Chicago, Ill., and Central High School, Cleveland, Ohio, 1896-1900; Dartmouth College, 1900-1 ; Dartmouth Medical School, 1901-3; M. D., Baltimore Med. College, 1905; Externe, Mary Hitchcock Hospital, Hanover, N. H., 1902-3; Surgical Externe, St. Vincent's Charity Hospital, Cleveland, Summer, 1902; Externe, Surgical and Genito-urinary Service, Lakeside Hospital, Cleveland, Summer, 1903; Resident Physician, Sibley Hospital, Washington, D. C., June to October, 1905. In general practice, Washington, since November, 1905. Member Med. Assn., D. C.; Therapeutic Society; Med. and Surg. Society, D. C.; A. M. A.; Lecturer Nurses' Training School, Sibley Hosp., since 1905; Associate Physician, General Medicine, Casualty Hospital, 1906-8; Associate Physician, Tuberculosis Dispensary, Associated Charities, since 1906.

APRIL 7, 1909

917. WILLIAM F. M. SOWERS—Born April 22, 1873, D. C. A. B., 1896, Princeton ; M. D., 1900, Johns Hopkins. Son of Dr. Z. T. Sowers, *supra.* Associate in Surgery, G. W. U. Med. School ; Associate in Surgery, Providence Hospital ; Visiting Surgeon, Freedmen's Hospital ; Instructor, Clinical Surgery, Howard Med. School.

918. GEORGE J. NEWGARDEN—Born June 25, 1864, Philadelphia, Pa. A. B., 1880; A. M., 1885, Central High School, Philadelphia, Pa.; M. D., 1889, Jefferson. Interne, Philadelphia Hospital (Blockley), 1890; Med. Examiner, Pension Bureau, Washington, D. C., 1890-1 ; Asst. Demonstrator, Operative Surgery, Jefferson Med. College, and Clinical Assistant, Medical Clinics, Jefferson Med. Coll. Hosp., 1891-2. Married, April 11, 1891, Margaret Woolever, of Allentown, Pa. First Lieut., Asst. Surgeon, U. S. A., Nov. 4, 1892 ; Captain, Nov. 4, 1897 ; Major and Surgeon, Nov. 23, 1905. Retired, for disability incident to service, April 24, 1907, with rank of Major. Served in various parts of the United States, in Cuba during the Spanish War (established the " Bloody Ford" dressing station on San Juan River, Santiago, Cuba, July, 1898), and in Philippine Islands.

919. BERNARD HOOE HARRISON—Born July 4, 1869, Houston, Texas. Attended High School and Conyngton Business College. Was in railroad work about three years. M. D., 1903, Howard. Since then has practiced in Washington. See Lamb's History, p. 246.

920. HENRY FENNO SAWTELLE—M. D., 1902, Coll. Phys. and Surg., Chicago. Deputy Health Officer, Washington, D. C.

921. WILLIAM MALCOLM—M. D., 1891, Med. Coll. Univ. City of N. Y.

922. ROBERT S. TRIMBLE—M. D., 1903, National Univ., D. C.

923. WILLIAM CABELL MOORE—M. D., 1902, Univ. Virginia.

924. MARTHA MARIA BREWER LYON—Born March 31, 1871, Peabody, Mass. Educated in Washington Public and Normal Schools. B. S., 1900; M. S., 1901, Columbian Univ.; M. D., 1907, Howard. Clinical Assistant in Ophthalmology, Howard Univ. Med. School, 1908-9. Married, Dec. 31, 1902, Dr. Marcus Ward Lyon, Jr. Teacher in Washington Public Schools, 1890-1902.

925. WILLIAM CLINE BORDEN—Born May 19, 1858, Watertown, N. Y. M. D., Columbian, 1883. Son of Daniel J. and Mary L. Cline Borden. Descendant of the Bordens who came from England in 1635 and settled in Providence Plantations, R. I., and of Jean of Bourdounay, of Normandy, who was with William the Conqueror, in the invasion of England. Educated in public schools, Adams Collegiate Institute, Adams, N. Y. Appointed Asst. Surgeon, U. S. A., in 1883; Captain, 1888; Brigade Surgeon and Major, 1898, in Spanish-American War; Major and Surgeon, U. S. A., 1901. Was in command of Army General Hospital, Key West, Florida; also commanded steamer transport hospital; Prof. Military Surgery, Army Med. School; Prof. Surgical Pathology and Military Surgery, Georgetown Med. School. Member A. M. A.; Assn. Military Surgeons; Fellow Micros. Society, England. Dean Med. Dept., G. W. Univ. Married, Oct. 23, 1883, Jennie E. Adams. Author of Photomicrographs, Columbus, Ohio, 1888-1891; Use of Roentgen rays by Med. Dept., U. S. A., in War with Spain, Washington, 1900 and 1902; Essay on Military Surgery, Washington, 1905. See Georgetown University, II, p. 108.

926. WILLIAM B. CARR—M. D., 1907, Columbian. Son of Dr. W. P. Carr, *supra*.

927. T. J. SULLIVAN—M. D., 1904, Georgetown.

928. WILLIAM J. FRENCH—M. D., 1905, Columbian.

929. RALPH A. HAMILTON—M. D., 1904, Georgetown. Son of Dr. J. B. Hamilton, *supra*.

The following changes in and additions to the above sketches should be made :

No. 81. J. E. MORGAN—The St. John's College named was at Frederick, Md.; from it he received the degree of A. M. in 1850.

No. 102. S. W. EVERETT—Was Demonstrator, not Professor, of Anatomy.

No. 153. W. H. TAYLOR—Was a member, but not President, of Med. Assn., D. C.

No. 229. W. J. CRAIGEN—Died July 17, 1909.

No. 315. C. W. FRANZONI—Add: member A. M. A. since 1872, and Biological Society, Washington, for twenty-five years.

No. 338. J. T. SOTHORON—Feb. 28 should be Sept. 28.

No. 373. S. S. ADAMS—Add: President, Amer. Pediatric Society, 1897, its Secretary since 1891. Educated in public schools of Washington and private schools, Alexandria Co., Va. Studied medicine with Dr. S. C. Busey, *supra*. Has been connected with Children's Hospital since 1876. Lecturer on Diseases Children, Georgetown Med. School, 1879-83 ; Prof. Theory and Practice Medicine, National Univ., 1883-94 ; Clinical Prof. Diseases of Children, Columbian Univ. Med. College, 1893-6 ; Prof. Diseases Children, Georgetown Med. School, 1896-8 (Georgetown was the second college in United States to establish a Professorship of Pediatrics, Harvard being the first); Prof. Theory and Practice Medicine and Diseases Children since 1898 ; Attending Physician, Wash. Home for Incurables; sometime Consulting Physician, Sibley Hospital, and President of Staff; Attending Physician, Children's Hospital, Secretary of Board of Directors. Chairman Committee Arrangements, First Pan-Amer. Med. Congress, 1893; Chairman Committee Arrangements, Third, Fourth and Fifth Cong. Amer. Phys. and Surg.; First Vice Pres. Section Diseases Children, Tuberculosis Congress, 1908; President two years, Wash. Obstet. and Gynecol. Society ; member Assn. Study Tuberculosis. Author, Diet after weaning, Keating's Cyclop. Diseases Children.

No. 450. E. L. MORGAN—President, 1899, Med. and Surg. Society, D. C.; an incorporator, but not President, Library Association, D. C.

No. 566. P. C. HUNT—The figures 1894-8 are incorrect ; the hospital was not then in existence. Dr. Hunt served several years.

No. 600. N. B. MORTON—Died July 19, 1909, Long Beach, Cal.

No. 613. W. M. BARTON—Is now Prof. Materia Medica, Georgetown Med. School.

No. 747. J. S. WALL—Is Prof. Physiology, Georgetown Med. School.

No. 788. B. R. SLAUGHTER (MORTON)—Is Chairman (National) Public Health Education Committee.

It will be observed that many of the foregoing personal sketches are very brief; this brevity, for many reasons, is much to be regretted. It is due, however, to the Committee on History, to state that abundant opportunity was given to the members of the Society to furnish the desired data or themselves to write up their own sketches. A preliminary circular, under date February 7, 1906, was sent to each member at that time, as also a blank form to be filled out and returned to the committee. From time to time, also, a notice appeared in the journal of the Society, the WASHINGTON MEDICAL ANNALS, reminding members of the necessity of sending their sketches and photographs for the use of the committee, and indicating the scope and character of the desired information.* More than three years elapsed, and as the time for publication approached, these reminders were made more urgent, and members of the committee took the trouble to personally urge the subject on the attention of the procrastinating ones. The number of sketches actually furnished to the committee was few; but, fortunately, many others were obtained from the biographical works named above on pages 210 and 211.

It should be understood that in the original sketches as furnished, and especially in those obtained from the books

---

* See WASH. MED. ANNALS, March, 1906, p. 63; May, p. 128; July, p. 187; September, p. 221; November, p. 309; January, 1907, p. 413; March, pp. 61–62; May, p. 173; July, p. 248; September, p. 324; March, 1908, p. 129; May, p. 190; July, p. 292; September, p. 324; November, p. 395; March, 1909, p. 80; May, p. 146; July, p. 218.

mentioned, there were more or less errors of fact; and to these others were inevitably added in the transcription. Some of these errors were eliminated in the reading of the proof, which was done by at least eight persons (the committee and Drs. S. S. Adams, J. D. Morgan and G. L. Magruder) besides the printer; what errors remain may be regarded as practically unavoidable and the percentage is doubtless small.

It seemed desirable that some facts brought out by an analysis of the sketches should be presented in a synoptical form; as, where members were born, where they graduated in medicine, where their non-medical education was obtained and who of them served in the military, naval or marine hospital services. As to the place of birth, the information is nearly complete and probably is approximately correct, although in a few cases a member in separate communications gave different dates of birth, or different places (sometimes far apart), and these discrepancies had to be corrected. As to the college of graduation in medicine, the information is more complete and probably correct, or nearly so. The table showing army, navy and marine hospital service is also in all probability nearly complete and correct. The list of non-medical educational institutions is probably far from complete, but as far as it goes is of interest.

TABLE I.*

PLACE OF BIRTH.

MAINE.—34, 85, 136, 142, 241, 319, 419, 441, 527, 549, 622, 659, 861.

NEW HAMPSHIRE.—78, 174, 177, 303, 312, 409, 443, 465, 597, 618, 677, 766, 777, 822, 829.

VERMONT.—538, 690, 713, 798, 897.

MASSACHUSETTS.—18, 21, 37, 107, 109, 117, 140, 175, 197, 199, 208, 259, 260, 276, 297, 310, 380, 381, 386, 404, 418, 430, 600, 616, 629, 803, 821, 858, 924.

RHODE ISLAND.—209, 495, 566, 692, 729.

CONNECTICUT.—83, 271, 452, 576, 702, 830, 834.

NEW YORK.—101, 124, 163, 167, 179, 182, 211, 228, 242, 262, 293, 294, 301, 314, 324, 348, 349, 398, 408, 421, 438, 460, 493, 503, 508, 512, 523, 537, 555, 575, 582, 594, 637, 646, 658, 688, 695 to 697, 704, 773, 792, 810, 845, 878, 907, 910, 925.

NEW JERSEY.—36, 39, 46, 53, 150, 231, 268, 423, 522, 535, 587, 624, 769.

PENNSYLVANIA.—25, 32, 38, 59, 67, 98, 128, 141, 153, 172, 213, 223, 230, 233, 238, 243, 257, 267, 272, 277, 278, 299, 332, 342, 362, 377, 385, 417, 433, 434, 447, 457, 458, 491, 525, 556, 573, 589, 593, 608, 627, 630, 666 to 668, 671, 689, 694, 722, 760, 778, 779, 786, 795, 811, 813, 817, 840, 848, 864, 865, 876, 877, 879, 883, 918.

DELAWARE.—244, 387.

MARYLAND.—1 to 3, 5 to 8, 12, 14 to 17, 20, 22, 24, 27, 29, 31, 42, 43, 45, 50, 51, 54, 56, 63, 70, 80, 81, 82, 87, 90, 91, 94, 95, 97, 99, 111, 113, 129, 137, 151, 154, 165, 178, 187, 191, 193, 195, 217, 220, 237, 245, 249, 283, 313, 317, 320, 327, 337, 338, 365, 366, 370, 389, 392, 395, 397, 400, 402, 405, 414, 425, 445, 453, 461, 468, 476, 484, 486, 499, 506, 511, 518, 524, 531, 534, 539, 542, 547, 548, 564, 569, 607, 614, 623, 625, 628, 634, 638, 648, 653, 665, 669, 670, 686, 693, 716, 718, 726, 728, 742, 749, 751, 752, 763, 775, 780, 790, 800, 814, 832, 836, 839, 847, 853, 856, 868, 871, 884, 888.

DISTRICT OF COLUMBIA.—23, 28, 44, 48, 49, 52, 58, 60, 61, 66, 68, 69, 71, 74, 75, 77, 79, 84, 86, 88, 93, 96, 100, 108, 112, 118 to 120, 122, 123, 125, 127, 133, 138, 143, 144, 147, 149, 155, 161, 162, 169, 170, 176, 180, 183, 185, 186, 188, 189, 192, 194, 196, 200 to 202, 206, 210, 212, 214, 219, 221, 222, 225, 235, 236, 251 to 253, 255, 263, 270, 280, 281, 284 to 289, 296, 298, 305 to 307, 311, 315, 316, 318, 326, 329 to 331, 334 to 336, 339 to 341, 343, 344, 346, 347, 357, 358, 368, 372 to 375, 383, 388, 391, 393,

---

* The figures in the tables are the serial numbers of the biographical sketches.

26

DISTRICT OF COLUMBIA.—Continued.

399, 403, 406, 407, 410 to 412, 415, 416, 420, 422, 426, 428, 432, 435, 437, 439, 442, 446, 448, 450, 455, 459, 464, 466, 467, 469, 471, 478, 482, 485, 489, 490, 492, 496, 497, 500, 501, 504, 505, 507, 509, 510, 514 to 516, 519, 528, 530, 532, 541, 543, 550, 557 to 560, 567, 568, 577 to 579, 584, 586, 588, 596, 598, 599, 602, 609, 610, 613, 619, 635, 647, 656, 657, 678, 679, 683 to 685, 687, 700, 703, 705, 706, 710 to 712, 714, 715, 717, 725, 732 to 735, 739, 741, 743, 744, 747, 756, 757, 759, 761, 767, 768, 774, 787, 789, 791, 794, 796, 797, 802, 804, 823, 825, 826, 833, 835, 846, 850, 859, 866, 869, 870, 872, 875, 885, 889, 893, 900, 917.

VIRGINIA.—4, 9, 13, 33, 40, 41, 47, 65, 92, 103, 105, 106, 116, 121, 130, 131, 134, 152, 156, 160, 166, 171, 181, 204, 229, 239, 258, 279, 291, 309, 323, 351, 356, 361, 364, 367, 371, 376, 379, 384, 390, 401, 427, 429, 431, 436, 440, 444, 454, 472 to 474, 479, 480, 483, 502, 513, 517, 520, 521, 529, 552 to 554, 570, 585, 590, 592, 606, 611, 620, 621, 631, 636, 639, 644, 649, 654, 655, 661, 663, 664, 672, 676, 681, 701, 707, 721, 724, 727, 731, 740, 746, 753, 788, 793, 799, 818 to 820, 824, 831, 851, 854, 860, 867, 873, 887, 896, 908.

WEST VIRGINIA.—282, 595, 612, 633, 754, 827, 901.

NORTH CAROLINA.—164, 234, 254, 275, 451, 488, 545, 565, 602, 650, 673, 772, 843, 915.

SOUTH CAROLINA.—157, 413, 571, 572, 603, 642, 776.

GEORGIA.—62, 135, 748, 882.

ALABAMA.—808.

MISSISSIPPI.—533, 784, 785, 806.

LOUISIANA.—494, 782, 841.

TEXAS.—838, 913, 919.

KENTUCKY—132, 145, 173, 250, 378, 481, 698, 815.

TENNESSEE.—266, 359, 709, 886.

OHIO.—148, 274, 449, 470, 546, 562, 580, 605, 640, 643, 680, 720, 736 to 738, 745, 750, 762, 765, 770, 783, 801, 805, 844, 855, 898.

INDIANA.—300, 322, 350, 540, 626, 674, 723, 758, 781, 916.

ILLINOIS.—352, 396, 536, 617, 632, 708.

MICHIGAN.—292, 498, 526, 812, 837, 894, 899.

WISCONSIN.—265.

MISSOURI.—218, 226, 462, 477, 816.

MINNESOTA.—574, 645.

IOWA.—475.

KANSAS.—682.

ARKANSAS.—382, 874.

CALIFORNIA.—857.

CANADA.—264, 463, 771.

WEST INDIES.—36.

CHILI.—224.

ENGLAND.—55, 102, 190, 205, 207, 248, 290, 295, 302, 363, 544, 563, 809, 849.

SCOTLAND.—110, 247, 273, 333, 394, 641.

IRELAND.—89, 114, 158, 159, 203, 304, 321, 353, 456, 591.

FRANCE.—115, 146, 354.

GERMANY.—64, 104, 126, 168, 184, 198, 227, 232, 240, 269, 308, 328, 345, 424, 581, 615, 652, 699, 807, 828, 852.

AUSTRIA.—216, 583.

ITALY.—651, 730.

SWITZERLAND.—719.

RUSSIA.—72.

INDIA.—487.

AUSTRALIA.—561.

TABLE II.

MEDICAL COLLEGES FROM WHICH GRADUATED. SOME MEMBERS GRADUATED
FROM MORE THAN ONE COLLEGE.

MAINE.

Medical Department Bowdoin College; Maine Medical School, Brunswick.—142, 264, 303, 319, 527, 659.

NEW HAMPSHIRE.

Medical Department, Dartmouth College, Hanover.—233.

VERMONT.

Castleton Medical College; Vermont Academy of Medicine; Academy of Medical Science, Castleton.—141, 418.

Medical Department, University of Vermont, Burlington.—369, 407, 455.

MASSACHUSETTS.

Harvard Medical School, Boston.—18, 21, 34, 37, 161, 310, 381, 409, 410, 441, 600, 616.

Berkshire Medical College, Pittsfield.—99, 199, 297.

New England Female Medical College, Boston.—629.

NEW YORK.

College Physicians and Surgeons; Medical Department, Columbia University, New York City.—101, 124, 207, 208, 261, 265, 355, 371, 411, 554, 594, 597, 610, 675, 702, 704, 716, 768, 828, 857, 897.

University City of New York.—86, 102, 131, 182, 360, 422, 426, 695, 808, 921.

Bellevue Hospital Medical College, New York City.—196, 201, 259, 293, 323, 359, 374, 492, 495, 612, 637, 796, 831, 915.

Woman's Medical College, New York City.—599.

Long Island College Hospital, Brooklyn.—198, 320, 491, 554, 786.

DISTRICT OF COLUMBIA.—Continued.

324, 327, 334, 335, 337, 341, 350 to 352, 357, 379, 380, 382, 383, 388, 393, 404, 408, 415, 417, 421, 430, 432, 433, 435, 436, 439, 442, 446, 448, 449, 454, 459, 461, 462, 466, 472, 475, 478, 479, 481, 482, 485, 489, 490, 497, 500, 501, 503, 513, 517, 519, 522, 523, 524, 526, 530, 534, 537 to 539, 541, 549, 553, 557, 559, 560, 565, 568, 570, 571, 576, 582, 587, 602, 604, 608, 615, 617, 620, 622, 628, 633, 635, 639, 640, 647, 651, 654, 656 to 658, 661, 665, 676, 678, 681, 684, 685, 693, 696, 703, 705 to 707, 710, 712 to 715, 718, 721, 722, 724, 727, 734, 736, 739, 741, 743 to 745, 748, 750, 753, 757, 758, 766, 771, 776 to 778, 782 to 784, 787, 790 to 794, 798, 812, 814 to 820, 832, 834, 836, 837, 840, 843, 845, 846, 848, 849, 851, 853, 855, 856, 859, 860 to 864, 868, 870, 872 to 876, 882 to 884, 888, 891, 894, 895, 899, 900, 904, 905, 909, 911 to 913, 926, 928.

Georgetown Medical School; Medical Department Georgetown University.—127, 130, 137, 143, 146, 158, 162, 163, 165, 167, 171, 173 to 175, 177, 180, 181, 186, 188, 193 to 195, 206, 209, 213, 214, 220, 221, 230, 235 to 238, 240, 241, 251, 253, 255, 256, 259, 260, 262, 263, 266 to 274, 277, 278, 280 to 282, 284, 285, 287, 288, 290, 292, 298, 300, 304, 305, 307, 311 to 314, 316, 318, 321, 322, 326, 328 to 332, 336, 338 to 340, 342, 343, 345, 347, 348, 349, 353, 354, 358, 363, 370, 372 to 375, 377, 378, 386, 391, 394, 395, 398 to 400, 403, 406, 412, 413, 440, 457, 460, 464, 467, 469, 471, 477, 496, 505, 507 to 510, 512, 514, 516, 518, 520, 531, 532, 540, 545, 547, 552, 555, 558, 561, 566, 567, 574, 575, 578, 579, 586, 589, 590, 591, 596, 598, 609, 613, 623, 626, 631, 634, 638, 646, 648, 664, 667, 689, 691, 708, 709, 717, 732, 733, 735, 747, 749, 759 to 761, 764, 765, 767, 773, 780, 789, 802, 822 to 826, 841, 842, 844, 850, 869, 878, 880, 887, 896, 901, 902, 907, 925, 927, 929.

Medical Department, Howard University.—333, 354, 419, 434, 438, 443, 453, 457, 465, 536, 546, 556, 562, 618, 625, 641, 669, 679, 683, 688, 694, 699, 708, 719, 728, 729, 738, 807, 849, 885, 888, 898, 919, 924.

Medical Department, National University, D. C.—437, 528, 529, 544, 588, 593, 636, 674, 711, 725, 756, 774, 799, 801, 838, 892, 922.

VIRGINIA.

Medical Department, University of Virginia, Charlottesville.—82, 366, 390, 422, 429, 444, 473, 474, 483, 521, 548, 592, 595, 603, 606, 644, 670, 731, 746, 775, 797, 831, 866, 867, 886, 908, 914, 923.

Medical College of Virginia, Richmond; Richmond Medical College.—145, 243, 401, 450, 584, 813, 854.

SOUTH CAROLINA.

University of South Carolina; Charleston Medical College, Charleston.—157, 542, 572.

LOUISIANA.

Medical Department, Tulane University, New Orleans.—785.

New Orleans School of Medicine.—355.

KENTUCKY.
    Medical Department, University of Louisville.—86, 431.
    Medical Department, Transylvania University, Lexington.—234.
    Louisville Medical College.—148, 361, 723.
    Hospital College of Medicine, Louisville.—698.
OHIO.
    Cleveland Medical College.—168, 463.
    Medical Department, Western Reserve University, Cleveland.—228,
        276, 470.
    Medical Department, Wooster University; Charity Hospital Medical
        College, Cleveland.—573, 580.
    Medical College of Ohio, Cincinnati.—299, 605, 671, 680.
    Columbus Medical College, Columbus.—720.
    Starling Medical College, Columbus.—770.
ILLINOIS.
    Rush Medical College, Chicago.—248, 396.
    Chicago Medical College.—367.
    College Physicians and Surgeons, Chicago.—920.
MICHIGAN.
    Medical Department, University of Michigan, Ann Arbor.—493.
MINNESOTA.
    Medical Department, University of Minnesota, Minneapolis.—662.
IOWA.
    Medical Department, University of Iowa, Iowa City.—581, 632.
MISSOURI.
    Ensworth Medical College, St. Joseph.—660.
CANADA.
    Medical Department, University Bishop's College, Montreal.—690.
    Medical Department, McGill University, Montreal.—890, 903.
MEXICO.
    Medical Department, University of Mexico, Mexico.—205.
ENGLAND.
    Royal College Surgeons, London.—159, 205, 239.
SCOTLAND.
    Medical Department, University of Edinburgh.—30, 487.
    Royal College of Surgeons, Edinburgh.—564.
IRELAND.
    Medical Department, Queen's College, Cork.—203.
    Medical Department, Queen's College, Belfast.—456.
    Rotunda Lying-In Hospital, Dublin.—159, 622, 730.
GERMANY.
    F. W. University, Berlin.—72, 184, 224, 383, 637, 828.
    Ludwig Max. University, Munich.—350.
    Julius Max. University, Wuerzburg.—424.

GERMANY.—Continued.
  E. K. University, Tübingen.—227.
  G. A. University, Goettingen.—126.
  University of Leipzig.—446, 652.
AUSTRIA.
  K. K. University, Vienna.—259.
  K. K. University, Prag.—216.
SWITZERLAND.
  University of Zürich.—104.
BELGIUM.
  University of Brussels.—564.
ITALY.
  University of Bologna.—730.

TABLE III.

EDUCATIONAL INSTITUTIONS ATTENDED; EXCLUDING PUBLIC SECONDARY SCHOOLS AND MEDICAL COLLEGES.

MAINE.
  Bowdoin College. Brunswick.—861.
  Colby College, Waterville.—419, 549.
  Gardiner Lyceum, Gardiner.—319.
  Westbrook Seminary, Woodfords.—527.
NEW HAMPSHIRE.
  Dartmouth College, Hanover.—140, 174, 233, 418, 677, 777, 829, 916.
  Appleton's Academy, New Ipswich.—175, 233.
  Strafford Academy, Strafford.—303.
  Wolfboro Academy, Wolfboro.—303.
  Crosby's Academy, Nassau.—354.
  Robinson's Female Seminary, Exeter.—443.
VERMONT.
  University of Vermont, Burlington.—190.
  Norwich University, Northfield.—226.
  Middlebury College, Middlebury.—897.
MASSACHUSETTS.
  Harvard University, Cambridge.—414, 441, 597, 616, 704, 768.
  Williams College, Williamstown.—538, 816.
  Amherst College, Amherst.—804.
  Holy Cross College, Worcester.—386.
  Smith College, Hatfield.—858.
  Winchendon Academy, Wichendon.—418.
  Phillips' Academy, Andover.—418.
  Groton Academy, Groton.—78.
  Round Hill School, Northampton.—62.

RHODE ISLAND.
 Brown University, Providence.—418, 452, 692.
 Wellesley College, Wellesley.—805.
CONNECTICUT.
 Yale University, New Haven.—62, 67, 135, 487, 702, 830, 834, 869.
 Trinity College, Hartford.—495, 603.
 Betts' Academy, Stamford.—226.
 Jones' Academy, Bridgeport.—226.
 Norwalk Academy, Norwalk.—350.
NEW YORK.
 Columbia University, New York City.—101.
 University of New York City.—821.
 Cornell University, Ithaca.—679.
 Syracuse University, Syracuse.—646.
 College St. Francis Xavier, New York City.—273.
 Manhattan College, New York City.—682.
 Union College, Schenectady.—23, 136, 697.
 Vassar College, Poughkeepsie.—599.
 Hobart College, Geneva.—522.
 Adams' Collegiate Institute, Adams.—925.
 Claverack College, Claverack.—716.
 Cooper Institute, New York City.—527.
 Arcade Seminary, Arcade.—294.
 Union Academy, Wayne County.—555.
 Genesee Wesleyan Seminary, Lima.—294, 493.
 Trumansburg Academy, Trumansburg.—591.
 Cazenovia Seminary, Cazenovia.—658.
NEW JERSEY.
 Princeton University, Princeton.—28, 36, 39, 46, 53, 86, 138, 144, 410,
  416, 438, 465, 466, 630, 680, 752, 835.
 Centenary Collegiate Institute, Hackettstown.—716.
 Belvidere Academy, Belvidere.—342.
 Freehold Academy, Freehold.—354.
 Edge Hill School, Princeton.—366.
 New Jersey State Model School, Trenton.—624.
PENNSYLVANIA.
 University of Pennsylvania, Philadelphia.—39, 109.
 Western University, Allegheny.—141.
 Bucknill University, Lewisburg.—260.
 Juniata College, Huntingdon.—457, 628.
 Jefferson College, Cannonsburg.—52, 151.
 Alleghany College, Meadville.—407.
 Washington and Jefferson College, Washington.—168.
 Dickinson College, Carlisle.—461.

PENNSYLVANIA.—Continued.

Pennsylvania College, Gettysburg.—198, 383, 653.

Lafayette College, Easton.—796.

Franklin and Marshall College, Lancaster.—786.

Philadelphia College Pharmacy.—722, 728, 879.

Temple College, Philadelphia.—894.

St. Mary's College, Northeast.—828.

Monongahela Academy, Monongahela.—282.

Huntingdon Academy, Huntingdon.—457.

Central High School, Philadelphia (confers degrees).—272, 918.

State Normal School, Millersville.—694, 817.

DELAWARE.

Delaware College, Newark.—387.

Milford Academy, Milford.—244.

Academy, Wilmington.—500.

MARYLAND.

Johns Hopkins University, Baltimore.—800, 836, 847, 850, 852, 871.

Mt. St. Mary's University, Emmetsburg.—94, 141, 384.

St. Mary's College, Baltimore.—56, 70, 111, 375.

Washington College, Baltimore.—151, 686.

St. James College, near Baltimore.—289.

St. John's College, Annapolis.—24, 29, 366, 392, 459, 500, 519, 623, 670, 808.

St. John's College, Frederick.—81.

St. John's College, Hagerstown.—123.

Mt. St. Joseph's College, Baltimore.—901.

Maryland Agricultural College, College Park.—832.

Rock Hill College, Ellicott City.—372, 391, 664, 726, 759.

Presbyterian College, New Windsor.—769.

Baltimore College Dental Surgery.—415.

Frederick College, Frederick.—468.

Rockville Academy, Rockville (McLeod's).—5, 127, 397, 420.

Frederick Academy, Frederick.—670.

Brookville Academy, Brookville.—65.

Upper Marlboro Academy, Upper Marlboro.—836.

Petersville Academy, Petersville.—313.

Bladensburg Academy, Bladensburg.—634.

Charlotte Hall School, Charlotte Hall.—42, 400, 484.

State Normal School, Baltimore.—669.

Glenwood Institute, Glenwood.—450.

DISTRICT OF COLUMBIA.

Abbott's Classical Seminary, Georgetown.—129.

Beck's Academy, 6th and H N.W.—180.

Breckenridge's Classical School, Harewood.—5.

INDIANA.
   University Notre Dame, South Bend.—589.
   Hanover College, Hanover.—754.
ILLINOIS.
   Mt. Vernon College, Mt. Vernon.—632.
   McCormick Theological Seminary, Chicago.—754.
MICHIGAN.
   University of Michigan, Ann Arbor.—335, 556, 894.
   Business College, Adrian.—641.
   Detroit College, Detroit.—765.
   Michigan Agricultural College.—899.
WISCONSIN.
   Page's Academy, Lancaster.—536.
KENTUCKY.
   Central University, Danville.—698.
   Kentucky University, Lexington.—913.
TENNESSEE.
   University of South, Sewanee.—494, 554.
MINNESOTA.
   University of Minnesota, Minneapolis.—803.
IOWA.   .
   University of Iowa, Iowa City.—557.
   Amity College, College Springs.—696.
MISSOURI.
   State Normal School, Kirksville.—556.
CALIFORNIA.
   Leland Stanford University.—808.
CANADA.
   Sackville College, Sackville, N. S.—264.
   Bailey's Academy, London.—463.
   St. Dunstan's College, P. E. I.—880.
ENGLAND.
   Bicester Diocesan School, Bicester.—190.
   Stonyhurst College, Lancashire.—353, 704.
   Burdis' Academy, Newcastle-on-Tyne.—544.
   Newnham College, Cambridge.—557.
SCOTLAND.
   University of Edinburgh.—17, 289.
   Anderson University, Glasgow.—394.
IRELAND.
   Trinity College, Dublin.—159.
   Jesuit College, Dublin.—89.
   Maynooth College, Maynooth.—321.
   Kilkenny College, Kilkenny.—353.
   Coleraine Institute, Coleraine.—456.

GERMANY.
Royal College, Münden, Prussia.—269.
Realschule, Alsfeld, Hesse.—328.
RUSSIA.
University of Dorpat.—72.

A. B.—28, 36, 39, 48, 52, 58, 60, 62, 71, 72, 78, 84, 86, 101, 109, 112, 120, 122, 123, 135, 140, 144, 149, 157, 159, 264, 272, 316, 319, 329, 335, 368, 373, 375, 383, 384, 386, 387, 410, 414, 418, 419, 438, 441, 442, 452, 461, 465, 466, 487, 492, 505, 517, 521, 522, 538, 549, 550, 562, 572, 589, 592, 595 to 597, 599, 603, 616, 617, 623, 644, 653, 664, 670, 677, 680, 692, 697, 701, 704, 754, 759, 768, 773, 776, 786, 800, 816, 828 to 830, 836, 847, 850, 852, 858, 861, 869, 871, 901, 917, 918.

A. M.—39, 46, 53, 60, 67, 68, 71, 75, 78, 81, 111, 112, 120, 122, 123, 127, 133, 136, 138, 140, 141, 149, 162, 168, 190, 200, 247, 259, 260, 271 to 273, 282, 288, 311, 316, 319, 321, 323, 329, 335, 353, 373, 375, 383, 384, 386, 387, 391, 392, 408, 410, 414, 416, 419, 438, 452, 459, 461, 465, 466, 470, 478, 495, 507, 522, 549, 550, 562, 578, 589, 596, 603, 630, 632, 653, 664, 670, 680, 682, 702, 752, 754, 759, 776, 786, 804, 815, 836, 897, 918.

B. S.—500, 530, 653, 682, 684, 696, 731, 738, 798, 803 to 805, 815, 821, 835, 848, 859, 860, 894, 899, 924.

M. S.—457, 798, 805, 832, 894, 899, 924.

Ph. B.—200, 315, 323, 341, 571, 605, 650, 834.

Ph. C.—894.

Ph. D.—159, 259, 269, 359, 368, 408, 589.

Ph. M.—605.

B. E.—628, 676, 817.

C. E.—731.

M. E.—457, 796.

L. B.—777.

LL. B.—242, 265, 288, 516, 556, 739, 761.

LL. M.—242, 516, 761, 849.

LL. D.—67, 94, 136, 190, 273, 307, 328, 376, 589.

D. D. S.—415, 593, 838.

Phar. G.—722, 879.

Phar. D.—65, 68, 403, 420, 453, 477, 508, 520, 540, 552, 577, 598, 636, 663, 780, 783, 824, 833, 845, 868, 872.

———

TABLE IV.

THE ARMY, NAVY AND MARINE HOSPITAL SERVICES.

Army (including all Military Organizations—United States, Confederate States, Foreign, and National Guard).—Sketches 3 to 5, 8, 11, 20, 22, 23, 29, 30, 32, 37, 40, 51, 59, 66, 67, 79, 81, 82, 88 to 90, 98, 101

APPENDIX.

CONSTITUTION AND BY-LAWS

AND CHANGES THEREIN.

The Society has printed its constitution, by-laws, etc., a number of times, namely, in 1820, 1839, 1854, 1861, 1867, 1870, 1882, 1894, 1897 and 1904. The first publication followed the first incorporation, the second publication followed the second incorporation.

The edition of 1820 contains the first charter, the constitution and by-laws, a list of twenty-eight resident members, of nine honorary members and of the officers, and the rules and regulations of professional etiquette. A copy was presented to the Society December 20, 1882, by Dr. John Frederick May, and is now in the library of the Surgeon General's Office. The edition of 1839 contains the second charter and the constitution and by-laws. That of 1854 contains the same, with the revision made to the constitution and by-laws January 2, 1854; also the Regulations of the Medical Association of the District of Columbia. The edition of 1861 contains the same with the revisions made July 12, 1859, July 1, 1860, and October 1, 1861; also a list of 106 members; and the Regulations of the Medical Association. The edition of 1867 contains the charter, etc., with the revisions made January 9 and 23 and July 5, 1865, and January 10 and July 2, 1866, and a list of resident members. The edition of 1870 contains the charter, etc., with revisions of January 5 and 12, 1870; lists of resident and honorary members and licentiates, and the Regulations of the Medical Association are bound up under the same cover. The edition of 1882 contains the charter, etc., with revisions made after the previous edition; also lists of resident and honorary members. The edition of 1894 the same, including revisions after the previous edition. The edition of 1897 the same, including revisions of January 4, 1897. The last edition is that of 1904, containing the same, with revisions of July 1, 1901, January 8, 1902, and January 13, 1904.

Revision of the constitution, by-laws and rules of order was usually the work of several months. For instance, July 1, 1850, a committee was appointed, consisting of Drs. T. B. J. Frye, Joshua Riley and H. Lindsly, to consider the propriety of a revision and also of petitioning Congress to amend the charter of 1838. Apparently this committee failed to do anything, because a new committee was appointed January 11, 1853, consisting of Drs. H. Lindsly, S. C. Busey and W. H. Saunders.

27

This committee evidently went to work, for we find that they reported a revision January 2, 1854, which was adopted and printed.

Again, March 14, 1864, a committee was appointed—Drs. Thos. Miller, Thos. Antisell and C. H. Liebermann—which reported September 5, 1866, when Drs. Antisell, Lovejoy and A. F. A. King were appointed to see to the publication, and it was published in 1867.

Subjoined appears in detail the original constitution, etc., the amendments thereto and the dates of adoption of the amendments :

CONSTITUTION.

Article I, Edition of 1820.—" This Society shall be called the Medical Society of the District of Columbia." There has been no change in this article. The title was, of course, fixed by the charters.

Article II, Edition of 1820.—" The object of this Society shall be the consideration and promotion of all subjects connected with medicine and the collateral branches of the science." The words of the charters are : " promoting and disseminating medical and surgical knowledge and for no other purpose whatever." Sections 3, 4 and 5 of both charters provided for a Board of Examiners for license to practice in the District ; the Board to be elected by the Society. The article, after the reincorporation, was changed by interpolating after the words "shall be," the words "the granting of licenses agreeably to the provisions of the charter." January 4, 1897, these interpolated words were struck out because Congress had passed a bill transferring the duty to the Commissioners of the District.

Article III, Section 1, Edition of 1820.—" The meetings of this Society shall be held quarter-yearly in the City of Washington, viz : on the first Mondays in January, April, July and October, and on its own adjournments." These stated meetings were required by the charter. The second charter, however, required only two meetings yearly, January and July, and the article was correspondingly changed after the reincorporation.

January 5, 1870, the wording of the paragraph was changed to read as follows : " There shall be two meetings of this Society annually, the first beginning with the stated meeting fixed by the charter on the first Monday in January, and the second beginning with the stated meeting on the first Monday in July." January 4, 1897, the words "fixed by the charter" were struck out.

Article III, Section 2, Edition of 1820.—" Special meetings shall be called by the President, or one of the Vice Presidents, on application being made in writing by three of the members." January 5, 1870, the following sentence was added : " The stated meetings shall be advertised by the Recording Secretary at least three times, and all special meetings at least once, in one or more newspapers of the District." January 4, 1897, this sentence was struck out.

January 5, 1870, a *section 3* was added : "During each session the Society may hold regular meetings for the promotion and dissemination of medical science." The first Monday in February, 1851, was appointed to receive and discuss medical subjects. The President was instructed to appoint members for the purpose. He appointed Drs. J. Borrows, W. P. Johnston and F. Howard. There is no record of any February meeting having been held. In the summer of 1864 meetings were held on Mondays when possible, and in the evening. January 23, 1865, Wednesday was selected for the regular meetings, and they have since been held on that day.

Article IV, Section 1, Edition of 1820.—"There shall be the following officers of this Society, viz : one President, two Vice Presidents, one Corresponding Secretary, one Recording Secretary, one Treasurer and one Librarian." This section is in the language of both charters, which named the individual officers and also the time they should be elected. There has not been any change in this section.

Article IV, Section 2, Edition of 1820.—"The officers of the Medical Society shall be chosen from the resident members, and be elected by ballot by a majority of the members present at the stated meetings (or meeting—printed both ways) in January in every year." July 12, 1859, this section was amended by interpolating after the word "Society" the words "and also delegates to the National Medical Association." January 10, 1866, the section was again amended to read "The officers of the Medical Society and delegates to the American Medical Association shall be chosen from the resident members as follows : the officers by ballot of a majority of members at the semi-annual meeting in January, the delegates to be selected by a committee appointed for the purpose, who shall present the names selected to the Society at an adjourned meeting in April. These names shall be confirmed by the Society by ballot as in the case of officers." January 5, 1870, the wording was again changed : "The officers of the Medical Society, the Board of Examiners and the delegates to the American Medical Association shall be chosen from the resident members, as follows : The officers and Board of Examiners by ballot of a majority of the members present at the annual meeting in January, the delegates by a ballot of a majority of the members present at a regular meeting in April." Again, January 4, 1897, the functions of the Board of Examiners having ceased and the Society having no longer representation in the American Medical Association, the section was simplified to read "The officers shall be chosen from the active members by ballot of a majority of the members present at the stated meeting in January." This again was changed January 13, 1904, to read "The officers shall be chosen from the active members at the stated meeting in January, and a majority of the votes cast shall be necessary for a choice."

Two new sections were added January 5, 1870. *Section 3*, "There shall also be a Board of Censors, consisting of three members, to be elected in the same manner as the officers." January 4, 1897, the word "also" was struck out and the number was increased from three to five. *Section 4*, "In case of the death, resignation or removal of any officer or member of either Board, an election may be held at any regular meeting to fill the vacancy." This section was amended January 4, 1897, by striking out the word "either" and adding after the word "Board" the words "of Censors," and was made *section 5* instead of 4; January 8, 1902, it became *section 6*.

Another *section 4* was added January 4, 1897: "There shall be appointed by the President, annually in January, a Committee on Public Health, consisting of seven active members; also a Committee on Legislation, consisting of nine active members; and also a Committee on Essays, consisting of three active members." January 8, 1902, this section became *section 5*, and the words "a Committee on Legislation" were struck out.

A new *section 4* was adopted January 8, 1902: "There shall be an Executive Committee, composed of fifteen active members, appointed by the President in January, 1902. Of the members thus appointed three shall serve for one year, three for two years, three for three years, three for four years and three for five years. The President, after his election at the stated meeting in January, 1903, and in each succeeding year, shall fill the vacancies on this committee by the appointment of three active members, who shall serve for five years. When a vacancy occurs on this committee by resignation or otherwise, the President shall appoint an active member to fill the unexpired term."

Article V, Section 1, Edition of 1820.—"The Society shall consist of honorary and resident members, and fellows." The words "and fellows," were struck out January 5, 1870, and, January 4, 1897, the word *resident* was changed to *active*, and the following words were added: "and members by invitation."

Article V, Section 2, Edition of 1820.—"Any person not residing in the District of Columbia who has obtained a degree in medicine or is eminent in the practice of physic or any of the branches thereof may be proposed as an honorary member. He shall be proposed by two members, at one stated meeting, balloted for at the next, and a majority of two-thirds of the members present shall be required for his admission." This section was amended July 2, 1866, by interpolating after the word "thereof" and in italics the words "or any resident medical man not engaged in practice, or who has grown old in the profession and retired from practice." For some reason, perhaps inadvertently, the word "stated" was omitted in the printing in 1867, but it was restored with emphasis January 5, 1870, where the sentence reads "He shall be proposed by two members at one of the stated meetings and may be balloted for at the next stated meeting;" and the word *required* was changed to *necessary*. A third sentence was added July 2, 1866 : "Honorary members removing to the District, as well as resident honorary members engaging in practice, will be required to pay the usual fee to the Treasurer and be proposed and elected as resident members." January 5, 1870, this sentence was struck out. January 4, 1897, the second sentence was amended by adding the words "but no nomination shall be acted upon until it has been reported upon by the Board of Censors. Honorary members shall have the privilege of attending all regular meetings of this Society held for the discussion of medical subjects, and of participating in such discussion ; but shall not have the right to attend the stated meetings, to hold office or to vote upon any subject connected with the management of the Society, or any of the elections." January 13, 1904, the words "three-fourths of the members present" were changed to "three-fourths of the votes cast."

Article V, Section 3, Edition of 1820.—" Resident members shall consist of medical gentlemen residing in the District of Columbia ; and for their admission it shall be necessary that they shall have received a diploma from some University or shall be considered respectable in the practice of medicine. They shall be proposed by two members, at least one stated meeting before being balloted for, and it shall then require the concurrence of two-thirds of the members present for their admission." After the reincorporation the wording of the second sentence was changed to read as follows : "They shall signify their desire to be elected, shall be recommended to the Society by the Board of Examiners at least one stated meeting before being balloted for, and it shall require the concurrence of two-thirds of the members present for their admission ; and every member so elected shall pay a fee of five dollars to the Treasurer."

July 1, 1860, the section was changed to read, "Resident members shall consist of medical gentlemen residing in the District of Columbia ; and all applications for membership shall be made to the President, who shall, on the applicant having exhibited satisfactory evidence of his qualifications, by the production of a diploma from a respectable medical college or a license from the Examiners of the Medical Society, and of his having paid the Treasurer a fee of five dollars, grant a temporary certificate of eligibility, and shall report the names of all such applicants to the next meeting of the Society, when they shall be balloted for, and the concurrence of two-thirds of the members present shall be necessary for their admission."*

---

*August 6, 1860, Dr. Wm. Marbury offered a resolution that no one should become a member of the Society who was engaged in any other than medical pursuits. The resolution, however, was laid on the table.

January 9, 1865, the reading was again changed : " Resident members shall consist of medical gentlemen residing in the District of Columbia ; and for their admission it shall be necessary that they shall have received a diploma from a regular medical college, or shall have received a certificate from the Examining Board of the Society. Candidates for membership shall be duly proposed to the Medical Society, and be recommended by the Board of Examiners, and may be balloted for at the meeting next after their proposal, when it shall require the concurrence of two-thirds of the members present for their admission ; and every member so elected shall have previously paid to the Treasurer of the Society an admission fee of ten (10) dollars." July 8, 1868, the words "every member so elected" were changed to "every non-licentiate so elected;" and after the words "ten dollars" were added "In the case of licentiates the fee for membership shall be one dollar."

Another change was made January 5, 1870: " Resident members shall consist of medical practitioners residing in the District of Columbia; and for their admission it shall be necessary that they shall have received a license from the Board of Examiners of the Society. Candidates for membership shall be proposed to the Medical Society upon the written request of the applicants, and only at the stated meetings in January and July; shall be recommended by the Board of Censors, and shall have been licentiates under the charter for the period of one year, at least, next preceding their election. They may be balloted for only at the first regular meeting in the ensuing April or October after their nomination, when it shall require the concurrence of three-fourths of the members present for their admission; and every practitioner so elected shall have previously paid to the Treasurer of the Society a fee of one dollar, and shall be received as a member on signing the constitution and laws of the Society." In the edition of 1882 this became *section 4*.

July 3, 1893, this section was amended to read that " Candidates for membership shall be proposed by two members, on the written request of the applicant, at the first regular meeting in any month ; shall be reported on by the Board of Censors, and shall be voted on not less than four weeks from the date of their proposal. Due notice of both proposal for membership and proposed vote shall be sent to each member of the Society by mail." [The amendment was never put in force.]

January 4, 1897, this section, still *section 4*, was amended in accordance with the new license law: "Active members shall consist of medical practitioners residing in the District of Columbia. Each candidate for such membership shall be proposed to the Medical Society, upon his written request, on a blank to be supplied by the Recording Secretary, at the stated meeting in January or July; shall be reported upon by the Board of Censors, and shall have been a licentiate under the charter, or a licentiate of the Board of Medical Supervisors of the District of Columbia for the period of one year, at least, preceding his election. Candidates may be balloted for only at the first regular meeting in the ensuing April or October after their nomination, when it shall require the concurrence of three-fourths of the members present for their admission; and each practitioner so elected shall pay into the treasury of the Society a fee of ten dollars, except such as are licentiates of this Society, who shall pay the sum of one dollar, and shall then be received as a member on signing the constitution and by-laws.''

July 7, 1902, the admission fee was reduced from ten to five dollars; and, January 13, 1904, the words ''three-fourths of the members present'' were changed to ''three-fourths of the votes cast.''

Article V, Section 4, Edition 1820.—'' In all propositions for the admission of honorary or resident members the names of the proposers shall be annexed to that of the candidate on the minutes.'' This section was struck out January 5, 1870, and a new section 4 substituted : '' None but resident members shall be entitled to attend the stated meetings, to hold office or to vote upon any subject connected with the management of the Society, or in any of the elections. Honorary members shall have the privilege of attending all regular meetings of this Society held for the discussion of medical subjects and of participating in such discussion.'' This new section became *section 5* (1882), and was amended January 4, 1897, to read : ''Active members only shall be entitled to attend the stated meetings, to hold office and to vote upon subjects connected with the management of the Society.''

Article V, Section 5, Edition of 1820.—''All those who have been resident members for the space of two years shall be considered as Fellows of the Medical Society ; and every honorary member who shall make a communication on any subject connected with medicine or the collateral branches of medical science, which communication being received and approved by the Society, may be elected a Fellow.'' June 2, 1866, this section was changed to read : ''All those who have been resident members for the space of two *years, and shall have written and defended a satisfactory thesis before the Society*, shall be considered as Fellows of the Medical Society ; and every honorary member who shall make a communication on any subject connected with medicine or the collateral branches of medical science, which communication being received and approved by the Society, may be elected a *Fellow; but should he become a resident practitioner he will be required, in order to enjoy the benefits of the Society, to pay the usual fee and be elected a resident member.*'' This entire section was struck out January 5, 1870.

In the *edition of 1882* a new section was inserted, numbered *section 3.* '' Members by invitation—Surgeons in the U. S. Army, Navy and Marine Hospital Service, temporarily residing in the District of Columbia, and not engaged in private practice—may, upon the nomination in writing by two members, at any regular meeting, be elected members by invitation. Such members by invitation shall have the privilege of attending all the meetings of the Society, of reading papers, presenting pathological specimens, and of participating in all the discussions before the Society on medical or scientific subjects, but shall not vote or hold office. No nomination shall be voted upon until it shall have been read at three successive regular meetings, and no physician shall be elected except by a two-thirds vote of the members voting." January 7, 1895, the words "and not engaged in private practice," were struck out; and, January 4, 1897, other changes were made, so that the section reads: "Surgeons in the U. S. Army, Navy and Marine Hospital Service, temporarily residing in the District of Columbia, and such members of the various scientific bureaus of the Government service as are engaged in work correlated to medicine, may, upon nomination in writing by two active members, at any regular meeting, be elected members by invitation; but no vote shall be taken upon such nomination until it shall have been reported upon by the Board of Censors, and no candidate shall be elected except by an affirmative vote of two-thirds of the members present. Members by invitation shall have the privilege of attending all regular meetings of the Society, of reading papers, presenting pathological specimens, and of participating in all of the discussions before the Society on medical or scientific subjects, but shall not vote or hold office." January 13, 1904, the words "members present" were changed to "votes cast."

Article VI, Edition of 1820.—"If any member be desirous of leaving the Society he shall signify it in a written communication, which, being read, shall lie over till the ensuing meeting, when, with the consent of the Society, his resignation shall be accepted; but he shall not be permitted to resign until he have discharged the arrears due from him to the Society." The word "have" was changed to "has" in the edition of 1861.

January 4, 1897, the following was added to this article: "Any member of the Society may be suspended from membership by a two-thirds vote of the members present at a regular meeting, and may be removed from membership by a two-thirds vote of the members present at any stated meeting; *Provided*, That any motion for the suspension or removal of any member shall be referred to and reported upon by the Board of Censors before being considered or acted upon by the Society." January 13, 1904, the words "two-thirds vote of the members present" were changed to "two-thirds affirmative vote."

Article VII, Edition of 1820.—"Members of the Society may prepare dissertations on subjects connected with medicine, or report in writing important cases in surgery or the practice of physic, which shall be directed to the President, who shall submit them to the Society for perusal. When permitted, the author, if present, shall read his own communication; otherwise it shall be read by the Secretary, and it shall be optional with the Society to enter into a general discussion of its merits." January 10, 1866, this article was struck out and another substituted : "The adjourned meetings of the Society for the advancement of professional knowledge shall be conducted through the medium of a committee of arrangements selected for the purpose, who will provide the facilities for the presentation of papers."

January 5, 1870, the article was much amended and divided into three sections, as follows :

Section 1. "The regular meetings of the Society for the advancement of professional knowledge shall be conducted through the medium of a Committee on Essays, consisting of three members, appointed by the President at the first regular meeting in January, who will provide the facilities for the presentation and publication of medical essays."

Section 2. "The Committee on Essays shall, at the commencement of each session, present the names of ten members agreeing to furnish essays on medical subjects. Such members, thus assenting, may provide a substitute."

Section 3. "Discussion on all medical papers presented under the foregoing provisions shall continue until a formal vote made to close the debate, which being carried, the author shall have the privilege of closing debate."

January 4, 1897, this entire article was struck out, its provisions appearing elsewhere in the constitution or by-laws.

Article VIII—(The edition of 1820 heads this, both as Article VIII and Section 3, which may be an inadvertence or have some other explanation, now impossible to arrive at.) "All propositions for altering the constitution shall lie over at least one stated meeting previous to being acted on, and shall then require the concurrence of two-thirds of the members present for their adoption." January 4, 1897, this became *Article VII;* and, January 13, 1904, the words "members present" were changed to "votes cast."

BY-LAWS.

(*Edition of 1820, Bye-Laws.*)

By-law 1. Of the President.—"The President shall preside at all meetings of the Society, to preserve order and decorum ; and may fine any member acting disorderly, in a sum not exceeding ten dollars, from whose decision the member incurring the fine may appeal to the Society." January 4, 1897, after the words "ten dollars," the following was added: "but the member incurring the fine may appeal to the Society. He [*i. e.*, the President,] shall also deliver an address during the month of

December of each year, the date being left to his convenience. He shall at the commencement of each year appoint essayists, one of whom shall read a paper before the Society on the first Wednesday in each month; and in event of the inability of any such essayist to so do, the President shall appoint a substitute as soon as practicable after becoming aware of such inability.''

[Just when the custom began of having the retiring President give a valedictory address it is impossible to state. This address was distinct from the annual oration which was given, with some irregularity as to time, by some member elected by the Society for the purpose, and was rather in the nature of an anniversary address, though not always so styled. The annual address in January, 1852, was given at the Smithsonian Institution. The next record of a Presidential address appears to have been March 8, 1865, when the President (Dr. Liebermann) was requested to make an address at the expiration of his term of office. We find that, January 3, 1866, he made an address as requested. Apparently, although President again, the next year he omitted to make any address, at least there is no mention of his having done so. This omission was probably the reason why the Society, January 6, 1868, made an order that the retiring President should deliver the valedictory address on the first Wednesday after the first Monday in January, that is, *not at* but *after* the annual stated meeting; and the annual festival was to be held on that day.

[November 15, 1871, however, it was ordered that the Presidential address should be made on the first Monday in January, at the stated meeting, and after the reading of the minutes, and that this should be a precedent. Accordingly, January 1, 1872, Dr. J. M. Toner, who was the retiring President, made an address. In 1897, as stated above, the President was required to give his address in December. It was given in December in 1890 and 1891. See "Anniversaries."]

The following members have served as President: Charles Worthington, 1817-29; Thomas Sim, 1830-2 (he died during his last term); Frederick May, 1833-48 (he also died during his last term); J. C. Hall, 1848-9; Alexander McWilliams, Sr., 1850; William Jones, 1851-8; Joseph Borrows, 1859-61 and 1864; there was no election during 1862 and 1863; Charles H. Liebermann, 1865-7; Thomas Miller, 1868-9; William P. Johnston, 1870; J. M. Toner, 1871; Grafton Tyler, 1872; J. E. Morgan, 1873; Johnson Eliot, 1874; J. W. H. Lovejoy, 1875; N. S. Lincoln, 1876; S. C. Busey, 1877 and 1894 to 1899; J. Ford Thompson, 1878; D. R. Hagner, 1879; Louis Mackall, 1880; W. G. Palmer, 1881; F. A. Ashford, 1882; A. F. A. King, 1883; A. Y. P. Garnett, 1884; W. W. Johnston, 1885; C. H. A. Kleinschmidt, 1886; J. Taber Johnson, 1887; T. C. Smith, 1888; C. E. Hagner, 1889; S. M. Burnett, 1890; D. W. Prentiss, 1891; William Lee, 1892; G. Wythe Cook, 1893; G. N. Acker, 1900; D. S. Lamb,

1901 ; S. S. Adams, 1902 ; G. M. Kober, 1903 ; C. W. Richardson, 1904 ; T. N. McLaughlin, 1905 ; J. D. Morgan, 1906 ; D. K. Shute, 1907; H. D. Fry, 1908 ; E. A. Balloch, 1909.

By-law 2. Of the Vice Presidents (1820).—"In the absence of the President his duty shall devolve on the Vice Presidents, so that they shall preside alternately at such meetings of the Society. And if neither the President nor a Vice President be present, a chairman shall be chosen from the members attending, who shall for that meeting exercise all the privileges and duties of the President."

This section stands just as printed in 1820.

The Vice Presidents have been as follows : Acker, 1890 and 1899 ; S. S. Adams, 1900 ; Antisell, 1865-8, 1878 ; Wm. Arnold, 1819 ; F. A. Ashford, 1876 ; Balloch, 1901 ; J. H. Blake, 1817-19 ; Bovée, 1896 ; C. Boyle, Sr., 1878 ; Bryan, 1896 ; Bulkley, 1875, 1879 ; Burnett, 1888 ; Busey, 1871 ; W. K. Butler, 1907 ; Causin, 1830, 1840 ; Chappell, 1902 ; Claytor, 1908 ; G. Wythe Cook, 1890, 1892 ; Cutbush, 1821, 1824-5 ; Dove, 1860 ; J. L. Eliot, 1893 ; Elzey, 1817-18 ; H. D. Fry, 1889 ; Garnett, 1877 ; C. E. Hagner, 1883, 1888 ; D. R. Hagner, 1872-4 ; J. C. Hall, 1846-7 ; J. B. Hamilton, 1886, 1891 ; F. Howard, 1869 ; Huntt, 1834-5, 1838 ; Hyatt, 1904 ; J. Taber Johnson, 1894 ; W. P. Johnston, 1867-8 ; W. W. Johnston, 1884 ; Jones, 1850 ; J. T. Kelley, 1908 ; A. F. A. King, 1877, 1880 ; Kleinschmidt, 1882, 1885 ; Kober, 1898 ; D. S. Lamb, 1887 ; F. Leech, 1906 ; Lincoln, 1872 ; H. Lindsly, 1851, 1859 ; Lovejoy, 1870 ; Lovell, 1826 ; McArdle, 1889 ; McLaughlin, 1895 ; A. McWilliams, Sr., 1834-5, 1838-9, 1841-9 ; L. Mackall, 1869, 1875 ; L. Mackall, Jr., 1904 ; G. L. Magruder, 1895 ; William Marbury, 1871 ; Fred May, 1819-20, 1822, 1825 ; Thos. Miller, 1848, 1864-6 ; E. C. Morgan, 1887 ; J. D. Morgan, 1897 ; Motter, 1905 ; Mundell, 1893 ; J. B. Nichols, 1907 ; Mary Parsons, 1901 ; Pool, 1903 ; D. W. Prentiss, Sr., 1881, 1883 ; Reyburn, 1876, 1894 ; C. W. Richardson, 1898 ; Joshua Riley, 1849, 1864 ; Rosse, 1892 ; Sewall, 1844-5 ; Shands, 1902 ; Shute, 1903 ; Sim, 1827-8 ; T. C. Smith, 1881 ; Sowers, 1899 ; I. S. Stone, 1897 ; W. H. Taylor, 1882, 1884-6 ; J. D. Thomas, 1905 ; J. Ford Thompson, 1873-4 ; William Thornton, 1820, 1823 ; J. M. Toner, 1870 ; Triplett, 1880 ; John Van Renssalaer, 1909 ; G. T. Vaughan, 1909 ; Warfield, 1830 ; Wellington, 1906 ; J. T. Winter, 1891 ; Woodward, 1900 ; J. T. Young, 1879 ; N. Young, 1839, 1861.

By-law 3. Of the Corresponding Secretary (1820).—"It shall be the duty of the Corresponding Secretary to manage all matters of correspondence in behalf of the Society ; to give notice to members and officers of their election; to write and answer letters, and respectfully to solicit from medical societies, faculties and individuals information calculated to benefit the science of medicine; all which correspondence he shall lay before the Society at the next succeeding stated meeting."

January 12, 1870, there was added after the word "meeting" the words "and shall be the custodian of the seal of the Society." The section was amended January 7, 1884, by adding the following : "Members shall be notified by mail by the Corresponding Secretary of the stated, regular and special meetings and of the title and author of the paper to be read."

November 19, 1890, the Society ordered that the Corresponding Secretary should furnish each member of the Society with a printed list of the names of all applicants for membership at least two days prior to the first Wednesday in April and October of each year, with the name of the college from which the applicant graduated and the time of graduation.

January 4, 1897, the section was rewritten, as follows: "The Corresponding Secretary shall conduct the correspondence of the Society, notify members and officers of their election, and forward by mail prior to each meeting, to each member entitled to attend, a notice of such meeting, specifying the business to come before it ; he shall furnish to each member, at least two days prior to the first Wednesday in April and October of each year, a printed list of the names of all applicants for membership, with the name of the college from which each applicant graduated and the date of graduation. He shall be the custodian of the seal of the Society."

The Corresponding Secretaries have been as follows : Antisell, 1864 ; Bohrer, 1830 ; Briscoe, 1872-4 ; Causin, 1834-5, 1838 ; G. Wythe Cook, 1888 ; Drinkard, 1870-1 ; H. P. Howard, 1865 ; Huntt, 1817-30; William Lee, part of 1872; Lovejoy, 1861, part of 1869; McArdle, 1881; McNally, 1869 ; J. M. Mackall, 1881-2 ; Louis Mackall, 1866-8 ; G. L. Magruder, 1876-7 ; Thomas Miller, 1844-7 ; Ross, 1875 ; Sewall, 1839-43 ; T. C. Smith, 1878-80, 1883-7, 1889 to 1909; Grafton Tyler, 1848, 1860. It is not known who served in 1831-3, 1836-7, 1849-59 and 1862-3.

By-law 4. Of the Recording Secretary (1820).—"The Recording Secretary shall attend each meeting of the Society ; call over the names of the members and take down the minutes, which he shall read at the next meeting and which, when corrected, he shall copy into a book kept for that purpose, and to which entry he shall sign his name. He shall also insert the reports of committees at full length ; he shall read all letters and papers relating to the business of the Society which do not particularly belong to the department of the Corresponding Secretary, and transcribe into a proper book such of them as the Society may think worthy to be preserved. He shall deliver to the Treasurer a correct statement of the fines incurred at each meeting. If he should be unable to attend a meeting of the Society he shall give due notice of it, by transmitting all the papers required at the meeting."

January 4, 1897, two changes were made ; the words "call over the names of members" were struck out, but after the word "minutes" was inserted "including the names of those present." The words "all the papers required at the meeting" were changed to "to the meeting all necessary papers."

[February 6, 1895, the Society created the office of "Assistant Recording Secretary," with a moderate salary. His duty should be "to make
a stenographic report of all medical discussions, and, after consultation
with the members concerned therein, to make the necessary corrections
in the report; these to be verified by a committee consisting of the President, Recording and Assistant Secretaries." February 2, 1898, the Assistant Recording Secretary resigned, and no one else was afterward
elected. The only person who ever served was Dr. H. L. Hayes.]

The following members served as Recording Secretary : S. S. Adams,
1887-98; J. B. Blake, 1826, 1834; Borrows, 1841-7; Causin, 1820-1; Cutts,
1886-7, resigned; Frye, 1848-51; Thomas Henderson, 1817-19, 1828;
Holmead, 1854-5; H. P. Howard, 1848, resigned; Richmond Johnson,
1834-5, 1838-9; W? W. Johnston, last half of 1870 and first part 1871, resigned; William Jones, 1840; A. F. A. King, 1865-8, resigned; Kleinschmidt, 1871-81; William Lee, 1868-70, resigned; Lippitt, 1859-60; Mc-
Ardle, 1881-6, resigned; Macatee, 1905 to 1909; F. P. Morgan, 1899-1905,
resigned; W. G. Palmer, 1865, resigned; J. C. Riley, 1856-8; Saunders,
1852-3; W. M. Tucker, 1861-4; Wilstach, 1824-7; N. W. Worthington,
1822-3. It is not known who served in 1829-33.

By-law 5. Of the Treasurer (*1820*).—"The Treasurer shall collect all
monies (afterwards spelled moneys) due to the Society, receive all donations of money which shall be made to the Society, and shall pay the
same agreeably to order certified to him by the President, Vice President,
or member who was in the chair when such order was made. He shall
keep a regular account of all monies received and paid by him as aforesaid; and once every year, or oftener, if required by the Society, shall
render a statement of the funds in his hands and of the disbursements;
and shall deliver up to his successor the books and all papers belonging
to the Society, together with the balance of cash; and for the faithful
discharge of his trust shall give a satisfactory security to the President
within one month after being appointed."

October 1, 1861, the words "which he shall deposit in bank to its
credit" were inserted after the words "shall be made to the Society;"
and "funds in bank" were substituted for "funds in his hands."

There have been but few changes in the treasurership. The following
have served: F. A. Ashford, 1871-4, resigned; Busey, 1850-4; Johnson
Eliot, 1848-9; Franzoni, 1874 to 1909; J. C. Hall, 1838-45; William Jones,
1817-25, 1846-7; H. Lindsly, 1834-5; William Marbury, 1860-70; T. C.
Scott, 1830; A. J. Semmes, 1855-9; Wilstach, 1826-7. It is not known
who served in 1828-9, 1831-3 and 1836-7.

By-law 6. Of the Librarian (*1820*).—"The Librarian shall take charge
of and preserve for the use of the Society all property, of whatever kind
it may be, money excepted, of which the Society may become possessed,
and keep a correct list of the same, together with the respective names of

the donors, in a book provided for that purpose, which book shall be laid before the Society as often as called for. The Librarian shall give such a receipt for everything committed to his care or charge as the Society may direct, and at the end of his term shall deliver up the same to his successor.''

In the edition of 1839 the following sentence was added : '' He shall report the state of the library to the Society at the annual meeting in each year.'' January 4, 1897, the word *state* was changed to *condition.*

The following members have served as Librarian : Craven, 1822-3 ; Grayson, 1860-1 ; Gunnell, 1824-34 ; Holmead, 1850-3 ; F. Howard, 1844-9 ; A. F. A. King, 1870-1 ; Lovejoy, 1867-8 ; Thomas Miller, 1835, 1838-43 ; E. L. Morgan, 1893 to 1909 ; J. E. Morgan, 1854-9 ; Mundell, 1884-92 ; Patze, 1873-84, resigned ; J. C. Riley, 1864-5 ; J. M. Toner, 1866, 1869, 1872 ; Weightman, 1817-18 ; N. W. Worthington, 1819-20. It is not known who served in 1821 or 1836-7.

By-law 7. Of Committees (1820).—'' The mode of appointing committees shall be as follows, viz : The President shall appoint one gentleman, who shall be considered as chairman of the committee ; he shall name the second, and so on, until the number agreed on shall be completed. But if the business be of an extraordinary or important nature, any member may move that the committee be chosen by ballot, which shall accordingly be done. The chairman of every committee shall appoint a time for its meeting before he leaves the Society.''

In the 1839 edition this section became *8* instead of *7* ; and was entirely struck out January 10, 1866.

January 4, 1897, a new section 8 was adopted, entitled '' 8. Of the Standing Committees.''

'' It shall be the duty of the Committee on Public Health to present to the Society an annual report upon the condition of the public health in the District of Columbia during the calendar year preceding.

'' It shall be the duty of the Committee on Legislation to discharge such duties pertaining to legislation as the Society may direct.

'' It shall be the duty of the Committee on Essays to secure and arrange for the presentation of medical essays and pathological specimens.''

January 8, 1902, the Committee on Legislation was replaced by an Executive Committee, with the following duties : '' It shall be the duty of the Executive Committee to keep informed in all matters concerning the interests of the medical profession generally and of this Society and its members in particular; to consider such resolutions as may be referred to it by the Society ; to suggest improvements in the conduct of the business of the Society; to consider and report upon matters requiring legislative action ; to represent the Society before Congress and the Commissioners of the District of Columbia, and to report its operations to the Society from time to time, as occasion may require, together with such recommendations as it may deem proper.''

Executive Committee.—Acker and S. S. Adams, 1902–9; R. W. Baker, 1909; E. A. Balloch, 1902–8; Bovée, 1902–9; G. Wythe Cook and W. B. French, 1902–5; Glazebrook, 1908–9; Hickling, 1902–9; W. W. Johnston, 1902; Kober, 1902, 1904–7; Louis Mackall, Jr., 1906–9; G. L. Magruder, 1902–3; J. D. Morgan, 1903–5, 1907–9; W. G. Morgan, 1902–6; McLaughlin, 1902–4, 1906–9; Neff, 1902–9; Reisinger, 1903–9; C. W. Richardson, 1902–3, 1905–9; Shute, 1906–7, 1909; Sowers, 1902–7; J. D. Thomas, 1907–9; Woodward, 1902–9.

Committee on Public Health.—Abbe, 1906–9; Balloch, 1898–1900; Briggs, 1906–9; Carr, 1895–7; Chappell, 1895–1909; Claytor, 1898–1901; J. T. Cole, 1902–3; Deale, 1898; Dowling, 1902; Dye, 1906–9; L. Eliot, 1902–3; Erbach, 1901; I. J. Heiberger, 1909; Holden, 1898–1901; Hyatt, 1895–7; G. W. Johnston, 1898–1901; W. W. Johnston, 1895–7; R. S. Lamb, 1902, 1904–9; D. O. Leech, 1895–7, 1899–1900; Frank Leech, 1904–5; McLain, 1901; Mayfield, 1895–7; J. D. Morgan, 1895–6; Rupert Norton, 1898; Robins, 1902–3; S. Ruffin, 1899–1901; Sprigg, 1904–5; Stoutenburgh, 1902–3; Wellington, 1904–5; A. A. Wilson, 1902–8; G. W. Wood, 1902–9; W. C. Woodward, 1897–8.

Committee on Legislation.—Busey, 1895–9; G. Wythe Cook, 1895–1901; L. Eliot, 1898; Hickling, 1900–1; W. W. Johnston, 1895–1901; Kleinschmidt and McLain, 1895–1900; G. L. Magruder, 1895–1901; W. G. Morgan, 1900–1; D. W. Prentiss, 1895; Reyburn, 1895, 1899, 1900–1; Sowers, 1895–9, 1901; C. G. Stone, 1895–7; Woodward, 1895–1901. The President of the Society was *ex officio* President of the Committee.

The Committee on Essays was called Committee on Evening Arrangements in 1867–8; the following served on it: Drinkard, 1868; Lovejoy, 1867; Peter, and J. Ford Thompson, 1867–8.

From 1869 to 1909, inclusive (excepting during 1875–8, when it was called Committee on Publication), the following have served: S. S. Adams, 1891; Charles Allen, 1869; F. A. Ashford, 1870, resigned; Balloch, 1905–8; N. P. Barnes, 1902–3, 1906–9; W. S. Bowen, 1892; Bryan, 1888, 90–1, 95; Busey, 1869–71; G. Wythe Cook, 1883–92; L. Eliot, 1892; Ford, 1870; H. D. Fry, 1889; Griffith, 1902–3; C. E. Hagner, 1873–4, 80; Hartigan, 1879; J. T. D. Howard, 1893; P. C. Hunt, 1909; W. W. Johnston, 1870–2; A. F. A. King, 1869–70, 73–4, 79, 81; William Lee, 1871; McLaughlin, 1904; L. Mackall, 1872; Murphy, 1880, 82; Mary Parsons, 1898–1901; Pool, 1893–1901; D. W. Prentiss, Sr., 1879; Schaeffer, 1881; Shute, 1904–5; T. C. Smith, 1884–91, 93–1909; Stanton, 1880; W. H. Taylor, 1882–5, resigned; B. Thompson, 1872–4; Triplett, 1880; R. Walsh, 1881; Woodward, 1894, 96–7.

By-law 7. Board of Examiners. Edition of 1839.—This new section 7 appears in the 1839 edition: "A Board of Examiners, consisting of five resident members, shall be elected by ballot at each annual meeting, whose duty it shall be to grant licenses, upon the payment of five dollars, to such medical and chirurgical gentlemen as they may, upon a full examination, judge qualified to practice the medical and chirurgical arts. No one shall be admitted to an examination until he shall, in conformity with the requisitions of the charter, produce a diploma from some respectable medical college or society, and shall furnish satisfactory evidence that he has studied physic and surgery three years, including one full course of medical lectures as usually taught at the medical schools, or four years without such a course of lectures. A majority of the Board shall constitute a quorum for business, and the senior practitioner shall be chairman. Any one of the Examiners may grant temporary licenses to practice during the intervals of the meetings of the Board. The Board shall keep a record of its proceedings, to be reported to the Society at its annual meeting."

This section is in accord with each charter, sections 3, 4 and 5. The edition of 1820 does not contain any corresponding provision in the by-laws, perhaps because the charter so fully covers the subject.

In the edition of 1867 the word *five* (dollars) is changed to *ten*. January 15, 1868, after the words "course of lectures" were added the words "provided always that nothing in this article shall be construed so as to imply that practitioners thus licensed shall be *de facto* members of the Society." July 8, 1868, the words "and shall furnish" were changed to "or shall furnish." January 12, 1870, the words "no one shall be admitted to an examination" were changed to "no one shall receive a license;" after the words "such a course of lectures" were added "and shall have passed a satisfactory examination before the Board of Examiners;" instead of "the senior practitioner shall be chairman," appeared "and shall elect their own chairman;" the sentence authorizing the granting of temporary licenses was struck out and the following was inserted: "The Board shall meet on the first Wednesday in every month, at such hour and place as they may determine."

January 4, 1897, in view of the passage by Congress of a Licensing Act, this section had become inoperative, and was therefore struck out.

The following served on the Board of Examiners : Acker, 1886–96 ; S. S. Adams, 1887–96 ; Antisell, 1869, resigned ; F. A. Ashford, 1870, 78 ; Austin, 1853–4 ; J. S. Beale, 1877 ; Bohrer, 1827–34 ; Borrows, 1838, 50–2, 65 ; W. S. Bowen, 1893–6 ; C. Boyle, Sr., 1858–61, 75 ; Bulkley, 1872–4, 77 ; Busey, 1872, resigned ; Causin, 1820, 30 ; A. C. Christie, 1872 ; George Clarke, 1820, 22 ; G. Wythe Cook, 1889 ; Cutbush, 1820–1 ; Cutts, 1887, resigned ; Dove, 1859 ; J. Eliot, 1860–1, 65, 67, 69, 72 ; L. Eliot, 1890–2 ; Fairfax, 1839 ; Ford, 1870–1 ; H. D. Fry, 1884, 6–8 ; Garnett, 1853–61, 68, 78 ; C. E. Hagner, 1875–7 ; D. R. Hagner, 1864, 67–8, 70–1, 75–6 ; J. C. Hall, 1838–9, 1850–2; Hartigan, 1878–81, 85; T. Henderson, 1822, 25; F. Howard, 1851–5, 72 ; Hyatt, 1881–2 ; H. L. E. Johnson, 1889–92 ; J. T. Johnson, 1878–80, 82–85 ; W. P. Johnston, 1844–9, 60 ; William Jones,

1826, 1848–9; A. F. A. King, 1869, 73–6; Kleinschmidt, 1879–81, 83–5, 87–96; Liebermann, 1856–61, 64–5; H. Lindsly, 1838, 40–50, 61, 66; Lovell, 1822, 25, 34–5; Lovejoy, 1866, 68, 73–4; McArdle, 1882–8; S. A. H. McKim, 1867; L. Mackall, Sr., 1865, 70–1; G. L. Magruder, 1881–3; G. W. May, 1826; Fred May, 1819; J. F. May, 1840–7; T. Miller, 1850–9; E. C. Morgan, 1886; J. E. Morgan, 1866, 69, 72; Murphy, 1877–8, resigned; Ober, 1893–6; W. G. Palmer, 1864, 70–1, 79–80; D. C. Patterson, 1881–5; Peter, 1873–4; D. W. Prentiss, 1878–80; J. C. Riley, 1869; J. Riley, 1827–35; T. C. Scott, 1827, 30; T. Semmes, 1819; Sewall, 1830, 35, 38–9; Shaaff, 1819; Sim, 1819–21, 23; T. C. Smith, 1877; Staughton, 1825–7; R. K. Stone, 1855–7; J. M. Thomas, 1840–9; B. Thompson, 1871–5; J. F. Thompson, 1866–9; J. M. Toner, 1864–5, 67; Triplett, 1875–6; G. Tyler, 1864, 66; L. Tyler, 1886; Warfield, 1820, 26; Washington, 1824, 30, 35; C. Worthington, 1819; N. W. Worthington, 1834–5, 38–43; J. T. Young, 1876; N. Young, 1839–58.

By-law 8. Of the Board of Censors. Edition of 1870.—This section was adopted January 12, 1870. "To the Board of Censors shall be referred the name of every person nominated for election as resident member or honorary member of the Society, and no election for resident member or honorary member shall be held until the said Board, after due investigation, shall report to the Society upon the character and qualifications of the person so referred. All charges of unprofessional or ungentlemanly conduct made to the Society against any member shall also be referred to this Board, who shall report thereupon."

January 4, 1897, the wording of the section was changed to read as follows: "To the Board of Censors shall be referred the name of every person nominated for election to any class of membership; said Board, after due investigation, shall report to the Society, on the night fixed for election, upon the qualifications of each person so referred, and no name shall be voted upon until such report has been received. All charges of unprofessional or ungentlemanly conduct made to the Society against any member shall be referred to this Board for investigation and report."

[NOTE.—Although there was no provision for Censors in the charters or constitution or the by-laws of the Society before 1870, there were Censors in its early years. Toner (1866) says: "It is perhaps to be regretted that the office of Censors in the Society has been discontinued. For many years three Censors were annually elected, whose duties were similar to those at present performed by the Censors of the Medical Association of the District, but in addition they also acted as the nominating committee for licentiates desiring to become members of the Society."]

The following have served on the Board of Censors: Acker, 1884–5, 1897–8; S. S. Adams, 1899; Antisell, 1877; Bohrer, 1819–20, 23; Borrows, 1873–4, Bovée, 1902; Bromwell, 1887; G. A. Brown, 1819–20, 23; Bulkley, 1882; Busey, 1873, 78; Chappell, 1901; G. Wythe Cook, 1885–7, 91, 99–

28

1900, 02; Deale, 1903–9; J. Eliot, 1875–81 ; Fenwick, 1882; W. B. French, 1897–1900; Friedrich, 1888, 1901; Garnett, 1876; Glazebrook, 1901 ; D. R. Hagner, 1883; F. R. Hagner, 1903–9 ; C. M. Hammett, 1888 ; Heiberger, 1901 ; Hoehling, 1883 ; Holden, 1886–7; J. T. Howard, 1888; Hyatt, 1886 ; E. F. King, 1893–7, resigned ; Kleinschmidt, 1897–1900; D. O. Leech, 1901–9 ; Liebermann, 1871–5 ; Lovejoy, 1876 ; McArdle, 1891–2 ; McLaughlin, 1900–2 : L. Mackall, 1872 ; G. W. May, 1819–20, 23 ; T. Miller, 1870–3 ; Moran, 1902–9 ; J. E. Morgan, 1875, 77–81 ; Murphy, 1879–81 ; Ober, 1889–90; C. W. Richardson, 1891–1900 ; Richey, 1882–4 ; Schaeffer, 1884–5 ; J. F. Thompson, 1870–1 ; J. M. Toner, 1874 ; Wall, 1903–9; J. T. Winter, 1889–90, 92–8 ; N. W. Worthington, 1819–20, 22.

By-law 8. Of Motions (1820).—"Any member may make whatever motion he thinks will tend to the benefit of the Society ; his proposal or motion must be given to the President in writing ; and it shall be immediately voted or balloted for, unless a majority of the members present wish it to lie over for consideration. In either case it shall be recorded on the minutes of the Society."

In the edition of 1839, this section became 9 instead of 8. January 4, 1897, the wording of the first part of this section was changed as follows : "Every motion must be given to the President in writing, and shall be immediately discussed and voted on unless," etc.

July 1, 1901, the wording of the first part was again changed to read "Every motion must be given to the President, and at his discretion the mover may be required to put the motion in writing, and it shall be immediately discussed," etc.

By-law 9. Of the Order of Debate (1820).—"No member shall interrupt the President, or any other member, while speaking ; every member shall stand while speaking, and address himself to the President."

This section, which became No. 10 in the edition of 1839, was struck out January 4, 1897.

By-law 10. Of Decorum (1820).—"No member or members shall be permitted to sit or stand with his or their heads covered."

This section became No. 11 in the edition of 1839 ; was struck out January 4, 1897.

By-law 10. Of Essays and Discussions. Edition of 1897.—January 4, 1897, the following section was adopted :

"Men eminent in medicine, not exceeding four in number, may be invited annually to address the Society ; the invitation to be made by a committee consisting of the President, the Corresponding Secretary and the Recording Secretary, and with the approval of the Society. (Originally adopted February 6, 1895.)

"No papers, essays, histories of cases or pathological specimens shall be read or presented to the Society for discussion if such papers, essays, histories or specimens have been read or presented to any other Society, or published or offered for publication in any medical journal. (Originally adopted February 25, 1891.)

"The discussion of any paper or pathological specimen, read or presented at a meeting of the Society shall not be continued to a subsequent meeting, except by an affirmative vote of two-thirds of the members present."

January 13, 1904, the words "members present" were changed to "votes cast."

July 1, 1907, the following amendments were adopted :

"That no paper read before the Society be allowed to consume more than twenty minutes in its delivery, and that the presentation of a case or of a pathological specimen be not allowed to consume more than ten minutes; that in the discussion of a paper, case or specimen, no member be allowed to speak more than ten minutes or to speak more than once, except the member reading the paper or presenting the case or specimen, who is entitled to close the discussion, and except in cases in which the regulation is waived by vote of the Society: *Provided*, that the foregoing restrictions do not apply to invited guests of the Society.

"That every member desiring to publish elsewhere than in the WASHINGTON MEDICAL ANNALS any paper that he has read before the Society, be required, unless he publishes his paper in regular order in the ANNALS, to furnish to the Editorial Committee an abstract of said paper within two weeks after it has been read."

By-law 11. Attendance of Meetings (1820).—"No member shall be permitted to retire after calling his name, without permission from the President, until the Society have adjourned."*

In the edition of 1839 this section became No. 13 ; January 12, 1870, the word *the* was inserted before, and *of* after *calling*, and *has* was substituted for *have*. January 4, 1897, the section was struck out.

By-law 12. Of a Quorum (1820).—"At each meeting of the Society any number, not less than seven, shall constitute a quorum."

In the edition of 1839 this section became No. 13. The minimum number, seven, was provided in the charters. January 4, 1897, the wording was changed to read "At the meetings of the Society seven active members shall constitute a quorum." July 1, 1907, the number was increased to fifteen.

By-law 13. Of Visitors (1820).—"Medical men, or men learned in the collateral branches of the science, on a visit to the District of Columbia, not members of this Society, may be permitted to attend meetings, on being introduced by a member of the Society."

This section became No. 14 in the edition of 1839 ; January 4, 1897, it

---

* The only record of a fine ever having been imposed is that of February 19, 1868 ; Johnson Eliot was fined by the President fifty cents for retiring without permission. Those who knew Dr. Eliot personally will appreciate the humor of the circumstance.

was made No. 12, and was changed to read "Non-resident medical men
and candidates for membership may be permitted to attend the regular
meetings on being introduced by an active member."

By-law 14. Routine of Business (1820).—"At each meeting of the Society, as soon as the President takes the chair and the meeting is constituted, the following shall be the order of proceeding : First, the roll shall
be called. Second, the minutes shall be read. Third, the election of
candidates for membership. Fourth, nomination of candidates for membership. Fifth, Report of Treasurer. Sixth, reports of committees.
Seventh, reports of the Corresponding Secretary. Eighth, medical
papers and essays read or presented for consideration."

This section became No. 15 in the edition of 1839; in 1866 it became
No. 14 again, and the order was amended by inserting as "eighth, Miscellaneous business." January 12, 1870, the section was made No. 15,
and the following was adopted as the order :

"At each regular meeting of the Society, as soon as the President takes
the chair and the meeting is constituted, the following shall be the order
of proceeding : First, the minutes shall be read. Second, the election
of candidates for membership (at the first regular meetings in April and
October). Third, nomination of candidates for membership (at the
stated meetings). Fourth, report of Treasurer (at the first regular meeting in each month). Five, reports of committees. Six, report of Corresponding Secretary. Seven, miscellaneous business. Eight, Pathological specimens. Nine, unfinished debates on medical papers. Ten,
medical papers and essays read or presented for consideration.

"All meetings of the Society shall commence at 8 o'clock P. M.

"By a rule of the Society [adopted January 23, 1865], thirty minutes
are allowed for all items in this routine of business up to the eighth.

"The regular business of the stated meetings shall not be suspended
for the consideration of any other matter; and if such business shall not
be concluded at the meeting on the first Monday in January or the first
Monday in July the stated meeting may be adjourned from day to day or
from week to week until that business is finished, when the stated meeting shall close and the regular meeting may commence. The regular
meetings shall be held on Wednesday of each week." (This last sentence
was adopted by the Society January 23, 1865, and again January 12, 1870.)

January 4, 1897, this section was made 13 instead of 15, and was much
changed in wording throughout : "The regular meetings of the Society
shall be held on Wednesday of each week, when the order of business
shall be as follows :

"First, introduction of visitors. Second, reading of the minutes.
Third, election of candidates for active membership (at the first regular
meetings in April and October). Fourth, report of Treasurer (at the
first regular meeting in each month). Fifth, report of Corresponding

Secretary. Sixth, reports of Committees. Seventh, miscellaneous business. Eighth, pathological specimens. Ninth, essay for the month, on evening assigned. Tenth, unfinished debates on medical papers. Eleventh, medical papers and essays.

"Only the business parts of the minutes shall be read, together with the title of papers and specimens read or presented, and the names of members engaged in their discussion. (Adopted February 6, 1895.) Not more than thirty minutes shall be allowed for the transaction of all business under articles numbered 1 to 7, inclusive.

"The order of business at any regular meeting shall not be suspended except by an affirmative vote of two-thirds of the active members present.

"The order of business at *stated meetings* shall be as follows: First, reading of the minutes of the previous stated meeting. Second, nomination of candidates for membership. Third, reports of officers. Fourth, reports of committees. Fifth, election of officers and censors. Sixth, miscellaneous business.

"The regular business of the stated meetings shall not be suspended for the consideration of any other matter, and if such business be not concluded on the first Monday in January or the first Monday in July such meeting may be adjourned from day to day or from week to week until that business is finished; nor shall the order of business be suspended except by an affirmative vote of two-thirds of the members present.

"All regular and stated meetings shall begin at 8 o'clock P. M."*

But few parliamentary rules were adopted by the Society until 1867, when, May 8th, a committee, consisting of the President, Secretary and Harvey Lindsly, was appointed to select from Jefferson's Manual and the Rules of the House of Representatives such rules as applied to the Society. May 15th, the committee reported a series of twenty rules, and May 22d these were adopted by the Society. Just what they were does not appear.

February 1, 1871, it was ordered that a manual of parliamentary law should be procured and placed in the library, but which manual was selected is not stated.

January 13, 1904, the following changes were made: "affirmative vote of two-thirds of the active members present" to "concurrence of two-thirds of the votes cast;" and "affirmative vote of two-thirds of the members present" in the same way.

By-law 15. Of Annual Contributions (1820).—"Each resident member shall pay annually to the Treasurer the sum of three dollars, for the use of the Society; which funds in the first place shall be appropriated to defray the current expenses of the Society, and the surplus shall be

---

* May 18, 1887, the chair (J. Taber Johnson) decided that one-fifth of the members present were necessary to call yeas and nays.

expended in purchasing medical books, under the direction of a committee appointed for the special purpose.''

In the edition of 1839 the number was changed to 16, the title simply '' of Contributions,'' and the wording as follows: ''The expenses of the Society shall be defrayed by the fees paid into the treasury, and by special assessments made upon the resident members from time to time as occasion may require ; and any member who shall neglect to pay his assessment for three years, except in case of absence from the District, shall forfeit his membership.''

January 12, 1870, the words '' any member '' became ''any resident member,'' and the number of the section 15 ; number 16 in 1894 ; 14 in 1897. The editions of 1882 *et seq.* say *two* instead of *three* years.

January 4, 1897, the section was changed to read '' The expenses of the Society shall be defrayed by an annual assessment upon the active members and by special assessments made from time to time as occasion may require ; and any member who shall neglect to pay any such assessment for two years shall forfeit his membership.''

Inasmuch as the expense of keeping up the Society must be provided for in some way, this Society at first established a yearly dues as the means of defraying expenses. In 1819 it fixed the annual dues at $3.00 ; this would appear a large sum for a Society having only four meetings a year, even though the membership was small, and therefore greater *per capita;* but the dues were intended also to buy books, that is, such sum as remained after paying other expenses.

It is presumed that this method continued until 1839, when the second charter was granted ; there is no record to the contrary. In 1839 it was provided that the expenses should be defrayed by the fees (*i. e.*, fees received from the Board of Examiners), and special assessments should be made when needed. This regulation continued unchanged until 1897, when the Board expired by law and fees from that source ceased. It was then provided that the expenses should be defrayed by annual assessments and by special assessments when needed.

From time to time one or more members were exempted from assessments, usually those who had been members a long time, or some other good reason seemed to justify such exemption. Under the rule such members if they failed to pay assessments would have been dropped. Sometimes new members were exempted for the year in which they were elected. At one time, November 15, 1865, the Society ordered that members who were not practicing, those who were out of the city, and those who had become members during the year, should be exempted. Again, February 7, 1866, exemption was given to new members and those not practicing. February 6, 1867, it was ordered that new members elected during the year should pay only so much of the yearly fee as corresponded to the portion of the year remaining from the time of their election.

March 4, 1868, it was ordered that members not practicing and members elected during the year should be exempted, and that a member who had removed from the city and afterward returned should be exempted for the year in which he returned. February 3, 1869, members elected during the year and those who removed and returned as just stated, were exempted. January 6, 1873, members elected during the year were exempted.

It is interesting to note that up to the year 1868, at least, it was customary, with more or less regularity as to time, to collect the assessments through some one member who lived in the "ward;" and as there were seven wards in Washington and two in Georgetown, and there was the "county" besides, these ten members made the collections.

February 3, 1875, it was ordered that members dropped for non-payment of dues should be required to pay up all arrears and apply again for membership. This action had already been taken in the case of S. S. Bond. The same question again arose March 20, 1878, and Dr. Busey recalled the order just mentioned. But Noble Young thought it would be better to have legal advice as to how far the Society as a chartered body could deprive a man of his membership. April 9, 1884, Vice President Taylor decided that a member dropped for any cause would need to go through the usual forms before reinstatement.

November 5, 1884, in the case of O. M. Muncaster, reinstated, and who had paid $1.00 initiation fee, the Society ordered the money refunded.

October 28, 1885, another question arose. J. C. Bird, who had been elected but had not signed the constitution and was dropped for non-payment of dues, contended that not having signed he was not therefore a member, and therefore could not be dropped. The Society, however, decided that he must again make formal application for membership.

By-law 16.—No section of this number in the edition of 1820.

By-law 17. Amendments.—There was no provision for amendments in the edition of 1820; in the year 1839 appears the following: "The preceding constitutional ordinance and by-laws, being adopted for the future regulation of the Society, all others not contained in this summary are hereby repealed; and all propositions for altering the foregoing shall lay over for one stated meeting at least before being acted upon."

January 12, 1870, the wording after the word "foregoing" was changed to read "Constitution or by-laws shall be made at one stated meeting and shall not be taken up for action until the next stated meeting; and such proposed amendments shall be read by the Recording Secretary. at each of the last three regular meetings preceding the stated meeting at which such action is to be had."

January 4, 1897, the number of the section became 15, and the wording was again changed to read: "The preceding constitution and by-laws being adopted for the future regulation of the Society, all rules and regulations not contained therein are hereby repealed ; all propositions for altering the same shall be made at one stated meeting and shall not be taken up for action until the next stated meeting ; and a copy of such proposed amendments shall be sent to each active member by mail, with the notice of the meeting at which they are to be acted upon.''

By-law 18. Edition of 1882.—'' The routine of business of the regular meetings shall not be suspended except by a vote of two-thirds of the members present.'' January 4, 1897, this was incorporated in section 13, and was therefore struck out as a separate section.

———

The following have served as *Vice Presidents of the Washington Academy of Sciences*, representing the Medical Society : S. S. Adams, 1902–3, 1905 ; Balloch, 1909 ; Busey, 1899–1901, died ; H. D. Fry, 1908 ; W. W. Johnston, 1901–2, died ; J. D. Morgan, 1906; C. W. Richardson, 1904; D. K. Shute, 1907.

Special Committees.—The following served as a special committee on Medical History and Statistics, appointed March 24, 1869 : J. M. Toner, William Lee, W. W. Johnston, D. W. Prentiss, Ford, W. E. Roberts, Croggon, Peter and Busey.

The following have served on the *Committee on Library :* May 10, 1869, Antisell, Drinkard, W. P. Johnston, Louis Mackall, Liebermann ; May 9, 1870, William Marbury, Mackall and Liebermann ; 1909, J. T. Howard; 1904–8, D. S. Lamb; 1904–9, E. L. Morgan; 1904–5, F. P. Morgan; and 1906–8, D. G. Smith.

Committee on Publication—The first committee consisted of J. H. Thompson, J. F. Thompson and William Lee, appointed in 1869.

From 1875 to 1878, inclusive, the Committee on Essays was called the Committee on Publication. The following served on the committee : Busey, 1875, resigned ; W. W. Johnston, 1875–6 ; A. F. A. King, 1875, resigned ; Kleinschmidt, 1875–8 ; William Lee and Murphy, 1877–8 ; Ross, 1875–6; B. Thompson, 1875, died.

From 1883 to 1909 the following served : S. S. Adams, 1885–96 ; Belt, 1893; Bovée, 1892; Burnett, 1889; G. Wythe Cook, 1894–6; Cutts, 1886–7; Edes, 1891 ; L. Eliot, 1898–1901 ; Fernald, 1888 ; H. D. Fry, 1885–8 ; G. B. Harrison, 1885–6; Hawkes, 1892; V. B. Jackson, 1902–4; W. W. Johnston, 1897–9, resigned; A. F. A. King, 1883, resigned; Kober, 1897–1901; D. S. Lamb, 1902–9; F. Leech, 1894–6; McArdle, 1883–6, resigned; J. D. Morgan, 1897–1900, resigned ; Motter, 1905–8 ; T. M. Murray, 1889–91 ; B. G. Pool, 1909 ; D. W. Prentiss, Sr., 1883–5, resigned ; C. W. Richardson, 1890 ; J. D. Thomas, 1899, 1901 ; Tompkins, 1893 ; W. A. Wells, 1902–6 ; C. S. White, 1908–9.

January 20, 1897, the name Committee on Publication was changed to the Committee on Editing the Transactions.

The following have served on the *Committee on Microscopy:* Acker, 1884–99; Balloch, 1893–7 ; G. B. Harrison, 1886 ; W. W. Johnston, 1877–83; A. F. A. King, 1876; D. S. Lamb, 1876–1900; Marshall, 1900–9; J. B. Nichols, 1900–8 ; D. W. Prentiss, Jr., 1902–9 ; Schaeffer, 1876–85, 1887–92; Vale, 1898–1901; W. W. Wilkinson, 1909.

The following have served as *Committee on Directory of Nurses:* S. S. Adams and H. H. Barker, 1891–1901 ; Burnett, 1883 ; G. Wythe Cook, 1889; H. Fisher, 1902; Griffith, 1904–9; Groover, 1906–9; H. L. E. Johnson, 1883, 1890–2, 1902–5 ; J. T. Johnson, 1901 ; G. W. Johnston, 1888 ; W. W. Johnston, 1884, 1887 ; Lovejoy, 1884–7 ; McArdle, 1883–91 ; McLaughlin, 1893–1901 ; Mundell, 1885–6 ; D. W. Prentiss, Sr., 1888–9 ; Ada R. Thomas, 1902–9.

The following have served on the *Milk Commission:* S. S. Adams, 1903–4, resigned ; E. A. DeSchweinitz, 1903, died ; Donnally and Hickling, 1905–9 ; J. H. McCormick and J. B. Nichols, 1903–5 ; E. Sothoron, 1905–9 ; Sprigg, 1903–9 ; Wall, 1904–9 ; Woodward, 1903, resigned.

The following have served on the *Committee on Entertainment:* F. R. Hagner and Jackson, 1905–8 ; L. H. Taylor, 1908 ; J. D. Thomas, 1905–7 ;

The following have served on the *Historical Committee:* A. F. A. King, 1902–6 ; Kleinschmidt and E. L. Morgan, 1902–5 ; D. S. Lamb, Franzoni, G. Wythe Cook and Holden, 1906–9 ; L. Eliot, 1908–9.

SUBJECT INDEX.

PERSONAL INDEX.

30